MAGNETIC RESONANCE IMAGING OF THE SPINE

Magnetic Resonance Imaging of the Spine

MICHAEL T. MODIC, M.D.
Professor of Radiology and Neurology
Case Western Reserve University School of Medicine
Head, Divisions of Magnetic Resonance Imaging and Neuroradiology
University Hospitals of Cleveland
Cleveland, Ohio

THOMAS J. MASARYK, M.D.
Assistant Professor of Radiology
Case Western Reserve University School of Medicine
University Hospitals of Cleveland
Cleveland, Ohio

JEFFREY S. ROSS, M.D.
Assistant Professor of Radiology
Case Western Reserve University School of Medicine
Neuroradiologist, University Hospitals of Cleveland
Cleveland, Ohio

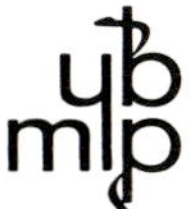

YEAR BOOK MEDICAL PUBLISHERS
CHICAGO • LONDON • BOCA RATON

3 4 5 6 7 8 9 0 KC 93 92 91 90 89

Library of Congress Cataloging-in-Publication Data

Modic, Michael T.
Magnetic resonance imaging of the spine / Michael T. Modic.
p. cm.
Includes bibliographies and index.
ISBN 0-8151-5956-0
1. Spine—Diseases—Diagnosis. 2. Spine—Imaging.
3. Magnetic resonance imaging. I. Title.
[DNLM: 1. Magnetic Resonance Imaging. 2. Spinal Diseases—diagnosis. 3. Spine—anatomy & histology. WE 725 M692m]
RD768.M63 1989
617'.3750757—dc19 88-27644
DNLM/DLC CIP
for Library of Congress

Sponsoring Editor: James D. Ryan
Associate Managing Editor, Manuscript Services: Deborah Thorp
Production Project Manager: Carol A. Reynolds
Copyeditor: Sally J. Jansen
Proofroom Manager: Shirley E. Taylor

To William C. Strittmatter,
for starting us all off.

CONTRIBUTORS

BONNIE D. FLANNIGAN-SPRAGUE, M.D.
Clinical Assistant Professor
Department of Radiology
UCLA Medical Center
Director of Neuroradiology and Magnetic Resonance Imaging
Valley Presbyterian Hospital
Van Nuys, California

E. MARK HAACKE, Ph.D
Assistant Professor
Radiology and Physics
Case Western Reserve University School of Medicine
University Hospitals of Cleveland
Cleveland, Ohio

MARK G. HUEFTLE, M.D.
Associate Radiologist
Washoe Medical Center
Reno, Nevada

BENJAMIN KAUFMAN, M.D.
Professor of Radiology
Division of Neuroradiology
Case Western Reserve University School of Medicine
Neuroradiologist, University Hospitals of Cleveland
Cleveland, Ohio

THOMAS J. MASARYK, M.D.
Assistant Professor of Radiology
Case Western Reserve University School of Medicine
Neuroradiologist, University Hospitals of Cleveland
Cleveland, Ohio

MICHAEL T. MODIC, M.D.
Professor of Radiology and Neurology
Case Western Reserve University School of Medicine
Head, Divisions of Magnetic Resonance Imaging and Neuroradiology
University Hospitals of Cleveland
Cleveland, Ohio

JEFFREY S. ROSS, M.D.
Assistant Professor of Radiology
Case Western Reserve University School of Medicine
Neuroradiologist, University Hospitals of Cleveland
Cleveland, Ohio

PREFACE

Since the introduction of MR, its potential for spinal imaging was obvious, but could not be immediately realized. The 15-mm thick, single-slice T_1-weighted images that took 8 minutes to acquire provided a glimpse into the multidimensional imaging world that MR would eventually achieve. T_2-weighted images provided the so-called CSF myelogram effect, but were time-consuming, taking between 20 and 40 minutes. Despite the cumbersome nature of the technique in the early days, the potential impact of MR provided a marked stimulus for development. Technical advances came rapidly in an effort to facilitate spinal exams. Multislice, multiecho techniques increased the area covered and improved the contrast available. Units with higher field strengths, surface coils, and sequence optimization increased signal-to-noise. This could be traded for smaller voxel elements and improved spatial resolution. Gradient-echo partial flip-angle imaging, cardiac gating, and refocusing pulses improved our control of contrast and intrinsic motion problems. Saturation pulses, half-Fourier imaging, and gradient-echo three-dimensional techniques provided artifact-free images in a shorter time with greater multidimensional reconstruction capability. Paramagnetic contrast agents have opened further avenues for both research and clinical applications by providing the ability to manipulate contrast in both normal and diseased tissues. Despite this progress, the modality remains in an evolutionary stage, with almost unlimited room for improvement.

What has resulted from these improvements is not just an imaging exam with superb morphologic accuracy, but a procedure that has provided us a view of the biochemical and pathophysiological changes at the heart of disease processes.

In our opinion, it is already the best first test for the majority of clinical situations requiring spinal imaging. But while providing more information than more conventional studies, it demands more in terms of understanding from its user. It is all too easy for technical imaging options to be ordered in a "cook book" fashion. Nevertheless, we should strive to maintain a cognitive rather than Pavlovian attitude, and should make an effort to understand the technical options available. To optimize the technical considerations and imaging protocols requires an understanding of the pathogenesis, presentation, and potential treatment options in various disease processes, as well as the normal anatomy and basic science aspects of the modality.

Hopefully, this text will serve all clinical scientists whose interest is the spine, no matter which discipline they call home. We have attempted to impart the present status of MR, both in terms of technique and clinical applications, in a logical fashion. It is our intention to integrate normal anatomy, disease process, basic science, and technical considerations in the performance of the MR exam. The first chapter deals with the basic principles behind imaging strategies and is followed by a chapter on normal anatomy that consolidates the technical principles with the anatomic substrate of the MR signal. The remainder of the book concerns itself with pathological processes, again integrating technical considerations with clinical conditions and suggesting reasonable imaging strategies. In this fashion we hope to address the major questions of spinal imaging, not providing dogmatic answers, but allowing informed choices.

It must be emphasized that MRI represents a tool for morphologic and biochemical analysis. In certain situations there may only be a moderate correlation between the imaging evidence of morphologic alteration and the presence of symptoms. The jump from the identification of an anatomic derangement to a symptom complex must be made with caution. The management of patients with spinal disorders must begin and end with a thorough clinical assessment, with imaging being an intermediate test that must be integrated into, rather than isolated from, that assessment.

Last, a critic might say that we do a disservice and perhaps even an injustice by focusing so strongly on MR as the primary diagnostic modality in the evaluation of the spine. That is their right, but this is our book.

Michael T. Modic, M.D.

ACKNOWLEDGMENTS

This text represents the direct and indirect contributions of many people without whose help it would never have been completed: Ms. Helen Kurz, whose organizational and word processing skills were severely tested but never broken; the technical staff, for their tireless devotion to excellence (when not behind schedule); our neuroradiology fellows, Mark Hueftle, Sarah Beale, David Berns, and Susan Blaser, who provided case material, suggestions, proofreading assistance, and, perhaps most important, physical support of our routine work during trying times. Joe Molter provided photographic support, while Anne Owens and Susan Weil provided their artistic skills. Eric Reinhardt, Klaus Hambueschen, and Gerhard Paetzel have been enthusiastic and instrumental in supporting our technical capabilities. Our chairman, Ralph J. Alfidi, provided the stimulus and atmosphere in which a book such as this could evolve. Last, and with our greatest gratitude, we thank our families, who never once raised the spectre of divorce or death (at least not out loud).

Michael T. Modic, M.D.

CONTENTS

The future's so bright you gotta wear — shades.

Tim Buk 3
The Future's So Bright

1

Image Behavior: Resolution, Signal-to-Noise, Contrast, and Artifacts

E. Mark Haacke, Ph.D.

INTRODUCTION

Magnetic resonance imaging (MRI) might well be classified as the most flexible imaging modality in medicine. The innate ability to massage the spins into the desired state and to enhance contrast almost at will leads to a myriad of practical sequences. Concomitant with this freedom is the large number of variable sequence parameters. Choosing the right sequence can be difficult, as the price to pay for certain advantages may be a reduction in resolution and contrast or an increase in imaging time. The astute user needs to address the following technical issues before acquiring the data: sampling interval, number of sample points, field of view (FOV), gradient strength, resolution, signal, contrast (and hence contrast resolution), slice thickness, field inhomogeneities, chemical shift, presence of metallic material and other potential artifacts inherent in a given sequence,[1–3] acquisition time, and sequence type. These issues will be presented qualitatively in the main text with the technical details relegated to subsections aimed at the interested reader. The technical details outlined in this chapter are an essential ingredient to the design of any MR imaging sequence. For those with little background in MR and for those practitioners desirous of a summary of current status, the text can serve as a primer; all of the qualitative features are summarized in the last section on clinical implementation. A brief reading is then possible by combining the last section on clinical implications and suggested protocols along with a study of the figures. In the conclusions, new suggestions generated as a result of the analysis presented in the body of the text are summarized.

SPIN BEHAVIOR

The MR image is obtained by encoding the spatial information in a specific manner, i.e., with applied magnetic gradients. To appreciate the anatomy of the experiment, the workings of magnetic resonance must be examined. A proton placed in a static magnetic field will precess (spin) about the field axis with a frequency proportional to the magnetic field strength (Fig 1–1). Specifically, the Larmor equation summarizes this behavior:

$$\omega = \gamma B_0 \tag{1}$$

The constant, γ, is the gyromagnetic ratio for the proton and in SI units is 2.67×10^8 rad/tesla(T)/second. This corresponds to 42.6 MHz/T for protons. Each element with spin has its own gyromagnetic ratio and Larmor frequency and will not interfere with proton imaging.

To detect a signal, the net nonzero bulk magnetization, M_0, generated by the static magnetic field, B_0, must be tipped into the plane perpendicular to B_0. Later, when the imaging concept is discussed, ρ will be used instead of M_0 to represent the local spin density. This transverse plane is usually chosen to be the xy plane. Applying an oscillating radiofrequency (rf) field along the y axis causes M_0 to be rotated about y until it is along x in the xy plane (Fig 1–2,*a* and *b*). It is then turned off, and we are ready to measure a signal. This is the simplest type of experiment and can be used to quantitate the total number of spins in the object being imaged. The signal will be detected by a coil whose design is such that any rotation of the magnetization in the xy plane is picked up as a flux change and hence induces a voltage (Fig 1–2,*c*). The resulting signal is Fourier transformed (i.e., we extract the different frequency components), and, of course, for a uniform static field, we find only a single component at zero frequency after demodulation of the signal (see equations 4 through 9). Note that no relaxation is assumed here, and it is the coupling of the rotating M_{xy} component that leads to detection, not the longitudinal decay of spins back along B_0.

Coils can be designed to transmit or receive in quadrature (the simultaneous transmission or detection of both x and y channels). The best approach is to drive the coils in a circular polarized mode (with equal components in the x and y directions but 90 degrees out of phase). The advantages for transmission are a more uniform rf field that penetrates the body and a factor-of-2 reduction in required power. For reception, the advantage is a factor of $\sqrt{2}$ improvement in the signal-to-noise ratio (S/N). Most units today still use linear polarized (driven in one direction only) coils and do not yet take full advantage of this potential.

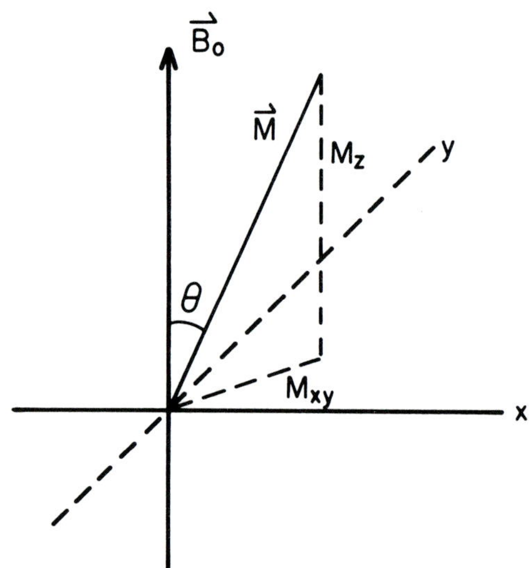

FIG 1–1.
A pictorial representation of the magnetization of a single spin in the presence of a static magnetic field along the z axis. The magnetic dipole of a spin precesses about B_o and has a nonzero M_{xy} component. A set or "isochromat" of spins has a uniform distribution of the phase of this M_{xy} component. Hence the bulk magnetization has $M_{xy} = 0$, and we "see" only a nonzero M_z component.

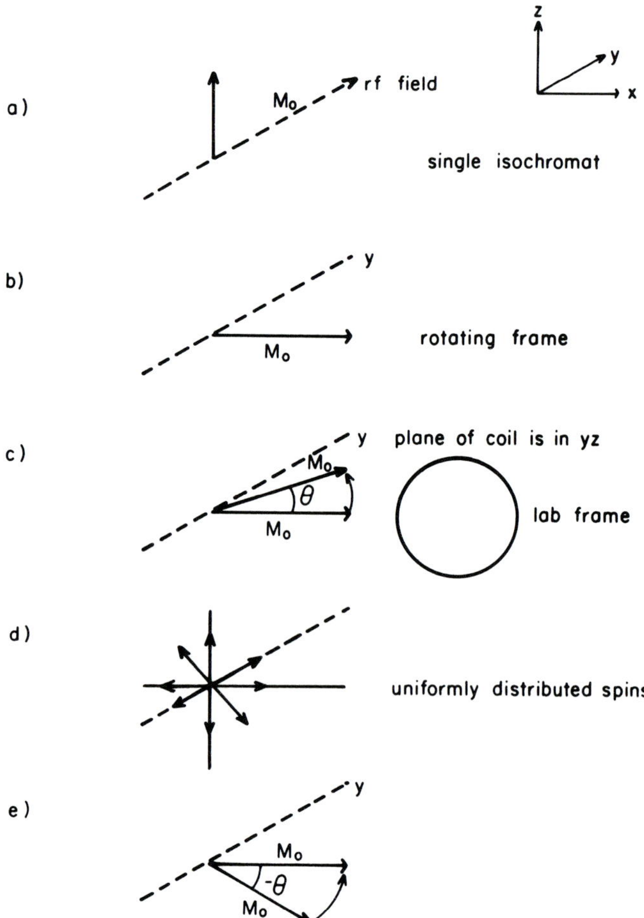

FIG 1–2.
The spin behavior of an isochromat *(a)* after reaching equilibrium and *(b)* after application of a $\frac{\pi}{2}$-pulse along the y axis in the rotating reference frame; *(c)* the same spins pictured in the laboratory frame at a time t ($\theta = \omega t$) rotating counterclockwise and inducing a voltage in the adjacent coil; *(d)* in a field with local inhomogeneities, the spins of the isochromat "dephase" so that the macroscopic signal M_{xy} goes to zero (this is the usual T_2 decay phenomenon); and *(e)* after rotation about x with a π-pulse, the spin at an angle θ becmes relocated at $-\theta$, and eventually it (and other spins too) refocus along x.

We assume that the spins start off aligned along the static field, B_0. They actually had to get to an equilibrium state first. They do this in a time frame determined by the longitudinal or spin-lattice relaxation time, T_1. The dependence of M_z on T_1 is expressed as

$$M_0(1 - e^{-t/T1}) \qquad 2$$

Here t is the time from when the M_z component was

zero. For t greater than $3T_1$, more than 95% of the equilibrium value has recovered. According to the simple experiment described above, M_{xy} is proportional to the starting value of M_z. Hence, the bigger M_z, the larger the flux change and the larger the signal.

Another relaxation phenomenon plays a significant role in imaging—the transverse or spin-spin relaxation, T_2. After spins are in the xy plane, if they interact with local fields, ΔB_0, so that the effective field that they see is not B_0 but $B_0 + \Delta B_0$, then neighboring spins will rotate at different frequencies. In that case, in a given local microscopic region, spins get out of phase (Fig 1–2,*d*). The effective magnetization is the vector sum of the spins, and when the spins have become uniformly distributed from zero to 2π, no signal will be left. The empirical behavior is found to be exponential in nature so that after a given $\pi/2$-pulse at a time t′ later, the signal has decayed by $\exp(-t'/T_2)$.

This dephasing can also occur on a macroscopic level and leads to additional dephasing apart from the intrinsic T_2 of the tissue. These other causes include local static field inhomogeneities such as those caused by metal implants, air/tissue interfaces, and any other susceptibility changes between tissues. Further dephasing effects can be caused by motion (see "Systematic Noise: Motion and Phase"). If the amount of dephasing in a pixel runs up to 2π (Fig 1–2,*d*), then no signal remains.

The spin-echo (SE) sequence (see "Sequence Structure and Contrast") was designed to refocus spins even in the presence of field inhomogeneities. If all spins are reversed about x by applying an rf pulse along x at a time τ then at 2τ they have all refocused. Similarly, when performing slice selection, the spins see different fields due to the gradient applied along the z axis (G_z). Figure 1–3 *a* through *d* shows the spins along z during and after the $\pi/2$-pulse and then again after refocusing the spins. For a π-pulse, no refocusing is required since the dephasing that occurs in rotating the first 90 degrees from the xy plane along $-B_0$ is exactly balanced by the continued rotation back to the xy plane along the opposite direction where the spins continue precessing in the same direction and hence refocus (Fig 1–3, *e–g*).

Relaxation-time dependence on frequency can be an important issue in choosing the ideal sequence. The changes in T_1 are fairly dramatic. For example, gray and white matter change from roughly 500 msec and 300 msec at 0.15 T to 1,000 msec and 600 msec at 1.5 T. The effects on T_2 are small, but the dependence of the T_2^* component due to static fields is linear with frequency. This can lead to significant signal loss for gradient echo sequences, which are more sensitive to T_2^* effects (see "Finite Sampling and Resolution").

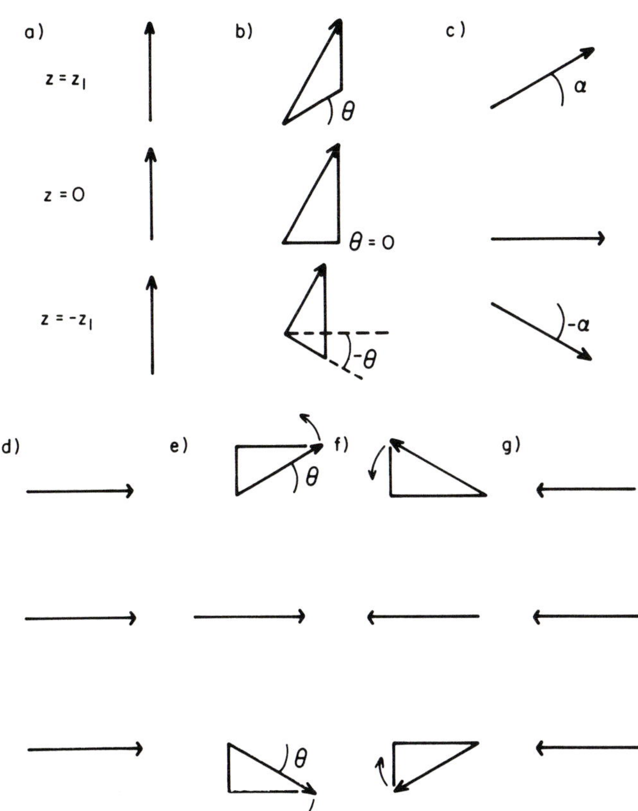

FIG 1–3.
When exciting a slice *(a)*, the gradient in the slice-select direction dephases the spins in the xy plane *(b)* throughout its rotation and in the final M_{xy} state *(c)*. For this reason, a rephasing gradient in z is applied to bring the spins back in phase *(d)*. Continuing the rotation with a π-pulse results in a similar dephasing *(e)*, but once the spins are past the 90-degree point *(f)*, any dephasing is automatically refocussed *(g)*.

THE IMAGING CONCEPT

Imaging a Line

The dependence of frequency on field strength suggests a simple way to discriminate an object's position along a line. Change the field along the line. This is done by introducing a magnetic field gradient, G, so that the frequency dependence is

$$f(x) = \bar{\gamma} G x$$

where $\bar{\gamma} = \gamma/2\pi$. The measured data then contain a sum of frequency components, in general, which can be separated by Fourier transformation. The amplitudies of the spectral components represent the spin density at that frequency or, equivalently, position.

Any extraneous noise at a frequency f′ would appear at the pixel associated with that frequency. The presence of a field inhomogeneity caused by diamag-

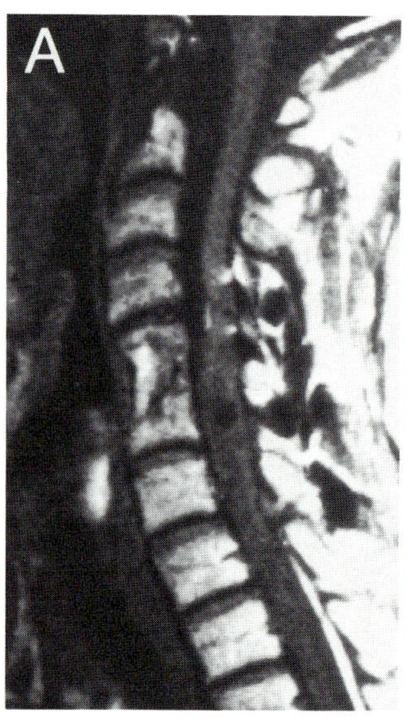

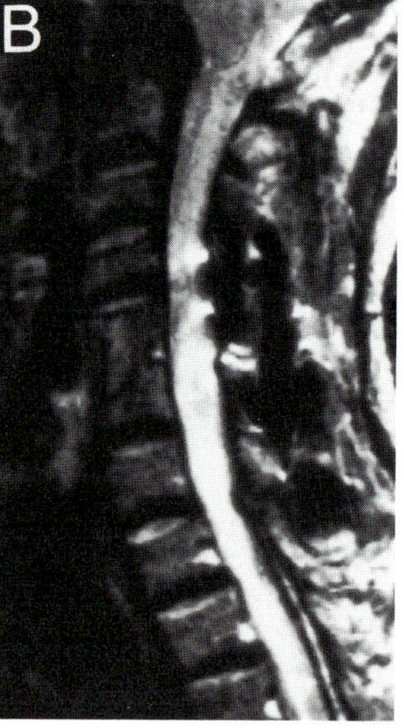

FIG 1–4.
An example of the distortion caused by a metal implant is shown for an SE sequence with TE = 20 msec (**A**) and TE = 90 msec (**B**). The latter was acquired with a lower read gradient (bandwidth optimized), and the distortion and chemical shift are accordingly worse. The associated inhomogeneities also cause changes in the slice profile. The effect of the field distortion near sinuses can leak into adjacent slices in a gradient echo (GE) sequence for similar reasons and cause significant darkening or dephasing.

netic (roughly several parts per million, ppm) or ferromagnetic material causes a shift in frequency. The effects from the latter can be so severe that local image intensity can be significantly affected (Fig 1–4).[1–4] Similarly, chemical shifts cause a pixel misregistration as shown in Figure 1–5.

The one-dimensional field dependence of a spin in a static gradient field is

$$B(x) = B_0 + Gx \tag{4}$$

where

$$G = \frac{\partial B_0}{\partial x} \tag{5}$$

is in the direction of the static field. The frequency dependence is

$$\omega(x) = \gamma Gx + \omega_0 \tag{6}$$

After demodulation,[5] (removing the central frequency),

$$\omega(x) = \gamma Gx \tag{7}$$

The frequency dependence in Hz is then

$$f(x) = \bar{\gamma} Gx \tag{8}$$

When a gradient is turned on in an imaging sequence, it causes a phase change in cycles equal to

$$\begin{aligned} \phi(x) &= \bar{\gamma} \int G(t)x(t)dt \\ &= \bar{\gamma} Gtx \end{aligned} \tag{9}$$

when G(t) and x(t) are independent of time. Hence, after the initial or dephasing gradient, if the gradient is switched, the phase reverses direction, and the spin echoes or refocuses when the second gradient has been on as long as the first (or when the integral of equation 9 gives exactly the same phase value of opposite sign). Unfortunately, switching the gradient does not cause spins rotating at the wrong frequency to be refocused. For a

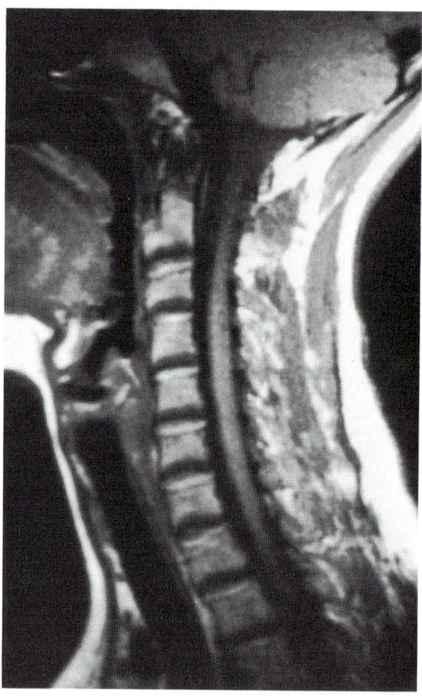

FIG 1–5.
Chemical-shift artifacts manifest themselves in two ways. First, fat shifts in the read direction by $G\Delta x/\delta B$ pixels where δ is the chemical shift in parts per million. This causes a loss of signal where it should be in one region and an increase in signal in the opposite direction (see the vertebral bodies/disk overlap). Unfortunately, there is a further complication; when fat and water overlap and the π-pulse is not properly centered with respect to the echo, some signal cancellation between water and fat occurs. When this cancellation is maximum, an opposed image is obtained, and regions where water and fat signals would otherwise have equal intensities now cancel. Signal from regions with intermediate combinations is appropriately reduced. Figure 1–32,*B* shows this for an opposed phase sequence designed with a shift in the π-pulse of 1.65 msec at 1.0 T.

spin-echo sequence, the π-pulse is applied at time TE/2 and rotates the spins from one side of the xy plane to the other about, say, the x axis. The phase is now $-\phi(x)$, and after an equal amount of time with a gradient of the same sign now, the phase refocusses at TE (see Fig 1–2, *c* and *e*). Note that even if the frequency is shifted by a field inhomogeneity, it still echoes. This is the reason for performing spin-echo sequences in many cases.

Now if a noise component has a frequency f it will appear at the position $x = f/\gamma G$. Likewise, if there is a field inhomogeneity $\Delta B(x)$, the information from x will appear at $x + \Delta B(x)/G$. The same type of dislocation occurs for a chemical shift, δ, where information is shifted by $\delta B(x)/G$.

Sampling

The data are sampled at uniform intervals in time chosen so as to avoid aliasing. Wrap-around, fold-over, or aliasing are synonyms for the misregistration of a frequency component when the sampling is not fast enough. For example, if you blink at time intervals of t when viewing a rotating disk and see a mark at the top, apparently unmoving, the disk may have rotated once, twice, three times, etc. Nevertheless, you will think it has the same period of motion as the rate at which you blink, i.e., t, (Fig 1–6). The Nyquist condition is then that

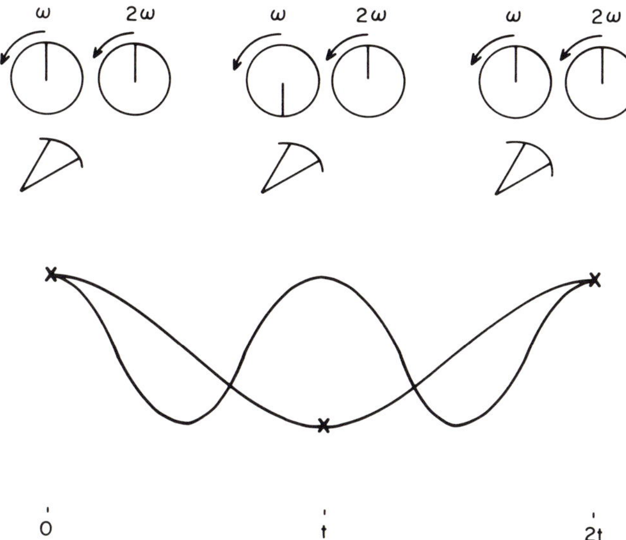

FIG 1–6.
Aliasing can be understood as an undersampling of the signal that contains some high-frequency components. Two spinning disks start at some phase, say 12 o'clock. After a time t, the slower disk appears at 6 o'clock, and the faster disk apparently has a frequency of 2ω, 4ω, or higher. At a time 2t, the slower dial has returned to 12 o'clock, and it is clear that it has a frequency ω. Frequencies that are higher than ω get aliased back modulo ω.

sampling rate at which no aliasing occurs or $1/\Delta t$. The maximum frequency range in the image, also called the bandwidth, must then be less than $1/\Delta t$. Some examples are presented in Figure 1–7.

The Nyquist condition for sampling sufficiently rapidly in time is

$$\Delta t = 1/\gamma GL \qquad 10$$

where t is the sampling interval, and L the field of view. Note γGL is the maximum frequency bandwidth occurring in the object being imaged. If n time points (or, equivalently, phase-encoded steps) are collected, the total sampling time, T, is

$$T = n\Delta t \qquad 11$$

and the spatial resolution, x, is defined as

$$\Delta x = L/n \qquad 12$$

Note that equation 10 can be rewritten several ways:

$$\gamma G = 1/T\Delta x \qquad 13$$

or

$$L = 1/\gamma G\Delta t \qquad 14$$

for example.

Image Reconstruction

Although no mathematical details of the Fourier transform (FT) or other reconstruction techniques will be given here (see reference 6), several general comments can be made. Initially, spectral estimates were obtained by reconstructing free induction decay (FID) data using cosine and sine transforms over n/2 positive time points only. When an echo occurs, a complex inverse Fourier transform is applied over n points. There is no improvement in resolution (since no new frequency information is obtained), but there is an increase in S/N of $\sqrt{2}$. This is all fine as long as $\exp(-TE/T_2)$ does not reduce the signal beyond $\sqrt{2}$ (unless a T_2-weighted image is desired). Today flow effects are recognized as being very sensitive to TE. Fast flow will have the lowest phase effects for the shortest TE. Likewise, for very short T_2 values, the shortest TE should be used. For these reasons, the FID sequence is likely to prove useful again.

When FID sequences are used, phases must be determined accurately in order to reconstruct an artifact-free image. For any data acquisition, sampling must be

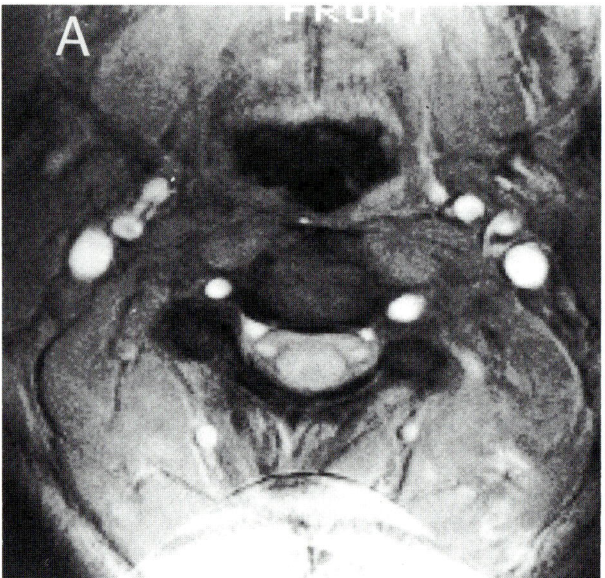

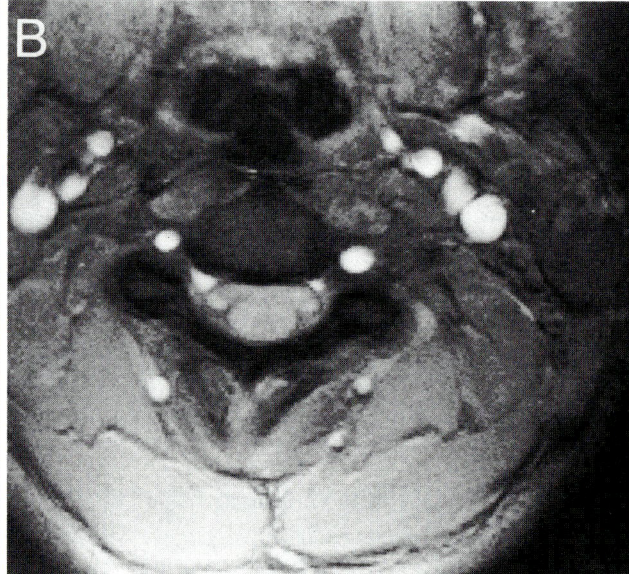

FIG 1–7.
Aliasing occurs when spurious frequency information is not filtered out and/or when the field of view (FOV) does not cover the whole object/subject. This is illustrated in the cervical spine. The read direction is along the vertical axis, and the FOV is 15 × 15 cm. Since the chin extends past 15 cm in the vertical direction, it folds back into the picture (**A**). By doubling the sampling rate, i.e., doubling the FOV in the read direction to 30 cm, the amount of information outside 30 cm due to coil fall off is negligible, and hence no aliasing occurs. Usually only the central 15 cm is displayed (**B**). (This could also have been accomplished with the perfect analog filter, but in practice there is a slight roll off at the edges). Another example of aliasing occurs in 3D imaging when the slice profile for a selective slab of interest is not ideal. Since an analog filter cannot be used in a phase-encoding direction to filter out unwanted material, the information from outside the slice will alias back into the 3D slices.

uniform if Fourier transform reconstruction is to be used. Techniques such as hybrid or echo-planar imaging collect data by nonuniform sampling. Nevertheless, it is still possible to reconstruct artifact-free images.[6]

SEQUENCE STRUCTURE AND CONTRAST

Radiofrequency Pulses and Region Selection

The use of gradients is not only for spatial localization for imaging a line but also for spatial selection of a region of interest. For example, applying a $\pi/2$-pulse with a gradient along z creates a region of spins in a slice transverse to z (Fig 1–8,*a*). Applying next a π-pulse at a time τ later with a gradient along y creates a slab of spins (Fig 1–8,*b*) that will refocus at 2τ. The usual π-pulse in a multislice sequence will be applied to excite the same region (see Fig 1–8,*a*) so that multiple pulses applied along the z axes will have the same T_1 behavior and less slice-to-slice interference. When contiguous slices are attempted with rf slice profiles so broad that slice overlap occurs, then saturation results in a significant signal loss (Fig 1–9).

Aliasing can be avoided in the read direction by the correct choice of analogue filter. To reduce the FOV by 2, simply cut the analogue filter in half. Unfortunately, the phase-encoding sampling is discrete, and unless projection reconstruction is used, there is no analogue filter to apply. Localization techniques are well known, however, from the desire to obtain spectroscopic information from a small region anywhere in the body. This is accomplished by changing the orientation of subsequent pulses in an SE experiment or just by introducing new "saturation" pulses. These concepts have reappeared as techniques also useful in imaging for avoiding aliasing with small FOV since only the region of interest is excited. For example, for a single acquisition and two orthogonal pulses, the excited region shown in the shaded volume of Figure 1–8, *b* can be obtained. Now the read direction lies along the lateral direction and can be analog filtered to allow very small-volume excitations.

The concept of a reduced FOV is, of course, identical to the proposed saturation schemes to reduce motion artifacts. The selected volume of interest is simply chosen to lie in a region where little or no motion occurs.[7] A review of volume localization appears in reference 8.

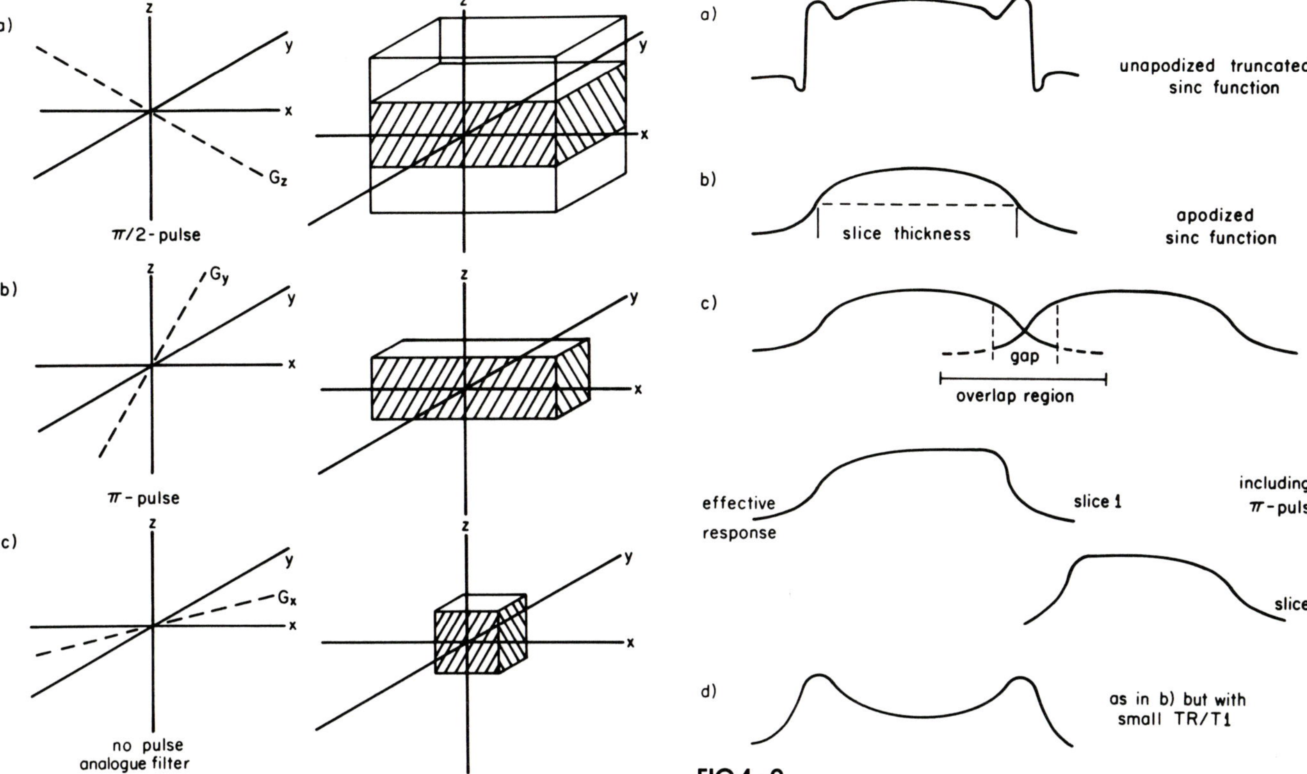

FIG 1–8.
Slice selection is accomplished by exciting a range of frequencies with an rf pulse applied while a gradient (or set of gradients) defines the axis perpendicular to the desired plane. A spin-echo sequence might have a $\pi/2$-pulse that selects a slab in the xy plane *(a)* followed by a π-pulse that selects a slab in the xz plane. Only the strip region remains *(b)*. During the read process, an analogue filter can be applied that then leaves signal from a selected volume of interest *(c)*. These saturation techniques are used in spatial localization for spectroscopy and motion suppression in imaging.

FIG 1–9.
The rf currents are usually applied to the coil for only a few milliseconds. A signal that is sin x/x in nature would normally produce a perfect square wave or set of frequencies to allow clean slice definition. When the signal is truncated, the frequency response is broadened *(a)*. If the signal is then filtered, the response is smoothed *(b)*. For multislice imaging, with a gap, the spins in a given slice may be multiply excited *(c)*. This extra saturation often causes a loss of signal (extra T_1 weighting). The first slice may be less affected, but subsequent slices will have a loss of signal (they are now effectively thinner). The best solution is to leave a larger gap or a full gap and interleave the slices. Even then, the effective TR in the overlap region is TR/2, and some signal loss still occurs. When short TRs are used, there is an optimal angle (see "Gradient Field Echo Sequences" and Figure 1–28), and the effective slice profile response is bilobed *(d)*.

Sequence Types

The free induction decay experiment described, via a single α-degree rf pulse (usually 90 degrees), can be used to image a line (Fig 1–10,*a*). Equivalently, if the object is in a uniform field and no gradient is applied, the Fourier transform will then give nonzero terms, which represent any chemical shift components. Usually these are so small in hydrogen imaging that they all lie in the same pixel (i.e., the shifts are only a small part of a pixel) except for the lipid components.

In the case when T_2 is small, the FID experiment is necessary because there is little time to collect the data before the signal is gone. In human imaging, tissue T_2 is usually long enough that there is time to apply a dephasing and rephasing gradient to create a gradient field echo sequence (Fig 1–10,*b*). This allows for an improvement of $\sqrt{2}$ in S/N because the number of sampled points has been doubled (although the image and pixel size remain unaltered). Gradient echo sequences can be made with very short TE values. This is useful to overcome field inhomogeneities and to obtain true spin-density or T_1-weighted images. Recall that if $T_2 = 80$ msec and TE $= 20$ msec 25% of the signal is still lost ($\exp[-TE/T_2] \approx 1 - TE/T_2$ for small TE). If no increase in gradient strength is required, then decreasing TE from 20 msec to 10 msec gives a 12.5% increase in signal. Of course, the shorter TE in an FID experiment allows for a slightly higher signal still.

When T_2^* is a problem, a T_2-weighted (or even a T_1-

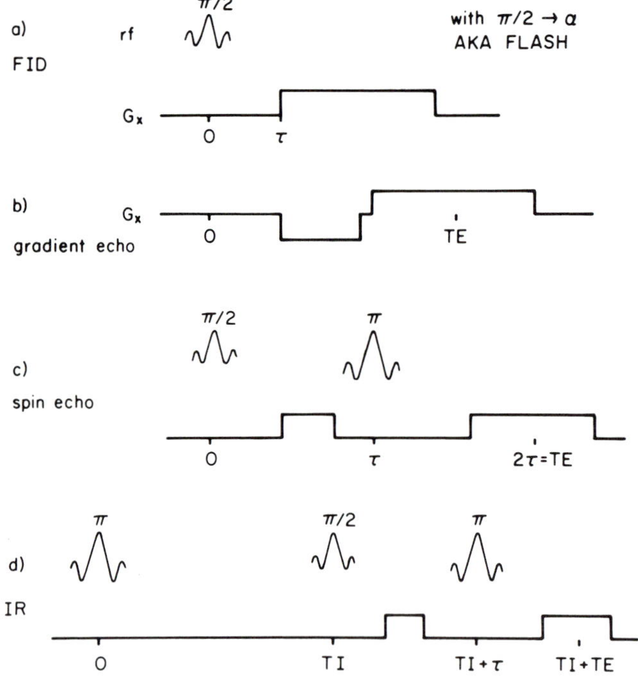

FIG 1–10.
The rf and gradient structure and timings for *(a)* a free induction decay (FID); *(b)* a gradient field echo (GFE); *(c)* a spin echo (SE); and *(d)* an inversion recovery (IR) sequence.

weighted sequence with TE = 20 msec or more) gradient echo sequence will be very poor. Hence a spin-echo sequence, which refocuses field inhomogeneities, is required. Otherwise, there would be little need for this specialized sequence as all T_1- and T_2-weighted properties are equally well represented by its gradient echo counterpart. The spin-echo sequence is a $\pi/2$-pulse followed by a π-pulse rotated about either the same axis (produces a negative echo) or the perpendicular axis (see Fig 1–10,*c*). By alternating multiple pulses in this manner, a multiecho sequence can be created. This is called a Carr-Purcell-Meiboom-Gill (CPMG) sequence.

The amount of T_1 weighting is determined (for the most part) by the repeat time for all of the previous three sequences and follows from equation 2 with t = TR (repeat time). An increase in T_1 contrast is possible with a variation on those pulse sequences by completely inverting the magnetization initially. Since it must grow back up to M_0, too, the z component behaves as

$$M_0\,(1 - 2e^{-TR/T_1}) \qquad 15$$

and hence, with respect to a given TR, it changes twice as fast as in the usual sequences (viz. equation 2). The more general inversion-recovery experiment allows for a reasonable recovery time, TI, before a $\pi/2$-pulse is applied after inversion to read out the data (see Fig 1–10,*d*). The image amplitude dependence then looks more like

$$M_0\,(1 - 2e^{-TI/T_1} + e^{-TR/T_1}) \qquad 16$$

Another useful aspect of this approach is the potential of exact cancellation of the signal from a specific tissue for the appropriate choice of TR and TI. This is the concept behind short TI inversion-inversion recovery (STIR)[9] to reduce motion artifacts by eliminating the signal from fat. This does not imply that this generates optimal contrast for discrimination between tissues or between diseased and normal tissue.

The usual image amplitude for a free induction decay sequence (Fig 1–10,*a*) is

$$\rho(1 - e^{-TR/T_1})\,e^{-\tau/T_2} \qquad 17$$

where M_0 has been replaced by ρ, the spin density. For a gradient echo sequence it is

$$\rho(1 - e^{-TR/T_1})\,e^{-TE/T_2} \qquad 18$$

Actually, the dependence is on T_2^* not T_2 where T_2^* contains filter and field inhomogeneity effects (see "Finite Sampling and Resolution" for more deails). When TR/T_1 is small, and TE = 0, the signal becomes

$$\rho\ TR/T_1 \qquad 19$$

This heavily T_1-weighted image can have its S/N increased linearly by only doubling its time to 2TR (if contrast so allows it). If TR/T_1 is very large, the image is only proportional to ρ.

However, the above equations are not complete when the flip angle is not 90 degrees because the spins are then acted on again when phase encoding is included. To account for this, several saturation cycles are run until equilibrium is attained. The actual equilibrium value reached when the transverse magnetization is zero prior to the next pulse for the gradient field echo (GFE) is

$$\frac{\rho\sin\theta\,(1 - e^{-TR/T_1})\,e^{-TE/T_2^*}}{1 - \cos\theta\,e^{-TR/T_1}} \qquad 20$$

and the maximum signal is obtained when

$$\theta = \cos^{-1}(e^{-TR/T_1}) \qquad 21$$

and is determined solely by TR/T_1. When the optimal angle is used and TR/T_1 is small, the image is proportional to

$$\rho\sqrt{TR/T_1} \qquad 22$$

Now doubling TR or taking two acquisitions gives identical results in terms of S/N. For larger angles, the image is T_1 weighted as usual, while for small angles, the image is proportional to $\rho\sin\theta$, i.e., spin-density weighted again but now for any TR/T_1.

An important modification of the above fast low-angle shot (FLASH) sequence is to refocus the phase-encoding gradient and not dephase the M_{xy} component. This sequence approaches equilibrium too, but now for TR << T_1, T_2 and alternating rf, the signal is

$$\frac{\rho\sin\alpha \; e^{-TE/T_2^*}}{1 + \frac{T_1}{T_2} - \cos\alpha\left(\frac{T_1}{T_2} - 1\right)} \qquad 23$$

The optimal angle is determined from

$$\cos\alpha = \frac{\frac{T_1}{T_2} - 1}{\frac{T_1}{T_2} + 1} \qquad 24$$

The shortest possible TR should be used for optimal S/N followed by, if time permits, an increase in the number of acquisitions. The signal then is proportional to

$$\rho T_2/2T_1 \qquad 25$$

This sequence is often called modified FISP (fast imaging with steady precession) or gradient-recalled acquisition in a steady-state mode (GRASS) or fast steady state (FAST).

For the spin-echo sequence, the exact expression is

$$\rho(1 - 2e^{-(TR - \tau)/T1} + e^{-TR/T_1})\, e^{-TE/T_2} \qquad 26$$

For τ/TR << 1, this reduces to equation 18.

The inversion recovery sequence is somewhat more complicated:

$$\rho(1 - 2e^{-TI/T_1} + 2e^{-(TR - \tau)/T_1} - e^{-TR/T_1})\, e^{-TE/T_2} \qquad 27$$

For τ/TI << 1, this reduces to equation 16.

Contrast Types

Three types of contrast are available with the described sequences. They are spin-density weighted, T_1-weighted, and T_2-weighted. The type of examination is likely to depend on both the anatomical region and the disease process. The relative increases (changes) in ρ, T_1, T_2, and T_1/T_2 all play a key role in the decision process.

Spin-density weighting generally requires a long TR so that TR/T_1 is large and a short TE so that TE/T_2 is small. The total effective contributing water content in tissues varies by only about 20%. If water (or cerebrospinal fluid [CSF]) has a normalized spin-density value of 1.0, other tissues have the relative values displayed in Table 1–1. The sequences best suited today to take advantage of this behavior are the GFE and SE sequences. The former can also be used with very short TR values and very small angles (see equation 17 and "Gradient Field Echo Sequences"). The available contrast is illustrated in Figure 1–11.

If long TR values again are used, T_2 weighting is best demonstrated by lengthening the TE value. Using two sequences with two different TE values, the ratio of the two images contains only T_2 weighting. Before taking the ratio, the images are both spin-density and T_2 weighted. Increases in T_2, often representative of disease, then lead to potentially enhanced contrast with surrounding tissues. The actual discrimination between the two images vs. an actual T_2-weighted image depends on the S/N and how many adjacent pixels are averaged. Figure 1–12 shows the contrast for the tissues of Table 1–1. As reviewed in the sections entitled "Finite Sampling and Resolution" and "Gradient Field Echo Se-

TABLE 1–1.
Tissue Parameters (at 1.5 Tesla)

Tissue*	T_1, msec	T_2, msec	T_2^*, msec	Spin Density (Relative)
CSF	3,000	2,200	2,200	1.00
VB	554	50	8	0.80
Disk	934	90	90	0.80
Cord	700	90	90	0.75
GM	955	95	95	0.90
WM	585	85	85	0.75
Fat	284	50	50	0.90
Muscle	758	45	45	0.75
Pathology	1,300	150	150	1.00

*CSF = cerebrospinal fluid; VB = vertebral body; disk = intervertebral disk, cord = spinal cord; GM = gray matter; WM = white matter.

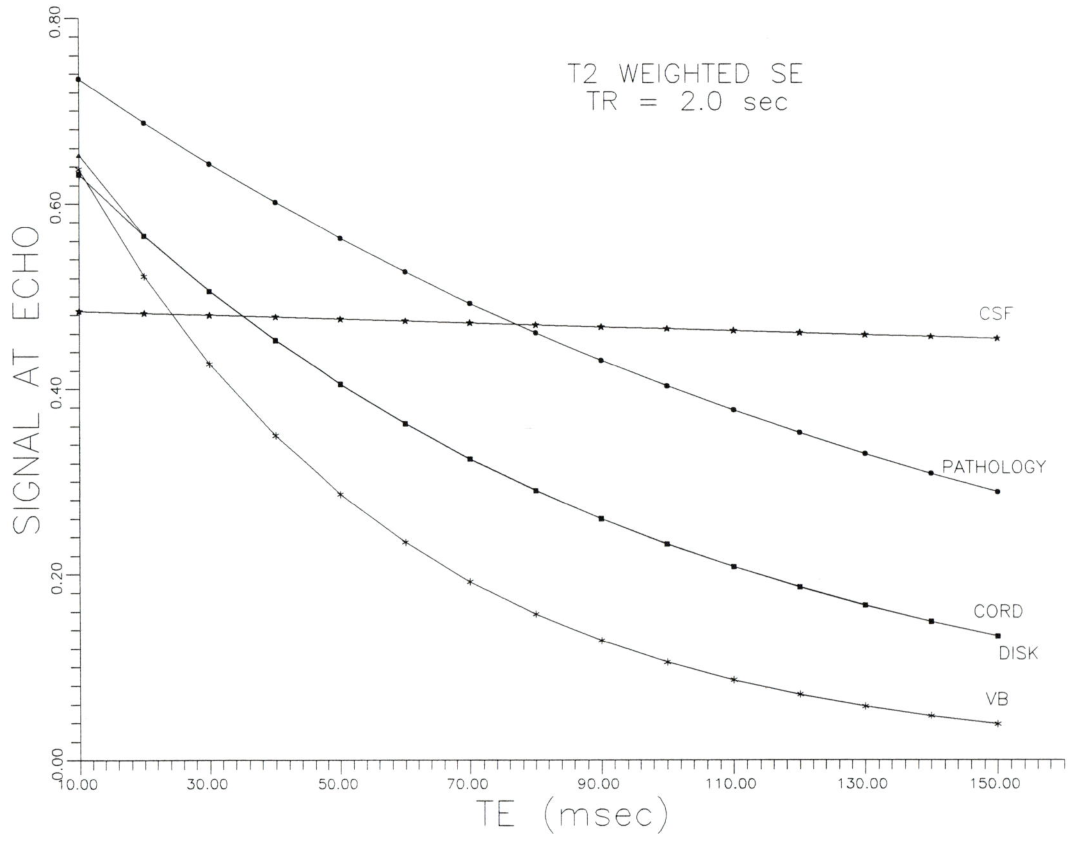

FIG 1–11.
Spin density (short TE) and T_2 (long TE) contrast example with TR = 2.0 seconds. For large TE, contrast reverses compared to the short TE portion. Note that the increase in contrast at large TE more than compensates the increase in scan time. CSF = cerebrospinal fluid; VB = vertebral body.

quences," gradient echo sequences are not appropriate for T_2-weighted images in fields with significant local field inhomogeneities.

The T_1 contrast discussed previously is best illustrated for the various tissues in Figure 1–13. The practical issue of S/N per unit time is an important one not properly revealed by Figure 1–13. For example, doubling TR gives only a small increase in actual contrast, whereas taking two acquisitions gives a $\sqrt{2}$ improvement in contrast to noise (C/N). Suggested parameter choices have been made for a variety of circumstances in several papers.[10–12]

MULTIDIMENSIONAL IMAGING AND EXAMINATION TIME

Two-Dimensional Imaging

Almost all the properties discussed in the one-dimensional (1D) imaging case carry over to 2D and 3D imaging. Two points are different: first, the sampling in the second and third direction is done by changing gradients; and second, the time required to improve resolution is no longer free as it was for extra sampling in the read direction by changing the analog filter to include only the central region of the image. This cannot be done in the other directions that are discretely sampled after the fact.

To encode the spins in the other directions, a special gradient is turned on to "phase encode" the spins. Each repeat time, the gradient is changed to encode the spins slightly differently. Just as sampling in time "catches" the spins along x at different phases, $\phi_x = \gamma G_x x t$, so each new phase-encoding step catches the spins in y at $\phi_y = \gamma G_y y t_y$. Three-dimensional imaging is accomplished by phase encoding in z (Fig 1–14) and 4D by also phase encoding in x. Note that the action of each gradient is independent, and each can be applied simultaneously. This does not apply to gradients that are on to select the slice of interest. In that case, gradients on in each direction would be used to select an oblique slice.

Of course, in 2D imaging, a slice-select gradient is applied to give a certain slice thickness. Since profiles

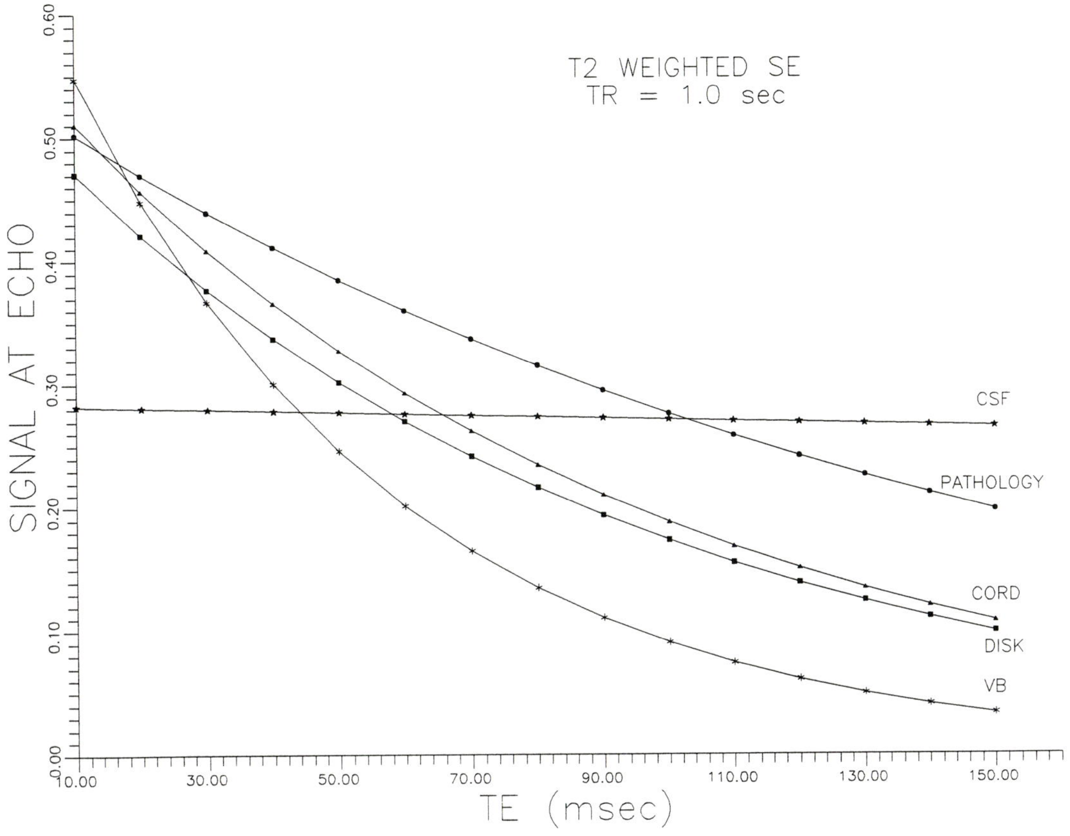

FIG 1–12.
T_2-weighted contrast curves for intermediate TR = 1.0 second. Although contrast is still good, to recover the same contrast to noise (C/N) as in Figure 1–11 at large TE = 90 msec, the scan would have to be repeated four times.

are not infinitely sharp, information from regions outside the desired slice all collapse to potentially confound image interpretation (partial voluming).[13–15] When multislice imaging is used, the interference between slice profiles can significantly decrease S/N and change expected contrast since some spins are more saturated than expected (see Fig 1–9). Two improvements include increasing the gap between slices or using gaps equal to the slice thickness and then interleaving back to fill in the gaps.

Three-Dimensional Imaging

As mentioned above, extra phase encoding along the slice-select direction allows for a 3D imaging technique. The real advantages of 3D imaging are efficiency; contiguous slices; short rf pulses for thick slices; higher signal-to-noise per unit time when multislice technique is not possible; a reduction of T_2^* effects when gradient echoes are used; and high-resolution, isotropic imaging. For fast imaging sequences with short repeat times, TR, 3D data sets can be collected in roughly 5 to 10 minutes. The single-slice equivalents, collected serially to avoid motion artifacts and maintain the same contrast characteristics, could also be done in the same time for the same number of slices as 3D phase-encoding steps, n, (or partitions) in the slice-select direction. Unfortunately, the single slices would suffer the usual rf profile difficulties, especially for thin slices, but even worse, the S/N would be $\sqrt{n}$ times lower. Three-dimensional imaging is more vulnerable to motion artifacts though, unless a reduced FOV and saturation pulses are used. When too few slices (or too small an n) are used, then the slice profile is effectively the point spread function of the finite window, and slice interference occurs due to Gibbs' ringing in this direction. The extra gradients associated with changes in permeability between different tissues or materials causes a lowering of T_2^* (see "Finite Sampling and Resolution"). Three-dimensional imaging can partially overcome this effect by collecting enough partitions so that the phase-encoding gradient exactly cancels the local induced gradient in that direction. Taking a few more steps past this then gives a signal in the slice-select direction that looks like an asym-

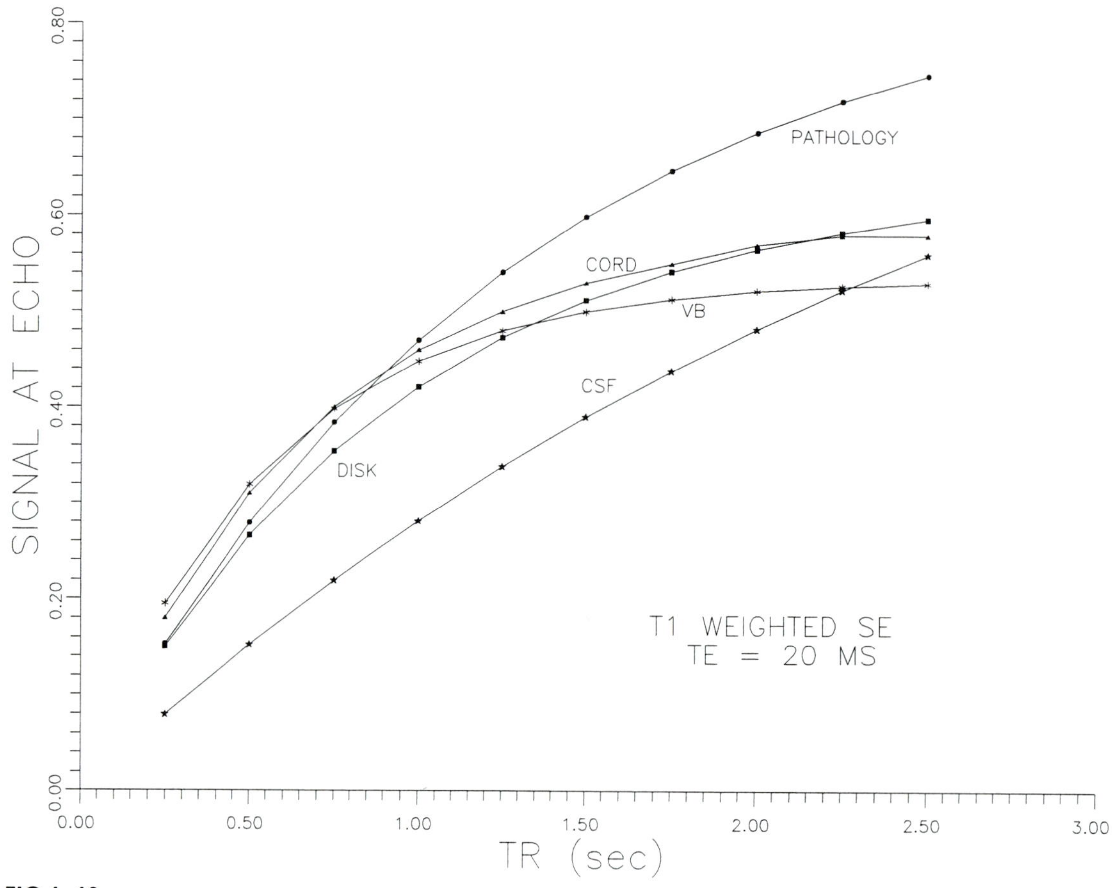

FIG 1–13.
T_1 contrast curves with TE = 20 msec. The optimal overall tissue contrast per unit time is for TR ≃ 0.5 sec. Large T_1 tissues appear very "black" or low in signal intensity.

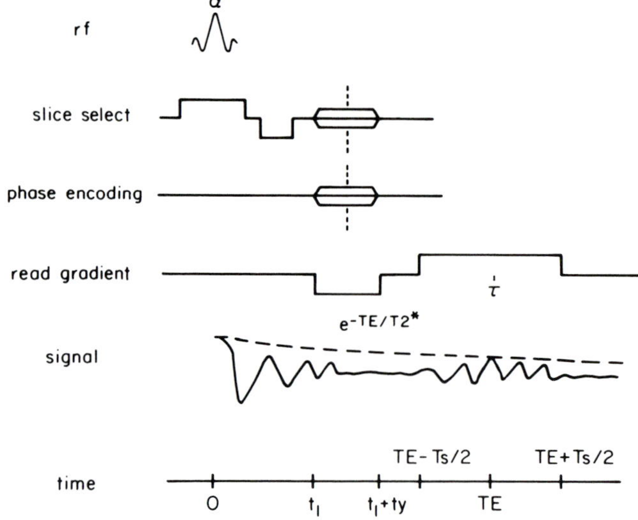

FIG 1–14.
The complete sequence structure for a 3D gradient echo sequence. Note that because of the independence of spin phasing, all three gradients can be applied simultaneously to accomplish the desired spin preparation.

metrically sampled echo. On Fourier transformation, the magnitude image has completely recovered its lost signal. This is demonstrated in Figure 1–15.[16] Dephasing still occurs in the read direction, and hence the smallest TE should still be used.

Four-Dimensional Imaging

Normally, the technique of phase encoding in all three directions and collecting the signal without a gradient is used for spectroscopic imaging. However, the 3D gradient echo images will still do poorly in the presence of metal implants due to large local gradients and T_2^*. By collecting 4D data, the frequency encoding distortion that remains can also be eliminated. After Fourier transformation, a set of 3D images with different frequency components will appear. Adding all of these together would then give an image without artifacts. With new fast imaging techniques, this may be very reasonable for in vitro high-field imaging if not for in vivo imaging.

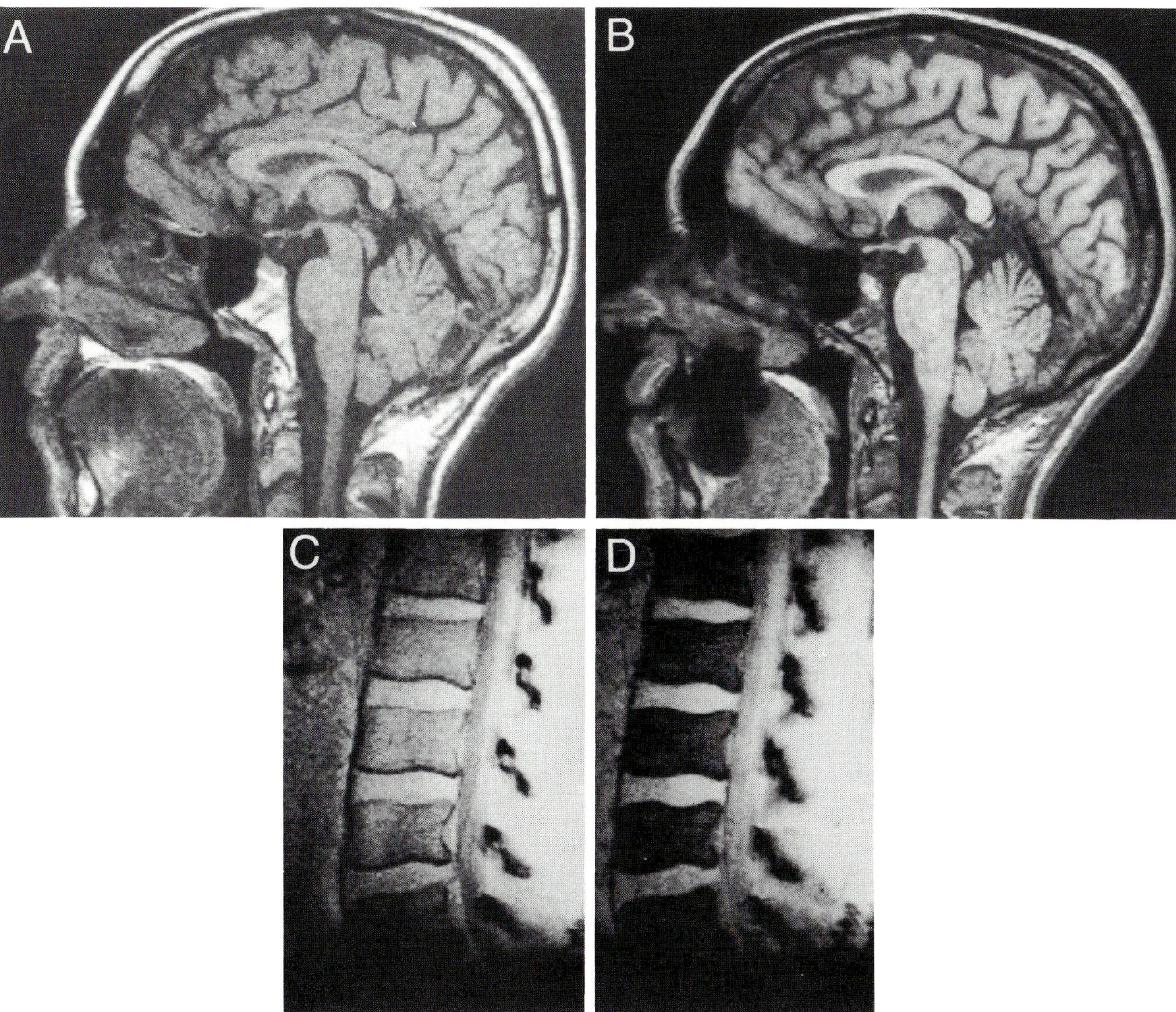

FIG 1–15.
Gradient echo imaging would be ideal for fast and slow imaging if field inhomogeneities did not cause low T_2^* and hence lead to poor quality T_2-weighted images. They would also be superior to spin-echo images because of poor rf slice profiles for the 180-degree pulses. Compare Figures 1–15,**A** and **B,** which are from a FATE (fast short TE spin echo sequence) and a GE TE = 15-msec sequence for n = 256 and FOV = 30 cm × 30 cm, respectively, at 1.0 T. The FATE image was acquired with 8 partitions with TE = 200 msec and the FLASH image with Nacq = 8 and TR = 100 msec. The slice thickness is 2 mm. However, if we increase TE to 30 msec, the loss of signal in the marrow and near bone or air spaces is deadly. This loss of signal is transparent in the air spaces and near metal such as in the teeth (**B**) and more subtly displayed as a type of false contrast in the lumbar spine. The lumbar spine example shows an opposed phase nature (**D**) even though it is in phase (TE = 10 msec). Reducing TE to 5 msec (**C**), also inphase, gives a much better result (higher marrow signal). By using 3D data acquisition, the shifting of the echo in the second phase-encoding direction can be reduced by acquiring enough partitions (phase-encoding steps in slice select).

In each imaging direction when gradient encoding is used, Nyquist's relation holds[17]:

$$\Delta k_x = \gamma G_x \Delta t = 1/L_x \qquad 28$$

and

$$\Delta k_y = \gamma G_y t_y = 1/L_y \qquad 29$$

Here t_y is the length of time that the phase-encoding gradient is on. The maximum spatial frequency is $k_{max} = 1/\Delta x$ and usually means that, unless we sample high enough in k, resolution will suffer. As before, $\phi_x = k_x x$ and

$\phi_y = k_y y$. Aliasing then is avoided when the change in phase across the FOV is less than 2π between sampled points.

Examination Time

The total examination time includes many unrelated imaging parameters such as patient handling, coil tuning, sequence loading, data handling, image reconstruction and display, decision making for alternate scans, and likely other points. For a given sequence, the first natural time constraints to be considered include TR, number of views (N), and number of acquisitions (Nacq). For each new imaging dimension, the time is increased according to the number of phase-encoding steps.

For new steady-state free precession (SFP) techniques, TR can be as low as 25 msec. This implies an imaging time of about 6 seconds for a 256 × 256 image for a single acquisition. By acquiring multiple slices or, equivalently, by collecting 3D images, a large and clinically useful region of the body can be imaged; however, beware of the reality—the total time to acquire 128 partitions is 13.7 minutes. True, isotropic data can be reoriented as you desire, but only one type of contrast can be obtained. Three such scans to obtain spin-density, T_1- or T_1/T_2-weighted images will take over 40 minutes. So much for the fast scans. To extract spin density, T_1 and T_2 will take further postprocessing.

FINITE SAMPLING AND RESOLUTION

When data are collected, only a finite number of sampled points are obtained. The maximum frequency is γGL, and hence the frequency interval that we can distinguish is

$$\Delta f = \gamma G \Delta x \qquad 30$$

with

$$\Delta x = L/n \qquad 31$$

To improve resolution, more points must be taken. As we shall see later, this causes a loss in S/N. Unfortunately, a Δx resolution is never quite realized.[17] This is because the reconstruction using Fourier transforms cannot precisely define sharp-edged objects, and finite sampling produces the infamous Gibbs' ringing or truncation artifact.[18–21]

Actually, if the object consisted of a set of uniformly spaced points, there would be no such artifact.[21] The discrete inverse Fourier transform assumes this model, and when it is violated, the artifact returns. Since tissue tends to be continuous, the effect is present unless a different reconstruction technique is used to accommodate the continuity. In practice, the effect stretches over many pixels, decaying only very slowly as 1/x and oscillating in nature (Fig 1–16). By increasing the sampling time (T_s), the Gibbs' phenomenon does not change in terms of the number of pixels covered. Since the artifact remains invariant in terms of the number of pixels, the distance over which it is serious is reduced linearly with increasing n. Decreasing the field of view by increasing the gradient again reduces only the distance over which the artifact travels, not the number of pixels. Sampling is usually symmetric about the echo to within a few sampling points. If the echo is shifted up to about $T_s/4$ from the echo, the image will still be reasonable, but some loss in resolution will occur.[17] Taking the magnitude image removes the linear phase error introduced by this mild form of asymmetric sampling. Gibbs' ringing will not be as bad as if only half as many points were acquired though. Short TE data can be collected this way, and the use of 512 points is worth considering.

The workings of MR are so intertwined that the identical information can be arrived at in two ways. For example, by decreasing G and increasing Δt, the phase, in radians,

$$\phi = \gamma G \Delta t x \qquad 32$$

remains constant. Decreased G also implies a reduced bandwidth and a reduction in noise. It is this approach that is used to optimize the signal-to-noise for a long TE where the sampling time can be longer without being affected by eddy-current problems. Of course, the ever present demons of field inhomogeneities and chemical shift must be lived with, and the number of pixel-shift artifact increases as G decreases. Further, if T_s is on the order of T_2, other artifacts occur.[17] The effects of field inhomogeneities can be reduced by increasing G without changing resolution, although the noise is once again increased (see the discussion associated with Fig 1–7).

Of course, it is taken for granted that sampling will be perfect, i.e., each Δt will be identical. For deviations of a few percent, an extra jitter is introduced into the signal, which is why 16-bit digital-to-analog (D/A) converters must be used in generating sampled points in the phase-encoding direction. Otherwise, systematic noise and ghosts may be the result. Similarly, if eddy currents cause a nonconstant gradient profile during sampling, image distortion will take place. This can be accommodated by either changing the sampling appropriately or changing the reconstruction.[21]

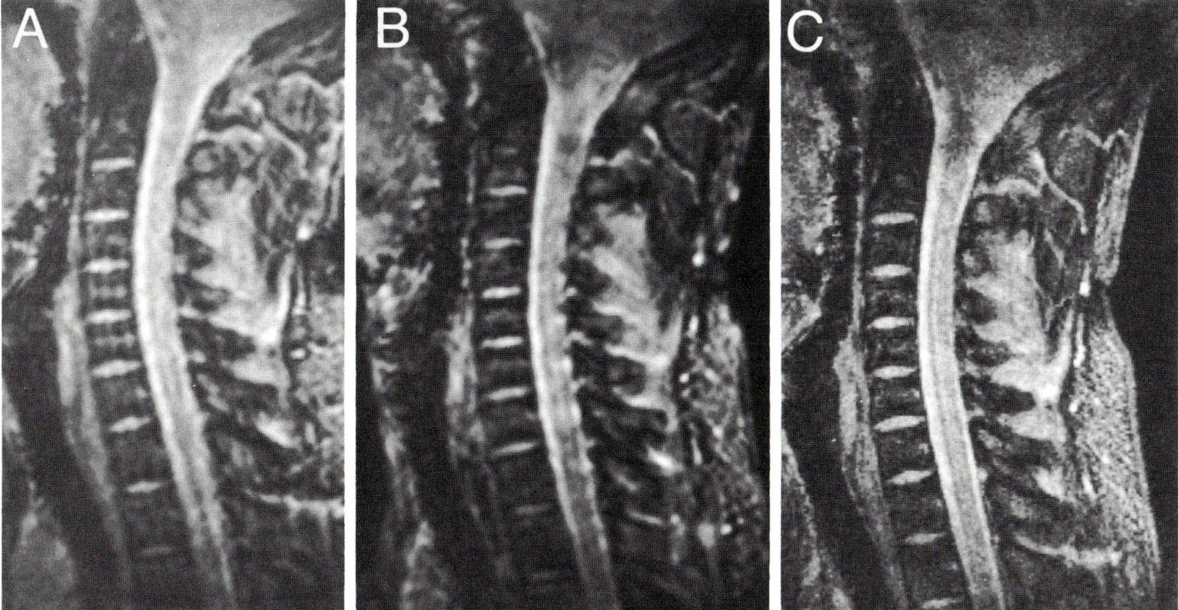

FIG 1–16.
Any sharp-edged object will produce ringing when an insufficient number of sampled points is used. By increasing the number of points, (i.e., opening the window), the number of pixels over which the artifact extends does not change, but the distance over which it affects the image (in this case infiltrating cord) diminishes linearly. **A** shows n = 128 with the read gradient in the vertical direction; **B,** n = 128 with the read gradient in the horizontal direction, and **C,** n = 256 points with the read gradient vertical. Note that the black-white alternating bands that penetrate the vertebral bodies in **A** are due to motion. Motion artifacts are eliminated in **B,** but Gibbs' artifact remains. Even with n = 256, a small Gibbs' artifact remains. When two edges are very close, constructive interference can occur between the artifacts from each edge, making the peaks and valleys more prominent. Note that doubling the FOV has the same effect, and with n = 128, but with a 15-cm instead of 30-cm FOV, the distance over which the artifact extends is reduced. Applying a Hamming filter eliminates the artifact but at the same time reduces resolution from the hoped for ideal of 2.4 mm to over 3 mm; no wonder 128 images acquired in this fashion are not considered acceptable.

Imagine a set of equally spaced points with a spin density equivalent of $\rho(x)$ generating a signal $s(k)$ from a spin-echo:

$$s(k) = \sum_{l=-N}^{N-1} \rho(x_l)\, e^{-i2\pi k x_l} \qquad 33$$

where we have used

$$k = \gamma G t \qquad 34$$

as the canonical or transform variable to x. The discrete inverse transform then gives exactly (i.e., no artifacts)

$$\rho(x) = \frac{1}{2N} \sum_{m=-N}^{N-1} s(k_m)\, e^{i2\pi k_m x} \qquad 35$$

where $s(k)$ has been sampled uniformly in k at points k_m. If $\rho(x)$ is continuous, then the effect of truncation depends on its shape and can be found from

$$\hat{\rho}(x) = \rho(x)*H(x) \qquad 36$$

where * implies convolution and

$$H(x) = \text{sinc}\,(\pi x/\Delta x) \qquad 37$$

where sinc is sin (xl/x). Now it is obvious that the ringing effect extends past $\rho(x)$ decaying in terms of pixels as $1/l$ where l means the lth pixel from the edge or feature causing the problem. Note that $H(x)$ is the Fourier transform of the boxcar function $h(k) = 1$ for $-\gamma GT_s/2<k<\gamma GT_s/2$, and 0 elsewhere. So k can be increased or the artifact reduced by increasing G or T_s.

The signal has already been written in discrete form in equation 33. If eddy currents, sampling errors, motion, or some other effect changes the assumed form of the signal to

$$s(k) = \sum_{l=-N}^{N-1} \rho(x_l) e^{-i2\pi G(k)kx_l/G} \qquad 38$$

then $\rho(x)$ can still be found. Rewriting the above equation in matrix notation gives

$$\hat{\vec{s}} = M\vec{\rho} \qquad 39$$

and hence

$$\hat{\rho} = M^{-1}\hat{s} \quad 40$$

Calculating M is not a problem, it is just more time consuming than the filtered Fourier transform (FFT).

The FOV is governed by both sampling rate and gradient strength. If either is not calibrated properly, then L_x and L_y may be different (i.e., the aspect ratio will not be unity), and the image will appear distorted.

Although the expected resolution is $\Delta x = L/n$, this is rarely realized. All of Gibbs' ringing, T_2 decay, the analogue filter (at the edge of the FOV), and any low-pass filter all prevent this. The effects of number of pixels and filtering can be appreciated in Figure 1–16. Gibbs' artifacts can manifest themselves as apparent dark or bright bands such as in the disks in the former case or in the CSF in the latter.

Resolution loss can occur due to pixel misregistration as in chemical shift or field distortion from metal implants or any local change in tissue permeability. In spin-echo imaging, filtering is the dominant source of resolution loss including finite sampling, exponential T_2 decay, analogue filters, and applied filters. The effect on resolution is[17]

$$\Delta\tilde{x} = (1 + \frac{\sqrt{3}}{\pi}\frac{T_s}{T_2} + T_s \sum_i F_i)\Delta x \quad 41$$

where F_i is the full width at half maximum (FWHM) of the ith filter, and the $\sqrt{3}$ includes the T_2 decay effects from the filter $\exp(-t/T_2)$.

For gradient echo imaging, we must add the dephasing effect of T_2:

$$\Delta\tilde{x}' = \Delta\tilde{x} + T_s\gamma\Delta B\Delta x \quad 42$$

For local in vivo changes in susceptibility, ΔB can be several ppm. For example,

$$\frac{1}{T_2^*} = \frac{1}{T_2} + \gamma\Delta B \quad 43$$

where ΔB is the change across half a pixel.

TABLE 1–2.
Imaging Parameter Effects

S/N	n	G_x	L	Δ_x
1	256	1	30	1
$\sqrt{2}$	128	1	30	2
2	128	0.5	30	2
0.5	256	2	15	0.5
0.707	512	1	30	0.5

The resolution can be improved by increasing G and for gradient echoes by shortening TE. Further improvements are possible by using 3D imaging, which allows almost complete recovery of the lost signal[16,22] (even though it may appear in the wrong location) thanks to the Fourier transform shift theorem.

SIGNAL-TO-NOISE

Imaging Parameter Effects

The amount of noise in an image is proportional to the square root of the bandwidth, $1/\Delta t$. As described earlier, increasing the gradient by a factor p and decreasing Δt by the same factor leaves the image unchanged but leads to a reduction in signal-to-noise of $\sqrt{p}$. The amount of noise in a pixel is also proportional to the square root of the number of sampled points. Usually, small fields of view are generated by increasing G by a factor q. This reduces the signal in each pixel by 1/q without changing the noise. However, by increasing n, which also changes the resolution (usually why a reduced FOV is used), only a factor of $1/\sqrt{q}$ is lost in the overall S/N. Increasing n can only be done until $n\Delta t \leq$ TE. Another alternative here is to reduce Gibbs' ringing by acquiring extra points in time and then averaging the adjacent points to recover lost S/N. Similarly, when a large zoom is used in a multiecho experiment, the second echo image S/N could be improved in the same way with the associated loss in resolution (which may be acceptable in many cases when Gibbs' ringing is not a problem). Table 1–2 summarizes these effects. This table also reveals that it is preferable to use 256 points and average adjacent points (giving S/N $= \sqrt{2}$) to have $\Delta x = 2$ rather than take $n = 128$, which has more severe truncation errors. Therefore, 128 phase-encoding steps can be taken to reduce acquisition time, but 256 time points should be used to reduce truncation error. This applies even if a lower G is used. When lower gradients are used ($T_s \leq$ TE), then S/N can be bandwidth optimized (Fig 1–17). Even if static field inhomogeneities are large, as long as a large zoom is used (i.e., maximum gradient strength) then optimal S/N will be attained with minimal distortion and chemical shift. Recall too that zooming will cause the Gibbs' phenomenon to be reduced in distance (not number of pixels) so that low S/N sequences can be modified with a low read gradient to allow improved S/N and throughput when smaller FOVs are desired. (The effects of field inhomogeneities are also fixed in number of pixels but reduced in distance when smaller FOV are used.) Often, for multiecho images, the second echo is much lower in S/N. In this case, *a 256 × 256 image can be reduced to a 128 ×*

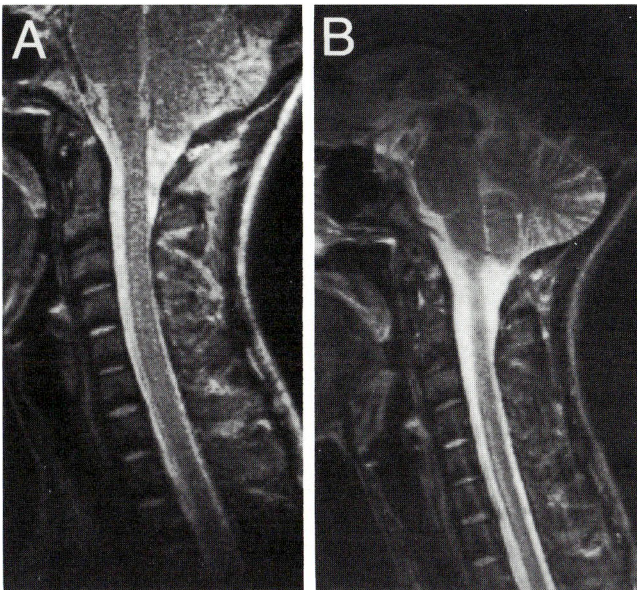

FIG 1–17.
The above images can be improved further by optimizing the bandwidth, that is, using the lowest gradient possible (so that $T_s = n\Delta t < TE$) without suffering too severe gradient distortions. The sampling rates, because of the TE restrictions, can also be different for different echoes, especially when the second echo is at large TE values. **A** shows a TE = 90-msec gated scan with Δt = 30 μsec, while **B** has Δt = 50 μsec ungated. Note the improved S/N in **B.** These two slices are somewhat offset from each other. They are both also flow-compensated sequences and show nicely improved CSF signal and contrast. The distortion from field inhomogeneities and chemical shift will be worse with lower gradients. Using a larger zoom can reduce the distance over which the artifacts act, but the number of pixels shifted remains the same. (See also Fig 1–22.)

128 image and then magnified by interpolation to give an image with two times higher S/N and with much less (by a factor of 2) Gibbs' ringing compared to the same scan acquired with 128 × 128 points.

Contrast will be lost if noise is too large. Sufficient contrast resolution is then the ability to discriminate two tissues at a given resolution for a given sequence in the presence of noise. What may be lost in a 256 × 256 image may be quite visible when displayed in a 128 × 128 extracted image. Contrast behavior depends on many parameters[11] including matrix size, TR, TE, sampling interval, sequence type, slice profile, and of course, spin density, T_1, and T_2.

As field strength increases, T_1 increases, and for a given short TR, the signal will drop as $1/T_1$ except for a fast low-angle shot (FLASH), which drops only as $1/\sqrt{T_1}$ at the optimal angle. If T_1 increases with field strength as $(B_o)^{0.33-0.5}$ for B_o between 0.5 to 2.0 T then longer repeat times are required to maintain contrast between tissues.[23] The need for larger gradients to reduce chemical-shift artifacts also leads to an increase in noise of $(B_o)^{0.5}$. Hence, depending on the squence timings, it may not be advantageous to use higher fields. In particular, the above analysis holds for T_1-weighted spin-echo images but not for sequences with long TR where the usual linear dependence on field strength is expected. Even though TR may be long, gradient echo sequences will still suffer severe T_2^* reductions, since $1/T_2^*$ varies linearly with field strength, and the signal decays exponentially for a fixed TE (see equation 43).

Radiofrequency Coil Parameter Effects

From a general perspective, all coils are normally assumed to have the optimal response. For the rf transmit coils, be they head or body, this means a uniform rf response, i.e., no penetration problems. This is usually true to within 10% up to 1.5 T. Even with this nonuniform response, the image is only affected by 1% to 2%.[24] At high fields, these effects are worse in the body and hence in the spine. Again uniformity is assumed for receive coils except for surface coils. Even the nonuniform receive distribution can be corrected.[25]

The S/N issue also relates to the coil response, particularly at high fields where magnetic losses dominate. What this means practically for coils is that the larger the excited area, the more noise is included (regardless of how much signal is excited). Hence, if a smaller coil can be used to receive signal only from the region of interest, the S/N ratio will improve accordingly. This potential is best realized nearest the coil where the coil response is the largest; hence, orbit and temporomandibular joint (TMJ) coils are very successful. Unfortunately, spine coils, cervical or lumbar, operate the same way, and we get optimal S/N for the fat! Some coil modifications are possible to move the region of maximum response in toward the region of interest. Although this does not appear to have been an optimal surface coil for the spine yet, new ladder designs do have the capability of allowing localization with improved S/N but all with one coil.[26] Figure 1–17 shows a bright fat signal with an S/N of 100:1, while 10 mm further in, it is only 20:1.

SYSTEMATIC NOISE: MOTION AND PHASE

Some forms of systematic noise have already been introduced, including, for example, poor generation of phase-encoding steps, nonideal sampling in time due to eddy currents, and finite sampling. Other phenomena that infest many images include motion and rf penetration. The latter can cause a loss of signal due to screening, and for high-conducting tissue, an increase in noise by $\sqrt{\sigma}$ where σ is the conductivity.[27] The former causes an incorrect sampling of k-space. Systematic sources of noise are best eliminated at the source. When this is not possible, the best way to acquire multiple acquisitions would then be to centrally weight the views until the systematic error in the central views is reduced to the same level as the background white noise.

Motion

We have shown that S/N and resolution are more than enough to produce excellent images in body tissues. Unfortunately, body motion changes all these ideal conditions and induces a systematic noise that has been enough to maintain skepticism on the part of physicians as to the utility of MRI in the abdomen. In the days when short TE values were 40 msec, respiratory motion artifacts were considered a serious impediment. This was initially blamed on motion between phase-encoding values,[28, 29] but in fact was not so much this motion but movement during application of the read gradients.[30–32] The subsequent dephasing caused severe phase variations at the echoes from view to view dominating the ghosting. Ironically, once this motion phase variation has been eliminated, the remnant respiratory ghosts become coherent and are significantly reduced in amplitude.[30] Even without gating, images are improved. Today the short TE values of 5 to 20 msec suffer less from those effects, and gating becomes necessary to remove the remnant artifact (approximately 10%) from phase changes due to motion between phase-encoding steps. Peristalsis is also a culprit leading to image degradation.

Complaints of motion artifacts also arise in conjunction with general spine imaging where blood flow, CSF pulsations, and respiration cause problems, and in cervical spine imaging where swallowing is also a problem.

Any technique that requires subtraction of two images, such as water/fat, is particularly susceptible to motion. This problem can be alleviated by interleaving the scans so that each phase-encoding value is repeated, i.e., once for the first scan type and once for the second. Both may well contain motion artifacts, but since the artifacts manifest identically in both cases, they should subtract out well.

The problem with motion artifacts would not be so severe if the artifacts remained localized near the source. In two-dimensional Fourier transform (2DFT) imaging, they appear throughout the image in the phase-encoding direction, sometimes coherent and sometimes incoherent, for reasons described earlier. To alleviate or remove the problem, the following concepts

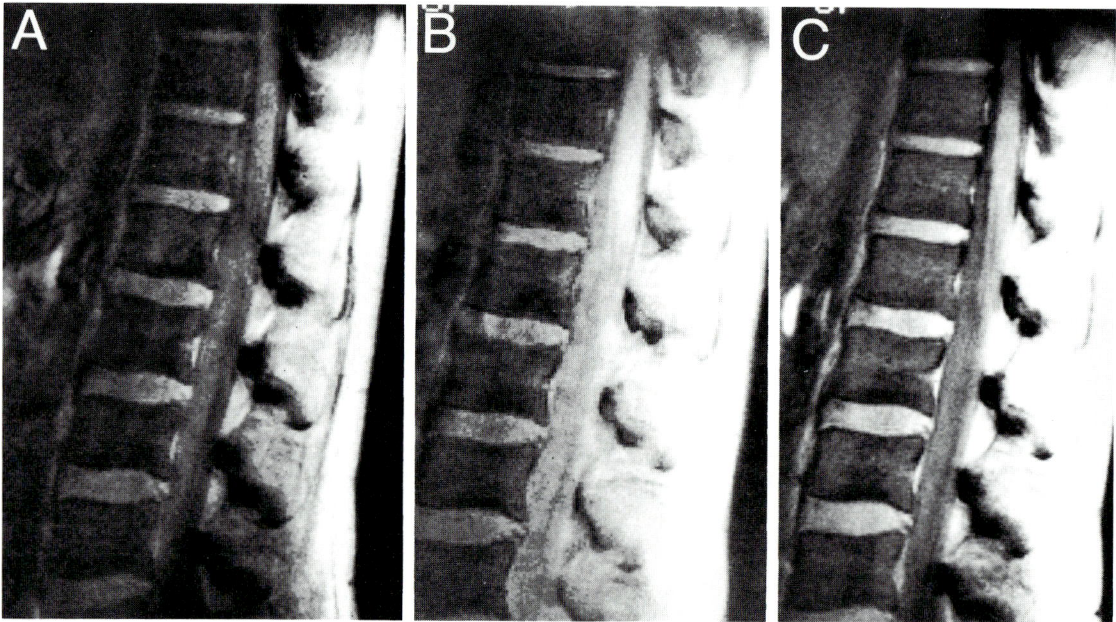

FIG 1–18.
Motion artifacts can be reduced by pseudogating (setting the number of acquisitions (Nacq) times TR to T or T/2 where T is the period of the motion). If TR is so short that nTR = T, then data should not be collected one phase-encoding view Nacq times but the whole data set serially Nacq times one right after the other. **A** shows a single acquisition with TR = 50 msec and **B** with TR = 200 msec. Note that acquiring TR = 25 msec 8 times (**C**) and averaging gives the same S/N as in **B** but much less artifacting (only a blur near the abdomen). The same holds true for vascular imaging.

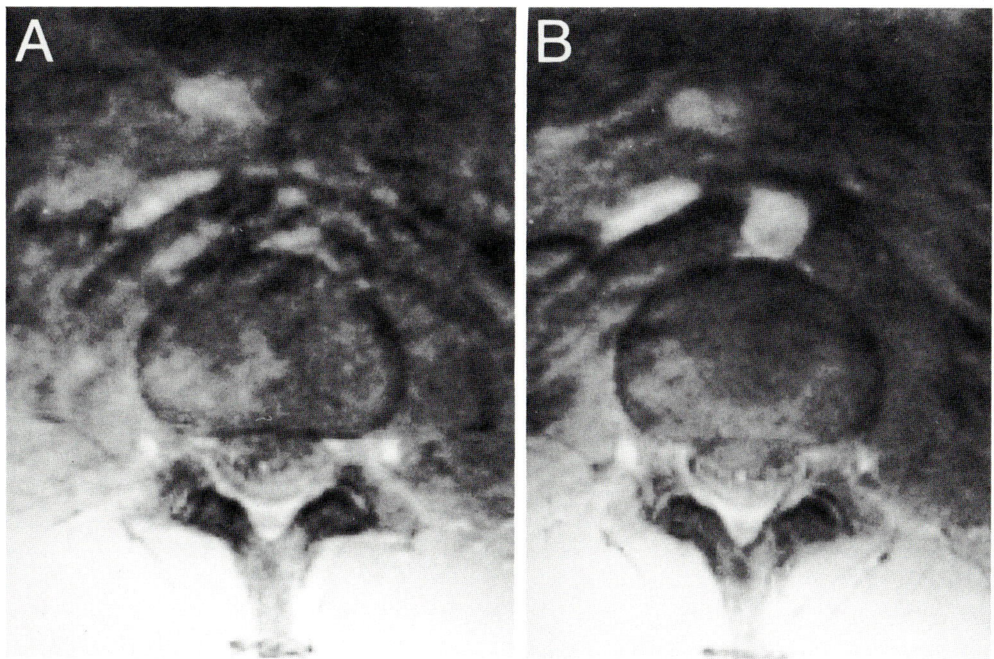

FIG 1–19.
An example of a lumbar spine with aorta flow artifact in the horizontal (**A**) and vertical (**B**) phase-encoding directions.

can be used: (1) stopping the motion (for example, applying a belt around the abdomen or administering glucagon); (2) triggering or gating the data at the same point in each cycle; (3) reordering the data[29, 33] to localize the scanning to within a pixel of the source; (4) applying scaling techniques[29] to correct for the motion-induced frequency and phase changes; (5) using reconstruction techniques accounting for the motion[29]; (6) pseudogating[34] (Fig 1–18); (7) centrally weighting the data; (8) switching the direction of read and phase-encoding gradients to put the artifact where it will not obscure the region of interest (Fig 1–19); (9) using fast imaging to acquire data in one breath (see Fig 1–18); (10) saturating moving tissues (Fig 1–20) so the artifacts that enter the region of interest are significantly reduced or eliminated[7]; or (11) rephasing moving spins with appropriate gradient compensation pulses.[30–32]

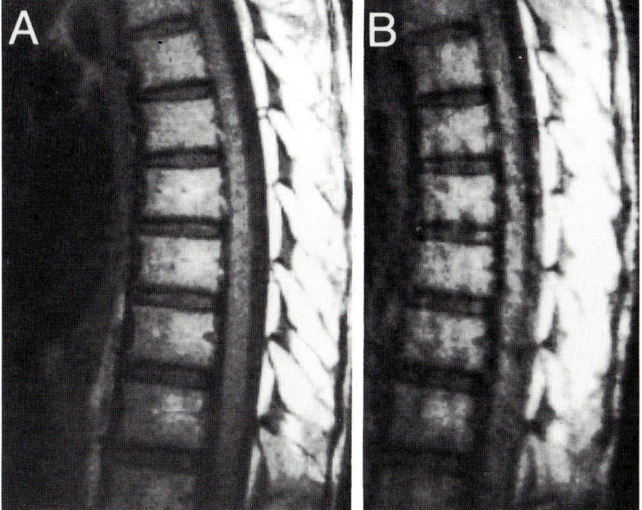

FIG 1–20.
Saturating the upper chest (**A**) removes the signal from tissue in the chest that normally blurs the region of interest (**B**). This can be employed with flow compensation sequences as well.

The latter two approaches have led to significant improvements in image quality even without respiratory gating. Saturation methods were discussed under rf pulses in the section entitled "Sequence Structure and Contrast." Rephasing methods have been extensively discussed in the literature under even echo rephasing, motion compensation gradients, and bipolar gradients.[30–32] The basic concept is that a moving spin will not refocus at the echo in the usual one- or two-gradient application in any axis. By introducing a third gradient both stationary and constant-velocity moving spins can be refocused. Introducing a fourth gradient, both constant velocity and acceleration effects can be refocused (Fig 1–21). The most important contributions are motion in read and slice-select direction. When spins moving in either direction are both rephased, the image quality dramatically improves.

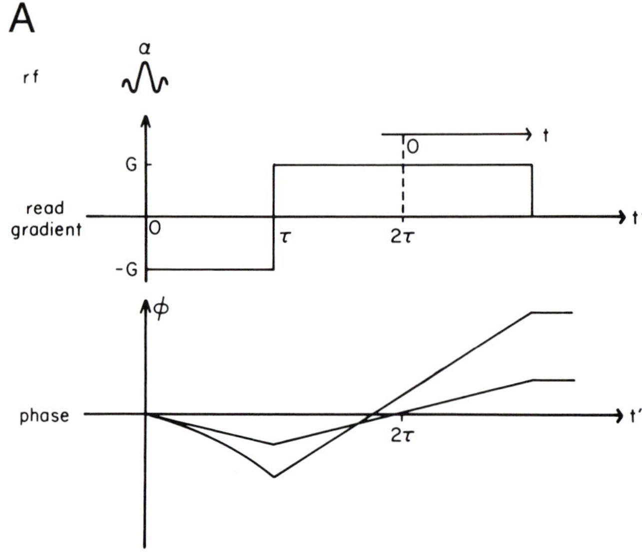

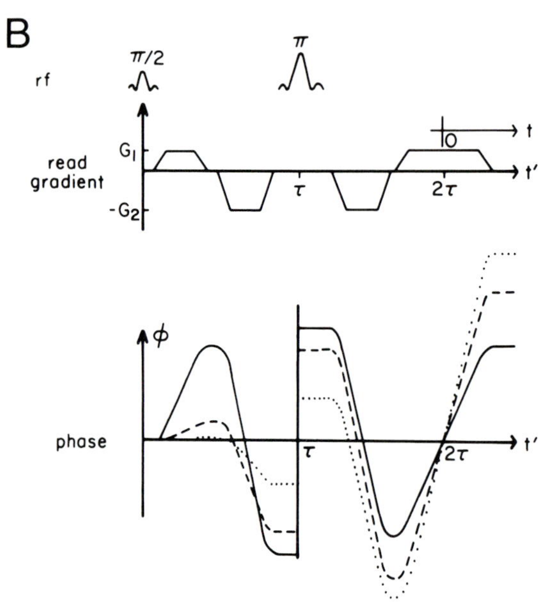

FIG 1–21.
Phase behavior for a gradient echo sequence with two gradients; the phase of stationary spins refocuses (*bottom solid line* in phase), and the phase of constant velocity moving spins is not focused (*upper solid line* in phase). With three gradients, constant velocity spins can be refocused (**A**). With four gradients, constant velocity and acceleration spins can be refocused (**B**). In the phase plot, the *dotted line* is for stationary spins, the *dashed line* for constant velocity, and the *solid line* for constant acceleration.

Flow

The random or periodic phase changes referred to earlier can be caused by flow equally well. Any fluid flow can lead to motion artifacts, including CSF, blood, and water in the bladder. Even very slow flow of CSF in the head (several millimeters per second or less) can cause significant signal loss[30] when long TEs are used (see Fig 1–17). (T_2 of CSF is about 2 seconds, but try and show this with a spin-echo sequence!) Higher flows of 1 to 10 cm/second in the cervical spine cause significant artifacts for everyday TE values. Blood flow of 10 to 100 cm/second and higher causes problems even for TE values less than 10 msec, as in imaging the carotid bifurcation. Many of these artifacts can be significantly reduced by using flow compensation sequences (see "Phase Images" for a detailed description). Qualitatively, the amount of dephasing is proportional to velocity (v) and TE for constant velocity moving spins. If flow void has not removed all signal, then that which remains will be significantly altered in phase each time the velocity changes. It is this change that leads to the ghosting.

Let us take a closer look at CSF flow effects in the spine. First we point out that a flow of 1 mm/second will cause ghosts as severe as respiratory motion of 1 cm for a TE of 90 msec. Hence with an uncompensated single-echo sequence, the image in the cervical spine may be severely degraded. When a properly designed even echo sequence with 45 and 90 msec is used the 90-msec image may be refocused, but the 45-msec image will still be poor. The best solution is to flow compensate both images, but if this is not possible, then use a very short TE, and flow compensate the 90-msec image. An example of such a sequence with TEs of 15 and 90 msec is shown in Figure 1–22. Sometimes slow flow can be distinguished from tumor by purposely dephasing the signal. This proves useful in the azygous vein in vascular imaging and to distinguish an arachnoid cyst from CSF in spine imaging.

The effects of uncorrected flow include dephasing or signal loss in a pixel (which in turn leads to a loss of edge definition) and ghosting. Cerebrospinal fluid flow is also pulsatile and as such can have ghosts even on transverse images if not cardiac gated.[35–40] This problem is caused by phase changes due to fast flow in systole that is not properly compensated. Cardiac gating alleviates the problem but at the expense of a longer scan. An intermediate solution is pseudogating[34] to the period of the heart. Combining both gating and rephasing of moving spins will give the best images (see Chapter 3). It is also important to recognize that when ghosts occur, the vessel may not appear bright where it actually belongs but may have a ghost below it bright and one above it black as well. This is a speical form of phase cancellation with stationary material. The original vessel appears low in signal because the ghosts have stolen the signal.

Some controversy remains over the increase in ap-

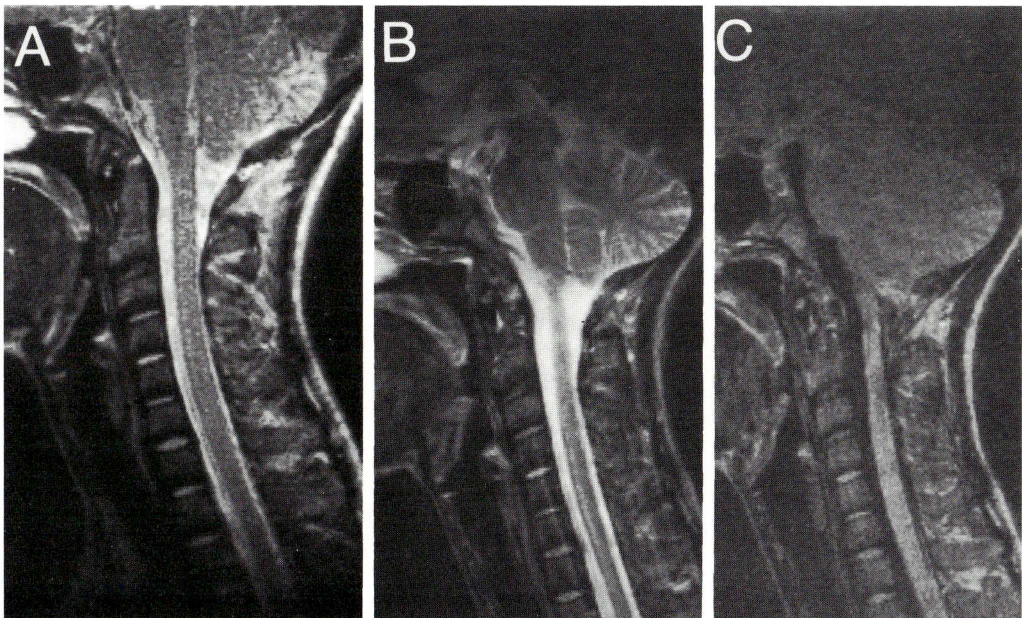

FIG 1–22.
Rephasing applied in the read direction for both gated (**A**) and ungated (**B**) CSF flow in the cervical spine. The gated image (**A**) is at a different slice location than the ungated optimized bandwidth image (**B**). (See also Fig 1–17.) The single, strong white flow artifact from the CSF that appears in the vertebral bodies in **B** has been eliminated by gating in **A.** When gating, diastole is always likely to give the best images in terms of edge definition. Another advantage of gated imaging is that the TE = 15-msec image, which is not easily rephased even though the TE = 90 msec image is, will have no ghosting. When no rephasing is applied, the spin dephasing is almost complete, ghosting is less, but no CSF appears (**C**).

parent ghosting in surface coil images. First, with improved S/N, the ghosts will be more evident. Second, motion in the region of high signal will propagate into regions of low signal and cause disproportionate ghosting intensity. Third, less averaging is done (usually only one excitation), and hence less artifacting is removed (averaging or pseudogating usually helps).[34] Fourth, a longer T_1 reduces the overall tissue signal, except for paradoxically enhanced blood, for example. Hence, since ghosting is proportional to the pristine signal, the artifact amplitude apparently increases at high fields.

Phase Images

When the initial frequency information is decoded by taking the inverse Fourier transform, both the amplitude (magnitude) and phase information are output. Since the phase information can be corrupted by rf penetration, eddy currents, sampling center location, π-pulse location, chemical shift, and field inhomogeneities, the magnitude is usually taken. If information about the aforementioned problems is desired, then the phase can be useful. Phase is also useful for distinguishing signal above noise since it is more robust to noise than the amplitude image. Recently it has been used to measure local field inhomogeneities, chemical shift between water and lipid components[41] (see "Water/Lipid Imaging"), and flow or motion. An example phase image of the CSF at different points in the cervical spine is shown in Figure 1–23. The CSF velocity is represented by the phase deviations from the stationary tissue. As expected, since the CSF is in a closed system, the velocity changes direction at different points in the cardiac cycle.

In a gradient echo sequence with the normal gradient structure, phase (in radians) for stationary spins during sampling behaves as

$$\phi(t) = \gamma Gxt \qquad (44)$$

whereas for spins moving with a constant velocity it is

$$\phi_v(t) = \gamma Gxt + \gamma Gv\left([t_2 - t_1][2\tau - t_2] + 2\tau t + \frac{1}{2}t^2\right) \qquad (45)$$

where t_1 is the starting time of G, and t_2 the time when G is turned off. This unexpected or incorrect phase behavior leads to position-shift artifacts, ghosts, and poor edge definition.[30] By using these gradients, the constant phase term can be removed to give

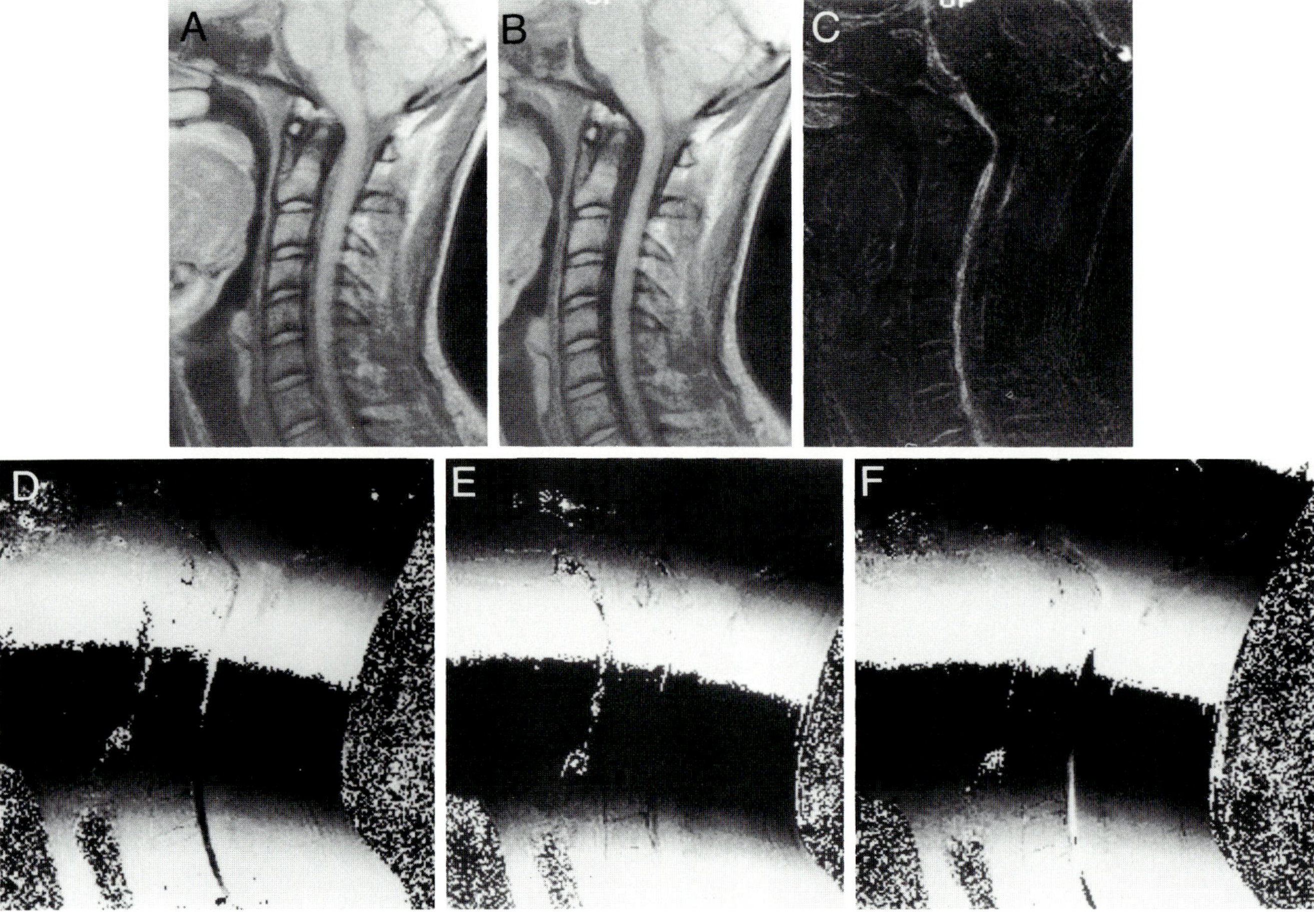

FIG 1–23.
An ungated example with TR = 1.0 second and TE = 34 msec. **A** is a refocused sequence and **B** a dephased sequence; **C** the scan was then repeated gated with only partial refocusing to illustrate phase and hence velocity behavior during diastole and systole. The three phase examples shown are TD = 250 msec (**D**), TD = 500 msec (**E**), and TD = 750 msec (**F**). Note the change in flow direction from TD = 250 msec to TD = 750 msec. The peak CSF flow can be as high as 5 to 10 cm/second and is the cause of CSF dephasing at long TE values and ghosting at shorter values unless the study is gated.

$$\phi_v(t) = \gamma G(x + vt)t + \frac{1}{2}\gamma Gvt^2 \qquad 46$$

This refocusing is illustrated in Figure 1–21. Obviously the phase information can be used to measure the velocity and hence direction of flow. Care must be taken to account for partial volume effects with stationary spins.

For a gradient echo sequence with a field inhomogeneity, the phase behavior is

$$\phi(t) = \gamma Gxt + \gamma\Delta B(x)(TE + t) \qquad 47$$

Of course, $\Delta B(x)$ can be caused by chemical shift as well. Hence, the phase serves as a measure of $\Delta B(x)$.

The measurement of the desired parameters can often be improved by subtracting two phase images so that spurious phase corruption is removed.

GRADIENT FIELD ECHO SEQUENCES

With the return of steady-state free precision (SFP) imaging and the subsequent advent of fast 3D imaging, gradient field echo sequences (GFE) have taken a major step forward. The reason for their success today is the improved field homogeneity and the very short TE values possible. Local in vivo susceptibility changes at tissue interfaces introduce field changes that cause a loss of signal and edge definition in these regions. Today TEs as low as 5 msec are available to essentially eliminate this problem. For example, a 1-ppm change in field across a pixel at 42.6 MHz leads to a T_2^* of 8 msec. If TE = 5 msec is used, 53% of the signal remains, while if TE = 15 msec is used, only 15% remains (see Fig 1–10). However, it may prove of interest to actually look for such effects through either magnitude or phase images. For example, hemorrhage can lead to a loss of signal due to local iron deposits, intracellular deoxyhemoglobin, and/or methemoglobin. A similar effect can be observed due to gas in the intervertebral disk secondary to degeneration (see "Contrast and Artifacts").

Fast Imaging

Earlier we introduced the gradient field echo sequences. These sequences can be run with a small-angle, α, rf pulse. When the equilibrium or steady state is reached by spoiling M_{xy} or making it zero before the next pulse, the sequence is called FLASH. If the M_{xy} is refocused in the phase-encoding direction before each pulse, the sequence is referred to as FAST, GRASS, or modified FISP. Notwithstanding the sensitivity to field inhomogeneities, short TR SFP imaging can yield data so quickly as to make 3D imaging practical. Repeat times as low as 10 to 20 msec are possible with some sequences. If a volume of 30 cm is desired with 1.2 mm resolution, it will only take 21 minutes with TR = 20 msec, TE = 5 msec, and a 256 × 256 matrix. This proves useful for a morphological analysis of the spine; nerve roots are very well delineated for example.

These rapid repeat times can lead to artifacts[42] if the transverse magnitization is not properly spoiled for FLASH (Fig 1–24) and not perfectly refocussed for modified FISP. Another serious problem in single slice or from slice to slice in volume imaging is that the image contrast is very sensitive to the rf profile[43] (see also Fig 1–9). What may give a uniform profile for long repeat times will not for short TR. The angular response changes the contrast at each point in volume imaging and must be integrated now in single or multislice images.[44, 45]

Motion during a FISP scan causes what would otherwise be a bright signal to dephase and become dark. Switching read and phase-encoding directions illustrates this point well (Fig 1–25). Unfortunately, rapid or turbulent flow may randomize the phase of the spins, which drastically reduces the signal. This is often true in the CSF in the spine where the usual bright CSF scan at 60 degrees in the ventricles is no longer seen.

Fast imaging may be a slight misnomer today. Single slices are taken faster, and motion artifacts can be reduced, but overall examination time is not likely to be reduced much below half an hour. This is because many single slices or a 3D data set must be acquired with sufficient S/N to be useful and to cover a large enough region of interest. Of course, the benefit of thin contiguous slices and motion reduction are maintained.

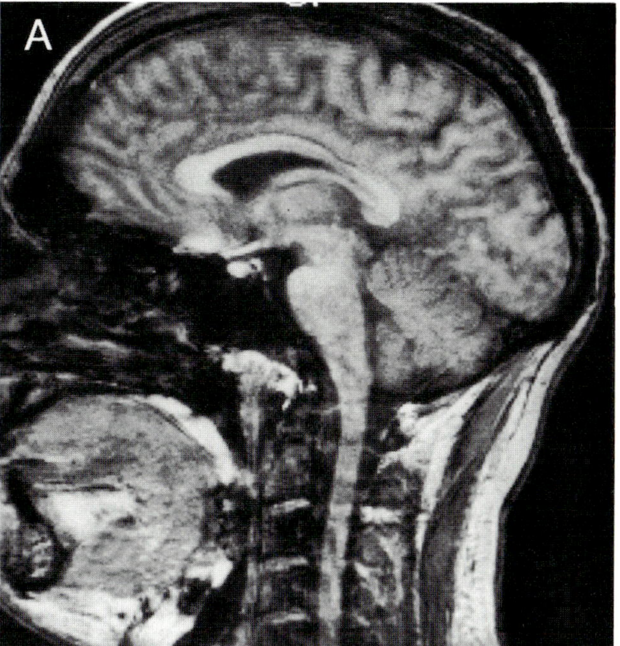

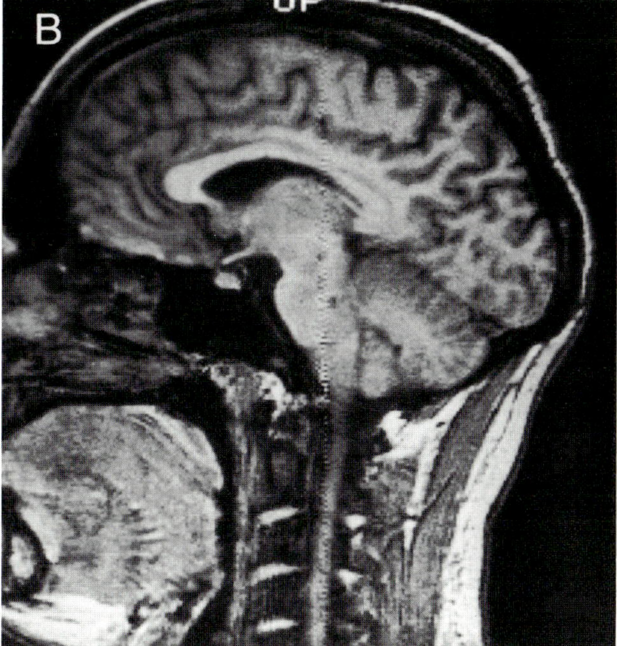

FIG 1–24.
A spoiled (**A**) and unspoiled (**B**) FLASH image. The resulting artifact is seen as a vertical line down the center of the image in **B.**

Contrast and Artifacts

Spin-echo T_2-weighted contrast has long been the benchmark of clinical detection of disease or abnormal pathology. In principle, however, any three scans are sufficient to extract ρ(spin density), T_1, and T_2 information. So why do we not do this? First, to accomplish

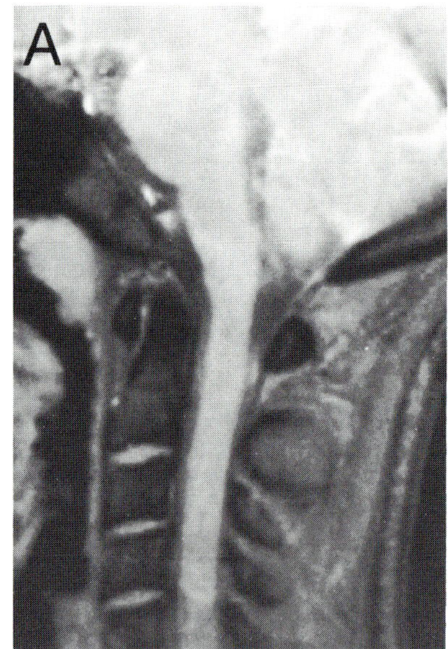

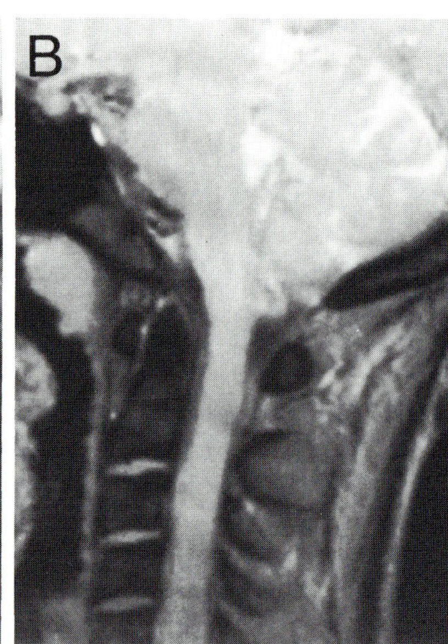

FIG 1–25.
Since FISP images require refocusing of the spins, any motion can disrupt the approach to equilibrium (**A**). Switching the read and phase-encoding directions so that the read direction is now horizontal illustrates this point in the craniovertebral region (**B**) and lumbar spine. The CSF in the cisterna magna and upper cervical canal is now much brighter, since the vertical motion no longer leads to dephasing along the read direction.

separation of the tissue parameters requires sufficient S/N. Second, postprocessing must be done immediately after all three images are acquired. Third, and most important, it takes too long to collect all three scans. Standard protocols usually acquire several short and long TE sequences but in different orientations. Also, slices are so thin that even when all three pieces of information are available, S/N is poor. Further difficulties arise in accounting for slice profile changes.[43]

Consider first the contrast curves for an SE sequence for signal vs. TR and several values of TE (10 msec, 40 msec, and 100 msec). The tissues considered are CSF, marrow (fat), disk, and cord; pathology is also considered. (See Figs 1–11 through 1–13 for spin-echo contrast.) Fast SFP imaging with FLASH and FISP allows for three rapid scans from which all information for tissue properties can be extracted. These images may not show the contrast available with T_2-weighted se-

A

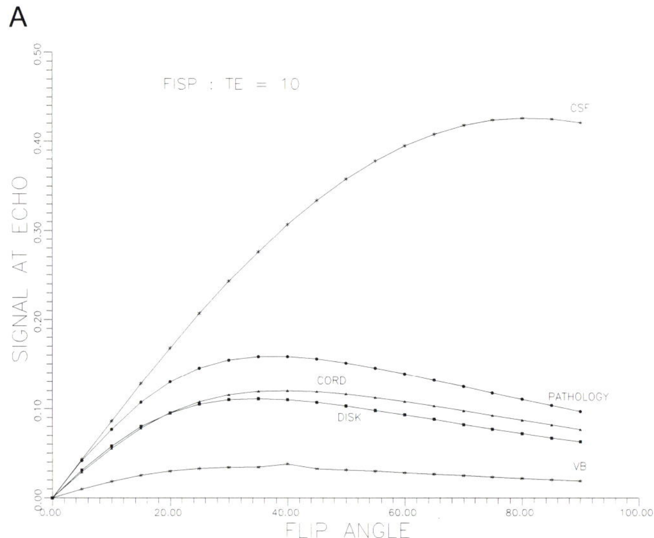

B

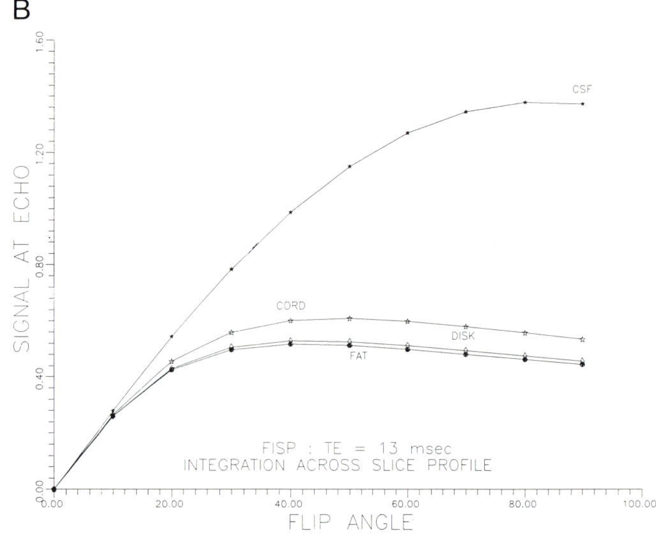

FIG 1–26.
Predicted contrast curves for different tissues for FISP image (**A**). The signal from tissues for which T_1/T_2 is small, e.g., cerebrospinal fluid *(CSF)*, increases dramatically at large flip angles. Due to poor slice profiles, the angles at which maximum contrast occurs are shifted higher than predicted with an ideal profile. Taking the slice profile into account yields the contrast curves in **B.** *VB* = vertebral body. The signal in **B** is scaled differently from that in **A**.

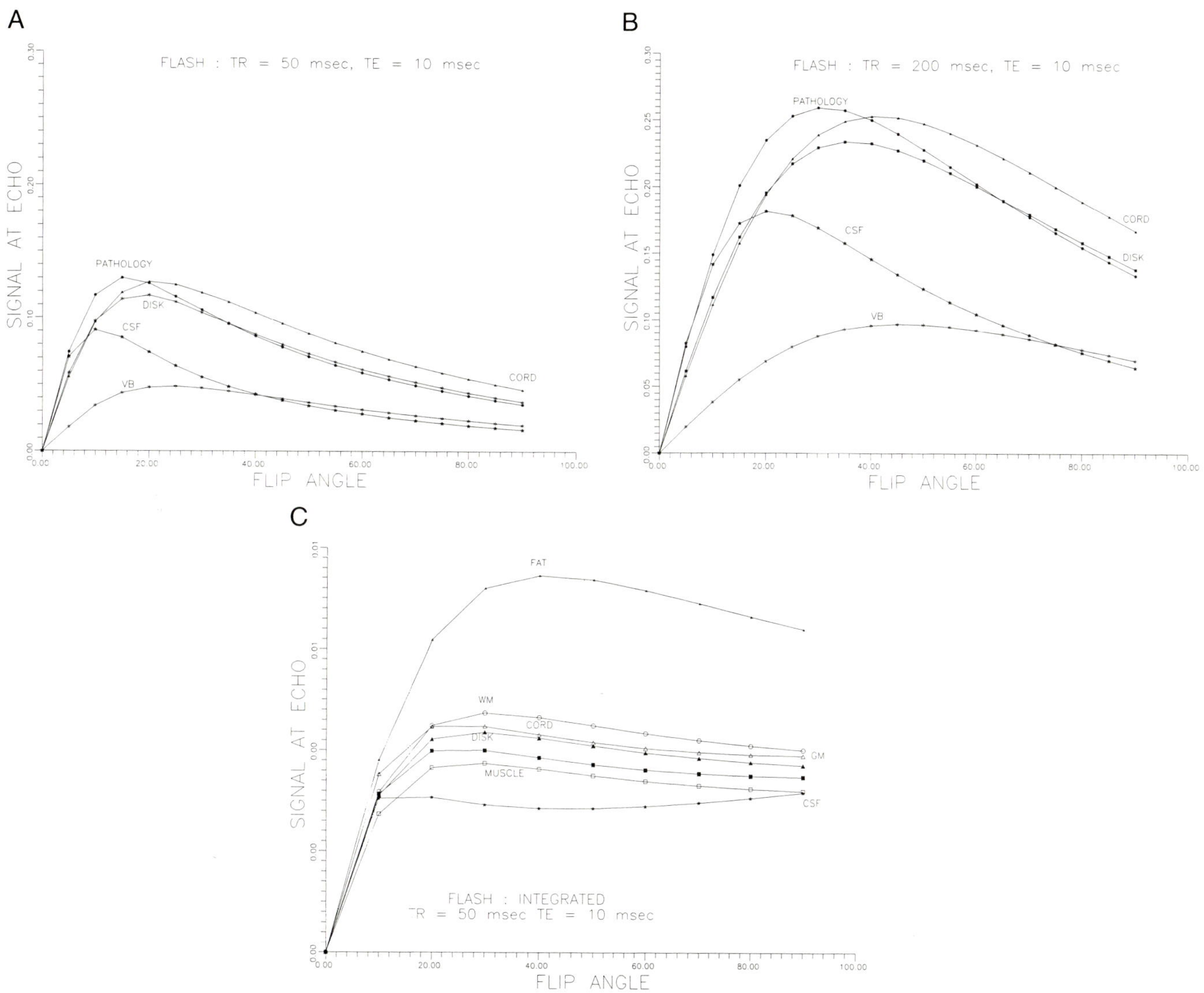

FIG 1–27.
Predicted contrast curves for different tissues for FLASH images for TR = 50 msec (**A**) and TR = 200 msec (**B**). Overall signal and the flip angles at which maximum signal is obtained are higher for all tissues at the longer TR. Taking the slice profile into account for TR = 50 msec yields the contrast curves in **C.** Notice that T_1 weighting is essentially the same for all angles greater than the optimal angle for fat. The signal in **C** is scaled differently from that in **A** and **B**.

quences,[46, 47] but the same information is in principle available with FISP (Fig 1–26). Next the signal is plotted vs. angle for a fixed, short TE and for two TR values (50, 200 msec) for FLASH (Fig 1–27). Note that the pathology example is for disease in gray/white matter and the ratio of T_1/T_2 is held fixed compared to white matter. The T_1 change is small, so contrast on a T_1-weighted image will be like gray/white contrast. On a FISP image, there will be little contrast, but because of the T_1 change, the isointensity in the FISP image is just as discriminating as a T_2-weighted spin-echo image since FISP behaves as T_1/T_2. Even more heavily weighted T_2, FISP-like images can be obtained with contrast-enhanced (CE)-FAST.[12] This sequence is similar to FISP, but the signal is read out just before the next rf pulse.

The short T_2s in tissues means that very short single-slice echo times are required to avoid signal loss near tissue boundaries, especially near the sinus or other regions with air. Volume fast imaging is a little more forgiving in that T_2^* signal loss is mostly recovered, although it may still be placed in the wrong slice. This

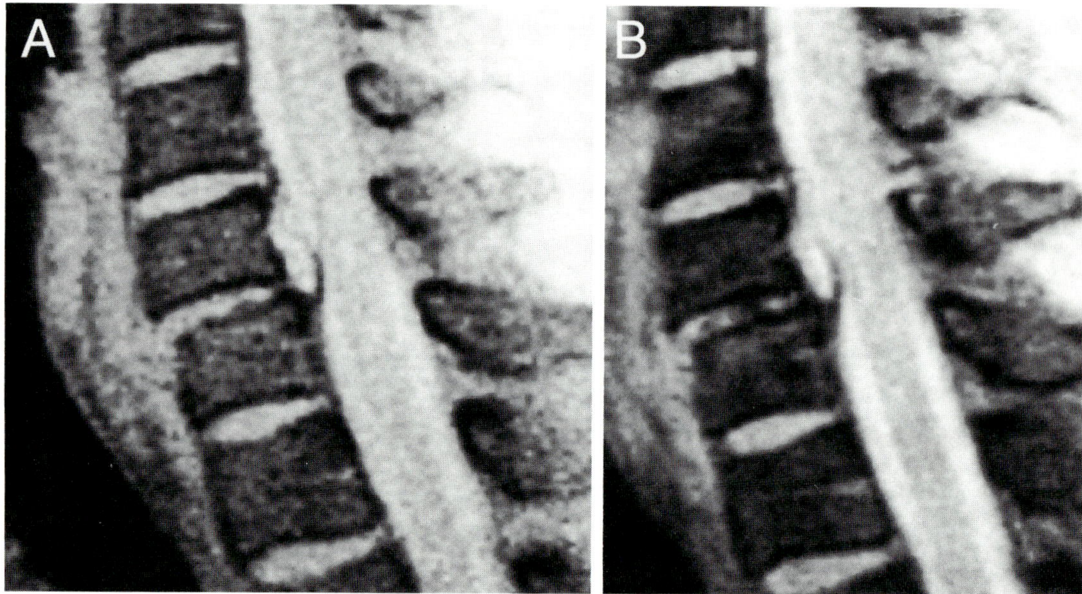

FIG 1–28.
A short TE = 5 msec (**A**) and long TE = 10 msec (**B**) GFE. Note the improved signal in the disk for TE = 5 msec due to the short T_2^* in the disk caused by local induced susceptibility.

can be understood as follows: the change in susceptibility leads to an induced field gradient in the slice-select direction; this acts to dephase the spins for a single-slice experiment; it further shifts the frequencies of these spins so that they may live in another slice; phase encoding in the slice-select direction may eventually exactly counter the induced gradient; hence the final signal has a shifted echo in the slice-select direction, and little overall signal is lost when short TEs are used. This slice-select shift will also occur for spin-echo experiments as will the frequency shift in the read direction, which also occurs in each slice.

An example of the short TE signal improvement is demonstrated in Figure 1–28. The loss of signal in the disk may be due to the existence of impurities in structure, such as bubbles. FATE is a sequence which, as a

FIG 1–29.
FLASH image (**A**) and FATE image (**B**) with TR = 200 msec, TE = 30 msec, α = 20°, 8-mm thick slice, Nacq = 2, 256 matrix with 23.1-cm FOV. Edge definition *(arrow)* is superior in the FATE image.

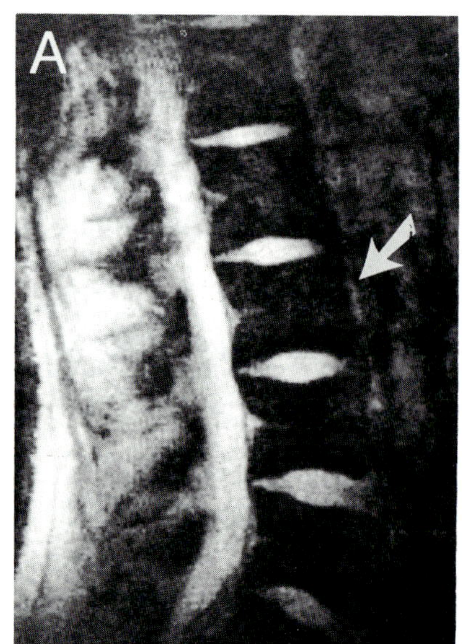

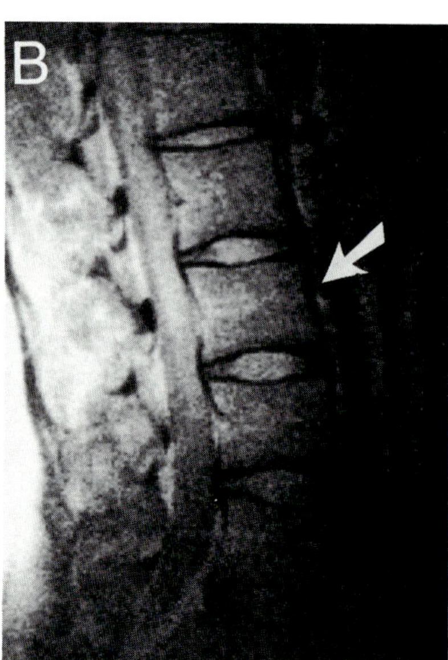

member of the spin-echo family, is also a good candidate for rapid imaging. Its contrast behavior is similar to FLASH.[47] An example comparison between the two is shown in Figure 1–29. Its utility is in regions where susceptibility changes hinder the performance of FLASH (near inhomogeneities in the disks, marrow, and near the pituitary and sinuses).

Hemangiomas have short T_1 that may be due to some increase in the fatty components. Another shortening of T_1 occurs in hematomas. When hemoglobin is changed to methemoglobins, the iron has an electron paramagnetic effect in the surrounding protons. After further buildup and production of hemosiderin, the local field is distorted, T_2^* is reduced, and signal rapidly vanishes. It may also be possible to detect small local calcium deposits via T_2^* signal loss.

Fast low-angle imaging has proven most useful for morphological studies (CSF, cord contrast as in Fig 1–30 with low-angle spin-density weighted images), extradural defect discrimination, real-time cine imaging and contrast-agent imaging.

Fast imaging sequences can be classified as T_1-, T_1/T_2-, or T_2- weighted. Fast low-angle shot imaging and FATE fall in the first category, and their signal varies as $\sqrt{TR/T_1}$ when the optimal angle is used. Hence, doubling TR is the same as taking Nacq = 2 for the original TR in terms of S/N. For FISP, GRASS, or FAST imaging, the signal varies as T_2/T_1 at the optimal angle. Hence, the shortest TR should be used for best S/N per unit time and to meet the criterion that TR be much less than T_2. Lastly, T_2-weighted FAST images, CE-FAST, have the extra behavior $\exp(-TR/T_2)$. All the above are, of course, also weighted by the infamous T_2^* term defined earlier. An example of T_2-weighted very short FISP sequence is demonstrated in Figure 1–31.

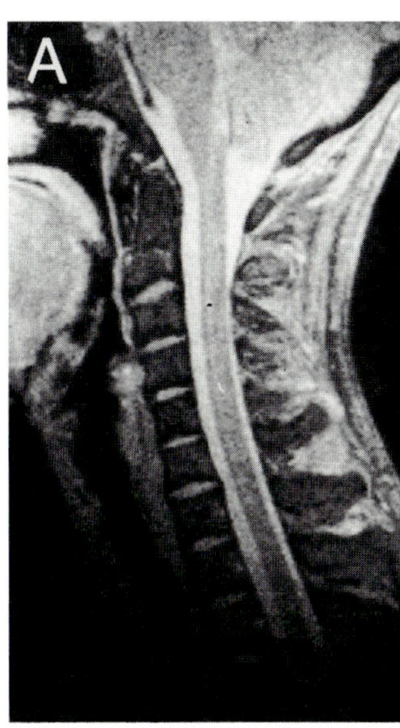

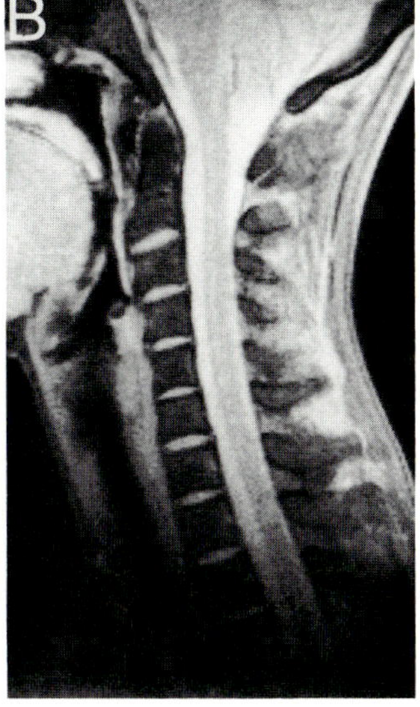

FIG 1–30.
Low-angle, spin-density, CSF cord contrast. **A,** shows a TE = 6-msec scan with Nacq = 2 and TR = 0.1 sec. **B** has TE = 9 and Nacq = 8. The edges are more sharply defined for the TE = 6 msec image, and the water/fat cancellation in the TE = 9 msec image is more pronounced. These two features and signal loss near inhomogeneities remains true even though the S/N in **B** is two times better.

WATER/LIPID IMAGING

Water/lipid imaging has been used on several occasions to ascertain the percentage content of water and fat components.[41] Figure 1–32,A shows an in-phase image and Figure 1–32,B an opposed image at TR = 1.0 second. Repeating this scenario at 0.5 second and using the fact that T_1 of fat is shorter than water allow the fat and water to be unambiguously separated as shown in Figure 1–32,C and D.

The amount of red marrow content may change either due to radiation or changes with age. We have noted on a study of 12 patients (all over 50 years of age) that each has a dominant lipid (yellow marrow) signal. On several younger volunteers (20 to 30 years of age), this was not the case; the spine was 70% water (red marrow) and 30% lipid. In one case of extensive radiation treatment on a patient with a tumor, the amount of lipid changed from 60% to 80% over a 4-month period. In a water/fat analysis of another patient, it was also shown that degenerative changes (type II) at the edges of the vertebral body (see Fig 1–32) were lipid. Similarly, for the osseous portion of vertebral hemangiomas,[48] the separation showed a dominant lipid contribution (Fig 1–33).

Perhaps future spectroscopic measurements of different spectra in hydrogen or carbon will reveal pathologic information. To date, chemical shift has only proved useful to quantify the effects of radiation in bone marrow[49] and to show disease infiltration in bone marrow.[50] As far as the utility of the actual discrimination between water and fat is concerned, the method is quite capable.

MICROSCOPY AND SUPER-RESOLUTION

Whole-body imaging systems can be used to image to 60 μm, albeit little signal remains in each pixel. The expected S/N for an ideal flat response coil for a 5-mm-thick slice with a repeat time of 1 second, a TE of 10 msec, a sampling rate of 30 μsec, a T_1 of 250 msec, a T_2

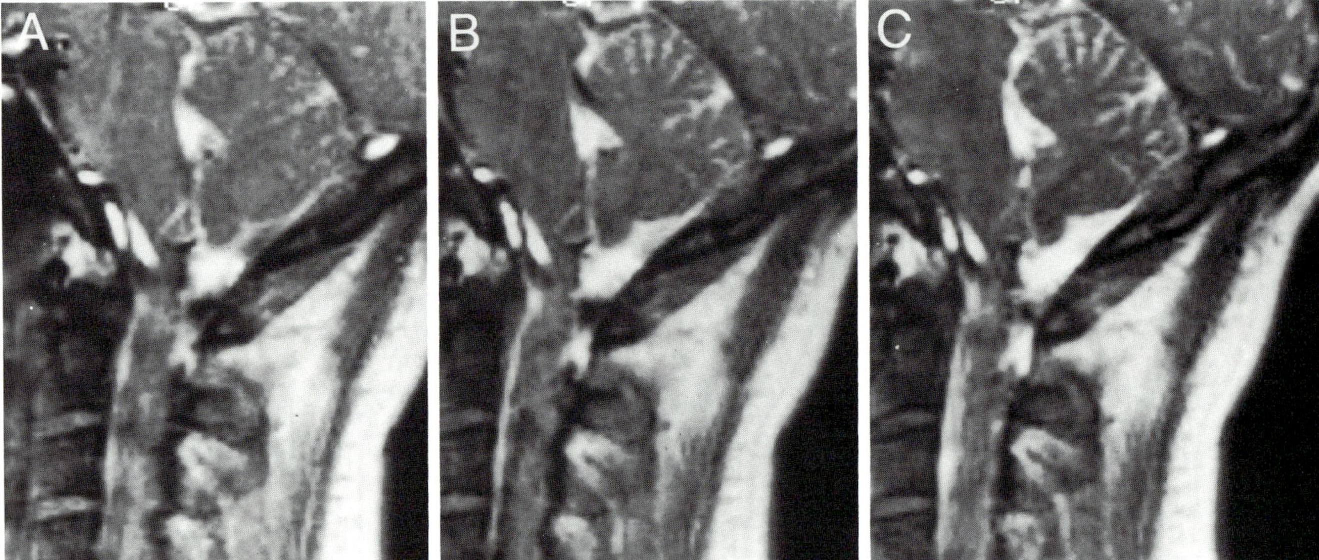

FIG 1–31.
A set of single-slice FISP images in the cervical spine for myelography. A very short TR must be used to allow the moving CSF to reach equilibrium. Compare TR = 50 msec (**A**), TR = 25 msec (**B**), and TR = 12 msec (**C**) in the cerebellar region.

of 20 msec is roughly 200:1 for an in-plane resolution of 1 mm. Increasing the number of points by four and changing the FOV in the y direction gives 250 μm resolution but only a S/N of 25:1. Even at this point, though, partial voluming effects over the 5-mm slice thickness are likely to dominate. Generally, further linear increases in resolution cause a linear loss in S/N.

For TE = 20 msec, G = 10 mT/m, and Ts = TE, the potential resolution is

$$x = 0.12\ (10/G)(20/TE) \text{ in mm} \qquad 48$$

The S/N for this one-dimensional analysis has a complicated dependence on all the parameters:

$$S/N \propto \left(\frac{G}{G_0}\right)^{1/2}\left(\frac{n_0}{n}\right)^{1/2}\left(\frac{B}{B_0}\right)\left(\frac{\Delta z}{\Delta z_0}\right) \qquad 49$$

As discussed earlier, for n sampled points and a FOV = L, the best expected resolution is $\Delta x = L/n$. However, if we assume that we know something about the object and that only m points characterize it, then if n is greater than m, we can be more precise in terms of both resolution and S/N by using this fact. For example, if an object is made up of m boxes, then m + 1 edges and m amplitudes characterize the object. If $n = p(2m + 1)$, then we have wasted $\sqrt{p}$ in S/N. This super-resolution scheme is referred to as constrained reconstruction or CORE.[20] Another advantage is that when it is no longer possible to increase n or G to improve resolution, and CORE is only limited by S/N, then simply taking more acquisitions is sufficient to improve resolution.

CLINICAL IMPLICATIONS AND SUGGESTED PROTOCOLS

In this section, the quantitative concepts of image optimization are put into a clinical perspective. The most important qualitative features are extracted as they relate to patient examination. The first step is the identification of the anatomical region and disease process suspected. The wide variation in the latter requires choosing an examination that covers the maximum number of differential considerations. Several suggested scan scenarios are included.

Qualitative Scan Features

The first practical issue is to achieve maximum S/N for morphological analysis and C/N for signal intensity characterization in view of time constraints. For spinal imaging, this necessitates the choice of an appropriate surface coil for maximum S/N. The smaller the coil, the less patient-generated noise is seen and the better the S/N that can then be traded off for smaller voxel elements and improved spatial resolution. The major disadvantage of surface coils is that the field of view is limited. This is usually not a problem in the cervical spine

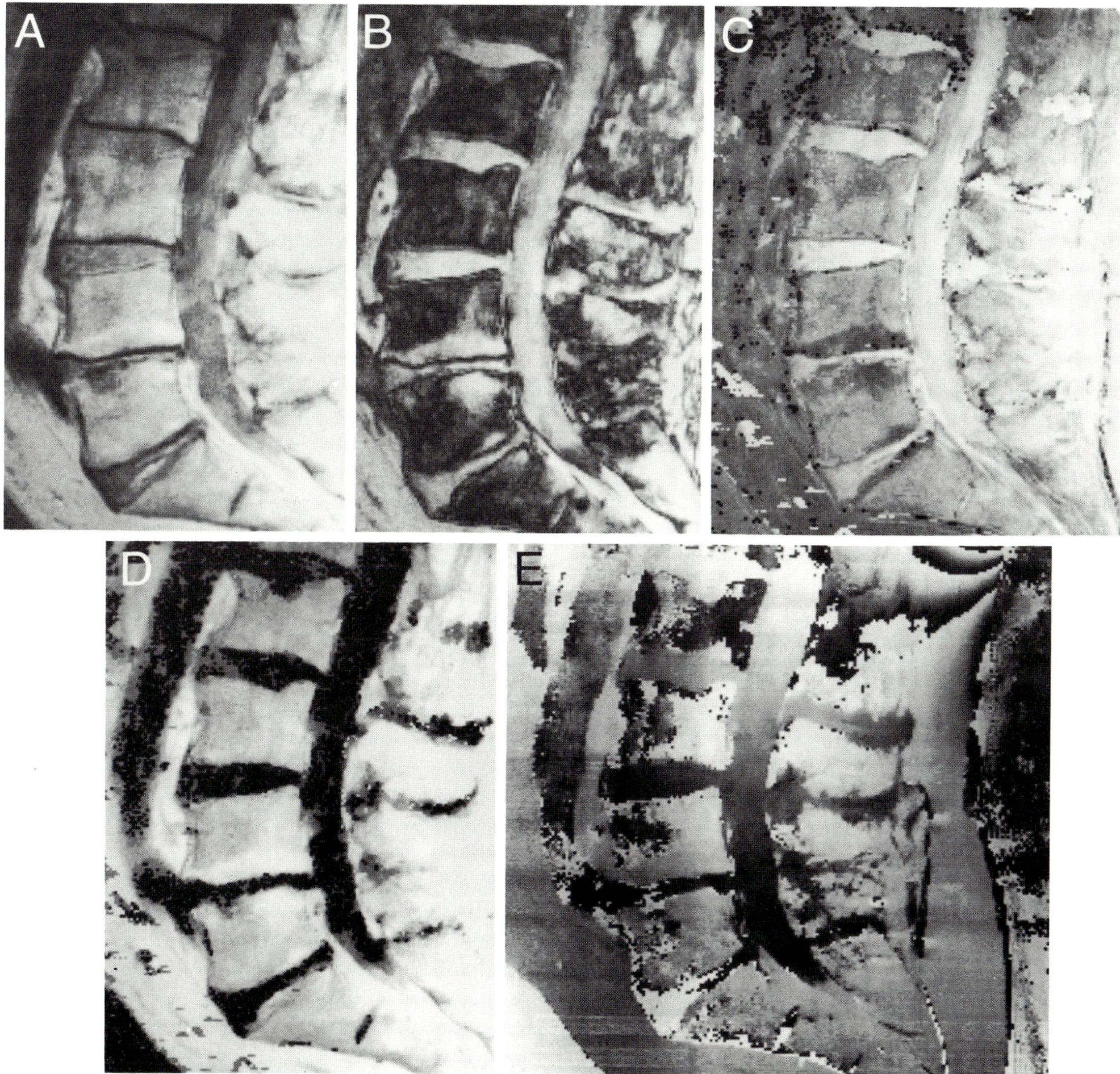

FIG 1–32.
Chemical-shift water/fat cancellations occur when the π-pulse of a spin-echo (SE) sequence is shifted by a time ϵ so that a 2π-shift at the echo causes the fat to be 180 degrees out of phase with respect to the water (called an opposed phase image). The usual SE sequence creates an inphase image (**A**). Note the lower signal in the marrow and fat in the opposed phase image (**B**). This is because the latter contains 20% water, while the former may contain up to 65% to 70% water in young healthy individuals. **C** and **D** show the separated water and fat images. Clearly the vertebral body lipid changes have significant fatty components. This is verified by examining the phase image in **E.** Note the CSF is black, 180 degrees out of phase with the vertebral body; hence, the vertebral body degeneration contains predominantly fatty components.

where the foramen magnum and C1 will almost always be in the field of view. In the lumbar region, identification of the L5-S1 interspace on the sagittal images can be difficult because lumbarization of S1 or sacralization of L5 can occur. Accurate verification is usually possible by obtaining a localized coronal scout view and assuming that the iliac crests are at the L4-L5 level. The coronal image also has an advantage in all areas by assessing the symmetry of the vertebral column, allowing repositioning for other planes if required. Sagittal and axial images are then correlated using a grid system on each image. In the thoracic spine, an initial scan with a body coil in

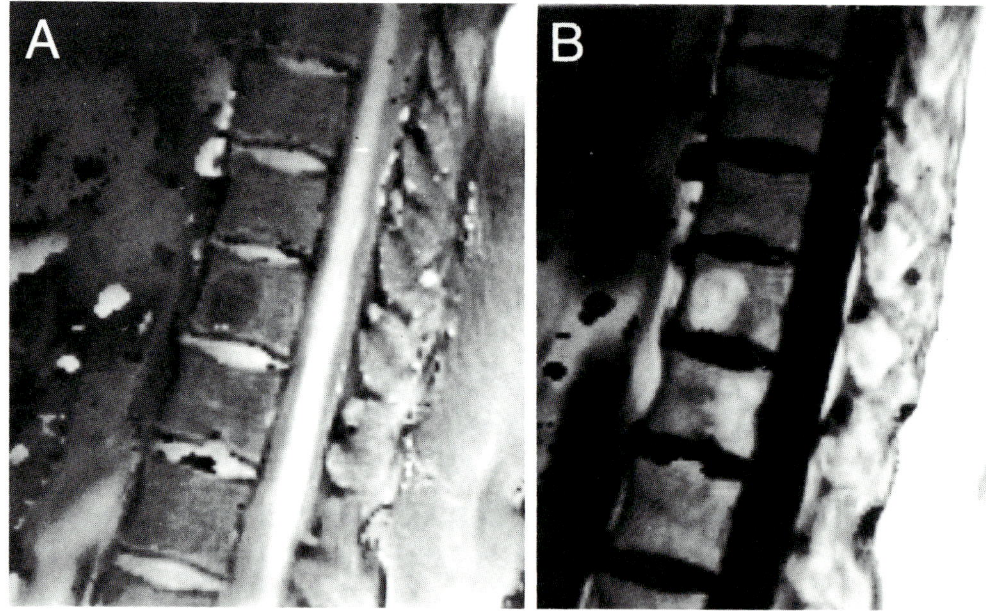

FIG 1–33.
Hemangioma presents itself as a low T_1, fat-like substance. It is absent in the water-separated image (**A**) and stands out in the fat image (**B**).

a large field of view (50 cm) may be required to localize the region of interest. This allows the identification of either C1 or the L5-S1 levels, allowing accurate localization on the surface coil studies with a grid system.

Signal-to-noise is also related to the following tissue properties: T_1, T_2, and spin density; and to the imaging parameters: TR, TE, number of acquisitions, voxel size, bandwidth, field of view, and flip angle; and to the physical phenomena: contrast agents, motion or flow, and metallic implants. Many of the imaging parameters are interlinked, and the final choice is mediated by contrast, resolution, and examination time consideration for various differential situations.

For the most part, tissue properties cannot be altered. They play a key role in image contrast as illustrated in Figures 1–11 through 1–13 for spin-echo experiments and Figures 1–26 and 1–27 for fast optimal-angle gradient echo sequences. Inherent tissue contrast can be enhanced by altering T_1 and/or T_2 relaxation times with a paramagnetic contrast agent such as Gd-DTPA.

Changing the imaging parameters gives a great deal of flexibility to MR and a myriad of choices for the operator. Generally, though, there are a few optimal choices that for the evaluation of the spine have been established as the workhorses of MR. A short TR and TE (500 msec or less and 30 msec or less, respectively) give a heavily T_1-weighted sequence and usually are adequate for a morphological examination. A long TR reduces T_1-weighted contrast and allows for a spin-density image when the first echo is a short TE (30 msec or less) and a T_2-weighted image when TE is long (60 msec or greater). These sequences with longer TEs allow more time for a lower bandwidth, which will improve S/N and motion compensation gradients, and/or cardiac gating, which will reduce CSF pulsation artifacts. Motion compensation coupled with cardiac gating[30] will give the sharpest edges. The CSF will be brightest relative to other tissues in the T_2-weighted sequence due to its long T_2 values.

Gradient echo techniques with partial flip angles are also useful. The contrast behavior in optimal-angle gradient echo techniques has a special dependence on the flip angle, as seen in Figures 1–26 and 1–27.

For low flip angles, the spin density will dominate, and a CSF myelogram-like scan can be obtained with either FLASH, FISP, or CE-FAST techniques. For FLASH imaging, angles above 30 degrees will provide more T_1-weighted images. The peak signal for repeat times between 50 and 200 msec lies between 30 and 40 degrees.

Once the appropriate contrast is established, S/N can be further adjusted by increasing voxel size or Nacq. Generally the pixel size should be kept as large as possible to maintain S/N and yet small enough to allow identification of the disease process of interest. Slice thickness is chosen in the same way. Doubling the slice thickness will double the S/N. In the above scenario, the conclusion is that doubling the voxel size doubles the S/N, and this can be accomplished in plane or in slice thickness. There is one additional variable that changes this interpretation and that is when the pixel size is changed by changing the size of the matrix. As the number of acquired points is doubled, then the pixel size is halved, but only a loss of $\sqrt{2}$ follows. A quadrupling of Nacq only gives a factor of two improvement in S/N. A halving of the FOV on the other hand gives a factor of four loss in S/N on conventional systems (since the FOV is changed in both in-plane directions).

Motion of the CSF (from a few millimeters per second to a few centimeters per second in systole), respiratory motion, blood flow, cardiac motion, peristalsis, and movement in general all lead to image degradation (see "Systematic Noise: Motion and Phase"). The CSF motion is caused by arterial pulsations in the brain resulting in a pumping action on the CSF. This drives the CSF caudally through the subarachnoid spaces surrounding the spinal cord. The motion causes loss of resolution, paradoxical enhancement, ghosting, and loss of signal from the moving tissue secondary to spin dephasing.

Paradoxical enhancement is an increase in signal intensity by the inflow of unsaturated spins. It can be seen best on the first or last slices, depending on the direction of the flow. It usually appears anterior to the cord. Cerebrospinal fluid pulsations also lead to ghosting, which is most evident on sagittal T_2-weighted images, where the high signal CSF ghosts can obscure both the intramedullary compartment and the CSF cord interface. This ghosting is caused predominantly by motion along the frequency-encoded direction. This same motion also leads to spin dephasing that reduces the signal intensity of the CSF and contrast and edge definition with the adjacent cord.

These problems are alleviated by motion compensation schemes (see "Systematic Noise: Motion and Phase") and by cardiac gating. The best results occur when both are performed together. Gating with even echoes is a form of a motion-compensated sequence. The reason cardiac gating alone is insufficient is that during systole CSF flows rapidly enough to cause spin dephasing although the signal is no longer ghosted. This, by necessity, limits the value of this technique in a multislice mode. Motion compensation gradients do limit the range of TE and bandwidths available, but it is possible to collect both the TE = 15 msec and a TE = 90 msec long TR image with high quality. Another scheme to reduce the motion artifacts is to switch the direction of the read and phase-encoded directions. This is useful when gradient compensated sequences are not available, but a potential for image aliasing exists depending on the field of view. This may also result in obscuration of extradural defects due to a redirection of the chemical-shift phenomenon. This can be avoided by switching the sign of the read gradient or using a sufficiently large gradient so that the chemical shift lies in one pixel.

The other forms of motion such as ghosting artifacts from the aorta and abdominal breathing artifacts in the lumbar and thoracic spine can be removed by applying special saturation pulses to remove signal from the unwanted regions that generate the noise.[7] This is also useful in the cervical spine, where swallowing can cause problems. The aliasing problems alluded to above can also be eliminated using this technique.

Optimal-angle gradient echo imaging has been referred to in a variety of applications above. It has been found most useful for producing the CSF myelogram effect. The short TRs possible with this technique also allow the potential for rapid 3D acquisitions for very thin effective slices. In addition to the obvious value of allowing reconstruction along the entire field of view in any plane, the 3D images suffer less from regions of field inhomogeneity and tissue susceptibility changes that plague the 2D techniques. These effects are most evident in the vertebral bodies where little signal remains at TEs of 10 msec and higher. Refer to "Contrast and Artifacts" for more details and to "Water/Lipid Imaging" for a comparison with water/fat and in-phase and opposed imaging.

In terms of disease processes themselves, the conventional categories of extradural, intradural, extramedullary, and intramedullary remain convenient for establishing basic protocols. It must be kept in mind, however, that the clinical presentation may be nonspecific and widespread for the disease process, mandating thorough coverage of all areas. While the following represent our recommendation for protocols, there exists more than one way to achieve comparable results.

Suggested Imaging Scenarios

Extradural and Intradural Extramedullary Imaging Protocols

In the extradural compartment and intradural extramedullary area, degenerative disease of the spine represents the overwhelming reason for referral for study. Trauma, neoplasms, congenital disorders, infection, and vascular abnormalities may involve either region. For most situations, T_1-weighted spin-echo sequences with some type of partial flip angle gradient echo scan (2D or 3D) will suffice. The most notable exceptions are vertebral osteomyelitis and trauma where T_2-weighted images for evaluation of disk extradural soft tissue and spinal cord signal intensity are critical.

1. Localizing or scout scan
   Coronal, short TR/TE (200–500 msec/15–30 msec) SE or FLASH 30–200 msec/6–13 msec/20–60 degrees
   Matrix: 128 × 128
   No. of acquisitions: 1
   Field of view: 30–50 cm
   Slice thickness: 10 mm
   Imaging time: 12 seconds to 1 minute

2. Definitive study
   a. Sagittal T_1-weighted SE (500 msec/15 msec) foramen to foramen
   Matrix: 256 × 256
   No. of acquisitions: 2–4
   Field of view: 24 cm
   Slice thickness: 3 mm
   Imaging time: 4–8 minutes
   b. Sagittal FLASH (50–200 msec/6–13 msec/5–10 degrees, cervical and thoracic; 40–60 degrees, lumbar); 2D or 3D
   Matrix: 256 × 256
   No. of acquisitions: 1–4
   Field of view: 24 cm
   Slice thickness: 3–4 mm 2D, 1.2–3 mm 3D (16–64 slices or partitions)
   Imaging time: 2D, 50–200 seconds; 3D, 3.5–14 minutes
   c. Axial T_1-weighted SE (500 msec/15 msec) through at least 3 disk levels
   Matrix: 256 × 256
   No. of acquisitions: 2–4
   Field of view: 24 cm
   Slice thickness: 3–4 mm
   Imaging time: 4–8 minutes

   or

   Axial FLASH (200/6–13/10 degrees, cervical and thoracic; 40–60 degrees, lumbar)
   Matrix: 256 × 256
   No. of acquisitions: 1–4
   Field of view: 24 cm
   Slice thickness: 3–4 mm, 2D; 1–2 mm, reconstructed 3D (16–64 slices)
   Imaging time: 2D, 50–200 seconds; 3D, 3.5–14 minutes

Other considerations for developing a protocol for extradural and intradural extramedullary disease are as follows:

1. Bandwidth optimization for S/N (given the ability to read through chemical-shift artifact)
2. Frequency oriented along spinal axis to reduce aliasing; frequency and phase-encoded direction may be interchanged to reduce ghosting through the area of interest
3. Refocusing in both read and slice to compensate for CSF ghosting
4. Saturation pulses anterior to the spine to reduce ghosting artifacts from outside the area of interest and posterior to spine to remove increased signal from fat that may adversely affect the gray scale setting
5. Three-dimensional imaging acquired sagittally to allow reconstruction through the entire field of view along the axis of the spine
6. Forty-five-degree oblique images in the cervical region for evaluation of the neural foramina (2D T_1-weighted images or 3D reconstructions)
7. Angled axial images through disk level

Intramedullary Imaging Protocols

The major considerations for intramedullary disease protocols include cystic lesions, neoplasms, cord trauma, demyelinating disease, ischemia, radiation injury, vascular malformations, and some developmental abnormalities. Exam considerations are essentially the same as extradural, but care must be taken not to obscure lesions with the surrounding CSF because of its decreased or increased signal depending on the sequence. This mandates using refocusing and/or cardiac gating and occasionally taking care to obtain both refocused and defocused sequences (e.g., suspected arachnoid cysts).

1. Localizing or scout scan
   T_1-weighted and/or FLASH sagittal and axial, plus

2. Definitive study
   Sagittal T_2-weighted SE (2000–2500 msec/60–90 msec)
   Matrix: 256 × 256
   No. of acquisitions: 1
   Field of view: 24 cm
   Slice thickness: 3–4 mm
   Imaging time: 8–10 minutes

CONCLUSIONS

The choice of MRI parameters allows high-resolution images to be obtained under a variety of conditions. In general, when TE is long and field inhomogeneities are small or not important (such as in vascular imaging), then low gradients and long sampling times or at least large n can be used to keep S/N high. When S/N is desired, but high resolution not required, then extra time points should be taken and averaged to produce a less artifacted, lower-resolution image.

Fast imaging schemes have begun to prove their utility in spine imaging. However, there are a variety of artifacts that can lead to poor image quality. These range from insufficient spoiling to the wrong flip angle for the desired contrast or to the loss of resolution and fake contrast associated with in vivo susceptibility effects. Nevertheless, 3D fast imaging has proven very useful for morphological studies when high resolution, contiguous slice imaging is required.

New methods to reduce motion artifacts such as motion compensation and saturation are also leading to further improvements in image quality. Coupled with high resolution and high S/N techniques, further refinements are still likely. The most promising approaches that can all be combined are ordered phase encoding, saturation of unwanted regions, and flow or motion rephasing sequences.

The existence of the many sequences and parameters is not a bane; on the contrary it is the strength of MR. Given this wide variety of choice, it will be necessary to create a utility map carefully illustrating the pros and cons of each sequence type relative to the particular disease, its location, the resolution required, and any other physical requirements and limitations. The material in this chapter should help answer some of these questions in the context of today's understanding as it relates to imaging the spine.

Acknowledgments

The work on chemical shift imaging was supported by Dr. Antonio Antunez in support of Todd Parrish who supplied the water/lipid separated images. My thanks to Dr. Jean Tkach for the contrast calculations and Dr. Michael Modic for his thoughts and suggestions on maintaining a clinical thrust with theoretical concepts.

REFERENCES

1. Bellon EM, Haacke EM, Coleman PE, et al: MR artifacts: A review. *AJR* 1986; 147:1271–1281.
2. Haacke EM, Bellon EM: Artifacts, in Stark DD, Bradley W (eds): *Magnetic Resonance Imaging.* St Louis, CV Mosby Co, 1987, Chapter 8.
3. Henkelman RM, Bronskill MJ: Artifacts in magnetic resonance imaging. *Rev Magn Reson Imaging* 1987; 2:1–126.
4. Ludecke KM, Roschmann P, Tischler R: Susceptibility artifacts in NMR imaging. *Magn Reson Imaging* 1985; 3:329–343.
5. Hinshaw WS, Lent AH: An introduction to NMR imaging: From the Bloch equation to the imaging equation. *Proc IEEE* 1981; 71:338–350.
6. Haacke EM: Solving for non-ideal conditions in two-dimensional Fourier transform magnetic resonance imaging using a generalized transform. *Inverse Problems* 1987; 3:421–435.
7. Felmlee JP, Ehman RL: Spatial presaturation: A method for suppressing flow artifacts and improving depiction of vascular anatomy in MR imaging. *Radiology* 1987; 164:559–564.
8. Aue WP: Localization methods for in vivo NMR spectroscopy. *Magn Reson Med* 1986; 1:21–72.
9. Young IR: Special pulse sequences and techniques, in Stark DD, Bradley W (eds): *Magnetic Resonance Imaging.* St Louis, CV Mosby Co, 1987, Chapter 6.
10. Hendrick RE, Newman FD, Hendee WR: MR imaging technology: Maximizing the signal-to-noise ratio from a single tissue. *Radiology* 1985; 157:749–752.
11. Hendrick RE, Kneeland JB, Stark DD: Maximizing signal-to-noise and contrast-to-noise ratios in FLASH imaging. *Magn Reson Imaging* 1987; 5:117–127.
12. Hendrick RE: Sampling time effects on signal-to-noise and contrast-to-noise ratios in spin-echo MRI. *Magn Reson Imaging* 1987; 5:31–37.
13. Bradley WG, Tsuruda JS: MR sequence parameter optimization: An algorithmic approach. *AJR* 1987; 149:815–823.
14. Bradley WG, Glenn BJ: The effect of variation in slice thickness and interslice gap on MR lesion detection. *AJNR* 1987; 8:1057–1062.
15. Feinberg DA, Crooks LE, Hoeninger JC, et al: Continuous thin slice multisection MR imaging by two-dimensional Fourier transform techniques. *Radiology* 1986; 158:811–817.
16. Haacke EM, Lenz GW: Short echo time, fast gradient echo imaging. *Radiology* 1987; 165(P):30.
17. Haacke EM: The effects of finite sampling in magnetic resonance imaging. *Magn Reson Med* 1987; 4:401–421.
18. Wood ML, Henkelman RM: Truncation artifacts in magnetic resonance imaging. *Magn Reson Med* 1985; 2:517–526.
19. Smith MR, Nichols ST, Henkelman RM, et al: Application of autoregressive moving average parametric modeling in magnetic resonance image reconstruction. *IEEE Trans Med Imaging* 1986; MI-5:132–139.
20. Haacke EM, Liang Z-P, Izen SH: Imaging with constraints: Overcoming the diffraction limit. *IEEE ASSP,* in press.
21. Bracewell RN: *The Fourier Transform and Its Applications,* ed 2. New York, McGraw-Hill Book Co, 1978.
22. Haacke EM: The need for very short echo times in fast magnetic resonance imaging, 1987 Topical Conference on Fast Magnetic Resonance Imaging. Cleveland, May 1987.
23. Bottomley PA, Hardy CJ, Argersinger RE, et al: A review of H nuclear magnetic resonance relaxation in pathology: Are T1 and T2 diagnostic? *Med Phys* 1987; 14:1–37.
24. Zypman FR, Haacke EM, Brown RW, et al: Radiofrequency

penetration at high frequencies in the human body. *Radiology* 1987; 165(P):130.

25. Fuderer M, van Est A: Surface coil intensity correction using homomorphic filtering, Society of Magnetic Resonance Imaging 6th annual meeting abstract book. New York, 1987, p 266.
26. Requardt H, Offermann J: Switched array coils: Multipurpose antennae with variable geometry. *Radiology* 1987; 165(P):344.
27. Gadian DG: *Nuclear Magnetic Resonance and Its Applications to Living Systems.* Oxford, England, Clarendon Press, 1982.
28. Wood ML, Henkelman RM: MR image artifacts from periodic motion. *Med Phys* 1985; 12:143–151.
29. Haacke EM, Patrick JL: Reducing motion artifacts in two-dimensional Fourier transform imaging. *Magn Reson Imaging* 1986; 4:359–376.
30. Haacke EM, Lenz GW: Improving image quality in the presence of motion by rephasing gradients. *AJR* 1987; 148:1251–1258.
31. Pattany PM, Marino R, McNally JM: Velocity and acceleration densitization in 2DFT MR imaging. *Magn Reson Imaging* 1986; 4:154–155.
32. Nishimura DG, Macovski A, Pauly JM: Magnetic resonance angiography. *IEEE Trans Med Imaging* 1986; MI-5:140–151.
33. Bailes DR, Gildendale DJ, Bydder GM, et al: Respiratory ordered phase encoding (ROPE): A method for reducing motion artifacts. *J Comput Assist Tomogr* 1985; 9:835–838.
34. Haacke EM, Lenz GW, Nelson AD: Pseudogating: Eliminating of periodic motion artifacts in magnetic resonance imaging without gating. *Magn Reson Med* 1987; 4:162–174.
35. Rubin JB, Enzmann DR: Imaging of spinal CSF pulsation by 2DFT MR: Significance during clinical imaging. *AJNR* 1987; 8:297–306.
36. Rubin JB, Enzmann DR: Harmonic modulation of proton MR precessional phase by pulsatile motion: Origin of spinal CSF flow phenomena. *AJNR* 1987; 8:307–318.
37. Rubin JB, Enzmann DR, Wright A: CSF-gated MR imaging of the spine: Theory and clinical implementation. *Radiology* 1987; 163:784–792.
38. Rubin JB, Enzmann DR, Wright A: Use of cerebrospinal fluid gating to improve T2 weighted images. *Radiology* 1987; 162:763–767.
39. Rubin JB, Enzmann DR: Optimizing conventional MR imaging of the spine. *Radiology* 1987; 163:777–783.
40. Kelly WM: in Brant-Zawadski M, Norman D (eds): *Image Artifacts and Technical Limitations.* New York, Raven Press, 1987.
41. Haacke EM, Patrick JL, Lenz GW, et al: The separation of water and lipid components in the presence of field inhomogeneities. *Rev Magn Reson Imaging* 1986; 1:123–154.
42. Frahm J, Hanicke W, Merbolt K-D: Transverse coherence in rapid FLASH NMR imaging. *J Magn Reson* 1987; 72:307–314.
43. Young IR, Payne JA: Slice-shape artifact changes with precession angle in rapid MR imaging. *Magn Reson Med* 1987; 5:177–181.
44. van der Meulen P, Groen JP, Tinus AMC, et al: Fast field echo imaging: An overview and contrast calculations. Submitted to *Magn Reson Imaging,* in press.
45. Sekihara K: Steady-state magnetization in rapid NMR imaging using small flip angles and short repetition intervals. *Proc IEEE* 1987; MI-6:157–164.
46. Wehrli FW: Fast-scan imaging: Principles and contrast phenomenology, in Higgins C, Hricak H (eds): *Magnetic Resonance Imaging of the Body.* New York, Raven Press, 1987, pp 23–38.
47. JA Tkach, Haacke EM: A comparison of fast spin echo and gradient field echo sequences. *Magn Reson Imaging,* in press.
48. Davis KR, Brady TJ: MR of hemorrhage: A new approach. *AJNR* 1986; 7:751–756.
49. Buxton RB, Wismer GL, Brady TJ, et al: Quantitative proton chemical-shift imaging. *Magn Reson Med* 1986; 3:881.
50. Remedios P, Colletti P, Raval J, et al: MRI of bone after radiation, Society of Magnetic Resonance Imaging 6th annual meeting abstract book. New York, 1987, p 155.

2

Normal Anatomy

Michael T. Modic, M.D.

LUMBAR SPINE

The lumbosacral spine, composed of vertebral bodies, lateral and posterior elements, together with adjacent soft tissues serves to carry the load of the upper body and transfer it to the lower limbs.

The bony lumbar spinal canal is formed by the vertebral bodies anteriorly, the pedicles laterally, and the lamina and base of the spinous process posteriorly (Figs 2–1 through 2–3). On T_1-weighted spin-echo (SE) sequences (short repetition time (TR)/short echo time (TE)), the cancellous hematopoietic portion of the osseous structures is of an intermediate signal intensity between paraspinal fat and muscle. The signal intensity is primarily a reflection of the marrow space with its lipid and hematopoietic elements. The relative signal intensity becomes brighter (diffusely, or in a focal spotty fashion) with increasing age secondary to an increase in the lipid component of the marrow space[1] (Fig 2–4). Occasionally, single focal areas of high signal intensity on T_1-weighted images with an intermediate signal intensity on T_2-weighted images are noted secondary to regions of focal yellow marrow.[2] The osseous structures are outlined by a thin low signal intensity from cortical bone. There is often a discrepant appearance of the superior and inferior end-plates secondary to chemical shift (see Fig 2–2).

The superior lumbar spinal canal is usually round or oval in shape with a transverse diameter that is equal to or greater than the anterior-posterior dimension. In the midlumbar and lower lumbar regions, the spinal canal takes on a more triangular configuration with the base projected anteriorly. Again, the transverse diameter is usually equal to or greater than the anterior-posterior dimension.

The transverse diameter of the lumbar vertebral body is larger than the anterior-posterior diameter. The vertebral bodies have a convex anterior and lateral margin with a flat or concave posterior margin. The superior and inferior vertebral body margins are flat or slightly concave. Basivertebral channels are usually present in the midportion of the vertebral body. These regions often have a high signal intensity on T_1-weighted images that is secondary to fat surrounding the basivertebral plexus and/or slow flow of venous blood (Fig 2–5).

The pedicles are bony pillars that project posteriorly and laterally from the superior aspect of the vertebral body and form the superior and inferior margin of the neural foramen. They are composed primarily of dense cortical bone but still contain enough marrow to approximate the signal intensity of the vertebral bodies on T_1-weighted sequences. The lamina are angled bony projections extending from the pedicles to the base of the spinous process. The superior aspect of the lamina lies anterior to its inferior margin.

The spinous process extends posteriorly and slightly inferiorly from the vertebral arch. The transverse processes extend laterally and slightly posteriorly from the junction of the pedicle with the lamina and are composed primarily of cancellous bone. The articular pillars include the bone at the junction of the lamina and pedicles. The superior and inferior articular processes arise from the articular pillars and in the transverse plane appear at the midlevel of the intervertebral foramen. The concave surface of the superior articular process and convex surface of the inferior articular process form the diarthrodial facet joints. The superior articular facet of the body below lies anterior and lateral and faces posteromedial to the inferior articular facet of the body above. At the inferior aspect of the intervertebral foramen, the superior articular facet becomes contiguous with the pedicle below and forms the posterior border of the lateral recess where the traversing nerve root lies

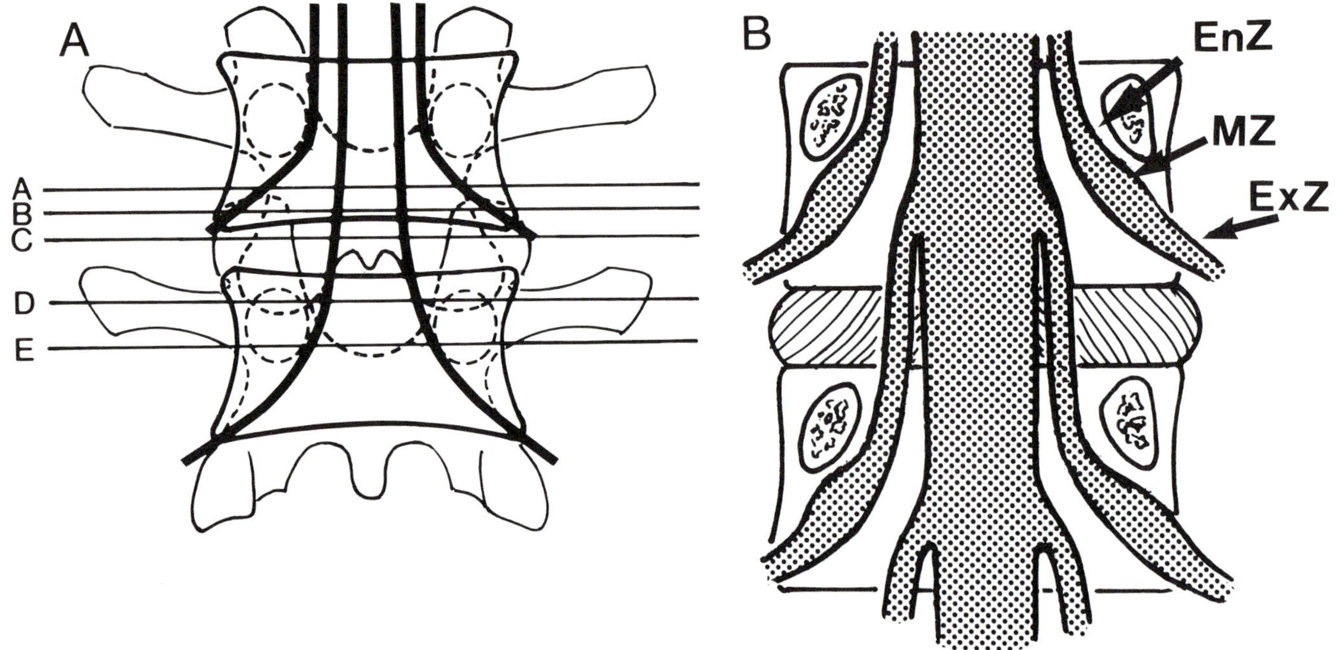

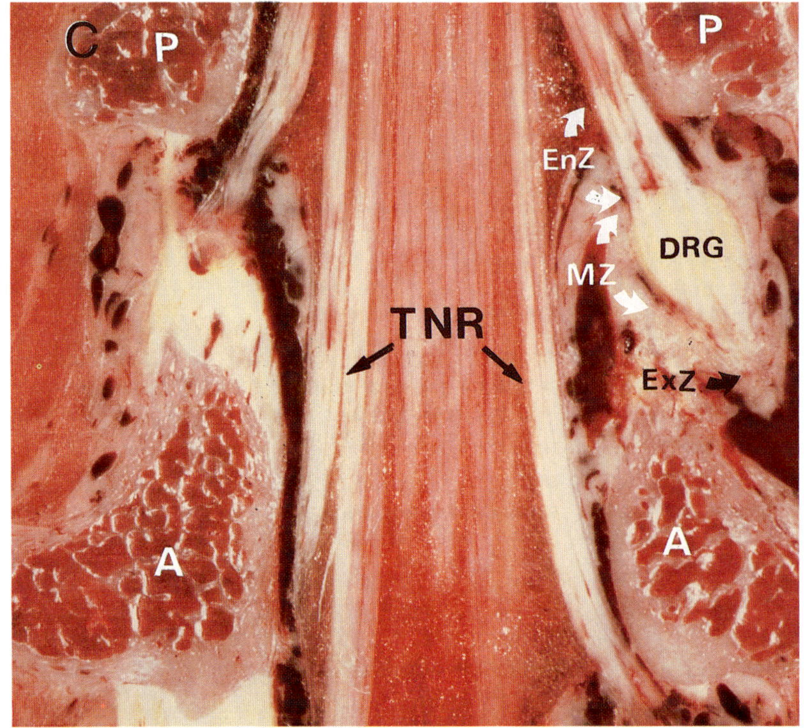

FIG 2–1.

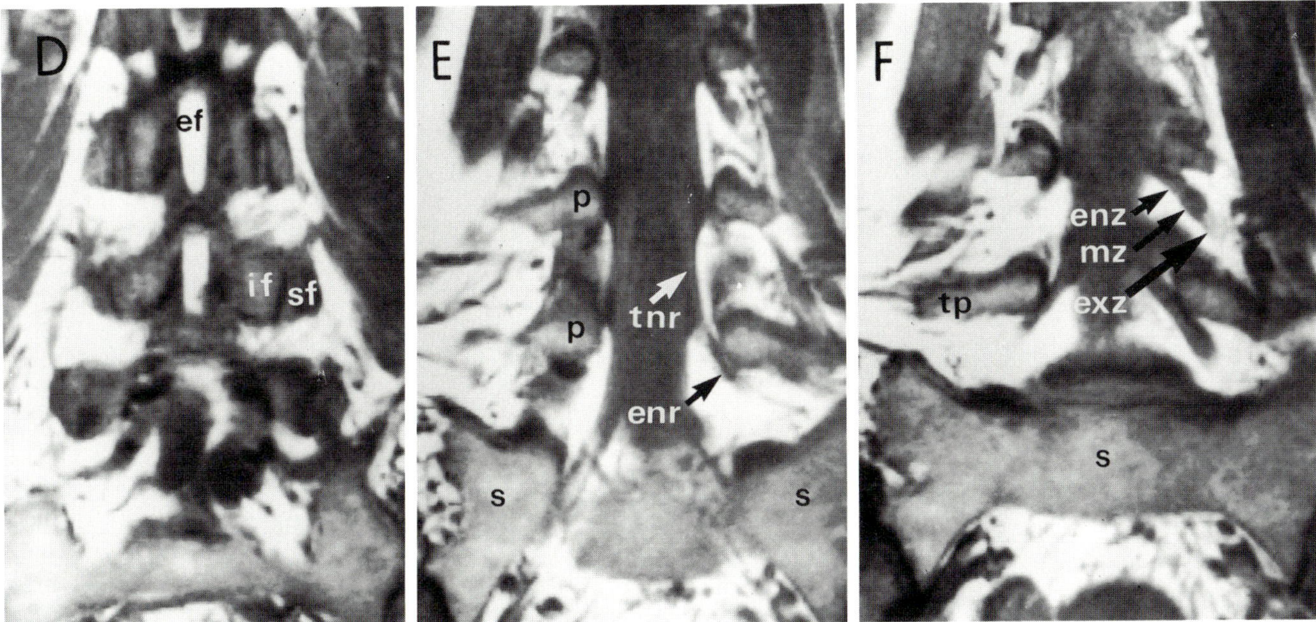

FIG 2–1.
A–F, coronal plane of the lower lumbar spine: Schematic diagrams, cryomicrotome anatomical section and T_1-weighted coronal MR images (500/17). *A* = articular pillar; *DRG* = dorsal root ganglion; *ef* = epidural fat; *en(r)* = exiting nerve root; *EnZ* = entrance zone; *ExZ* = exit zone; *if* = inferior facet; *MZ* = midzone; *P* = pedicle; *s* = sacrum; *sf* = superior facet; *tp* = transverse process; *TNR* = traversing nerve root.

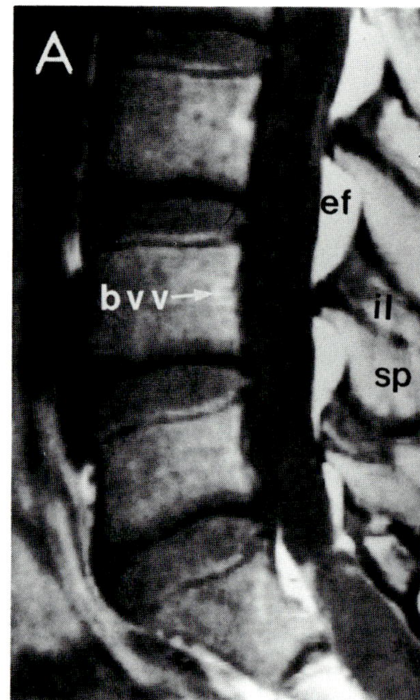

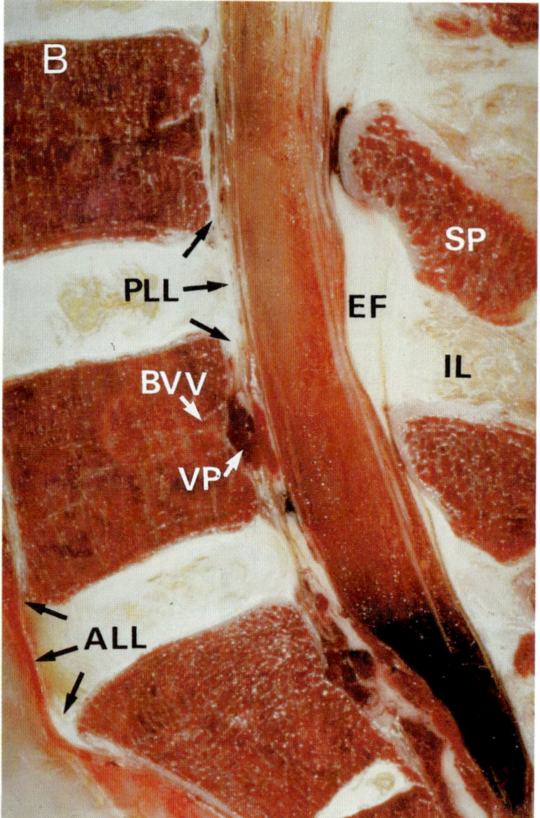

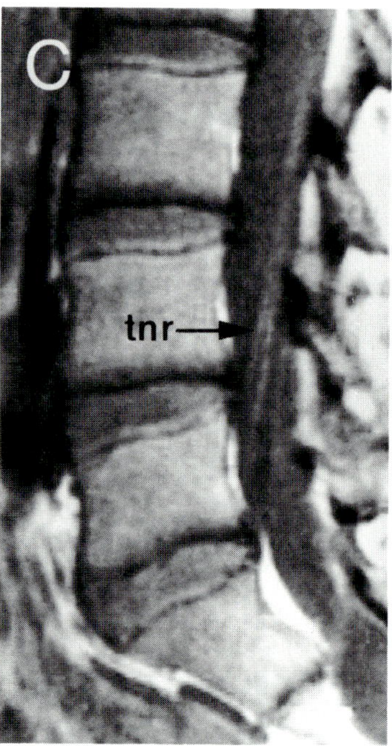

FIG 2–2.

A–C, sagittal plane of the lumbar spine: Cryomicrotome anatomical sections and T_1-weighted MR images (500/17). *A* = articular process; *ALL* = anterior longitudinal ligament; *BVV* = basivertebral vein(s); *D* = disk; *DRG* = dorsal root ganglion; *EF* = epidural fat; *EN(R)* = exiting nerve root; *IF* = inferior facet; *IL* = intraspinal ligament; *LF* = ligamentum flavum; *LR* = lateral recess; *P* = pedicle; *PLL* = posterior longitudinal ligament; *SF* = superior facet; *SP* = spinous process; *TNR* = traversing nerve root; *VP* = venous plexus; *VSR* = ventral spinal root. *(Continued)*

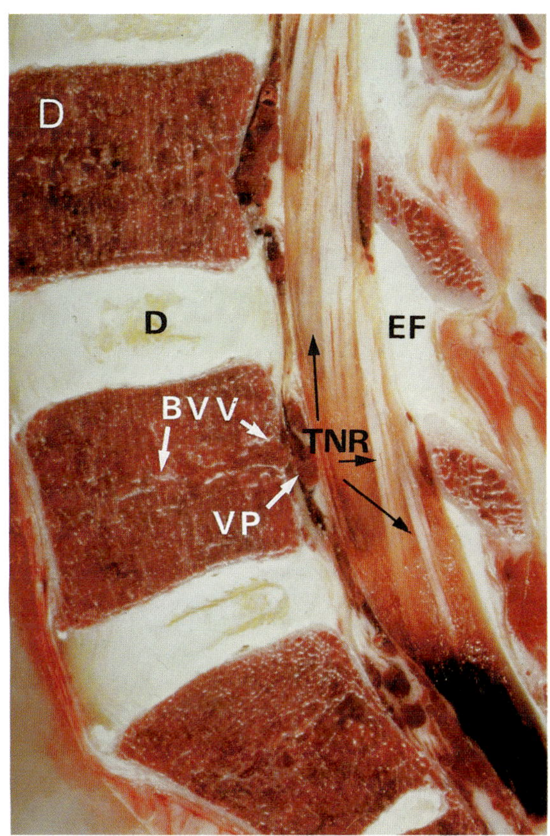

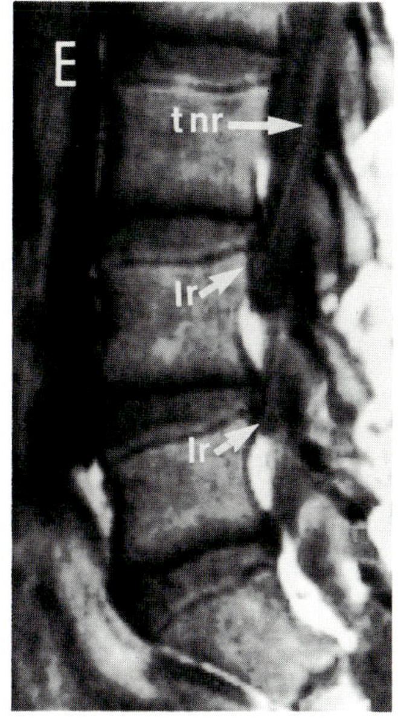

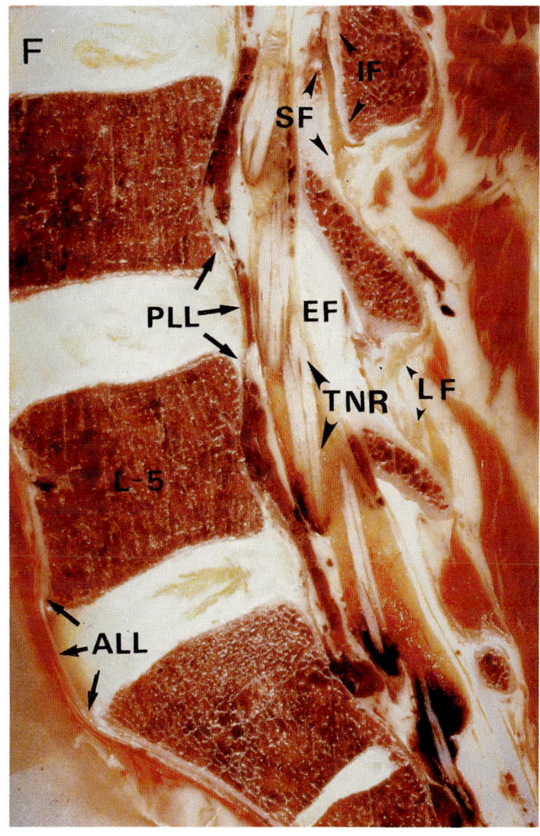

FIG 2–2 (cont.).
D–F, sagittal plane of the lumbar spine: Cryomicrotome anatomical sections and T_1-weighted MR images. (See p. 38 for explanation of abbreviations.) *(Continued)*

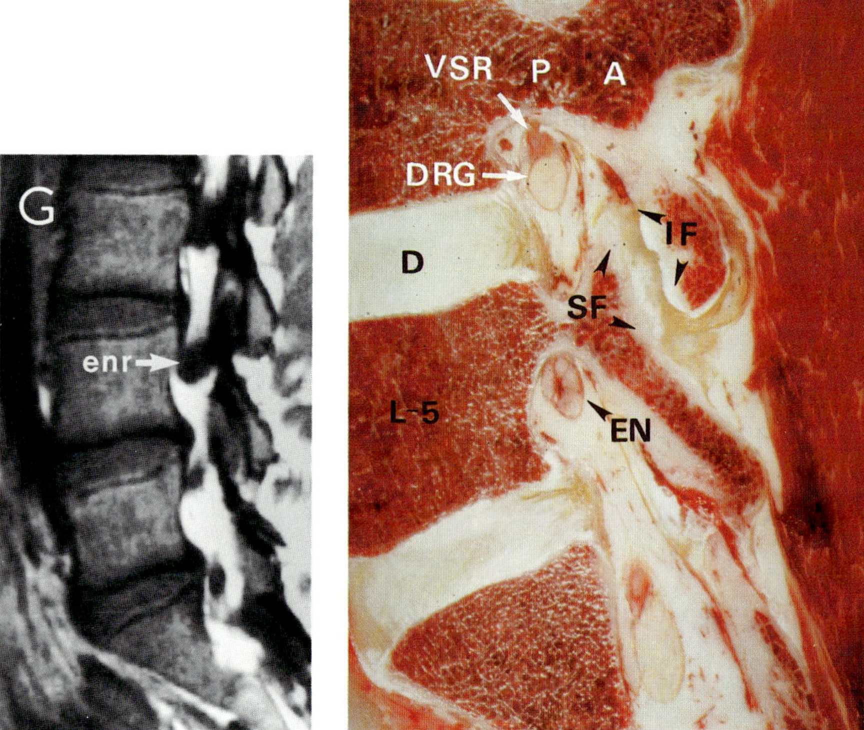

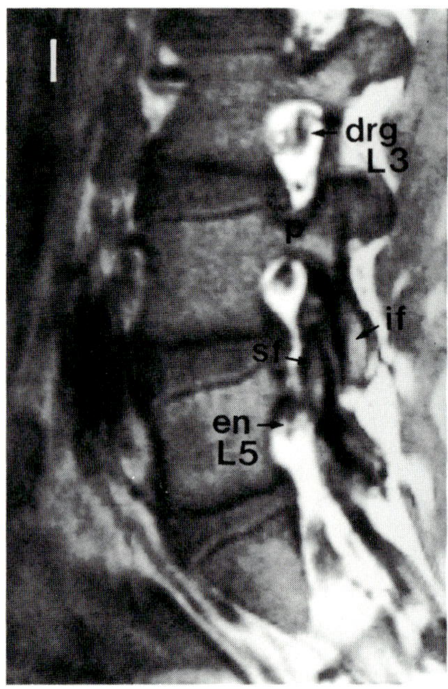

FIG 2–2 (cont.).
G–I, sagittal plane of the lumbar spine: Cryomicrotome anatomical sections and T_1-weighted images. (See p. 38 for explanation of abbreviations.)

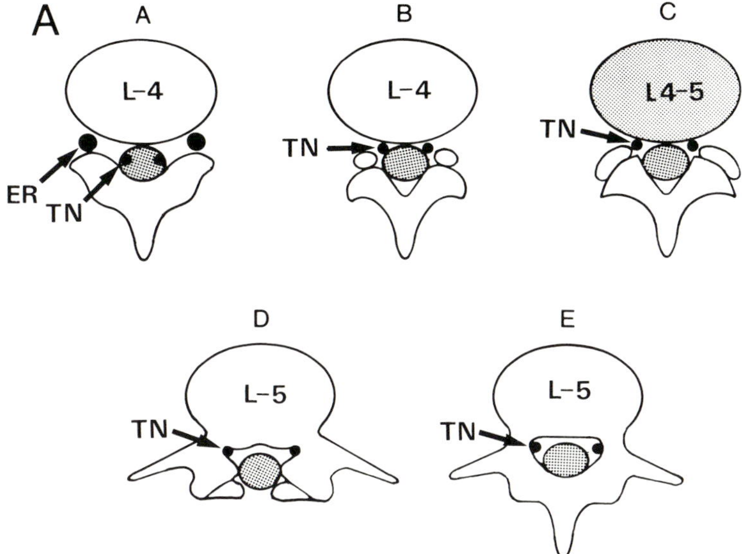

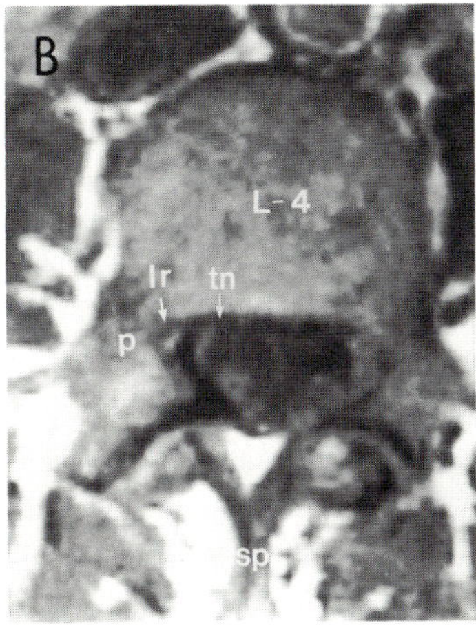

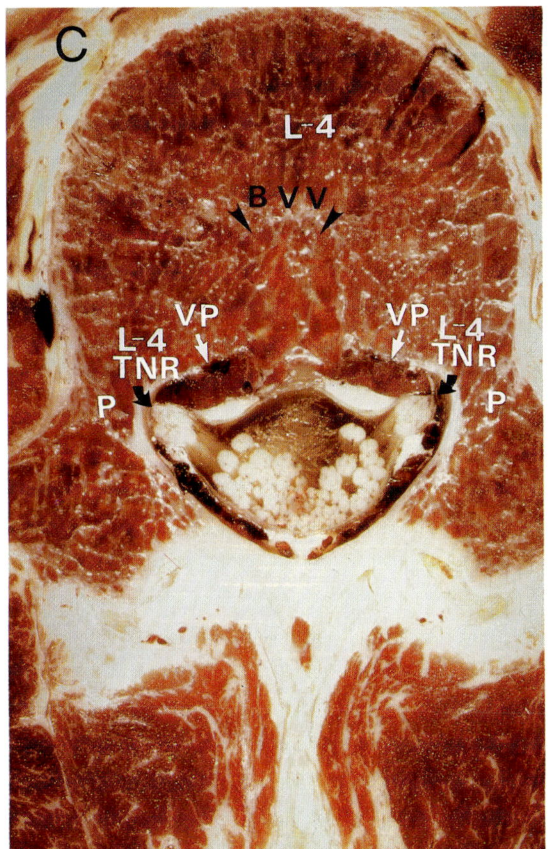

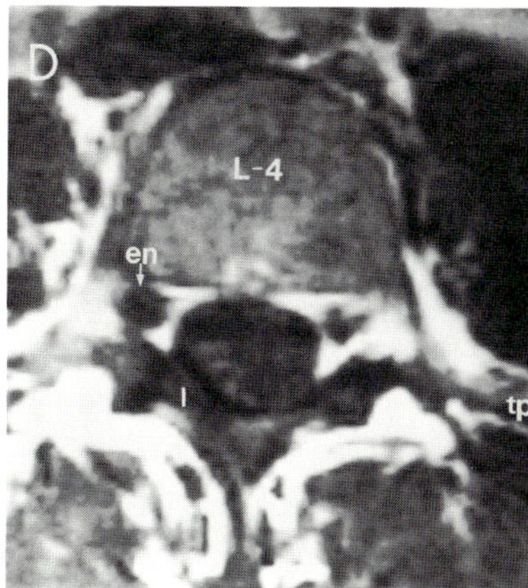

FIG 2–3.

A–D, axial plane of lumbar spine: Schematic diagram, cryomicrotome anatomical sections, and T_1-weighted MR images (500/17). *AF* = anulus fibrosis; *BVV* = basivertebral veins(s); *CE* = cartilaginous end plate; *DRG* = dorsal root ganglion; *EF* = epidural fat; *EN(R)* = exiting nerve root; *if* = inferior facet; *LF* = ligamenavum; *LR* = lateral recess; *NF* = neural foramen; *NP* = nucleus pulposus; *P* = pedicle; *sf* = superior facet; *SP* = spinous process; *TN(R)* = traversing nerve roots; *tp* = transverse process; *VP* = venous plexus. *(Continued)*

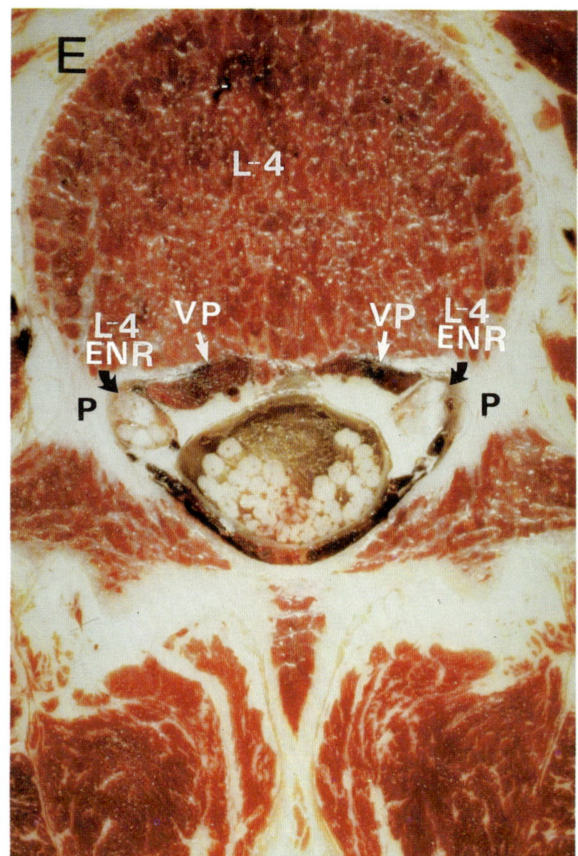

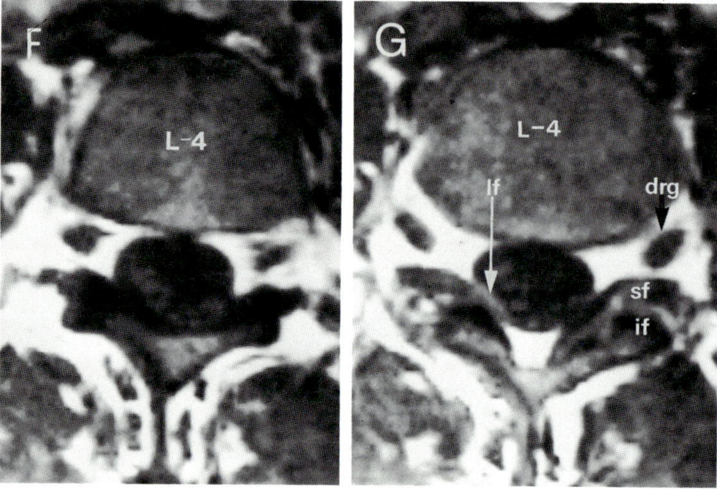

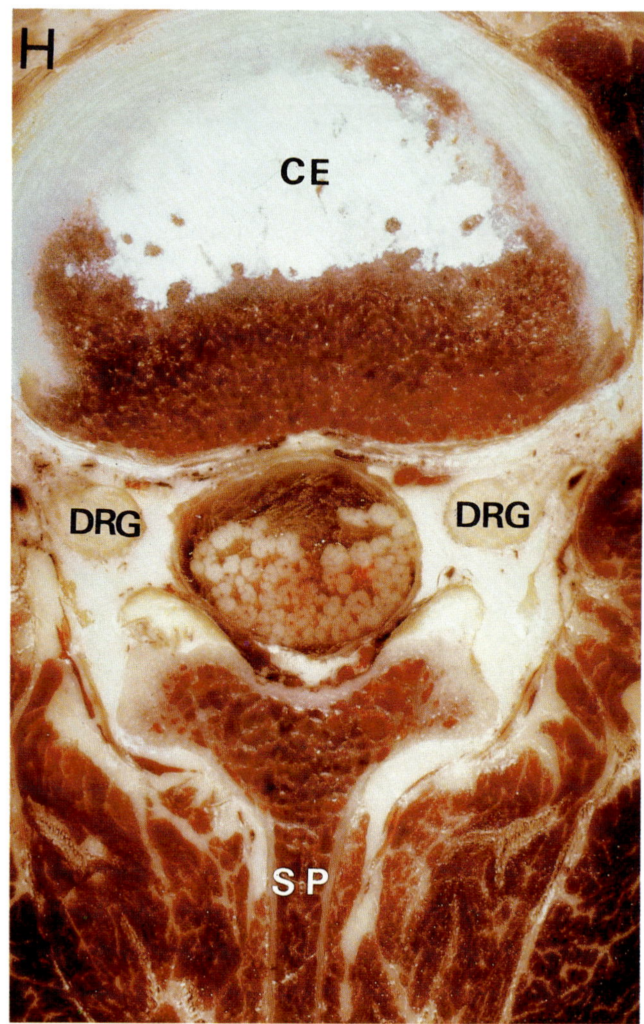

FIG 2–3 (cont.).
E–H, axial plane of lumbar spine: Schematic diagram, cryomicrotome anatomical sections, and T_1-weighted MR images. (See p. 41 for explanation of abbreviations.) *(Continued)*

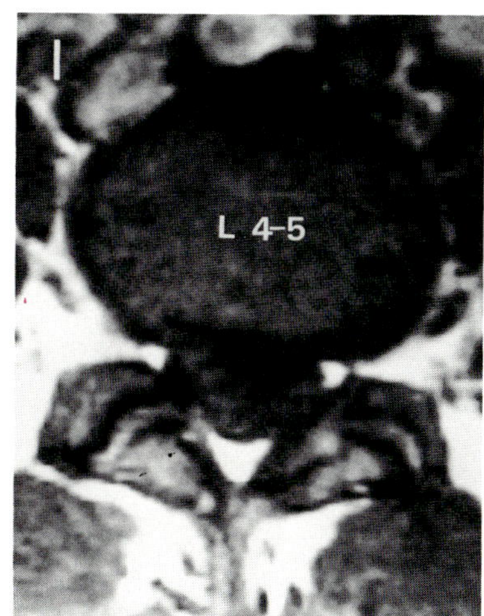

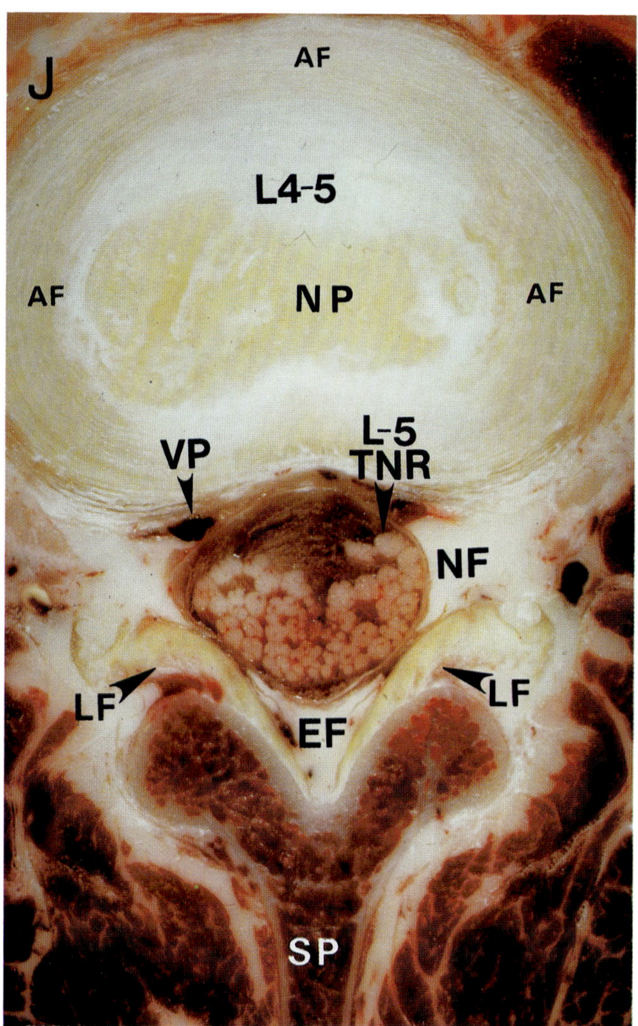

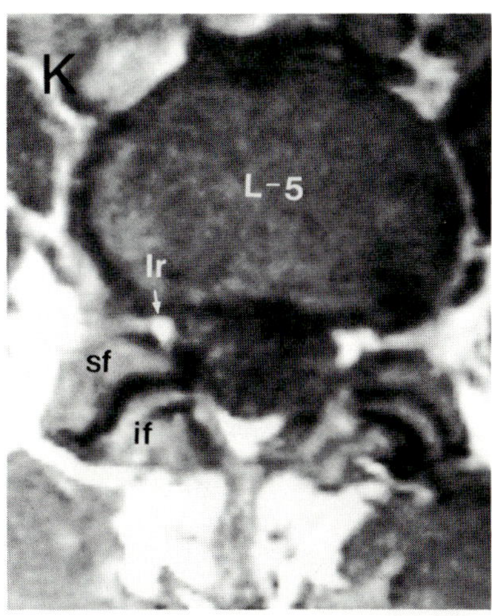

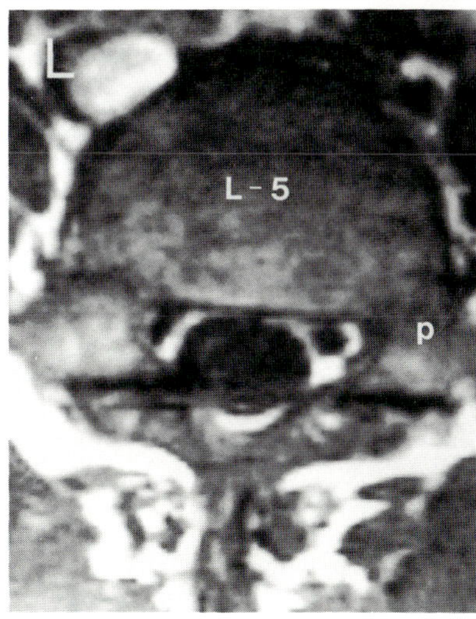

FIG 2–3 (cont.).
I–L, axial plane of lumbar spine: Schematic diagram, cryomicrotome anatomical sections, and T_1-weighted MR images. (See p. 41 for explanation of abbreviations.)

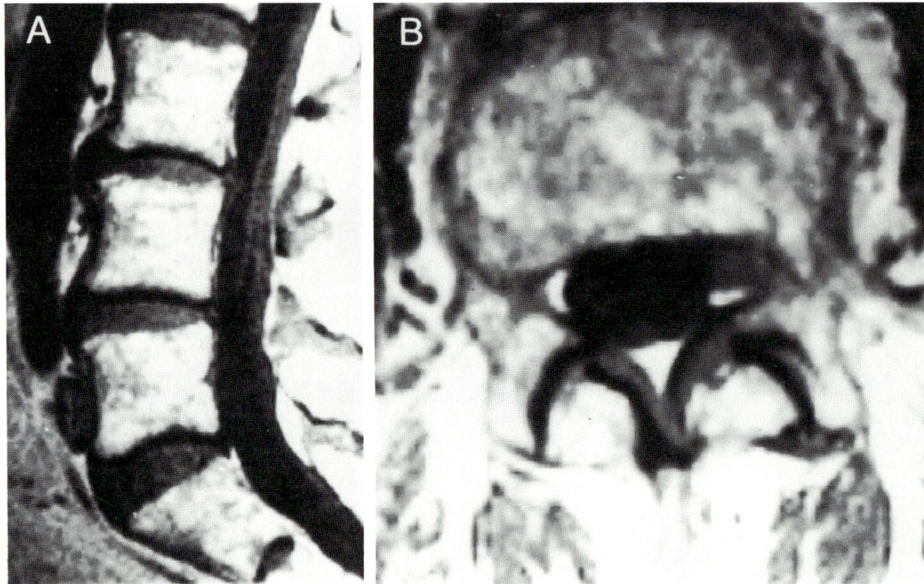

FIG 2–4.
Sagittal (**A**) and axial (**B**) T_1-weighted spin-echo (500/17) images through the lumbar spine. The "spotty" high signal intensity of the vertebral body marrow is secondary to an increased lipid content that is common with advancing age.

medial to the pedicle, anterior to the superior articular facet, and posterior to the vertebral body and disk.[3–6]

Hyaline cartilage covers each facet and varies in thickness from 2 to 4 mm. Medial and lateral fibroelastic capsules enclose the joint. On the medial surface, the capsule is reinforced by the anterolateral attachment of the ligamentum flavum. The superior and inferior aspect of the capsule contain synovium and fat, both of which can extend between the facets, even in normal subjects.[7–10] The facets and intervening joints, while seen in the sagittal plane, are best visualized in the axial plane. While the cartilage can be identified on spin-echo images, it is best seen on gradient echo scans where its increased signal stands out sharply against the decreased signal of the adjacent cortical bone. Chemical shift artifact, depending on the direction of the readout gradient

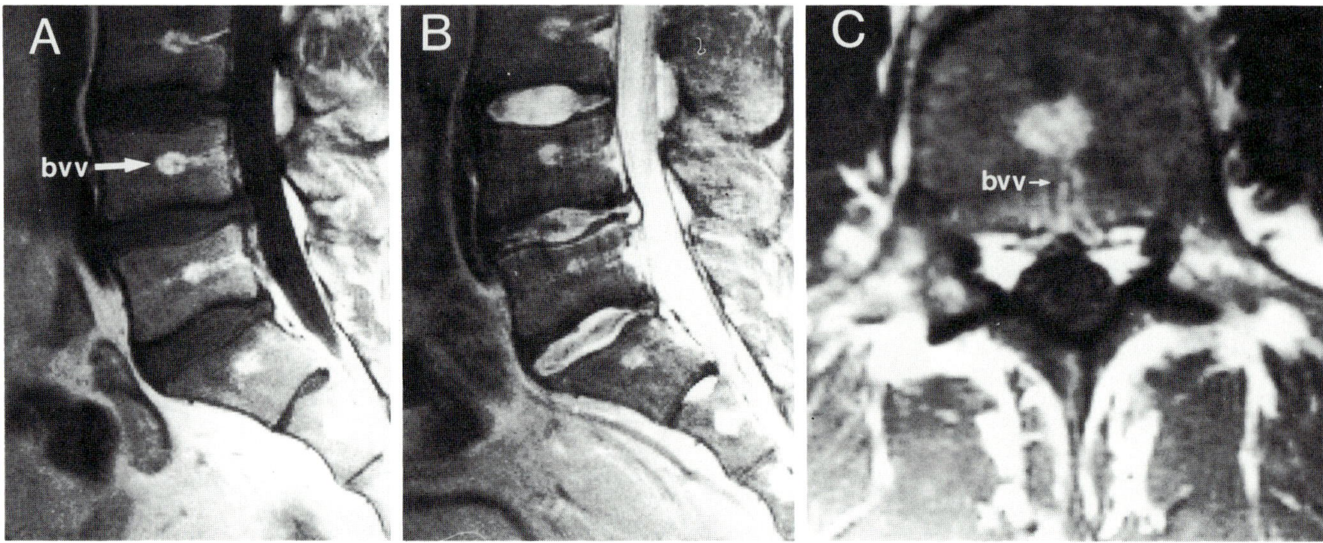

FIG 2–5.
Basivertebral vein. **A,** sagittal T_1-weighted SE (500/17). **B,** sagittal T_2-weighted SE (2000/90). **C,** T_1-weighted axial SE (500/17). Note the high signal intensity secondary to represent either increased lipid content and/or slow flow within the basivertebral vein (bvv)*(arrows).*

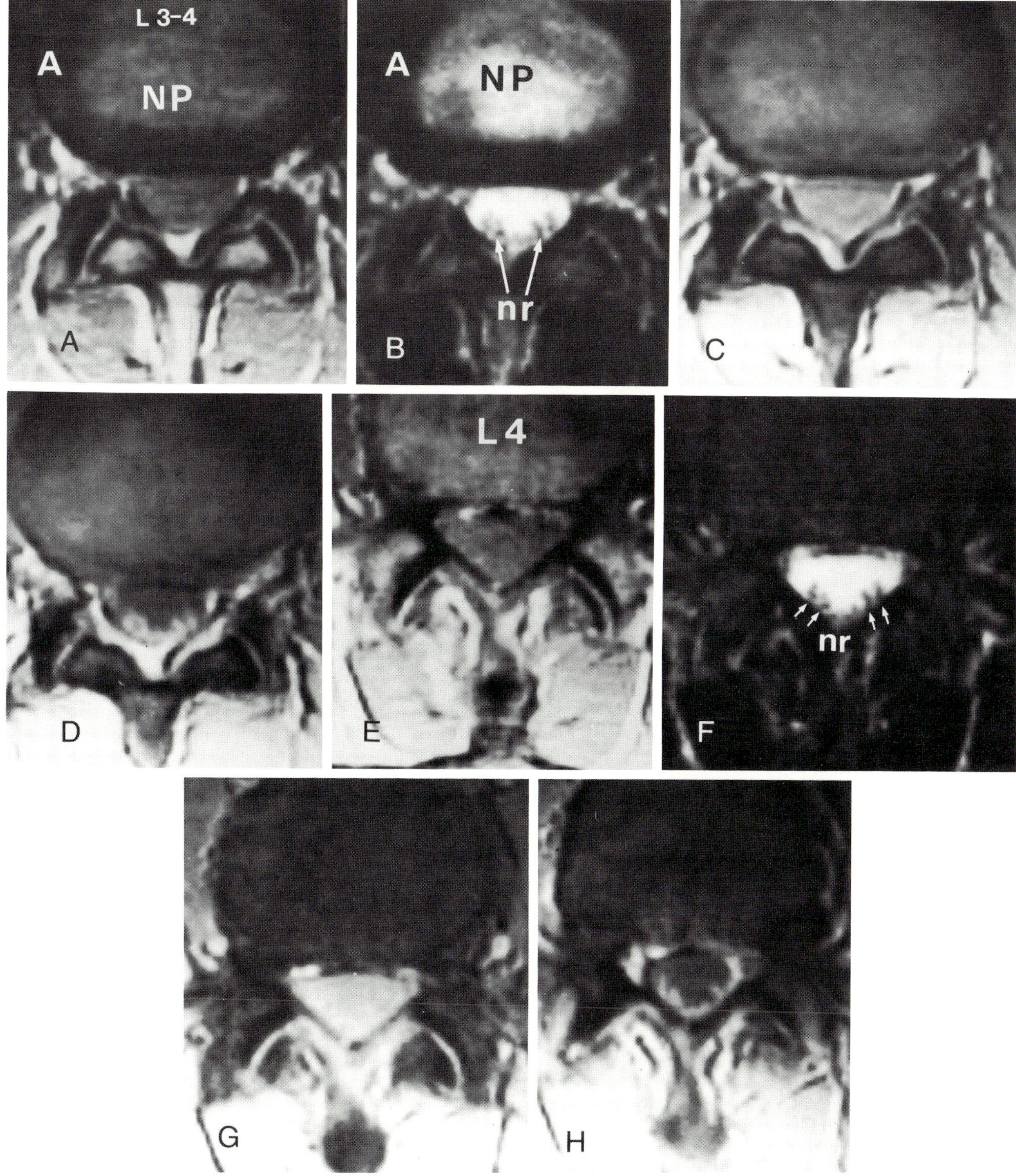

FIG 2–6.
Normal axial T_1-weighted SE (500/17), T_2-weighted SE (2000/90), FLASH 50/13/10 degree, FLASH 50/13/60 degree images through the L3-4 disk and L4 body. **A** and **E** are T_1-weighted SE; **B** and **F** are T_2-weighted SE; **C** and **G** are FLASH 10-degree flip angles; and **D** and **H** are FLASH 60-degree flip angles. Note the high signal intensity of the articular cartilage within the facet joints on the FLASH images. *Arrows* indicate nerve roots within the thecal sac. A = articular pillar; NP = nucleus pulposus; nr = nerve root.

can cause apparent asymmetry of the cortical thickness[7] (Fig 2–6).

The epidural space lies between the dura and the bone confines of the spinal canal. Its contents include epidural fat, ligaments, nerves, and blood vessels. The epidural fat has a high signal intensity on T_1-weighted sequences and lies anterior and anterolateral to the dura and posterior and medial between the ligamentum flavum. Epidural fat is usually not seen in this latter region at the L5-S1 level where the dural sac enlarges and usually lies in direct contact posteriorly with the ligamentum flavum and intraspinal ligament. The signal intensity of the ligamentum flavum on T_1-weighted sequences is slightly higher than other spinal ligaments and the adjacent osseous elements (see Fig 2–3). It also has a higher signal intensity on fast gradient echo low flip-angle scans similar to that of articular cartilage within the facet joints (see Fig 2–6). This increased signal intensity has been speculated to be secondary to its higher elastin (80%) and low type I collagen (20%) content. Conversely, the low signal intensity of the other ligaments may be due to a higher type I collagen content.[7] The ligamentum flavum forms the anterior lining of the interlaminal interval. The ligaments insert on the anterior surface of the lower edge of the superior lamina and the posterior surface of the inferior lamina and are usually 3 to 5 mm in thickness. The anterolateral extension of the ligamentum flavum serves to reinforce the medial portion of the facet joint capsule with which it fuses laterally. Its thickness in the axial plane in normal subjects has been measured at 4.5 ± 0.97 mm.[7]

The posterior longitudinal ligament is a fibrous structure that is continuous from the base of the skull to the sacrum. It is tightly adherent to the anulus fibrosis and inferior and superior margins of the vertebral bodies but not to the midposterior surface of the body. In this latter area, the posterior longitudinal ligament is stretched across the concave posterior osseous surface, allowing vascular structures to enter and leave.[11]

The anterior longitudinal ligament is a strong band of fibers that is continuous from the occipital bone to the first sacral segment and provides a wide continuous covering of the anterior vertebral body and disk. It is relatively narrower in the cervical region and expands in width in the thoracic and lumbar regions. It is composed of three sets of fibers: (1) deep fibers that span one intervertebral articulation, (2) intermediate fibers that unite two or three levels, and (3) a superficial layer that connects four or five vertebral bodies. While the anterior longitudinal ligament is loosely attached to the connective tissue band that encircles the anulus, it is most firmly attached to the osseous surface of the vertebral body itself above and below the diskovertebral junction.[11,12] Both the anterior and posterior longitudinal ligament have a decreased signal intensity on magnetic resonance imaging (MRI) that blends with the decreased signal intensity of the peripheral portion of the anulus and the cortical bone of the vertebral bodies.

The dura is a dense fibrous tissue extending distally to the S2 segment. The lateral outpouching of the dura at the level of the nerve roots also contains arachnoid that forms the neural sheath. The arachnoid is loosely attached but separated from the dura by a normally small subdural space. These structures are usually indiscernible from the underlying cerebrospinal fluid (CSF).

The spinal cord lies within the subarachnoid space with its terminal portion, the conus medullaris, at the level of L1-2 (Fig 2–7). The conus medullaris has a variable appearance at the T11-12 level. It can be oval or, less commonly, round, occasionally with a rounded eminence posteriorly. At the mid-T12 level, the posterolateral margins are often linear. At the T12-L1 level, two constant features are noted. The anterior median fissure is seen as a small groove on the central aspect of the cord, and a small conical projection is present on the dorsal aspect.[13–14] These are often effaced by intramedullary tumors. The neural elements within the subarachnoid space have an intermediate signal intensity similar to that of the intervertebral disk on T_1-weighted sequences but are decreased in signal intensity relative to the disk and CSF on more T_2-weighted examinations (see Fig 2–7). The filum terminale represents the fibrous filament that extends inferiorly from the conus to the distal sac. While it has a signal intensity similar to or less than that of the neural elements, in approximately 5% of normal cases, it can contain variable amounts of fat that stand out as a high signal intensity (Fig 2–8). The cauda equina refers to the downward passing lumbar and sacral nerve roots at the level of the conus. The nerve roots of the cauda equina descend alongside the conus medullaris and are more densely packed into ventrolateral and dorsolateral bundles. The appearance of the nerve roots at the conus—from whence they descend inferiorly—is often described as "spider-like" on axial sections[14] (see Fig 2–7). At the L2 level, the roots are seen as a mass of soft tissue signal in the dependent portion of the thecal sac. The roots assume a smooth crescentic appearance following the curvature of the thecal sac. The most common pattern of the nerve roots at the L3 level is one of a group of roots that mass posteriorly (dependent position), which may be crescentic and smooth or more globular and irregular in appearance. The roots about to exit the dural tube are located anterolaterally in a symmetrical pattern. At the L4 level, the roots are often dispersed enough that they are seen as separate delicate entities, arranged in a symmetric

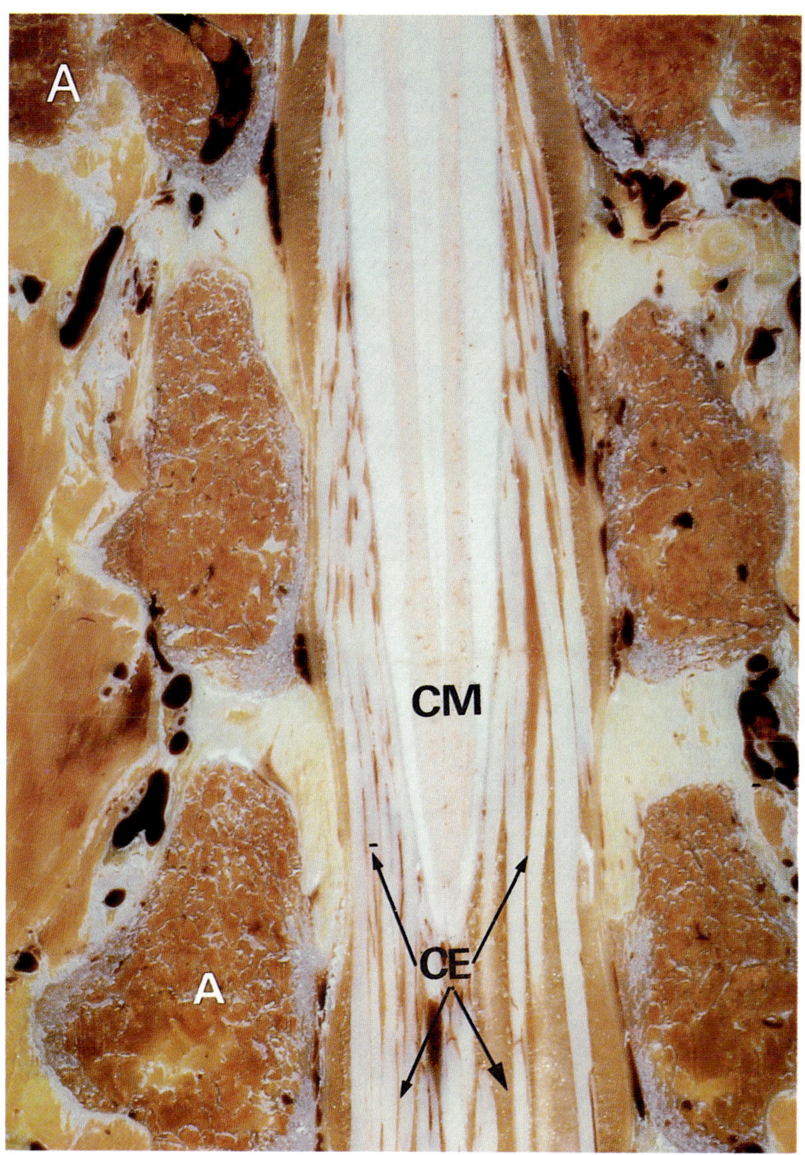

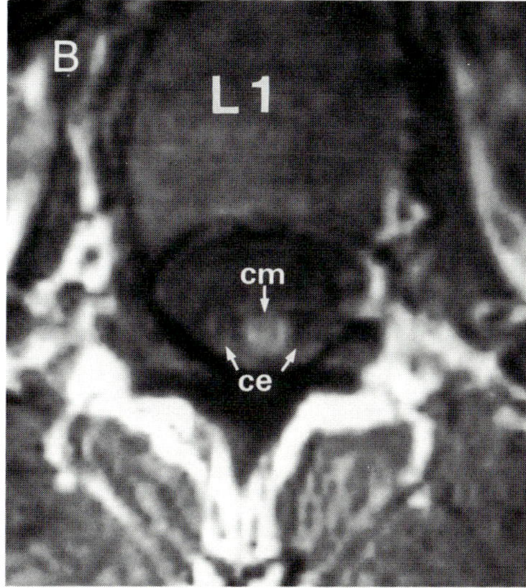

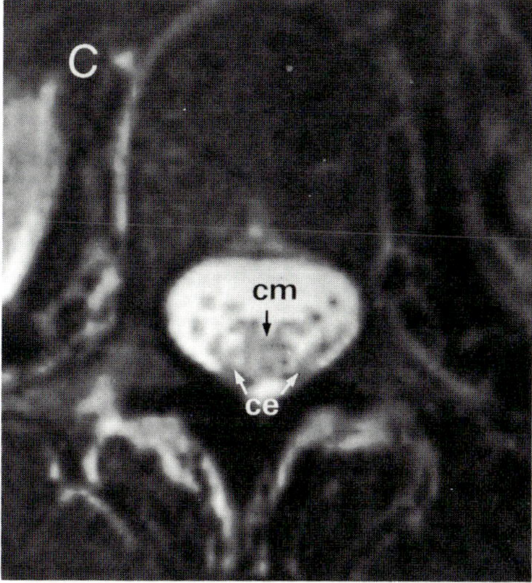

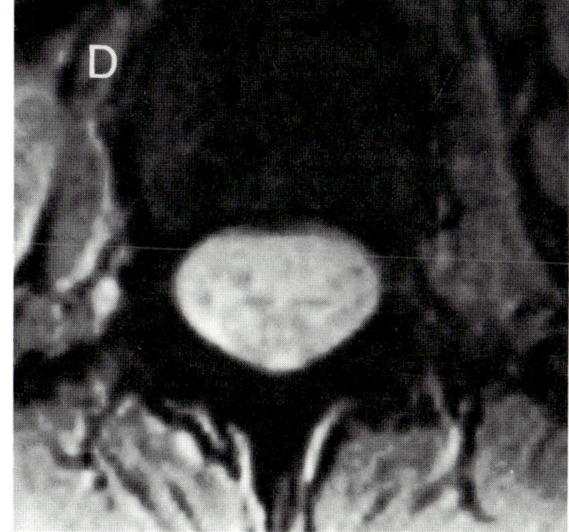

FIG 2–7.

Normal conus medullaris and cauda equina. **A,** coronal cryomicrotome section through the distal thoracic cord, conus medullaris, and proximal cauda equina. **B,** axial T_1-weighted SE (500/17). **C,** axial T_2-weighted SE (2000/90). **D,** axial FLASH (50/13/10 degree) image through the conus medullaris. *CM* = conus medullaris; *CE* = cauda equina; *A* = articular process.

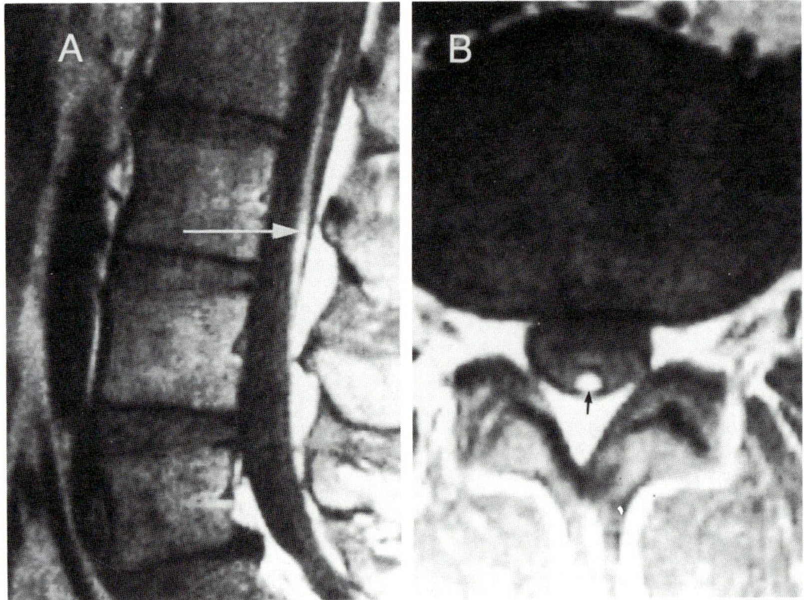

FIG 2–8.
Fat in the filum. **A,** sagittal midline T_1-weighted SE (500/17). **B,** axial T_1-weighted SE (500/17) through the lower L3 vertebral body level. *Arrows* denote high signal intensity of fat within the filum terminale.

pattern within the CSF. By the L5 level, the few roots present are equally spaced from each other within the thecal sac. A pattern of conglomeration within the center of the thecal sac is conspicuously lacking at this level (Fig 2–9).[15] Midline sagittal images show the roots as a single linear area of intermediate signal intensity following the posterior thecal sac. The roots gradually taper from the conus to the L4 level. More parasagittal images demonstrate the roots dispersing in a fan-shaped manner as the roots travel in a posterior-superior to anterior-inferior direction (see Fig 2–2). The appearance of the neural elements in relationship to the CSF differs on fast gradient echo variable flip-angle scans, depending on the flip angle employed. At lower flip angles, the signal intensity of the nerve roots is less than that of the surrounding CSF but gradually increases in signal as the flip angle approaches 90 degrees (Fig 2–10).

The traversing portion of the nerve root is that segment that passes downward from the conus within the dural sac (see Figs 2–1 through 2–3). They pass anteriorly and laterally at the level of the disk above. The traversing portion of the nerve root at the level below lies in the lateral recess that is formed where the superior articular facet becomes contiguous with the pedicle below. The nerve root sleeve usually ends ventrally near the medial border of the superior articular facet at the inferior portion of the neural foramina of the level above. This area is also referred to as the "entrance zone." The traversing nerves become exiting nerves when they pass laterally underneath the pedicle and into the foramen. There they enlarge to become the dorsal root ganglion. This region is referred to as the midzone. From this point, the peripheral nerve distal to the ganglion passes laterally out of the foramen, known as the exit zone. The boundaries of the neural foramen are (1) the pedicles above and below, (2) the posterolateral as-

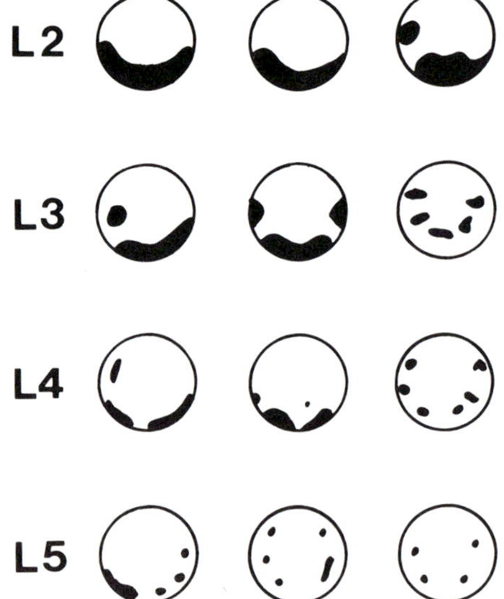

FIG 2–9.
Diagrammatic representation of the variable MR axial appearance of lumbar nerve roots.

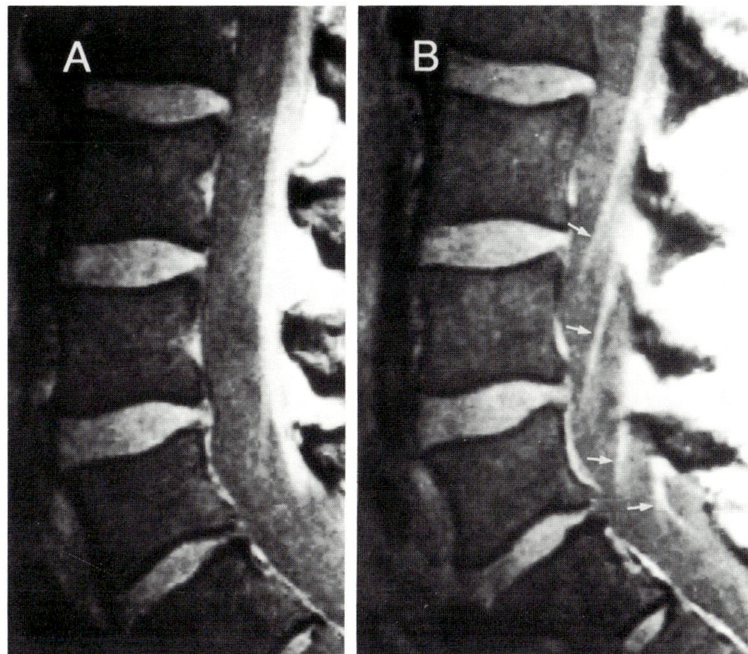

FIG 2–10.
A and **B,** traversing nerve roots in the sagittal plane on FLASH images (200/13/60 degrees). **A,** midline. **B,** parasagittal image 1 cm to the left of midline. Note the high signal intensity of the traversing nerve roots within the thecal sac on **B** *(arrows).*

pect of the vertebral body laterally, (3) the intervertebral disk anteriorly and medially, and (4) the superior articular facet joint posteriorly and laterally (see Figs 2–1 through 2–5).[3,4] On both axial and parasagittal T_1-weighted SE images, the nerve roots are noted as areas of decreased signal intensity surrounded by epidural fat beneath the pedicle. Occasionally two or more nerve roots will be conjoined and exit from the same foramen (Fig 2–11). Epidural veins appear as areas of decreased signal intensity, usually located superior and anterior to the nerves (see Figs 2–1 through 2–3).

The intervertebral disk is composed of three distinct parts: the cartilaginous end-plate, anulus fibrosis, and nucleus pulposus.[16–19] As a structural unit, the intervertebral disk is designed to alleviate shock and transmit forces applied to the spine from every conceivable combination of vectors. The lumbar disks are reniform, and the lumbar lordosis is due to the equivalent increase in the differential between the anterior and posterior thickness of the disk, a situation that makes the lumbosacral disk the most wedge-shaped.[12]

The cartilaginous end-plate is composed of hyaline cartilage that covers the inferior and superior vertebral body surfaces central to the site of fusion of the previous epiphyseal ring (Fig 2–12, A). It serves a key role as a biomechanical and metabolic interface between the vertebral body and nucleus pulposus.[20] While the end-plate contains numerous blood vessels at birth, in the adult the disk remains the largest avascular structure in the body. Nevertheless, it remains metabolically active, and the end-plate serves as the major site of diffusion from the vertebral body spongiosa.

The anulus fibrosis serves as the limiting capsule of the nucleus pulposus (Fig 2–12,B). Its collagenous fibers are short and stout, providing greater strength anteriorly than posteriorly, where they are thinner, fewer in number, and more closely packed. The anulus is completely circular and attaches superiorly and inferiorly into the vertebral body at the site of the fused epiphyseal ring by Sharpey's fibers as well as to the longitudinal ligaments anteriorly and posteriorly. Its purpose is to resist radial tension induced by axial loading of the disk through confinement of the nucleus pulposus as well as to resist stresses from torsion and flexion.[16–19] The hydration of the anulus fibrosis is approximately 80% in the young. Type I collagen predominates in the peripheral anulus and type II collagen in the inner anulus and nucleus pulposus. The tensile strength of the anulus is attributed to the type I collagen fibers as is found in tendons elsewhere in the body. The type II collagen fibers in both the inner anulus and nucleus pulposus provide compressive protection and are abundant in hyaline articular cartilage, present on surfaces where compressive forces are high.[21] Examination of the col-

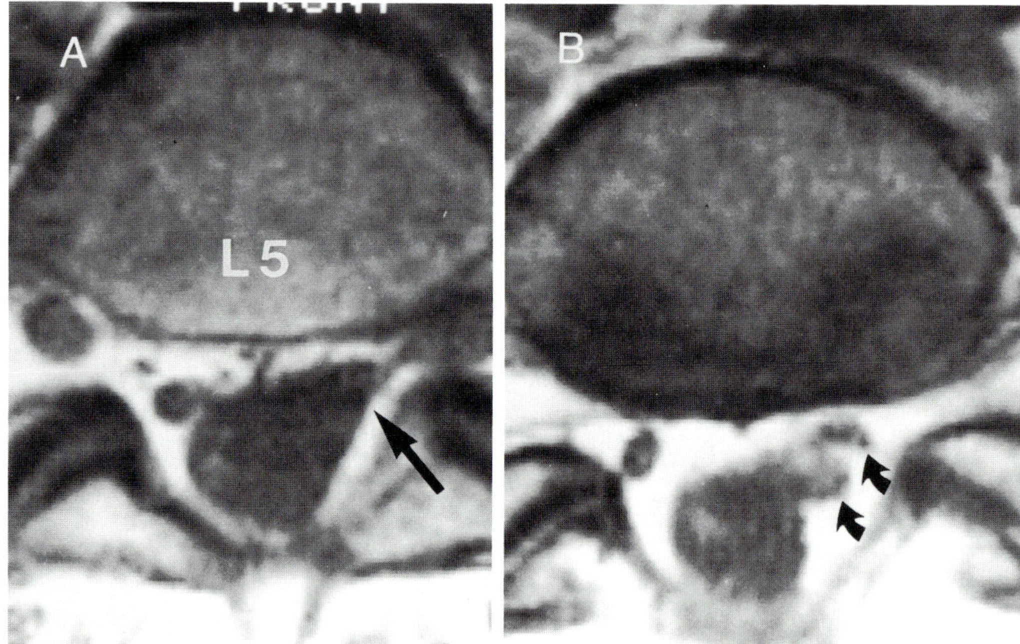

FIG 2–11.
Conjoined nerve root. Axial T_1-weighted SE images through the lower L5 vertebral body (**A**) and the L5-S1 superior end plate (**B**). *Arrows* demarcate asymmetry of the thecal sac caused by conjoined nerve roots on the left.

lagen within the disk suggests that the type II collagen fibers may be more hydrated than the type I fibers, with covalent cross-linking perhaps determining their behavior.[20]

The nucleus pulposus represents the definitive remnant of embryonal notocord and is normally composed of well-hydrated, loose, delicate fibrous strands forming an incompressible gelatinous matrix (see Fig 2–12,A). Peripherally it blends imperceptibly with the anulus fibrosis with no clear demarcation between the two. Collagen and proteoglycans comprise the major macromolecular constituents of the nucleus pulposus and anulus fibrosis. The nucleus is richer in proteoglycans than the anulus; chondroitin-6-sulfate, keratan sulfate, hyaluronic acid, and chondroitin-4-sulfate have all been noted.[22, 23] The hydrostatic properties of the disk arise from its high state of hydration. The nucleus consists of 85% to 90% water and the anulus 80% water. The hydrophilia of the disk is not strictly biochemical as diurnal variations in the disk height indicate water can be expressed via pressure.[20]

On T_1-weighted images, the central portion of the disk has a slightly decreased signal intensity when compared to the peripheral portion, which then blends with an area of even greater decreased signal intensity representing the outer layers of the anulus fibrosis at its confluence with the longitudinal ligaments[24] (see Figs 2–1 and 2–3). A similar appearance is also noted on T_2-weighted images, although the signal intensities are reversed. On T_2-weighted spin-echo sequences, the normal disk has a central portion of high signal intensity and a peripheral portion of decreased signal intensity (Figs 2–6 and 2–13). Anatomical correlation suggests that there is no clear separation of the nucleus pulposus and anulus fibrosis but rather an inner region representing the nucleus pulposus as well as inner portion of the anulus fibrosis, and a more peripheral region representing the outer layers of the anulus and its confluence with the longitudinal ligaments.[25] It is tempting to suggest that the signal intensity differences are related to the differences in hydration between the inner nucleus anulus and outer complex, reflecting a longer T_1 and T_2 centrally and shorter relaxation times more peripherally. How this relates to the degree of hydration of type I and type II collagen, proteoglycan distribution, and aggregation is as yet not understood.

On more T_2-weighted images there is often an area of variable size and decreased signal intensity within the central portion of the disk, creating a notched to biconcave appearance of the disk similar to that seen at diskography. While not immediately apparent on gross inspection, histologic studies indicate it represents a more fibrous tissue than the surrounding nucleus pulposus and is almost universally seen after 30 years of age (see Fig 2–13).[26] In other regions of the spine, most notably the thoracic, a band of decreased signal intensity repre-

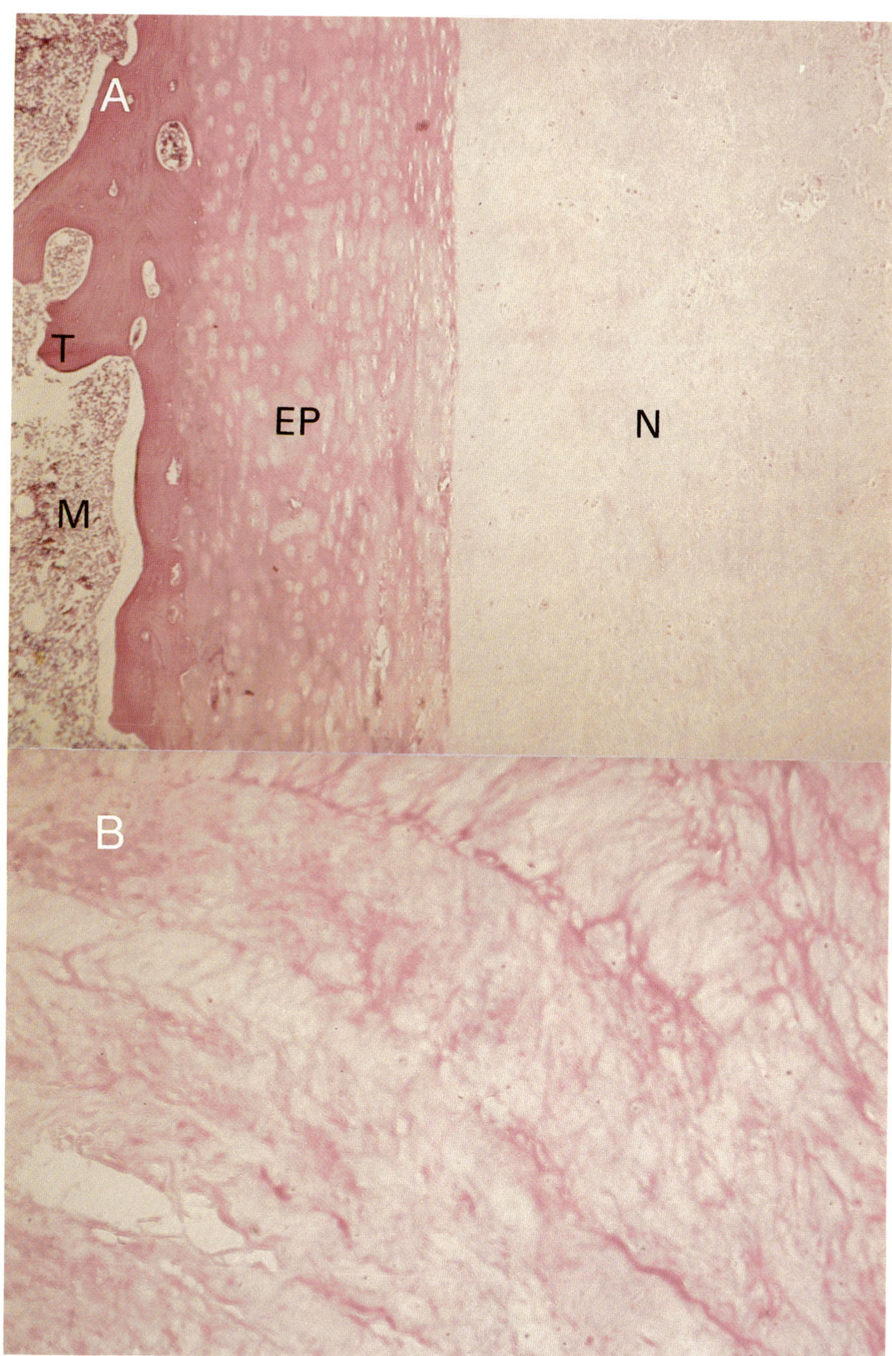

FIG 2–12.

A and **B,** normal histology of the intervetebral disk from a 36-year-old male (hemotoxin and eosin). **A,** low power of the end plate at its junction with the nucleus pulposis in the central portion of the disk. *EP* = end plate; *M* = subcortical vertebral body marrow; *N* = nucleus pulposus; *T*=trabeculae. **B,** high power of the anulus fibrosis. The anulus fibrosis is composed of pink-staining collagenous fibers that transcend both an oblique and spiral course.

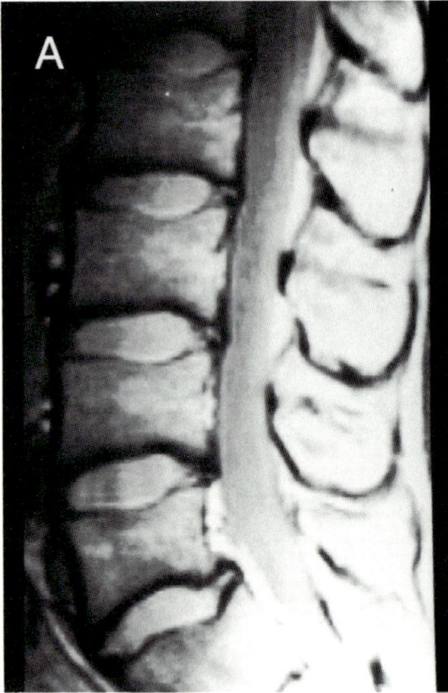

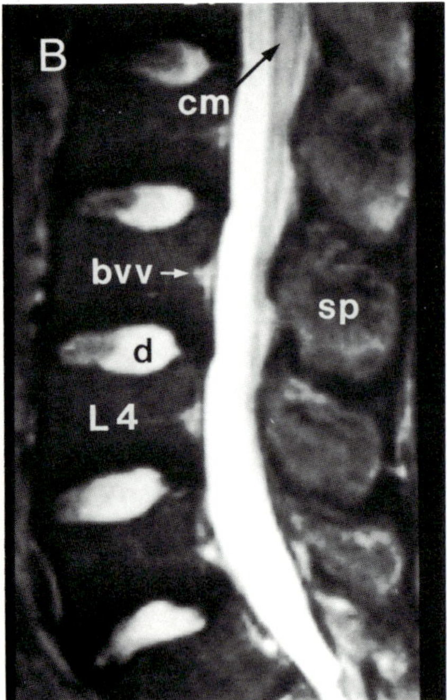

FIG 2–13.
A and **B,** normal sagittal. **A,** intermediate 2000/20 msec SE and T_2-weighted SE (2000/90 msec) sagittal images through the lumbar spine. Note the normal high signal intensity of the central portion of the intervertebral disk on the 90-msec TE image. Anteriorly an area of decreased signal intensity is identified bisecting the disk. *bvv* = basivertebral vein; CM = conus medullaris; *d* = disk; sp = spinous process.

senting a truncation artifact may be seen that, unlike the lumbar finding, will disappear with changes in the imaging matrix and/or phase-encoded direction.

The appearance of the disk and vertebral body on gradient echo images will vary depending on whether lipid and water components are in phase or opposed (dependent on TE), and on the TR and flip angle employed.[27] The signal intensity of the normal disk is usually higher than adjacent vertebral body and quite homogeneous (Fig 2–14).

The signal intensity of the CSF is decreased relative to the extradural elements on T_1-weighted images secondary to its long T_1 and T_2 (see Fig 2–2). With increasing TE and TR, the signal intensity will increase. In gradient echo images, the signal intensity is highest relative to extradural structures with low flip angles (see Fig 2–14). Its appearance, however, is variable, depending on the degree of CSF pulsations and the pulse sequence parameter employed.[28, 29] In the lumbar region, the problem most often encountered on T_1-weighted sequences is a variable signal intensity masquerading as an intradural mass or arachnoiditis. This is presumably secondary to either slow flow or variable flow in different portions of the CSF. On T_2-weighted images, loss of signal secondary to spin dephasing and ghosting artifacts can also occur.[15] Ghosting artifacts can not only be projected outside the spine from the CSF but over the spine from the adjacent abdominal vessels or secondary to excessive abdominal breathing (Fig 2–15). A more in-depth discussion of the variability of the signal intensity and its causes has been discussed previously[28, 29] (see Chapter 1).

The blood supply of the lumbar spine consists of paired segmental lumbar arteries that arise from the posterior aspect of the abdominal aorta at the first four lumbar levels. The fifth lumbar arteries are more variable in origin and often arise from the sacral artery. The arterial supply of the dural sac and its contents is provided by segmental radiculomedullary branches of the segmental lumbar arteries (Fig 2–16), the most important of which is the artery of Adamkiewicz, which usually arises from the intercostal branches of the lower thoracic aorta (typically T9 on the left) and less frequently the upper lumbar arteries.[12]

The venous anatomy consists of spinal radicular veins (intervertebral veins) that interconnect the anterior internal vertebral veins and the ascending lumbar veins. The intervertebral veins course laterally through the neural foramen above or below the pedicle to join the segmental lumbar veins. From here, the venous drainage extends anteriorly through the anterior external plexus into the common iliac vein. The posterior-

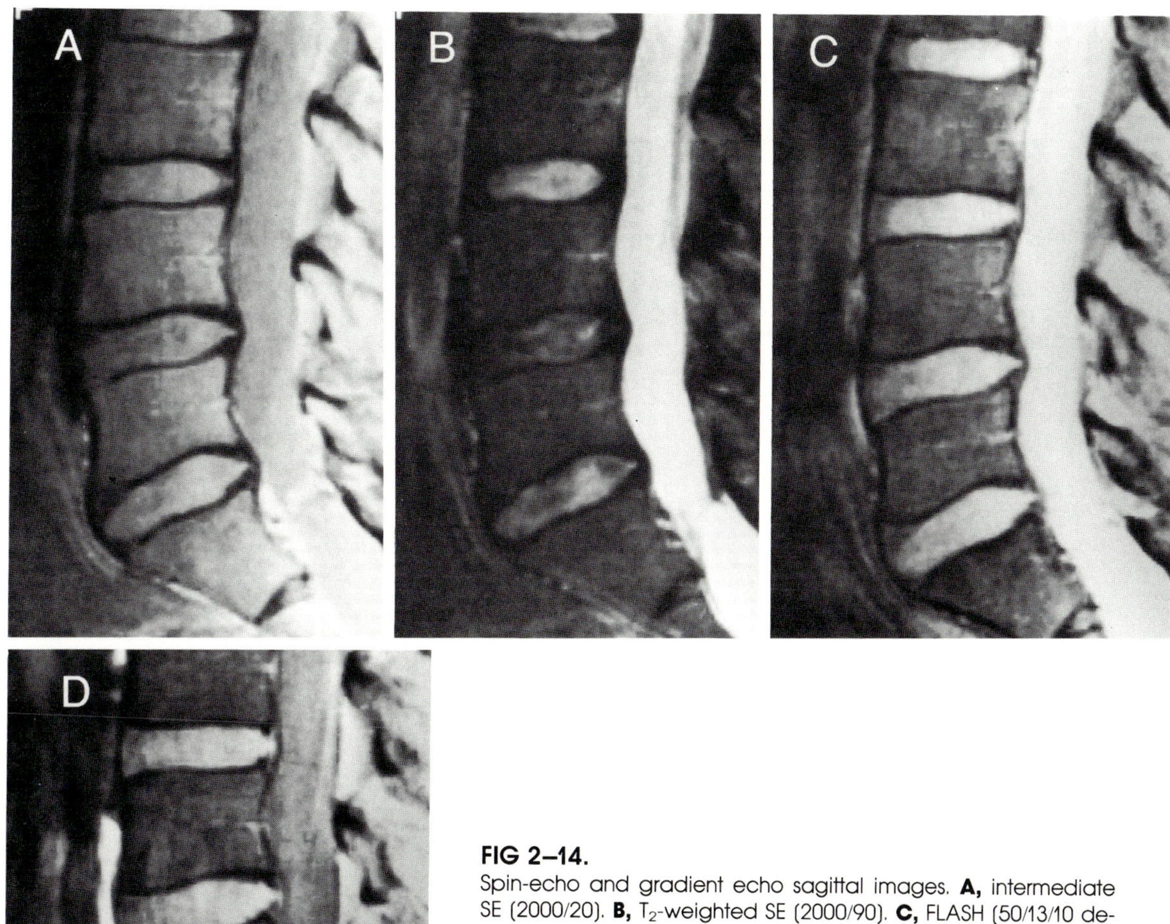

FIG 2–14.
Spin-echo and gradient echo sagittal images. **A,** intermediate SE (2000/20). **B,** T_2-weighted SE (2000/90). **C,** FLASH (50/13/10 degrees). **D,** FLASH (50/13/60 degrees). **B,** shows decreased signal in the L4-5 and L5-S1 disk consistent with degeneration. **A** and **B** were performed with refocussing gradients that have essentially eliminated all CSF ghosting artifacts (compare with Fig 2–15). Note the high signal intensity of the CSF on the 10-degree flip-angle images compared with the 60-degree.

inferior venous plexus also communicates with the intervertebral veins. The basivertebral veins (single or paired) are formed by radiating venous channels within the vertebral body. They communicate posteriorly with the anterior internal vertebral veins in the midportion of the vertebral body. The anterior internal vertebral veins are usually paired and lie on either side of the midline, coursing longitudinally behind the vertebral bodies and intervertebral disks in the epidural space[12] (Fig 2–17). Inferiorly, they begin in the sacral canal and pass superiorly the entire length of the spinal canal to become continuous with the clival venous plexus at the craniovertebral junction. Their size and appearance are inconstant and may occasionally be represented by a plexus or smaller venous channels rather than the usual paired structures. They anastomose extensively with the posterior internal venous plexus and ascending lumbar veins via the intervertebral veins. They are most prominent on transverse imaging at the L5-S1 level and less so at the L4-5 level. The signal intensity of the arterial structures is usually decreased secondary to the velocity of the blood flow. The appearance of the epidural venous

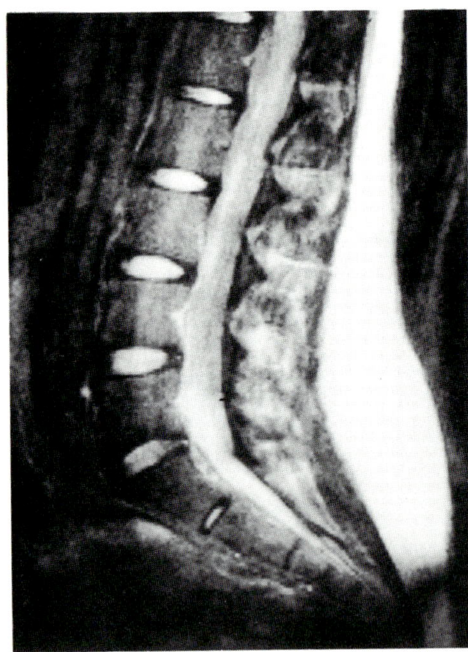

FIG 2–15.
CSF ghosting artifacts. Sagittal T_1-weighted SE (2000/90), one excitation study without cardiac gating or refocussing. Note the prominent ghosting artifacts secondary to the CSF pulsations (compare to Fig 2–14,B).

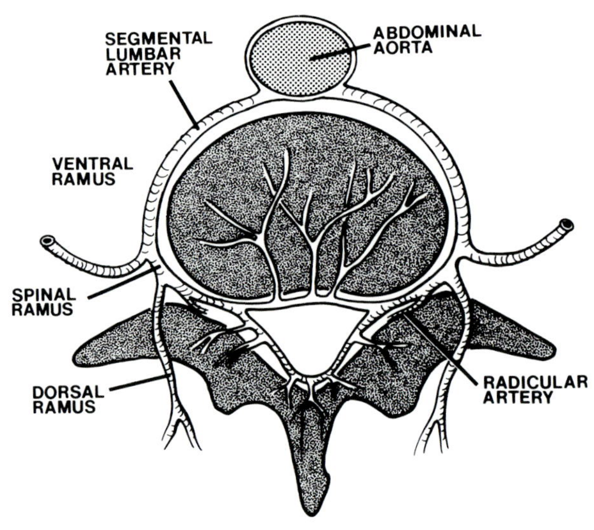

FIG 2–16.
Arterial supply of the lumbar spine.

structures, however, is more variable, and the full gamut of signal intensities may be seen (reflecting the often slower velocities and potential for even echo rephasing on certain sequences). As with computed tomography (CT), when prominent, they may blend in signal intensity with the adjacent intervertebral disks, especially at the L5-S1 level.

The classically described patterns of peripheral nerve distribution have been based on the segmental aspects of vertebral development.[12] Clinical observation, however, has shown substantial individual variation from the theoretically expected system of innervation, particularly in the lumbosacral region. These atypical neurologic patterns are attributed to peculiarities in plexus formation, intrathecal alterations in the level of spinal nerve origin and vertebral exits, or anomalous connections between adjacent nerve roots. In addition, more recently a previously described intersegmental system of axons has been observed on the ventrolateral surface of the conus medullaris. While these axons usually unite with the rootlets of a more caudal spinal nerve, they have been observed combining with others to form grossly visible ectopic rootlets that can be traced

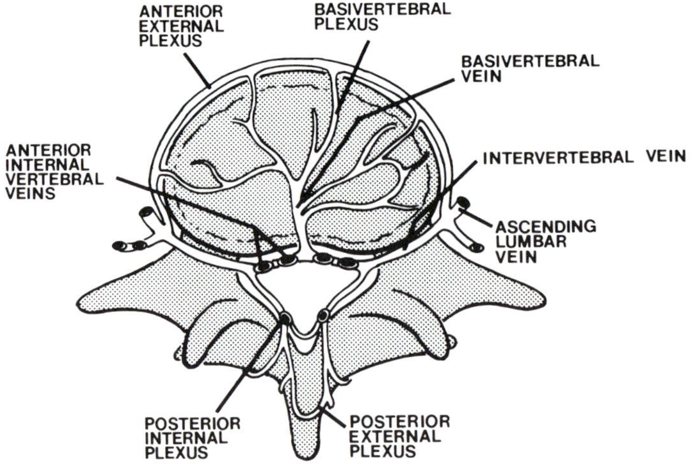

FIG 2–17.
Venous drainage of the lumbar spine.

to where they join a typical spinal nerve root one to several segments caudal to their level of origin.[30]

Classically, the innervation of the lumbar canal is ascribed to the sinu-vertebral nerve, a branch of each spinal nerve that passes back through the intervertebral foramen to supply fibers to the articular connective tissue, periosteum, meninges, and vascular structures associated with the vertebral canal. The nerve originates distal to the dorsal root ganglion (Fig 2–18) and passes backward through the foramen, curving upward around the base of the pedicle and dividing to give superior and inferior branches that approach the posterior longitudinal ligament. Branches are distributed to the periosteum, the posterior longitudinal ligament, and the dural and the epidural vessels with a pattern of branching that roughly corresponds with the arterial distribution. The posterior primary ramus innervates the facet joints at this same level and usually innervates the level above. This ramus also innervates the soft tissues in the lower back in the first three lumbar segments. Anatomical work has revealed anastomotic connections at each level; the existence of those of adjacent segments provides an explanation for the mutual overlapping of segmental sensory nerve distribution and suggests that diskogenic pain from a single level may involve more than one recurrent branch of the spinal nerve. Free nerve endings and complex unencapsulated pain terminations are demonstrable in the posterior and anterior longitudinal ligaments, the periosteum of the vertebral body, and the synovial capsules of the articular facets. The lack of neural elements within the nucleus pulposus and inner lamella of the anulus is accepted, but the presence of nerve endings within the outer lamella has been both demonstrated and denied by various investigators. The point is moot, however, as the relationship of this structure to well-documented innervated areas is clearly accepted, particularly in the case of the posterior longitudinal ligament and central disk herniation.[12]

THORACIC SPINE

The MR signal intensity of the osseous, soft tissue, and fluid structures of the thoracic spine is similar to that in the lumbar region (Figs 2–19 through 2–21).

The thoracic spinal canal is defined by the vertebral bodies and disks anteriorly, the pedicles laterally, and the lamina and base of the spinous processes posteriorly.[4–6, 31] The thoracic spinal canal has a relatively constant size throughout its length with equal transverse and anterior posterior dimensions with a rounded configuration.

The bodies are convex anteriorly and concave posteriorly with an approximately equal transverse and anterior-posterior dimension. There is a progressive increase in the size of the thoracic vertebral bodies moving rostral to caudal.

The pedicles arise from the upper half of each vertebral body and pass posterolaterally and slightly inferior to the articular pillar and posterior neural arch. They form the upper and lower boundaries of the intervertebral foramen. The lamina are broad and short and pass from the articular pillars in a medial and posterior direction and overlap. The spinous process is longer and more slender than in the lumbar region and again passes downward and posteriorly. The transverse processes extend outward, upward, and posteriorly from the articular pillars. They are closely related to the heads, necks, and tubercles of the corresponding ribs. The pedicles arise from the upper half of each vertebral body and pass posterolaterally and slightly inferiorly to the articular pillars and posterior neural arch.

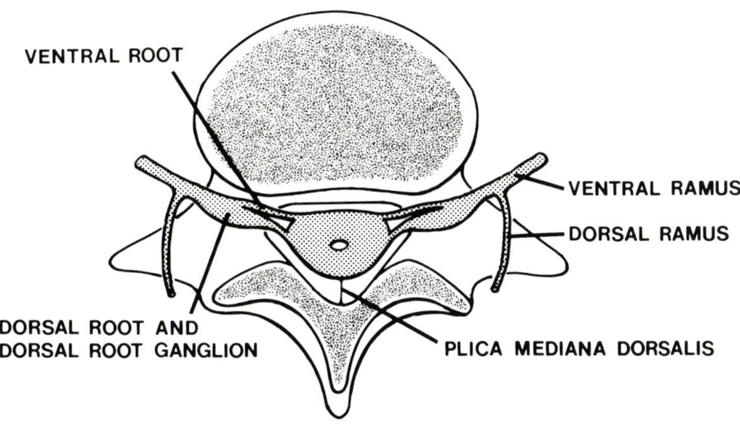

FIG 2–18.
Innervation of the lumbar spine.

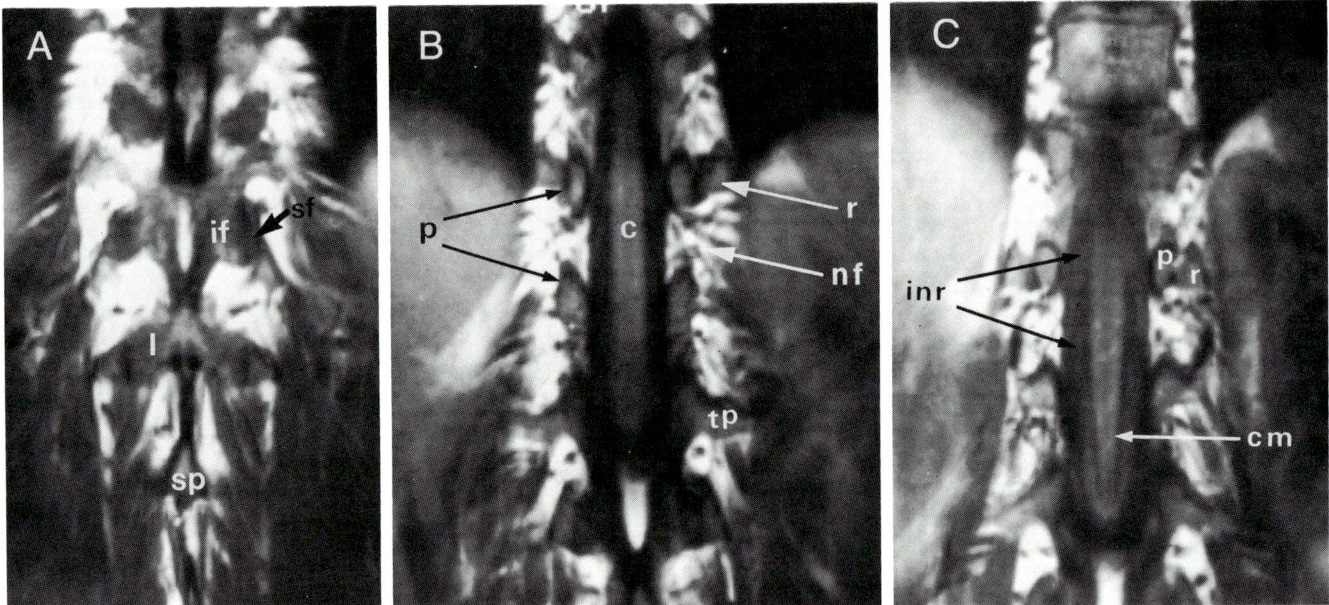

FIG 2–19.
A–C, normal thoracic T_1-weighted SE MR anatomy (500/17). *c* = cord; *cm* = conus medullaris; *if* = inferior facet; *inr* = intradural nerve root; *L* = lamina; *nf* = neural foramen; *p* = pedicle; *r* = rib; *sf* = superior facet; *sp* = spinous process; *tp* = transverse process.

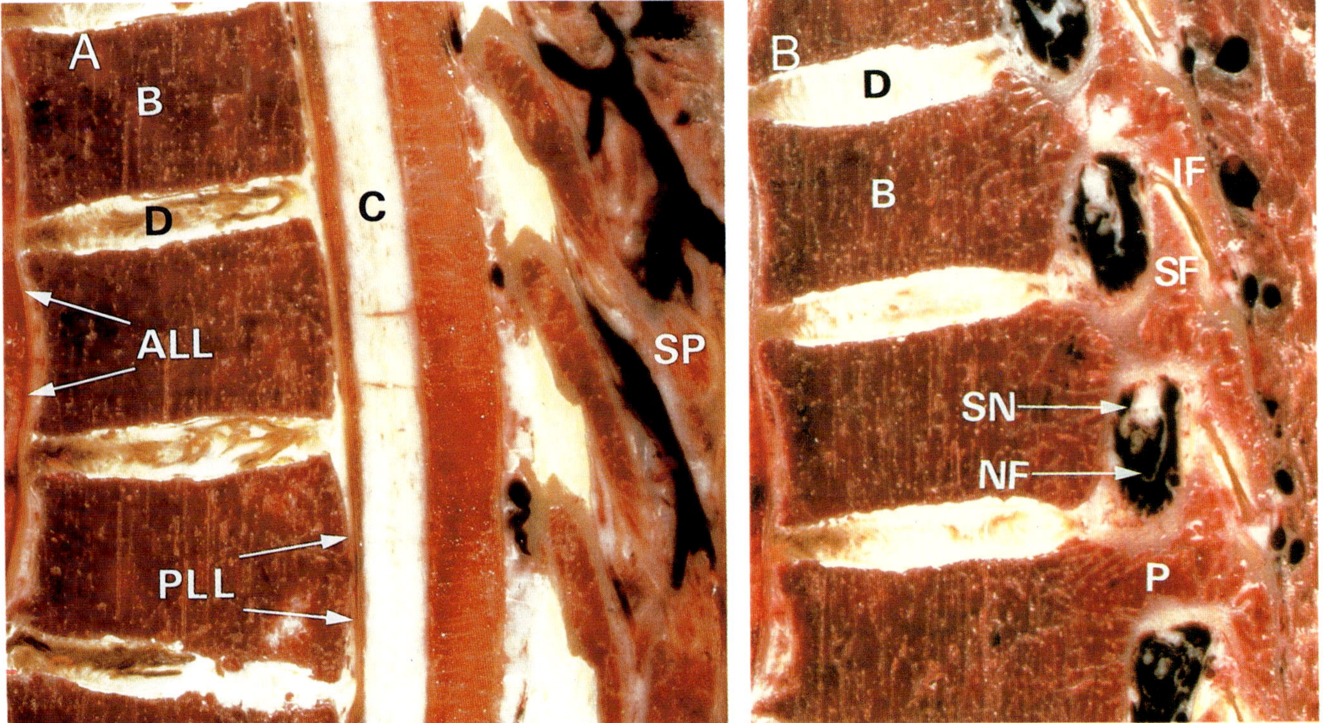

FIG 2–20.
Normal sagittal thoracic cryomicrotome and MR anatomy. **A,** midline cryomicrotome section in the sagittal plane in through the upper thoracic cord. **B,** parasagittal cryomicrotome section through the neural foramina at the same level as **A.** (See p. 58 for explanation of abbreviations.) *(Continued)*

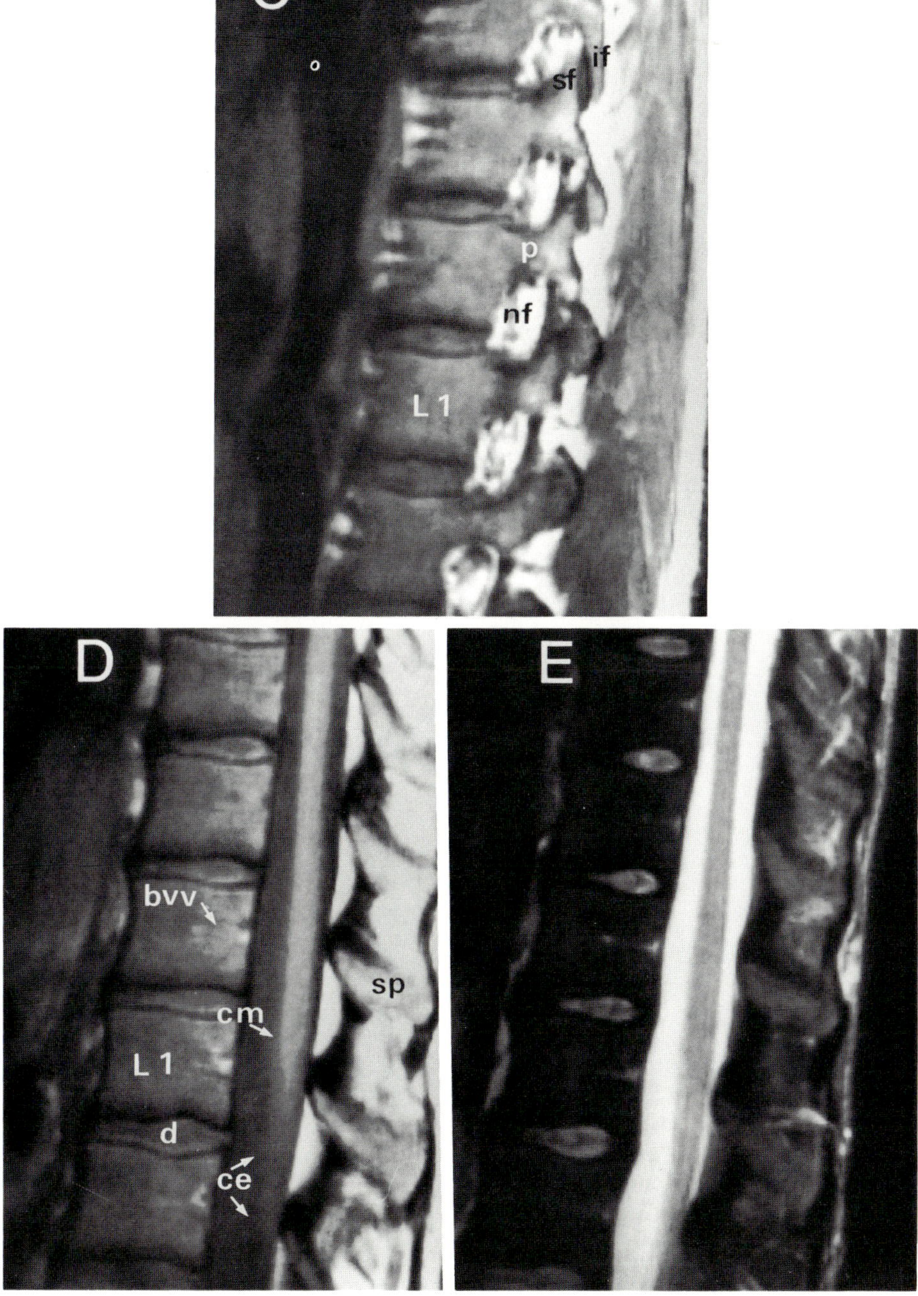

FIG 2–20 (cont.).
Normal sagittal thoracic cryomicrotome and MR anatomy. **C,** parasagittal T_1-weighted SE (500/17) image through the neural foramen. **D,** midline sagittal T_1-weighted SE (500/17) through the distal thoracic cord and conus medullaris. **E,** midline sagittal T_2-weighted SE (2000/90) image through the same plane as **D.** (See p. 58 for explanation of abbreviations.) *(Continued)*)

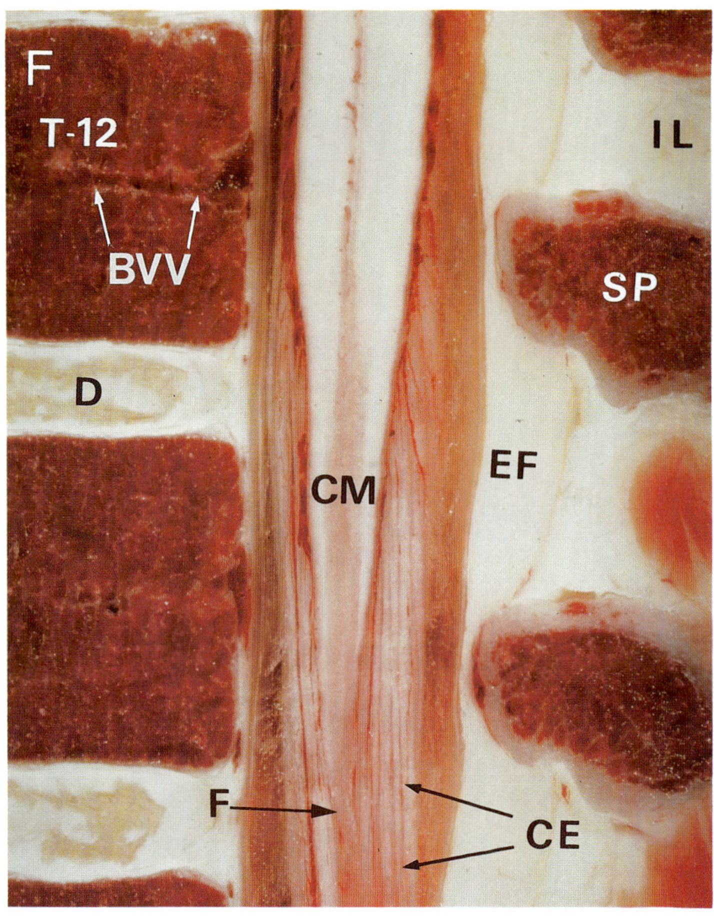

FIG 2–20 (cont.).
Normal sagittal thoracic cryomicrotome and MR anatomy. **F,** midline cryomicrotome section in the sagittal plane through the distal thoracic cord and conus medullaris. *All* = anterior longitudinal ligament; *B* = body; *BVV* = basivertebral vein; *C* = cord; *CE* = cauda equina; *CM* = conus medullaris; *D* = disk; *EF* = epidural fat; *F* = filum terminale; *IF* = inferior facet; *IL* = intraspinous ligament; *NF* = neural foramen; *P* = pedicle; *PLL* = posterior longitudinal ligament; *SF* = superior facet; *SN* = spinal nerve; *SP* = spinous process.

The superior articular processes project superiorly from the junctions of the pedicles and the lamina on each side. The facets are directed posteriorly and slightly laterally. The portion of the neural arch at the junction of the pedicle and lamina and between the articular facets is called the articular pillar. At the lateral portion of the lamina, the inferior articular process projects inferiorly and anteriorly.

The intervertebral foramen is directed laterally at the inferior half of the vertebral body. The superior-inferior margin is formed by the pedicles with the neck of the rib anterolaterally, the vertebral body anteriorly, and the facet joints posteriorly. The foramina for the thoracic spinal nerves lie in a higher position relative to the intervertebral disk than those of the cervical vertebral bodies.

The ribs of the 12 thoracic vertebral bodies are opposed posteriorly to the transverse process and vertebral body of the same number. There is a smaller articulation with the lower aspect of the next higher body. The crest of the head of the rib is joined at the intervertebral disk by an intra-articular ligament and lies parallel to the plane of the intervertebral disk.

The epidural space and contents are similar to those in the cervical and lumbar regions. There is abundant epidural fat posteriorly between the neural arch and the dura and laterally in the intervertebral foramen. There is less epidural fat in the anterior half of the epidural space than in the lumbosacral region. The anterior longitudinal ligament is thicker in the thoracic region than in the cervical or lumbar region and is more prominent opposite the bodies. The posterior longitudinal ligament

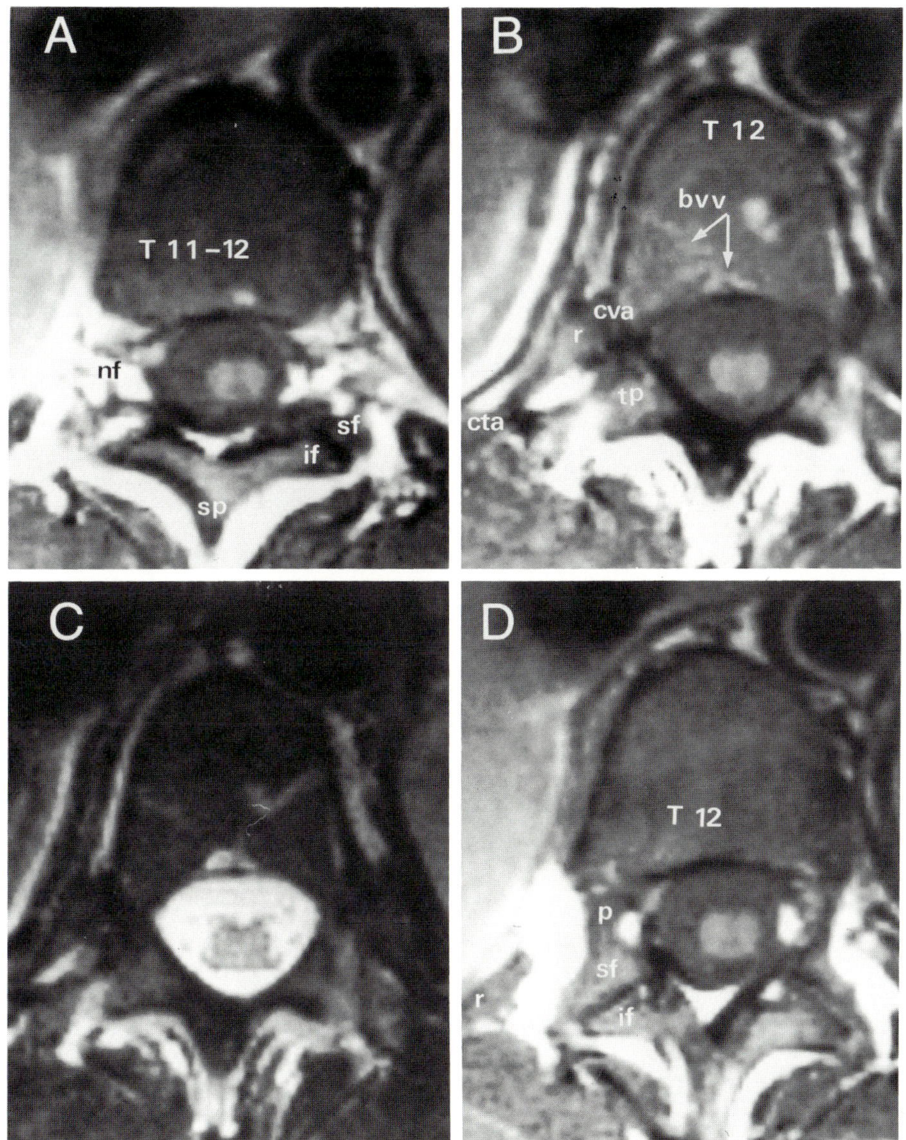

FIG 2–21.
Normal axial T_1-weighted (500/17) and T_2-weighted SE (2000/90) images from the T11–12 through the T12–L1 disk. **A, B, D, F, H,** T_1-weighted SE. **C, E, G, I,** T_2-weighted SE. (For explanation of abbreviations, see p. 60.) *(Continued)*

extends along the posterior aspect of the vertebral bodies and is thicker again than in the cervical or lumbar region.

The thoracic dural sheath is significantly larger than the spinal cord. The dural sheath extends along the nerves for a shorter distance than in the lumbar region. The thoracic cord, dorsal and ventral thoracic nerve roots, radicular veins, and spinal arteries are surrounded by the cerebrospinal fluid and occupy the intradural compartment. The thoracic spinal cord is more rounded than the usual elliptical appearance of the cervical cord. An anterior median fissure indents the ventral surface of the cord. The posterior intermediate and posterolateral sulci in the dorsal surface of the cord are shallow. In the upper thoracic spine, the cord segment is two levels lower in number than the corresponding vertebrae (e.g., cord segment four lies at the level of the vertebral canal at the second thoracic vertebrae). In the lower thoracic spine, there is a difference of three levels between the cord and vertebrae. Thus, depending on location, the dorsal and ventral thoracic nerve roots must descend two to three vertebral body segments in

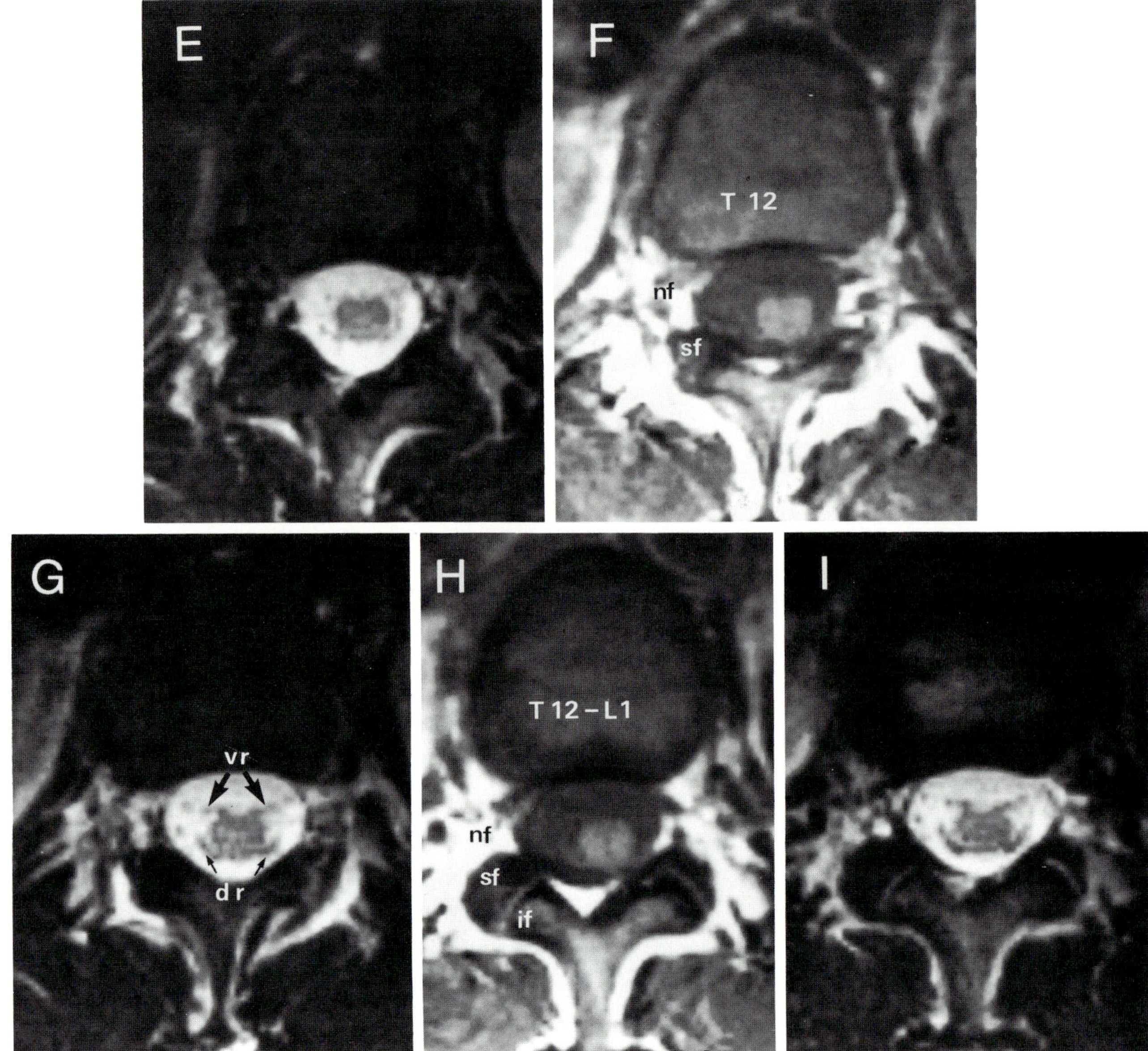

FIG 2–21 (cont.).
Normal axial T_1-weighted (500/17) and T_2-weighted SE (2000/90) images from the T11–12 through the T12–L1 disk. **A, B, D, F, H,** T_1-weighted SE. **C, E, G, I,** T_2-weighted SE. *bvv* = basivertebral vein; *cta* = costotransverse articulation; *cva* = costovertebral articulation; *dr* = dorsal root; *if* = inferior facet; *nf* = neural foramen; *p* = pedicle; *r* = rib; *sf* = superior facet; *sp* = spinous process; *tp* = transverse process; *vr* = ventral root.

the subarachnoid space to exit through the appropriate intervertebral foramen. The upper six pairs are larger than their caudal counterparts. Both groups, however, are significantly smaller than their cervical, lumbar, or sacral counterparts.[5, 6, 31]

The thoracic disks are somewhat heart-shaped on section, the nucleus pulposus being more centrally located than in the lumbar region. The intervertebral disks are thinner vertically than their cervical or lumbar counterparts, but larger in volume than the cervical disk. The end-plates of the vertebral bodies are flat. Both the thickness and horizontal dimensions of the thoracic disk increase caudally with the corresponding increase in size of the vertebral bodies. The normal thoracic kyphosis results from a disparity between the anterior and posterior heights of the vertebral bodies as the disks are of uniform thickness.[12] The intervertebral disks are confined anteriorly and posteriorly by the longitudinal ligaments with an attachment to the crest of the ribs posterolaterally. The area of decreased signal intensity seen within the high signal intensity of the disk on T_2-weighted sequences is not as constant as in the lumbar region.

The CSF signal intensity is more variable than in the lumbar region because of more prominent CSF pulsations. On T_1-weighted axial images, this may be manifested as areas of relatively intermediate signal intensity that may be curvilinear or oval and appear both anterolateral and posterior to the cord. On T_2-weighted images, ovoid areas of decreased signal intensity may be noted (Fig 2–22). Again, these areas most likely reflect differences in the velocity of the CSF in different portions of the canal and are to some degree produced by the exiting nerve roots and septum posticum.

Problems with signal loss and ghosting of the CSF on more T_2-weighted images are also more prominent than in the lumbar region secondary to the greater pulsatile flow. In addition, overlying cardiac and respiratory motion can severely obscure the extradural, intradural, and intramedullary interfaces. This latter problem can usually be addressed with saturation pulses placed so that the signal intensity of these artifacts is decreased.[28]

The arteries and veins to the thoracic region are similar to those in the cervical and lumbar regions.

CERVICAL SPINE

In the sagittal plane, the cervical spine has a slightly lordotic curvature, and the bodies become broader and gradually increase in size from C3 to C7[5, 6, 32] (Figs 2–23 and 2–24). The first and second cervical vertebrae are unique in configuration. C1 (the atlas) is devoid of a body and spinous process and is comprised of a posterior arch joined by two lateral masses that support the weight of the skull. C2 (the axis) has a bony protuberance that projects rostrally from the body—the dens or odontoid process. Unlike the remaining portions of the cervical spine, the dens can demonstrate a decreased signal relative to the other vertebral bodies, presumably secondary to partial volume averaging. A persistent remnant of the subdental synchondrosis is often recognized on sagittal MRI as a horizontal dark band at the base of the odontoid process, which is a normal feature and should not be mistaken for a fracture. Approximately midway between the end-plates, the vertebral bodies are penetrated by the basivertebral veins similar to those in the thoracic and lumbar regions.

The cervical pedicles are paired, short cylindrical structures filled with cancellous bone marrow and surrounded by a compact cortical bone rim. The pedicles connect the vertebral body to the articular pillars midway between the superior and inferior articular processes. Axial sections through the pedicles reveal the spinal canal completely surrounded by bone. The laminae (originating from the articular pillars) are two struts of bone that join in the midline at an obtuse angle to form the spinous process. The cervical vertebrae are characterized by a foramen within each transverse process (foramen transversarium) that transmits the vertebral artery and small veins. The transverse foramina of C2 through C6 are round or oval and slightly larger on the left than on the right.

The uncinate processes are bony ridges that project superiorly from the lateral margin of the vertebral bodies. These ridges fit into corresponding notches laterally and posterolaterally in the lower end-plates of the upper vertebrae. While in the same plane as the disk superiorly, they can usually be separated by the increased signal from the vertebral marrow. Oblique clefts in the disk following the medial contour of the uncinate process give the impression of true articulations commonly referred to as the uncovertebral or joints of Luschka.

The configuration of the cervical spinal canal is triangular with the apex posterior. The spinal canal decreases in size from C1 to C3 and has a fairly uniform dimension from C3 through C7. The anterior-posterior (AP) diameter of the normal cervical canal has a lower limit of 12 mm in the lower cervical spine, 15 mm at C2, and 16 mm at C1 in both males and females. The seventh cervical vertebra is a transitional vertebra. Its spinous process is longer, thicker, and has a more inferior tilt than the more rostral cervical spinous process.

The facet joints are diarthrodial joints formed between the superior and inferior articular processes of adjacent neural arches. The joints are characterized by the facets being more oblique than in the thoracic and lumbar spine and the joint capsules more lax than in other levels to allow a gliding motion. The joint surfaces lie in a plane approximately halfway between the axial and coronal planes. The lining of each of the surfaces is articular cartilage. Menisci are present within the cervical facet joints and have a variable appearance depending on the level and subject age. Their purpose is the uniform distribution of pressure.[33] In the adult, they are usually small and triangular but in children may be large and flat. Surrounding the joints is a fibrous capsule with a synovial membrane on its inner aspect.

The joints between the dens and atlas, the occipital condyles and atlas, and the atlas and axis are synovial joints. The pivot joints between the odontoid process and the atlas and axis usually contain two small synovial cavities, one anteriorly between the anterior arch and the dens and the other between the dens and the transverse ligament. The most posterior one together with the transverse ligament and prominent venous structure

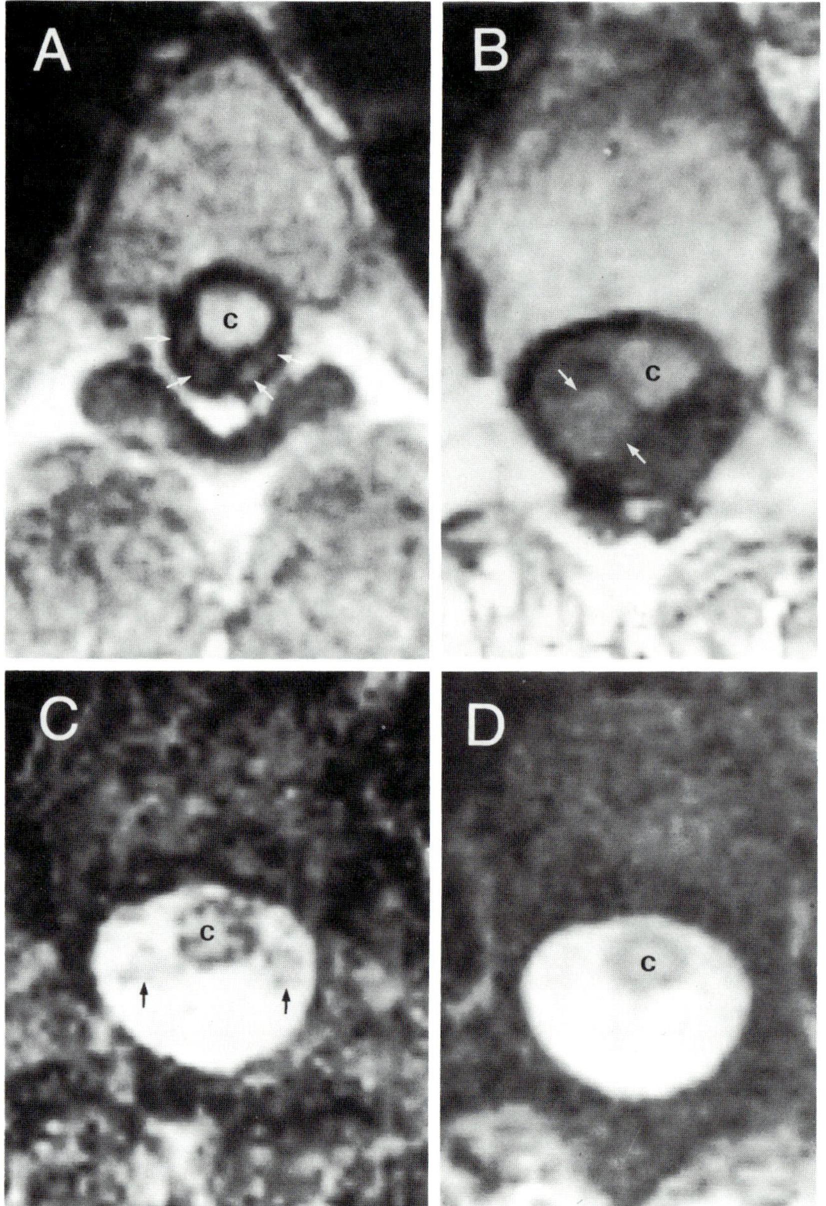

FIG 2–22.

Thoracic CSF pulsation artifacts. **A,** axial T_1-weighted (500/17) SE image through the midthoracic spine. Note that the small ovoid areas have increased signal intensity compared to the adjacent CSF surrounding the posterior and lateral aspect of the cord *(white arrows)*. These regions represent areas of relatively slower CSF flow and pulsations and should not be mistaken for intradural masses. **B,** T_1-weighted SE (500/17) image through the midthoracic spine. An ovoid area of signal intensity similar to that of the adjacent cord *(c)* is noted posteriorly and laterally on the right. **C,** axial T_2-weighted SE (2000/90) ungated or refocussed image. Note on this image two areas of relatively decreased signal intensity approaching that of the adjacent cord laterally and posteriorly *(black arrows)*. This is at the same level as **B.** The variations of signal intensity in these areas on both T_1- and T_2-weighted SE images are secondary to variations in the CSF flow and as seen in **D** are not seen on an axial FLASH (200/13/10 degree) image.

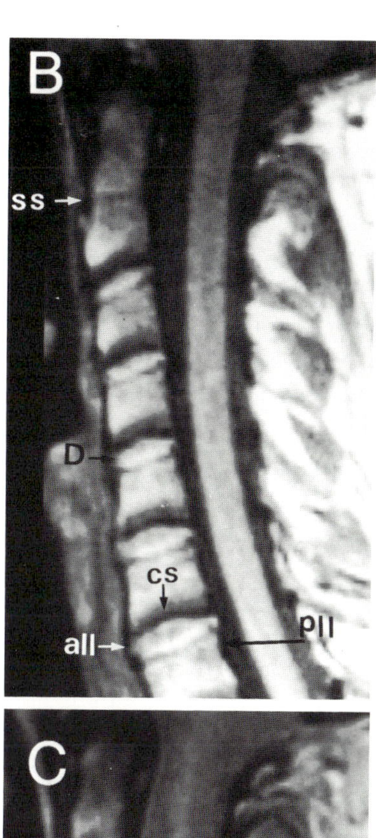

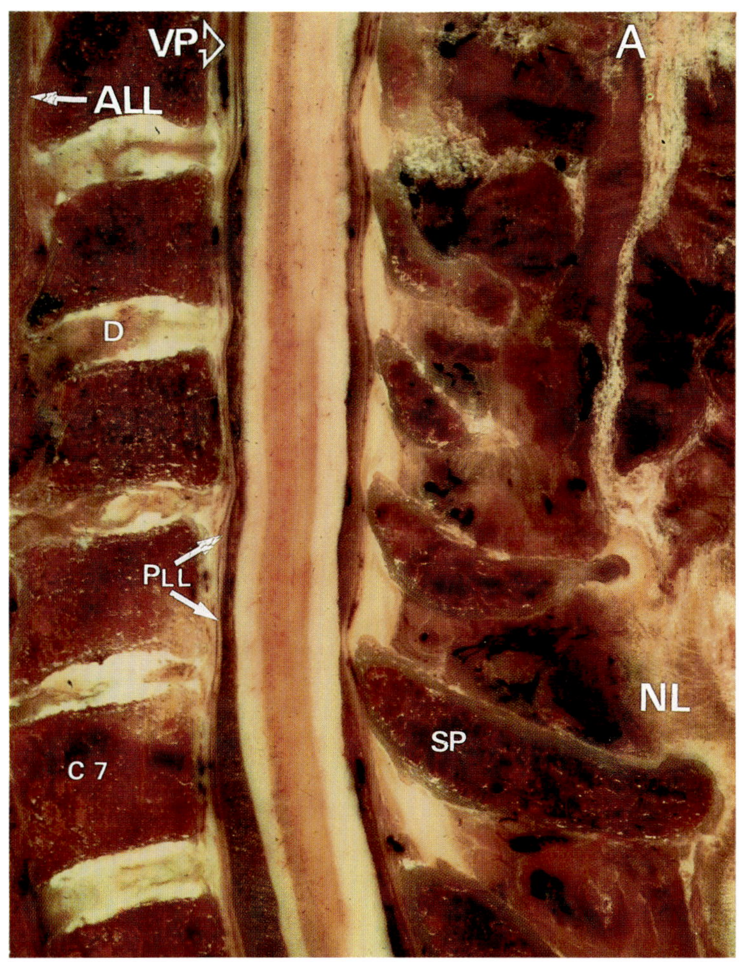

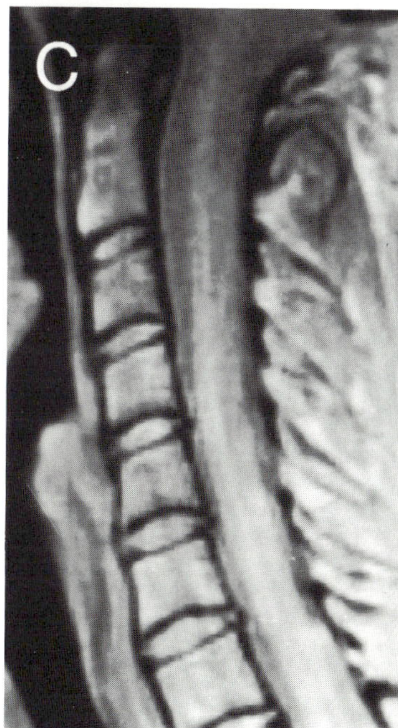

FIG 2–23.
Normal cervical anatomy. **A,** midline cryomicrotome section through the cervical spine. **B,** midline sagittal T_1-weighted SE (500/17). **C,** midline sagittal intermediate SE (2000/20). (For explanation of abbreviations, see p. 64.) *(Continued)*

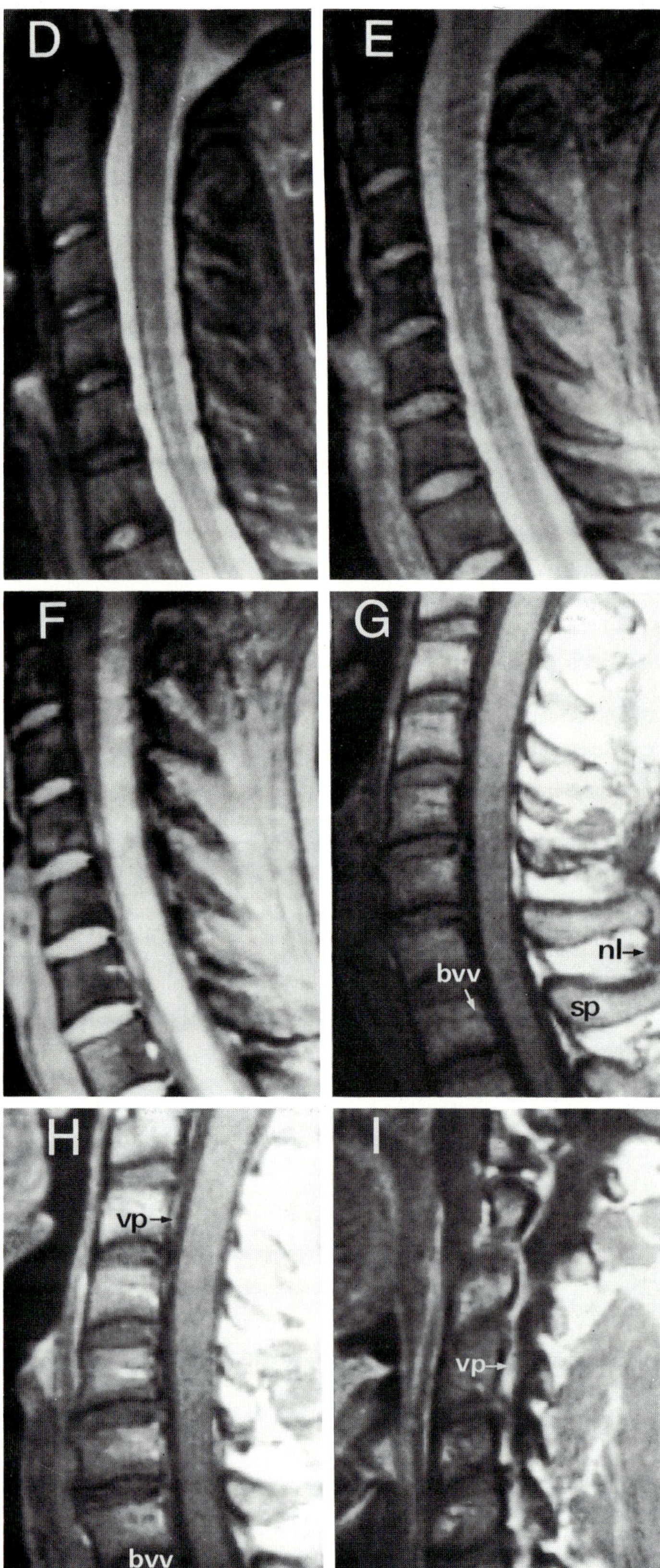

FIG 2–23 (cont.).
Normal cervical spine anatomy. **D,** sagittal midline T_2-weighted (2000/90) refocussed image. **E,** sagittal midline FLASH (200/13/10 degree) image. **F,** sagittal midline FLASH (200/13/60 degree) image. **G,** sagittal midline T_1-weighted SE (500/17) before administration of gadolinium diethylenetriamine penta-acetic acid (Gd-DTPA). **H,** sagittal midline T_1-weighted SE (500/17) following the intravenous administration of 0.1 mmole/kg of Gd-DTPA. Note that there is some enhancement of the basivertebral veins, but little enhancement is noted in the midline posterior to the vertebral bodies. **I,** parasagittal T_1-weighted SE (500/17) following the administration of 0.1 mmole/kg of Gd-DTPA. Note that there is now enhancement in the anterior longitudinal epidural venous plexus. *ALL* = anterior longitudinal ligament; *bvv* = basivertebral vein; *CS* = chemical shift; *D* = disk; *PLL* = posterior longitudinal ligaments; *SP* = spinous process; *ss* = subdental synchondrosis; *VP* = venous plexus.

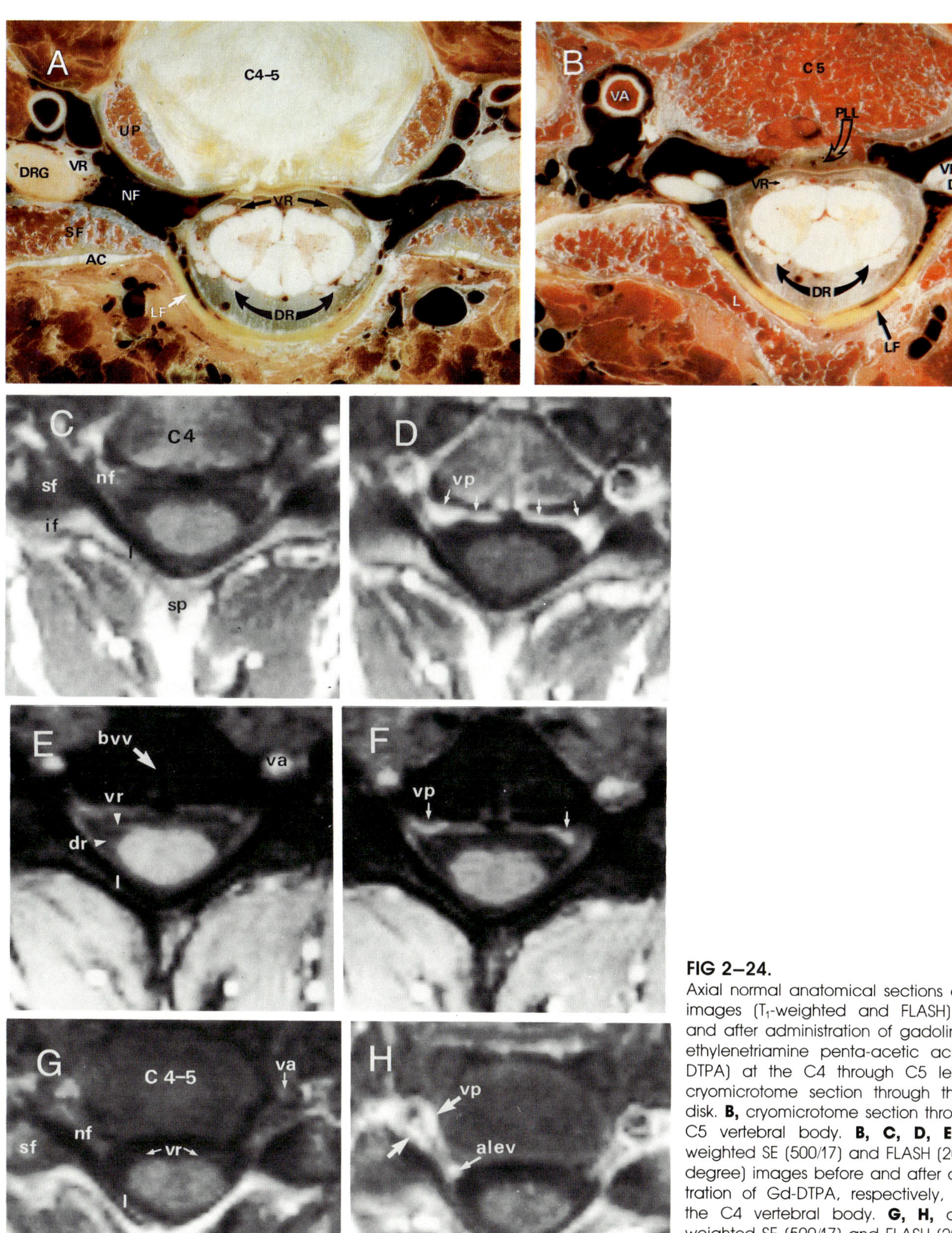

FIG 2–24.

Axial normal anatomical sections and MR images (T_1-weighted and FLASH) before and after administration of gadolinium diethylenetriamine penta-acetic acid (Gd-DTPA) at the C4 through C5 levels. **A,** cryomicrotome section through the C4-5 disk. **B,** cryomicrotome section through the C5 vertebral body. **B, C, D, E, F,** T_1-weighted SE (500/17) and FLASH (200/13/60 degree) images before and after administration of Gd-DTPA, respectively, through the C4 vertebral body. **G, H,** axial T_1-weighted SE (500/17) and FLASH (200/13/60 degree) images before and after administration of Gd-DPTA, respectively, through the C4-5 disk. (See p. 66 for explanation of abbreviations.) *(Continued)*

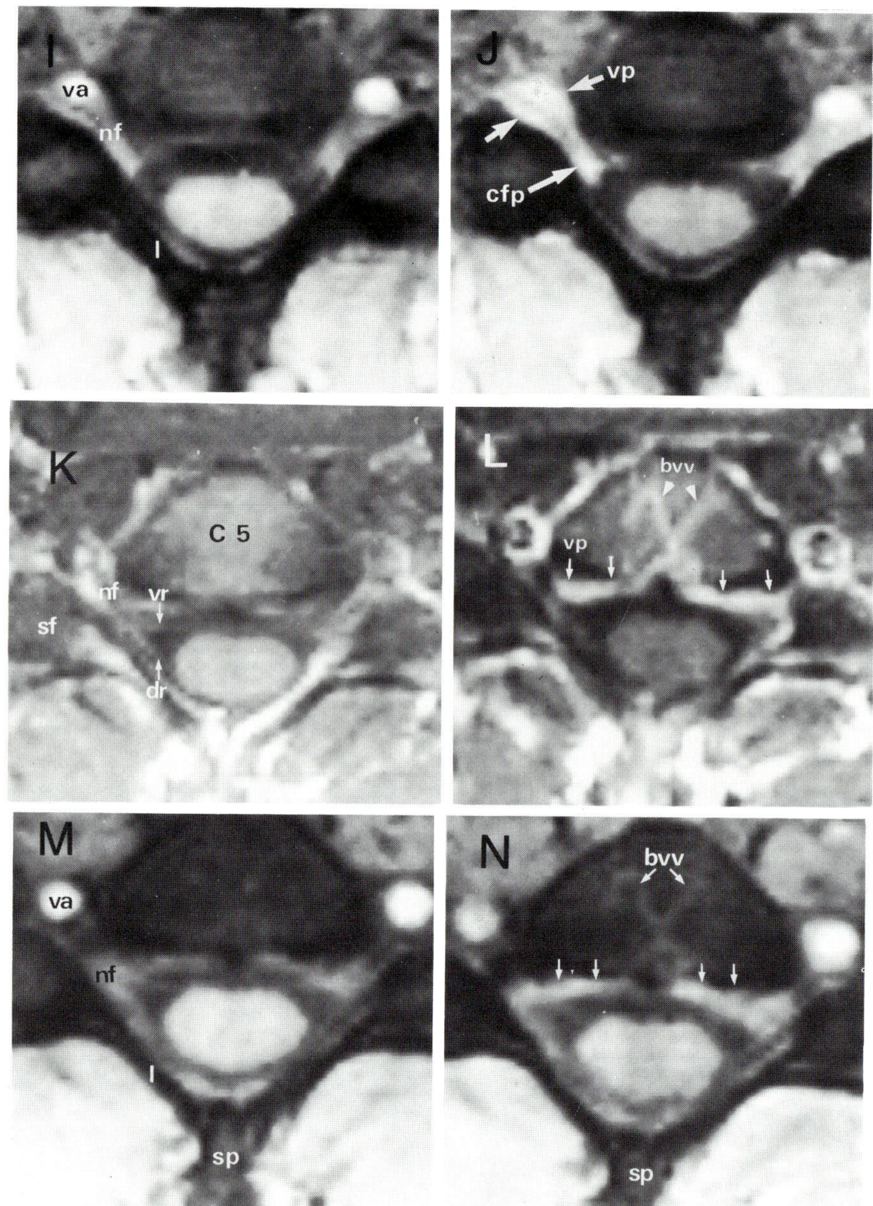

FIG 2–24 (cont.).

Axial normal anatomical sections and MR images (T_1-weighted and FLASH) before and after administration of gadolinium diethylenetriamine penta-acetic acid (Gd-DTPA) at the C4 through C5 levels. **I, J,** axial T_1-weighted SE (500/17) and FLASH (200/13/60 degree) images before and after administration of Gd-DPTA, respectively, through the C4-5 disk. **K, L, M, N,** axial T_1-weighted SE (500/17) and FLASH (200/13/60 degree) images before and after administration of Gd-DPTA, respectively, through the C5 vertebral body. *AC* = articular cartilage; *alev* = anterior longitudinal epidural vein; *BVV* = basivertebral vein; *cfp* = communicating foraminal plexus; *DR* = dorsal root; *DRG* = dorsal root ganglion; *iF* = inferior facet; *l* = lamina; *LF* = ligamentum flavum; *NF* = neural foramen; *pll* = posterior longitudinal ligaments; *SF* = superior facet; *SP* = spinous process; *UP* = uncinate process; *VA* = vertebral artery; *vp* = venous plexus; *VR* = ventral root.

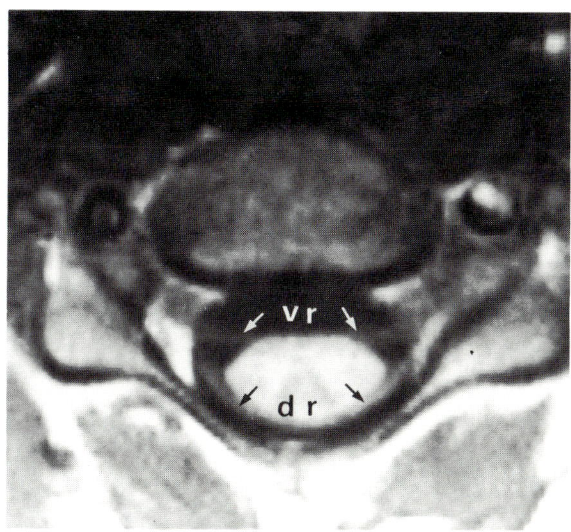

FIG 2–25.
Normal nerve roots. Axial T_1-weighted SE (500/17) image through the C5-6 level. Note the ventral *(vr)* and dorsal *(dr)* roots highlighted by the low signal intensity of the adjacent CSF.

forms a small protruberance of intermediate signal intensity.

The cervical epidural space that surrounds the thecal sac contains neurovascular and connective tissue elements. The cervical vertebrae are connected by the anterior and posterior longitudinal ligaments. The anterior longitudinal ligament covers the anterior lateral aspect of the disks and vertebral bodies. It extends from the anterior margin of the foramen magnum to the sacrum. The posterior longitudinal ligament extends over the posterior aspect of the vertebral bodies from the posterior surface of the body of C2 to the sacrum. Its fibers diverge at each disk level and blend with the anulus fibrosis and adjacent margins of the vertebral bodies. At the midvertebral level, the ligament is narrower and lies 1 to 2 mm behind the body posterior to the retrovertebral venous plexus. A rostral extension, the tectorial membrane, extends to the foramen magnum. The tectorial membrane merges into the basiocciput at the level of the hypoglossal canal inside the skull.

The superspinous ligament connects the tips of the spinous processes, while the intraspinous ligament extends between them. The ligamentum flavum is situated in the posterior aspect of the spinal canal and attaches to the laminae of the adjacent neural arches. The elastic fibers within it give it a yellow color in anatomical section. The signal intensity of the ligamentum flavum on T_1-weighted spin-echo images has an intensity less than fat and equal to or slightly greater than muscle.

Beneath the tectorial membrane lies the crural ligament. The most important component of this structure is the transverse ligament that extends across the ring of the atlas to enclose the odontoid process. The inferior and superior longitudinal bundles extend from the transverse ligament down to the body of the axis and up to the basiocciput, respectively. The accessory atlantoaxial ligaments extend from the basis of the lateral masses at the atlas to merge into the base of the dens and the body of the axis. These ligaments may be significant because of arteries they support, that is branches of the vertebral artery that provide the dens with a portion of its blood supply. At the apex of the dens is a small apical ligament that attaches to the anterior rim of the foramen magnum. It is flanked by two alar ligaments that pass out to the lateral margin of the foramen magnum.[5, 6, 32]

The cervical spinal cord is nearly elliptical in cross section, and the vertically oriented dentate ligaments tether the cord laterally. The dentate ligament takes the form of a serrated ribbon that is attached along the lateral surface of the cord midway between the dorsal and ventral roots. The spinal cord is enlarged in two regions for innervation of the limbs. The rostral enlargement extends from C4 through T1. The corresponding spinal nerves join in the brachial plexus to provide the nerve supply of the upper extremities. Eight pairs of spinal nerves arise from the cervical cord. Each one consists of a dorsal (sensory) and ventral (motor) root. The nerve roots fuse just beyond or lateral to the dural sheath to form the spinal nerves. The dorsal root ganglion is located in the neural foramen just proximal to the point of union of the dorsal and ventral roots. The roots of each spinal nerve from C1 through C7 leave the spinal canal through the intervertebral foramina above the corresponding vertebrae. The first and second cranial nerves lie on the vertebral arches of the atlas and axis, respectively. The eighth cervical nerve passes through the foramen between the seventh cervical and first thoracic vertebrae, there being eight cervical cord segments and seven cervical vertebrae.[5, 6, 32]

The size and contour of the spinal cord are well depicted on T_1-weighted images, where the cord has a higher signal intensity than CSF, allowing maximum cord-CSF contrast. On fast gradient echo scans, the cord has a decreased signal intensity with flip angles of 5 to 15 degrees relative to the signal intensity of the CSF, with an isointense crossover at approximately 20 degrees (see Fig 2–23). With increasing flip angles, the CSF loses signal intensity relative to the cord. On T_2-weighted spin-echo images with refocusing or cardiac gating, the signal intensity of the CSF again is high relative to the cervical cord[31] (see Fig 2–23).

Sagittal images through the cervical cord often reveal linear regions of altered signal intensity that can cause problems by obscuring anatomy and simulating pathologic conditions such as syrinx formation. These appear decreased on T_1-weighted images and may appear increased on more T_2-weighted images. This appearance is created by sampling-related effects (truncation errors) that can be predicted to occur at high-contrast anatomical boundaries. These can be reduced or eliminated by increasing the number of phase-encoded steps, interchanging the phase-encoded direction with the frequency direction or filtering. These are usually not a problem when a 256 × 256 matrix or a smaller field of view is used[34,35] (see Chapter 1).

Axial sections through the cervical cord often reveal internal structure, e.g., gray-white architecture, as well as external surface anatomy (see Figs 2–24 and 2–25). The ventral and dorsal nerve roots are identified coursing through the subarachnoid space on route through their respective neural foramina (see Fig 2–25). In the anterior lateral recesses of the neural foramina, a high signal intensity is often visualized surrounding the nerve roots that represents the extensive venous network in the anterior cervical epidural space and foramina.[36] There is a paucity of fat in the cervical epidural region in contrast to the lumbar region.

Cross-sectional imaging is best performed with acquisitions oriented parallel and orthogonal to the area of interest. This allows complete evaluation by means of two views differing by 90 degrees. In the cervical spine, transverse and sagittal views are complementary in the central portion of the neural canal and obviate some of the disadvantages of partial volume averaging. The routine parasagittal images, however, are not optimally oriented for the neural foramina, which forces one to rely on the axial image. The additional acquisition of oblique MR images oriented perpendicular to the true course of the neural foramina facilitates the identification of disease laterally by providing a second orthogonal imaging plane in relationship to the diseased area.[37,38] Anatomical studies have described the cervical neural foramen as a 4- to 5-mm-long bony canal through which the cervical nerve roots pass anterolaterally at approximately a 45-degree angle with respect to the coronal plane and downward 10 degrees with respect to the axial plane. This is best depicted by oblique T_1-weighted images where the ventral and dorsal nerves are identified in the inferior portion of the neural foramen at or below the disk level[37] (Fig 2–26). Each foramen is outlined by a dark line corresponding to the compact cortical bone of the inferior pedicle cortex superiorly, the superior pedicle cortex inferiorly, the posterior cortical bone of the vertebral bodies anteriorly, and the cortical bone of the posterior elements posteriorly. The uncinate process appears as a small, triangular osseous projection.[37] The visual integration of oblique and axial images decreases the problem of partial volume averaging and the potential problem created by an interspace gap; it allows one to distinguish disk from bone accurately and to determine the relationship of both the neural structures. The oblique plane can be oriented to include all of the cervical neural foramina but must be interpreted on contiguous images as the foramina do not all lie in the same superoinferior plane.

The cervical intervertebral disks are similar in composition to but smaller than the thoracic and lumbar disk. Their lateral extent is less than that of the corresponding vertebral body because of the uncinate process. In the cervical spine, as in the lumbar region, the intervertebral disks are wedge-shaped, the greatest width being anterior. This produces the normal cervical lordosis.[12] Their signal intensity on various pulse sequences is again similar to that in the lumbar region but not as well appreciated because of their smaller volume.

The effect of physiologic parameters on the behavior of CSF is greatest in the cervical region on MR. Here again changes in the signal intensity may be related to flow-related enhancement, ghosting, and/or spin dephasing. Flow-related enhancement is most obvious in the cervical region where it usually occurs at the entry slice secondary to a wash-in of the unsaturated spins produced by the pulsatile motion of the CSF[29] (Fig 2–27,A). This is less commonly seen as an exit slice phenomenon secondary to the pulsatile to-and-fro nature of the CSF motion. Ghosting and spin dephasing can also degrade the quality of the examination and at higher field strengths where one excitation is the rule (Fig 2–27,B), and thus refocusing and/or gating are usually employed (Fig 2–27,C and D). As mentioned previously, an additional trick to reduce ghosting in the area of interest is the utilization of saturation pulses, which reduces the signal of these ghosting artifacts, or to exchange the read and phase direction so they are oriented away from the area of interest (Fig 2–27,E and F).[28]

The transverse foramina transmit the vertebral arteries and veins in a plexus of sympathetic nerve fibers. The vertebral artery usually enters the foramen at the C6 level but may enter at C5 or C7. The vertebral arteries exit from the foramina transverse area of the transverse process of the atlas and wind around the lateral masses, passing in a group just posterior to the superior articular facet from the cranial surface to the posterior arch. The arterial supply of the spinal cord is from branches of the vertebral, thyrocervical, and costocervical arteries that enter the spinal canal through the intervertebral foramina.[36]

The cervical epidural venous plexus is an extensive

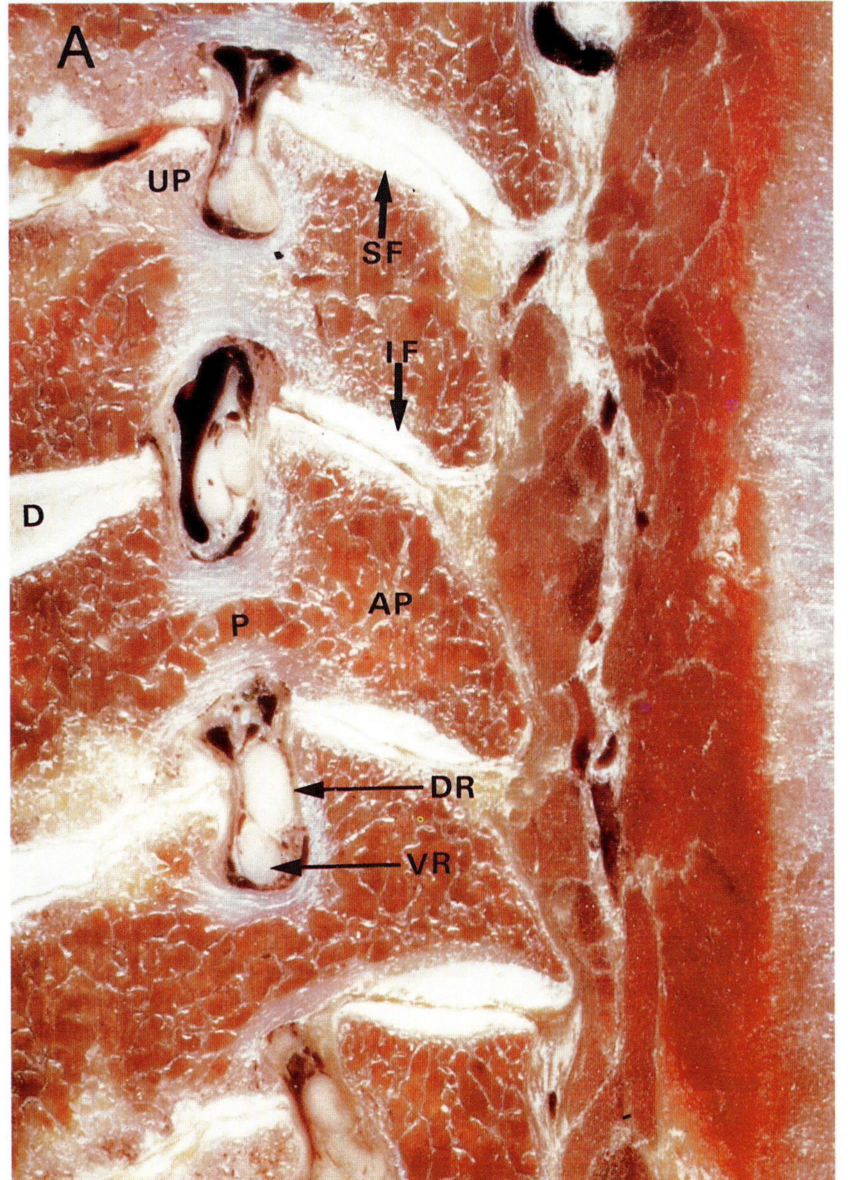

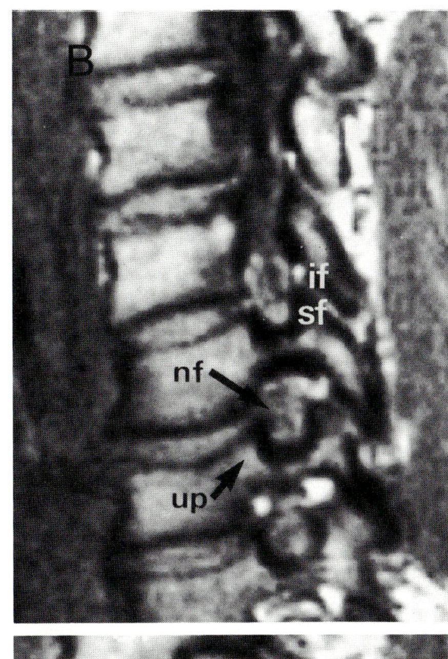

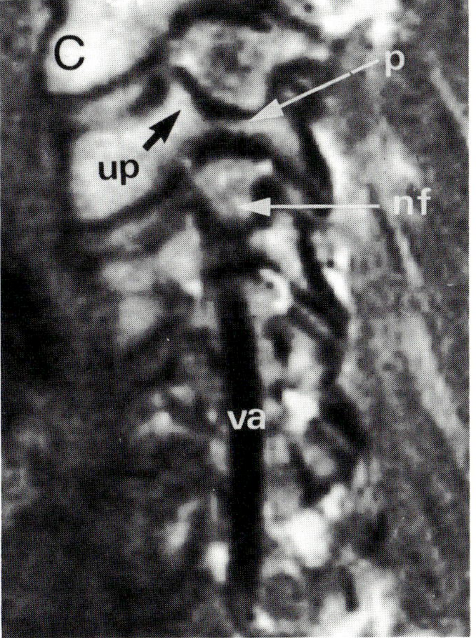

FIG 2–26.
Anatomy of the cervical neural foramen in the oblique plane. **A,** cryomicrotome section through the cervical neural foramen in a 45-degree oblique plane. **B** and **C,** contiguous T_1-weighted SE (500/17) oblique images through the neural foramen. *AP* = articular pillar; *D* = disk; *DR* = dorsal root; *IF* = inferior facet; *nf* = neural foramen; *P* = pedicle; *SF* = superior facet; *UP* = uncinate process; *va* = vertebral artery; *VR* = ventral root.

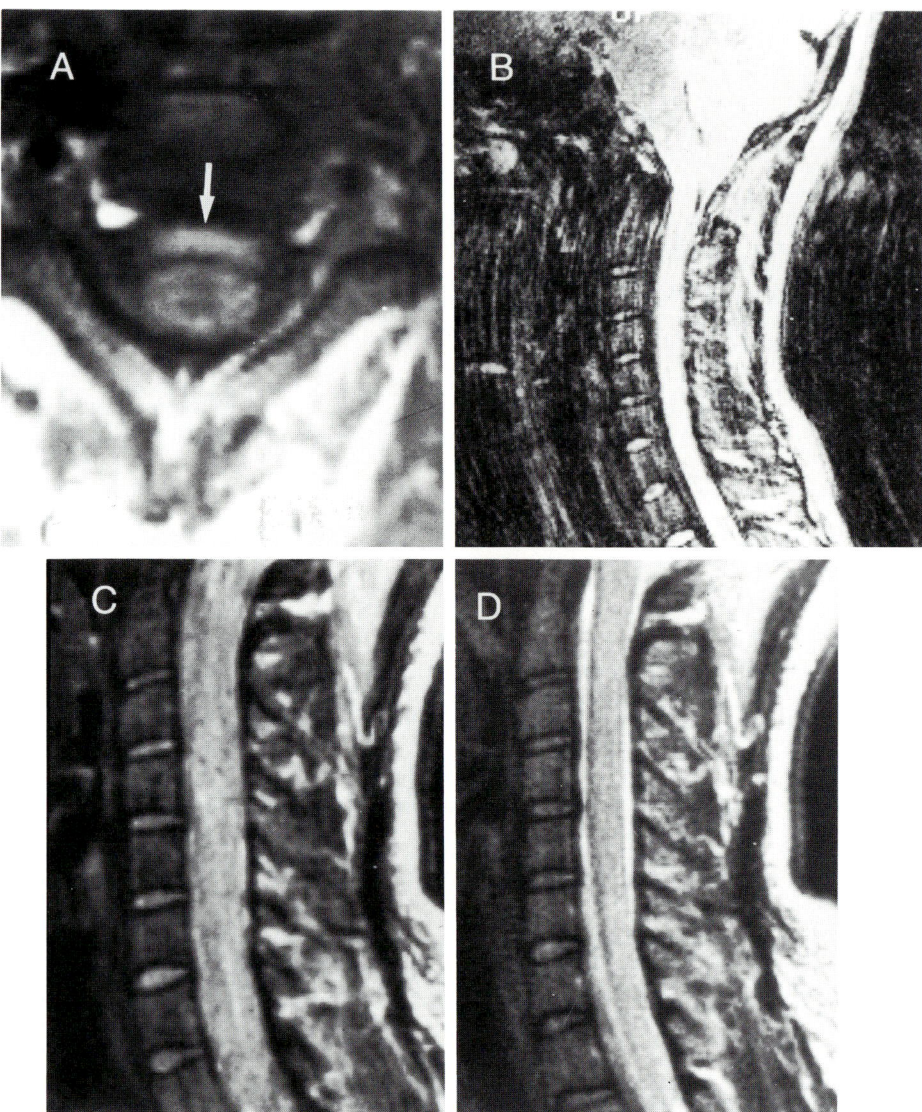

FIG 2–27.
CSF pulsations and refocusing. **A,** axial T_1-weighted SE (500/17) image that is the first slice of a multislice series. The increased signal intensity anterior to the cord demarcated by the *white arrow* represents the entry slice phenomenon that is secondary to the entry of unsaturated CSF into the imaging volume. **B,** midline sagittal T_2-weighted SE (2000/90) unrefocused or gated image. Note the extensive CSF ghosting artifacts on this long TE image with only one excitation without gating or refocusing. **C,** sagittal midline T_2-weighted SE (2000/90) partially refocused image. Even with one excitation, this long TE image shows little if any CSF ghosting. The refocusing, however, is partial, and there is no clear separation between the CSF and the cord indicating that there is still some blurring of margins. **D,** sagittal midline T_2-weighted SE (2000/90) image with more carefully calibrated refocussing in the same plane as **C.** With better calibrated refocussing, there is now a clear separation of the CSF cord interface as well as elimination of CSF ghosting artifacts. *(Continued)*

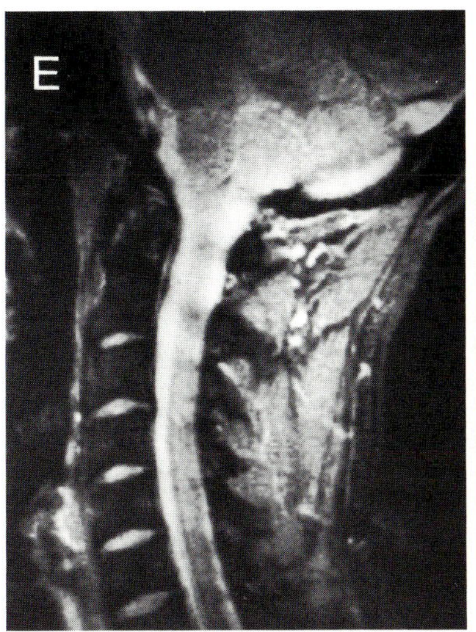

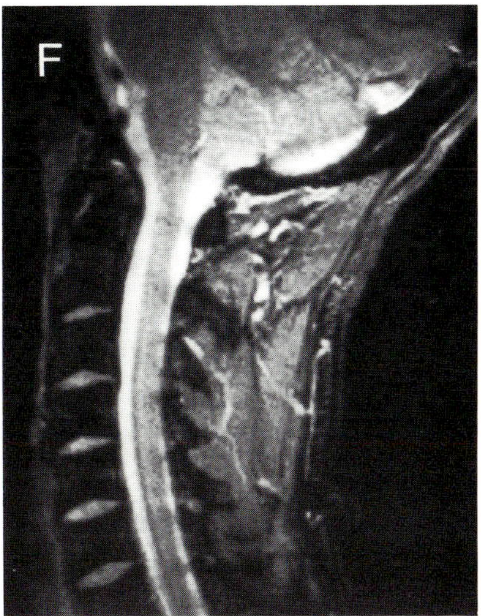

FIG 2–27 (cont.).
CSF pulsations and refocusing. **E** and **F,** sagittal midline FLASH (200/13/10) image before (E) and after (F) the application of a saturation pulse over the anterior neck and face. Notice the decreased signal in the region anterior to the spine on **F.** A technique such as this will reduce the signal intensity of ghosting artifacts from motion in the more anterior structures providing a more artifact-free image of the region of interest.

sinusoidal network in the cervical epidural space[36] (Figs 2–23, 2–24, 2–28, and 2–29). The plexus is particularly prominent at the level of C2. The epidural venous system consists of medial and lateral longitudinal channels located in the anterolateral portion of the epidural space. These two channels are connected behind each vertebral body by retrocorporeal veins (like rungs on a ladder) that communicate with the basivertebral venous system at the midportion of each vertebral body. Posterior internal veins lie ventral to the vertebral arches and

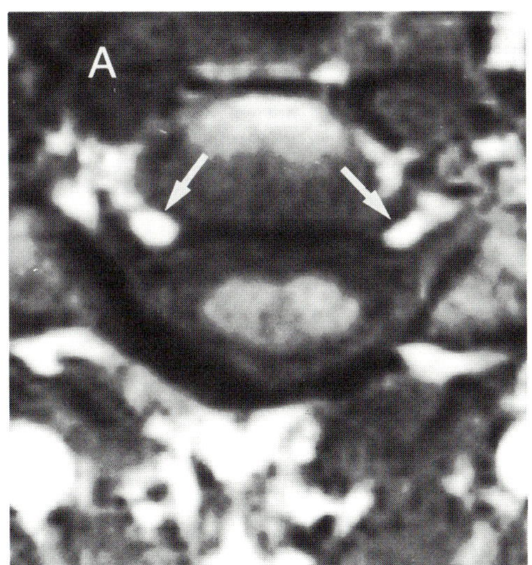

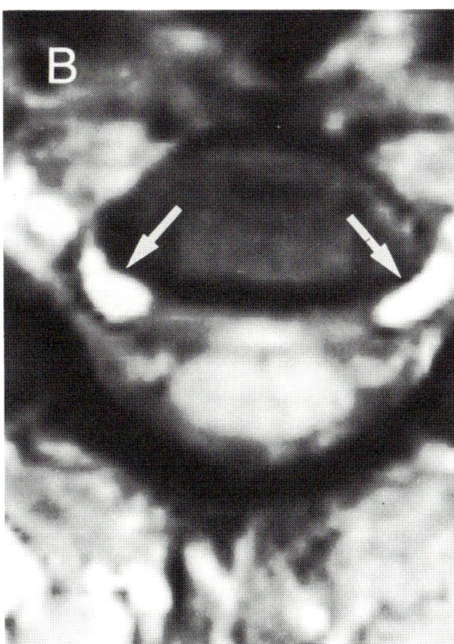

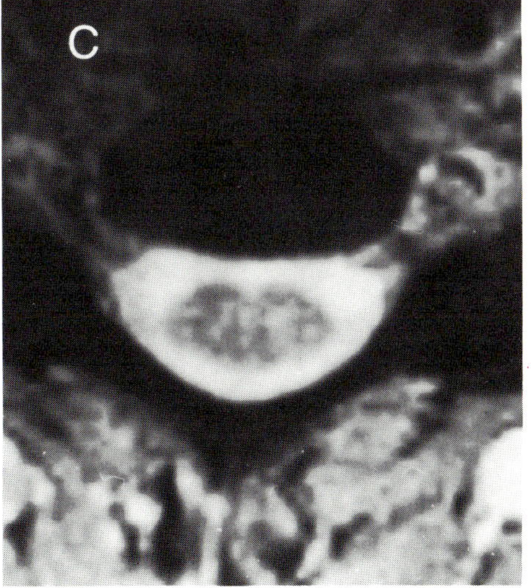

FIG 2–28.
Variable epidural venous signal. **A,** axial T_1-weighted SE (500/17) through the region of the neural foramina at C4-5. Note the high signal intensity of the epidural veins and proximal portion of the neural foramen as outlined by the *white arrows.* **B,** axial FLASH 200/13/60 degrees. Again high signal intensity is noted in the epidural venous plexus and the lateral aspect of the neural canal and proximal portion of the neural foramen. **C,** axial FLASH (200/13/10 degree) image that shows no increased signal intensity in the epidural venous plexus in the same plane as **A** and **B.** This variable signal intensity is related to multiple factors that include pseudogating, the TR, and velocity of blood within the venous plexus and epidural veins. Signal intensity of the blood within the epidural veins and plexus is related to the TE, TR, and slice position as well as to any physiologic gating.

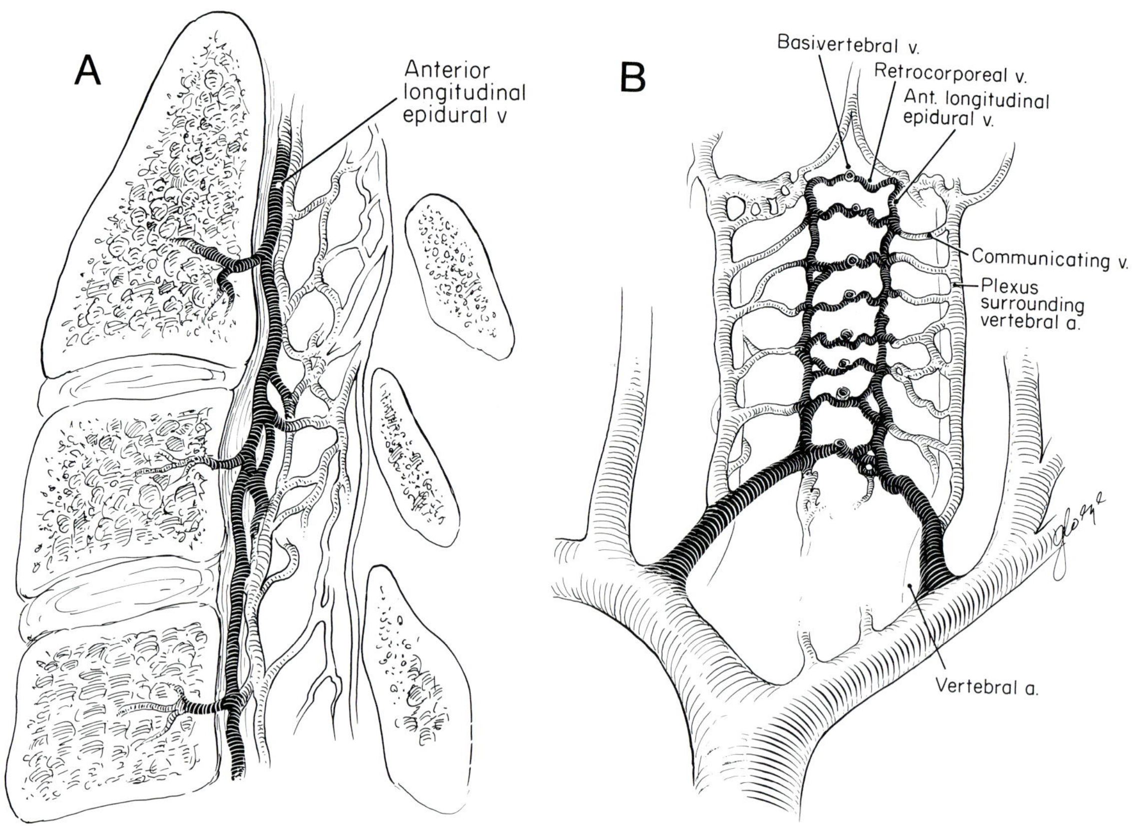

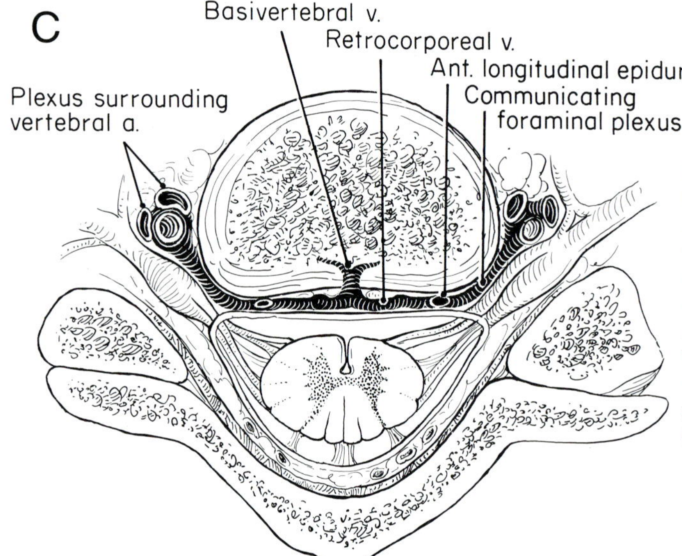

FIG 2–29.
Diagrammatic representation of the cervical vertebral venous anatomy in the sagittal (**A**), coronal (**B**), and axial (**C**) planes. Note that the retrocorporeal veins pass behind the vertebral body, and at the disk level itself, the most prominent structures are the anterior longitudinal epidural veins that are off the midline. (From Flanagan BD, Lufkin RB, McGlade C, et al: MR imaging of the cervical spine: Neural vascular anatomy. *AJNR* 1987; 8:27–32. Used by permission.)

ligamenta flava and receive veins from these structures. The anterior internal veins lie behind the vertebral bodies and receive veins from the ventral dura and vertebral bodies. The external venous plexus lies outside the vertebral channel along the surface of the vertebral bodies and communicates with the internal plexus through veins in the neural foramina. The longitudinal channels communicate with the foraminal venous plexus that extends anteriorly to surround the vertebral artery on each side. This system is an intricate lattice-like network composed of slowly flowing blood. These veins can be seen on both sagittal and axial images as areas of increased signal intensity. Parasagittal views best demonstrate the segmented longitudinal bandlike channels in the anterior lateral recess of the cervical spinal canal (see Fig 2–23). Increased intensity is representative of slow to stagnant venous flow. Axial sections demonstrate the veins as areas of high signal intensity in the anterolateral recess of the spinal canal (see Fig 2–28). While often seen on nonenhanced contrast studies, the appearance of the epidural venous plexus can be confusing depending on the direction and velocity of blood flow. They are more consistently and accurately depicted following the administration of gadolinium diethylenetriamine pentaacetic acid (Gd-DTPA), which produces a uniform high signal intensity of these epidural venous structures outlying the extradural space, particularly along the anterolateral aspect of the spinal canal and neural foramina (Figs 2–23 and 2–24).

References

1. Kricun ME: Red-yellow marrow conversion: Its effect on the location of some solitary bone lesions. *Skeletal Radiol* 1985; 14:10–19.
2. Hajek PC, Baker LL, Goobarg JE, et al: Focal fat deposition in axial bone marrow: MR characteristics. *Radiology* 1987; 162:245–249.
3. Dorwart RH, Sauerland EK, Haughton VM, et al: Normal lumbar spine, in Newton TH, Potts DG (eds): *Computed Tomography of the Spine and Spinal Cord*. San Anselmo, Calif, Clavadel Press, 1983, pp 93–114.
4. Latchaw R, Taylor S: CT of the normal and abnormal spine, in Latchaw R (ed): *Computed Tomography of the Head, Neck, and Spine*. Chicago, Year Book Medical Publishers, 1985, pp 595–618.
5. Daniels DL, Haughton VM, Williams AL: *Cranial and Spinal Magnetic Resonance Imaging*. New York, Raven Press, 1987.
6. Schnitzlein HN, Murtagh FR: *Imaging Anatomy of the Head and Spine*. Baltimore-Munich, Urban & Schwarzenberg, 1985.
7. Grenier N, Kressel HY, Schiebler ML, et al: Normal and degenerative posterior spinal structures: MR imaging. *Radiology* 1987; 165:517–525.
8. Lewin T, Moffet B, Viidik A: The morphology of the lumbar synovial intervertebral joints. *Acta Morphol Neerl Scand* 1962; 4:299–319.
9. Schellinger D, Wener L, Ragsdale BD, et al: Facet joint disorders and their role in the production of back pain and sciatica. *RadioGraphics* 1987; 7:923–944.
10. Harris RI, McNab I: Structural changes in the lumbar intervertebral disks: Their relationship to low back pain and sciatica. *J Bone Joint Surg [Br]* 1954; 36:304–322.
11. Resnick D: Degenerative diseases of the vertebral column. *Radiology* 1985; 156:3–14.
12. Parke WW, Schiff DCM: The applied anatomy of the intervertebral disc. *Orthop Clin North Am* 1971; 2:309–324.
13. Grogan JP, Daniels DL, Williams AL, et al: The normal conus medullaris: CT criteria for recognition. *Radiology* 1984; 151:661–664.
14. Monajati A, Wayne WS, Rauschning W, et al: MR of the cauda equina. *AJNR* 1987; 8:893–900.
15. Ross JS, Masaryk TJ, Modic MT, et al: MR imaging of lumbar arachnoiditis. *AJNR* 1987; 8:885–892.
16. Coventry MB, Ghormley RK, Kernohan JW: The intervertebral disc: Its microscopic anatomy and pathology. I: Anatomy, development and physiology. *J Bone Joint Surg Am* 1945; 27:105–112.
17. Coventry MB, Ghormley RK, Kernohan JW: The intervertebral disc: Its microscopic anatomy and pathology. II. Changes in the intervertebral disk concomitant with age. *J Bone Joint Surg Am* 1945; 27:233–247.
18. Coventry MB, Ghormley RK, Kernohan JW: The intervertebral disc: Its microscopic anatomy and pathology. III. Pathological changes in the intervertebral disc. *J Bone Joint Surg Am* 1945; 27:460–474.
19. Coventry MB: Anatomy of the intervertebral disk. *Clin Orthop* 1969; 67:9–15.
20. White AA, Gordon SL: Synopsis: Workshop on idiopathic low back pain. *Spine* 1982; 7:141–149.
21. Adams P, Eyre DR, Muir H: Biochemical aspects of development and aging of human intervertebral discs. *Rheumatol Rehabil* 1977; 16:22–29.
22. Lipson SJ, Muir H: Experimental intervertebral disc degeneration: Morphological and proteoglycan changes over time. *Arthritis Rheum* 1981; 24.
23. Lipson SJ, Muir H: Proteoglycans in experimental intervertebral disc degeneration. *Spine* 1984; 6:194–210.
24. Modic MT, Pavlicek W, Weinstein MA, et al: Magnetic resonance imaging of intervertebral disc disease. *Radiology* 1984; 152:103–111.
25. Pech P, Haughton VM: Lumbar intervertebral disk: Correlative MR and anatomic study. *Radiology* 1985; 156:699–701.
26. Aguila LA, Piraino DW, Modic MT, et al: The intranuclear cleft of the intervertebral disk: Magnetic resonance imaging. *Radiology* 1985; 155:155–158.
27. Winkler ML, Ortendahl DA, Mills TC, et al: Characteristics of partial flip angle and gradient reversal MR imaging. *Radiology* 1988; 166:17–26.

28. Edelman RR, Atkinson DJ, Silver MS: FRODO pulse sequences: A new means of eliminating motion, flow, and wraparound artifacts. *Radiology* 1988; 166:231–236.
29. Rubin JB, Enzmann DR: Imaging of spinal CSF pulsation by 2D FTMR: Significance during clinical imaging. *AJNR* 1987; 8:297–306.
30. Parke WW, Watanabi R: Lumbosacral intersegmental epispinal axons and ectopic ventral nerve root outlets. *J Neurosurg* 1987; 67:269–277.
31. McMasters DL, deGroot J, Haughton VM, et al: Normal thoracic spine, in Newton TH, Potts DG (eds): *Computed Tomography of the Spine and Spinal Cord*. San Anselmo, Calif, Clavadel Press, 1983, pp 79–92.
32. McMasters DL, deGroot J, Haughton VM, et al: Normal cervical spine, in Newton TH, Potts DG (eds): *Computed Tomography of the Spine and Spinal Cord*. San Anselmo, Calif, Clavadel Press, 1983, pp 53–78.
33. Yu S, Sether L, Haughton VM: Facet joint menisci of the cervical spine: Correlative MR imaging and cryomicrotomy study. *Radiology* 1987; 164:79–82.
34. Levy LM, Di Chiro G, Brooks RA, et al: Spinal cord artifacts from truncation errors during MR imaging. *Radiology* 1988; 166:479–483.
35. Bronskill MG, McVigh ER, Kucharczyk W, et al: Syrinx-like artifacts on MR images of the spinal cord. *Radiology* 1988; 166:485–488.
36. Flanagan BD, Lufkin RB, McGlade C, et al: MR imaging of the cervical spine: Neural vascular anatomy. *AJNR* 1987; 8:27–32.
37. Daniels DL, Hyde JS, Kneelon KN, et al: The cervical nerves and foramina: Local coil MR imaging. *AJNR* 1986; 7:129–133.
38. Modic MT, Masaryk TJ, Ross JS, et al: Cervical radiculopathy: Value of oblique MR Imaging. *Radiology* 1987; 163:227–231.
39. Daniels DL, Grogan JP, Johansen JG, et al: Cervical radiculopathy: Computed tomography and myelography compared. *Radiology* 1984; 151:109–113.

3

Degenerative Disorders of the Spine

Michael T. Modic, M.D.

Degenerative disorders of the spine are among the most common causes of impairment in both males and females and are among the leading cause of disability in the working years. Surveys have shown that 60% to 80% of adults suffer from back pain at some time in their life and up to 25% of working men are affected in any given year. The economic impact can further be appreciated from statistics that indicate that 2% of the population consults a doctor each year because of low back pain.[1–3]

Deterioration of the osseous and soft tissue structures of the spine is a normal consequence of the aging process and can be predisposed to or accelerated by a variety of developmental and/or acquired factors. The manner of degeneration of the various components of the spine is mediated and manifested by the specific structure involved. The consequences and symptom complex with which patients present usually involve instability and malalignment abnormalities, intervertebral disk degeneration and/or herniation, spinal stenosis, and facet disease.[4]

Of the multitude of symptoms that may result from degenerative diseases of the spine, the three most important in attempting to localize a lesion and develop an etiologic differential are pain, sensory changes, and weakness.

Pain is the most important symptom by virtue of its frequency and as a common cause of debilitation. Pain may be divided into local, referred, radicular, and secondary arising from muscular spasm. Local pain is usually caused by a process that involves the sensory nerve endings. This therefore requires innervation of a structure. For instance, a large amount of destruction of a vertebral body may occur without pain, whereas small lesions involving the periosteum, anulus fibrosis, ligaments, or facet joint capsule may cause extreme pain.

Referred pain refers to that which is projected from or to the spine into or from other structures lying within the same dermatome. Pain from diseases of the upper part of the lumbar spine is usually referred to the anterior aspects of the thighs, legs, or lower part of the back. Pain produced in the lower part of the lumbar spine is usually referred to the lower buttocks due to irritation of the lower spinal nerves, which also activate regions in the posterior thigh and calves. Conversely, abnormalities of the abdominal or pelvic bursae may be projected back into the spine.

Radicular pain is similar to referred pain but is usually of greater intensity, with the distal radiation confined to the territory of the irritated nerve root. Radiculopathy refers to pain, weakness, or dysesthesias in the distribution of the spinal nerve with or without reflex changes due to compression of a nerve root. In the lumbar region, the symptom is often referred to as sciatica, that is, pain radiating in the distribution of the sciatic nerve. Radicular pain nearly always emanates from a central position near the spine to some part of the lower extremity and is usually superimposed on a dull referred pain.

Pain from muscle spasm usually occurs in relationship to local pain and is reflexive to guard the diseased portions against motion.

In addition to pain, other symptoms of spinal degenerative disease, especially when the cord itself is involved, include weakness of the extremities, spasticity, and/or a sensory deficit. Myelopathic symptoms such as these, particularly in the cervical and thoracic regions, can be caused by extrinsic spinal cord compression from degenerative or neoplastic disease, or by intrinsic causes such as cysts, neoplasms, multiple sclerosis, amyotrophic lateral sclerosis, and myelitis.[5] The role of imaging is to sort out these differential considerations, a task for which magnetic resonance (MR) is well designed. At the outset, however, it must be emphasized that because there is a morphological abnormality does not mean that it is necessarily responsible for the patient's symptomatology or that it must be symptomatic.[6, 7]

MALALIGNMENT

Traditionally the evaluation of malalignment abnormalities has consisted of a combination of plain radiographs and tomography with flexion and extension films for the evaluation of abnormal motion. This may still provide the most rapid cost-effective way of evaluating the bony spinal canal for malalignment. While MR can be used with both flexion and extension views, its major role has been in the evaluation of the overall spinal canal contour and alignment in the sagittal, coronal, and axial plane as well as in evaluation of the intervertebral disks, ligaments, and neural foramina. This can best be accomplished by a T_1-weighted spin-echo (SE) sequence or fast variable flip-angle gradient echo scan in the axial and sagittal planes. Oblique views may be necessary for the evaluation of the pars interarticularis and the neural foramina in the cervical region.

Various types of alignment abnormalities can exist alone or in combination, but the two most frequent are segmental instability and spondylolisthesis.

Segmental Instability.—Degenerative changes involving the invertebral disk, vertebral bodies, and facet joints can impair the usual pattern of spinal movement, producing motion that can be irregular, excessive, or restricted.

Spondylolisthesis.—This condition results when one vertebral body becomes displaced in relationship to the next most inferior vertebral body (Fig 3–1). The most common types include degenerative, isthmic, iatrogenic, and traumatic. Degenerative spondylolisthesis is usually seen with an intact pars interarticularis and is primarily related to degenerative changes of the apophyseal joints and is most common at the L4-5 vertebral level, presumably because the more sagittal orientation of the facet joints makes them more prone to anterior displacement. Degenerative disk disease may predispose to or exacerbate this condition secondary to narrowing of the disk space, which can produce subsequent malalignment of the articular processes leading to rostrocaudal subluxation. Retrolisthesis is more common in the cervical and lumbar regions, which are more mobile. Isthmic spondylolisthesis occurs secondary to a defect in the pars interarticularis that results in a subluxation of the vertebral bodies. Iatrogenic spondylolisthesis can occur secondary to surgery, especially with concomitant facetectomy that produces a loss of stability. This may also occur above levels of fusion secondary to stress fractures because of abnormal motion. Traumatic spondylolisthesis can result from fractures of the neural arch and/or facet dislocation. This latter entity is more common in the lower thoracic and cervical regions but has been identified in the lower lumbar spine. Various miscellaneous entities may also result in spondylolisthesis. These would include rare congenital abnormalities such

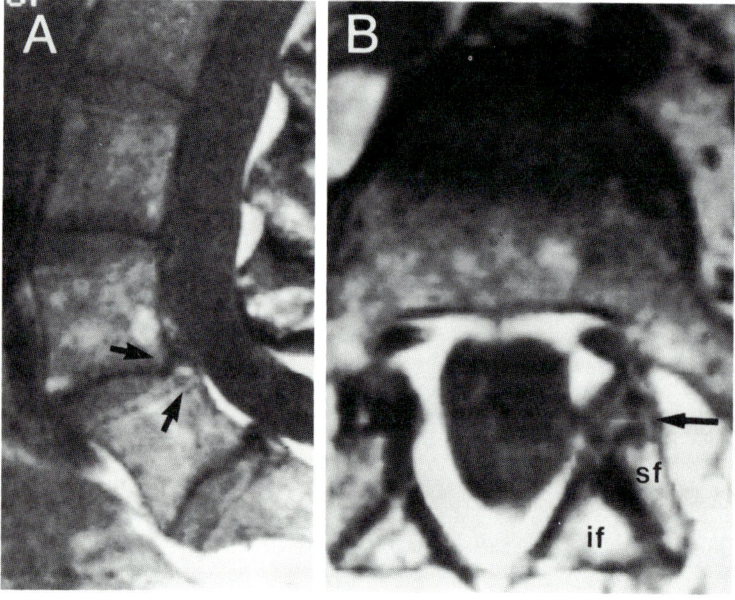

FIG 3–1.
Spondylolisthesis. **A,** sagittal midline T_1-weighted SE (500/17) that demonstrates a grade I spondylolisthesis of L4 on L5 *(arrows).* **B,** axial T_1-weighted SE (500/17) through the pars of L5. *Black arrow* denotes the region of spondylolysis. *sf* = superior facet; *if* = inferior facet.

as dysplastic spondylolisthesis and certain pathologic bone diseases such as Paget's or metastatic disease, which can result in pathologic changes predisposing to abnormal motion.[8]

Sagittal T_1-weighted images provide the most accurate means of identifying the spondylolisthesis, but axial and oblique images are needed to define the elements of the motion complex, the facet joint, the pars, and the neural arches.

DEGENERATIVE DISK DISEASE

Degeneration of the intervertebral disk complex is a process that begins early in life and is a consequence of a variety of environmental factors as well as normal aging. The pathophysiology of this disorder is complicated and poorly understood. It has been stated "the term 'degeneration' as commonly applied to the intervertebral disk covers such a wide variety of clinical, radiological and pathological manifestations that the word is really only a symbol of our ignorance."[9]

The sequelae of disk degeneration remain among the leading causes of functional incapacitation in both sexes and are an all too common source of chronic disability in the working years. In accordance with its incidence, morbidity, and socioeconomic impact, there have been extensive research efforts into the epidemiology, anatomy, biomechanics, biochemistry, and neuromechanisms of degenerative disk disease.[10] Correspondingly, advances in imaging have been applied both in vivo and in vitro in an effort to facilitate a better understanding of the cause of disk degeneration as well as of its impact on clinical symptomatology and therapy. Again, it is important to stress that imaging studies traditionally have been tools for morphological analysis.[6,7] By the age of 50 years, 85% to 95% of adults show evidence of degenerative disk disease at autopsy,[11] and thus the jump from the identification of an anatomical derangement to symptom complex must be taken with caution, as to date there is only a moderate correlation between imaging evidence of disk degeneration and symptomatology.[10]

A variety of biochemical and structural changes take place during the process of both aging and degeneration that are similar enough that the process of degeneration itself can be thought of as a normal phenomenon of senescence over time.

During the aging process, the cartilaginous end-plate becomes thinner and more hyalinized. Fissuring, regenerating chondrocytes, and granulation tissue may be noted in the severely degenerated disk within the end-plate (Fig 3–2, A), as well as in the anulus fibrosis and nucleus pulposus, indicating attempts at healing.[12]

With degeneration and aging, type II collagen increases outwardly in the anulus, and there is a greater water loss in the nucleus pulposus than the anulus. This results in a loss of the hydrostatic properties of the disk with an overall reduction of the hydration in both areas to about 70%. The individual chemical structures of the proteoglycans are not changed with degeneration, but their relative composition is. The ratio of keratan sulfate to chondroitin sulfate increases, and there is a diminished association with collagen that may reduce its tensile strength. The decrease in water-binding capacity of the nucleus pulposus is felt to be related to the decrease in the molecular weight of its nuclear proteoglycan complexes (aggregates). Aggregating proteoglycans then may be a sign of health as they are seen to decrease with both aging and degeneration. The disk becomes progressively more fibrous and disorganized, with the end stage represented by amorphous fibrocartilage with no clear distinction between nucleus and anulus fibrosis[13–16] (Fig 3–2, B).

The etiology of disk degeneration is as yet unknown. Multiple factors have been implicated such as autoimmune reaction, genetic makeup, reabsorption, and biomechanics. The immunology of collagen has been studied in some detail, and at least ten different types of collagen have been noted. Some investigators have demonstrated the ability of disk tissue to stimulate lymphocytes in regional lymph nodes, but there is no evidence of circulating antibodies or inflammatory infiltrates in the disk itself. While this issue is by no means resolved,[17–19] autoimmune reaction is not currently considered a major factor in disk degeneration.[10]

Genetic predisposition has been suggested by animal models that consistently develop degenerative disk disease at an early age,[20] as well as by reports of familial osteoarthritis and lumbar canal stenosis in humans.

It is known that the volume of the intervertebral disk tissue decreases with degeneration. The lumbar disk may decrease in volume from 15 cu cm to 1 cu cm. Disk herniation explains only a minor part of this process. A study of intervertebral disks based on a 160 postmortem examinations showed that anular radial rupture often occurs early in the process of degeneration and can be followed by prolapse of disk tissue through the fissure. The herniated mass consists of nucleus pulposus as well as anulus fibrosis. It appears that disk tissue may be "digested" and absorbed as it reaches the surface. At pathology, closely connected with necrotic degenerated portions of disk tissue, loose granulation tissue is sometimes noted, providing a potential mechanism of absorption. Whether this is an etiologic factor or a second-

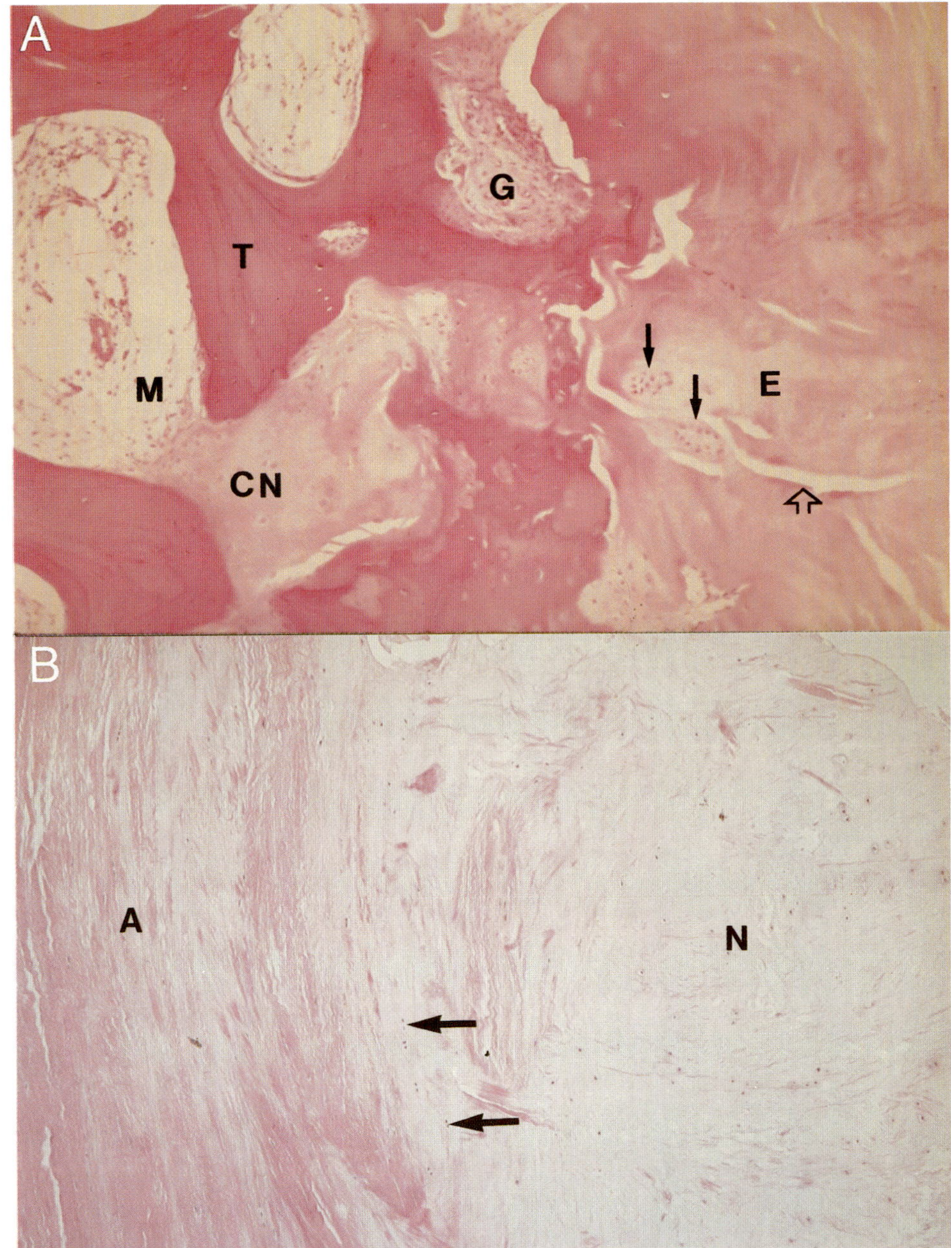

FIG 3–2.
Histology of a degenerated intervertebral disk. **A,** the end-plate *(E)* shows cracks and fissures *(open arrow)* as well as areas of pale staining. Packets of chondrocytes *(black arrows)* and granulation tissue *(G)* are present that are characteristic of regeneration and degeneration. A cartilaginous node *(CN)* is seen protruding between thickened trabeculae *(T)*. The adjacent marrow space *(M)* shows an increase in lipid elements (hematoxylin-eosin, low power). **B,** the transition zone between the degenerated nucleus pulposus *(N)* and anulus fibrosis *(A)* shows evidence of fragmentation, fissuring, and sequestration of collagen in both regions with a loss of normal architecture. Several multinucleated chondrocytes *(arrow)* are indicative of regeneration (hematoxylin-eosin, low power).

ary phenomenon in disk degeneration is as yet unclear.[21]

Failure of the human lumbar intervertebral disk occurs more frequently in that part of the spine subjected to the heaviest mechanical stress. Under high vertical loads, postmortem specimens of disks burst superiorly or inferiorly, while radial rupture of the anulus fibrosis was uncommon.[22–24] Torsional or flexion stresses appear to be more damaging to the anulus fibrosis.[22, 23, 25]

Results of animal studies suggest that degeneration

takes place in response to a loss to the confined fluid state rather than to a primary defect in the proteoglycans as the etiologic cause. The anulus may begin to fragment resulting in radial and concentrically oriented fissures that can predispose to degeneration and subsequent herniation of the nucleus pulposus both into and through the anulus fibrosis. Degeneration always follows herniation. It seems likely, then, that the anulus fibrosis determines the fate of the disk, allowing it to adapt to axial loading, or to decompensate, resulting in biochemical changes within the disk itself.[15, 16]

The contrast sensitivity and multiplanar imaging capability of proton MR places the modality in a position to provide a unique noninvasive means of imaging the intervertebral disk. The implementation of surface coil technology,[26] cardiac gating,[27] gradient refocussing,[28] and paramagnetic contrast agents[29] has done much to improve visualization of the intervertebral disk and surrounding tissue, as well as to increase MR's sensitivity to and specificity for disease. More recent innovations and pulse sequence designs such as saturation pulses[30] and gradient echo volume imaging are likely to further refine the utility of MR imaging of degenerative disk disease.

When a combination of imaging planes and pulse-sequence parameters is used, the anatomy of the intervertebral disk, spinal nerves, dural sac, and adjacent structures can be clearly depicted. From a morphological aspect, MR imaging may be the most accurate means of evaluating the intervertebral disk. Accordingly, most research to date has been clinically directed towards optimizing anatomical image display in a fashion similar to that of CT for assessment of disk contour.[31–37] Unlike CT and conventional radiography, which are dependent on information related to electron density, proton MR signals are influenced by the T_1 and T_2 relaxation time, and proton density providing greater tissue contrast. Thus, its role may go beyond gross anatomical appraisal to actual tissue characterization of pathology and biochemical change.[38]

The relationship among the vertebral body, endplate, and disk has been studied by using both the de-

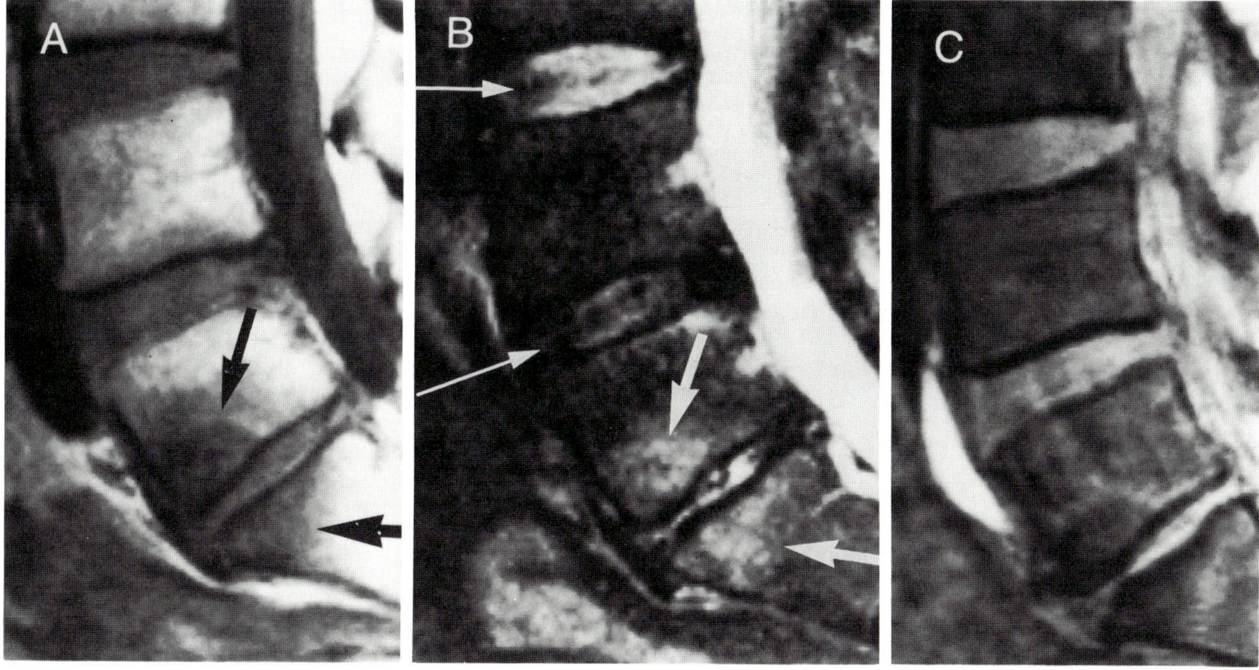

FIG 3–3.
MR of the degenerated lumbar disk and type I marrow change from a 38-year-old female. **A,** T_1-weighted sagittal SE (500/17) 4-mm midline section. There is mild narrowing at the L4-5 interspace and moderate narrowing at L5-S1. There is a decreased signal intensity of the adjacent anterior portion of the L5-S1 vertebral bodies *(arrows)* indicative of type I change. **B,** T_2-weighted sagittal SE (2000/90) 4-mm midline section. The L3-4 disk has a normal configuration and signal intensity. There is a decreased signal intensity of the degenerated L4-5 disk and increased signal intensity of the adjacent portions of the L5 and S1 vertebral bodies *(large white arrows).* Note the linear regions of decreased signal bisecting the L3-4 and L4-5 disk *(arrows).* The high signal intensity within the disk space at the L5-S1 level is presumably secondary to fluid within the cracked and fissured L5-S1 disk. Note also the increased signal within the disk anteriorly and posteriorly, most likely representing tears in the anulus fibrosus. **C,** fast low-angle shot (FLASH) sagittal (50/13/50 degrees) 4-mm section. The signal intensity difference between the normal L3-4 and degenerated L4–5 disk space is reduced when compared to **B.**

generated and chymopapain-treated disks as models.[39–42] Signal intensity changes in vertebral body marrow adjacent to the end-plates of degenerative disks is a common observation in MR imaging. These appear to take three main forms. Type I changes demonstrate a decreased signal intensity on T_1-weighted images and an increased signal intensity on T_2-weighted images and have been identified in approximately 4% of patients scanned for lumbar disease (Fig 3–3). Type I changes are also seen in approximately 30% of chymopapain-treated disks, which may be viewed as a model of acute disk degeneration.[42] Type II changes are represented by an increased signal intensity on T_1-weighted images and an isointense or slightly hyperintense signal on T_2-weighted images (Fig 3–4). These were seen in approximately 16% of cases. In both types, there was always evidence of associated degenerative disk disease at the level of involvement.[40] Histopathologic sections of disks with type I changes demonstrate disruption and fissuring of the end-plate and vascularized fibrous tissues within the adjacent marrow producing prolongation of T_1 and T_2 (Fig 3–5). Disks with type II changes also show evidence of end-plate disruption with yellow marrow replacement in the adjacent vertebral body resulting in a shorter T_1 (see Fig 3–5). There appears to be a relationship between these as type I changes have been observed to convert to type II with time, while type II changes seem to remain stable. To date no attempt has been made to correlate the marrow changes with clinical symptoms or to determine whether they are related to specific biomechanical derangements such as instability.

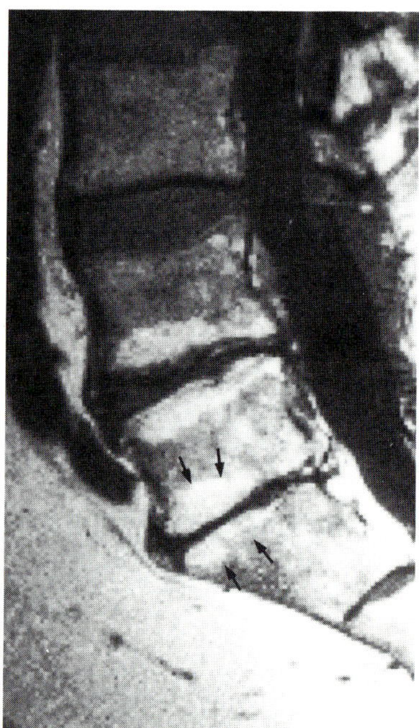

FIG 3–4.
MR of type II vertebral body change in a 56-year-old male. T_1-weighted sagittal (500/17) 4-mm midline section. High signal intensity is noted within the vertebral body marrow at the adjacent portions of the L4-5 and L5-S1 *(small black arrows)* disk spaces.

A third type is represented by a decreased signal intensity on both T_1- and T_2-weighted images that appears to correlate with extensive bony sclerosis on plain radiographs. The first two types show no definite correlation with sclerosis seen at radiography, which is not surprising when one considers the histology. The sclerosis on plain radiographs is a reflection of dense woven bone within the vertebral body rather than of the marrow elements. The MR signal intensity is more a reflection of the marrow elements, normal hematopoietic tissue, fibrovascular tissue, and lipid (or lack there of) between trabeculae. The lack of signal in the type III change no doubt reflects the relative absence of marrow in areas of advanced sclerosis. While the signal intensity changes of type I may be similar to those seen in vertebral osteomyelitis, the distinguishing factor (at least in the adult population) is the involvement of the intervertebral disk, which shows an abnormal high signal intensity and abnormal configuration on T_2-weighted images of infection.[43]

As mentioned previously, the anulus fibrosis is thought to play a key role in the pathophysiology of disk degeneration. Initially, MR characterization of anulus changes before gross disruption was limited because of spatial resolution and a signal intensity similar to that of the adjacent longitudinal ligaments. Recently, however, it has been shown that T_2-weighted spin-echo sequences may be able to identify and characterize radial, transverse, and concentric tears on T_2-weighted images.[5, 53a]

Preliminary work using T_2-weighted spin-echo sequences further suggests that MR is capable of detecting changes in the nucleus pulposus and anulus fibrosis relative to degeneration and aging based on a loss of signal presumed to be secondary to the known changes of hydration that occur within the intervertebral disk[38] (see Fig 3–3). However, correlation is not straightforward as differences in signal intensity appear to be somewhat exaggerated for the degree of water loss noted with degeneration (e.g., ~ 15%).[5] At this time, the role that specific biochemical changes (e.g., proteoglycan ratios and aggregating complexes) play in the changes of signal intensity is not well understood. In the case of severely degenerated disk, where the overall signal intensity is decreased, there may be linear areas of high signal intensity on T_2-weighted spin-echo images that are thought to represent free fluid within cracks or fissures of the degenerated complex[44] (Fig 3–6).

On MR, the vacuum phenomenon and calcification

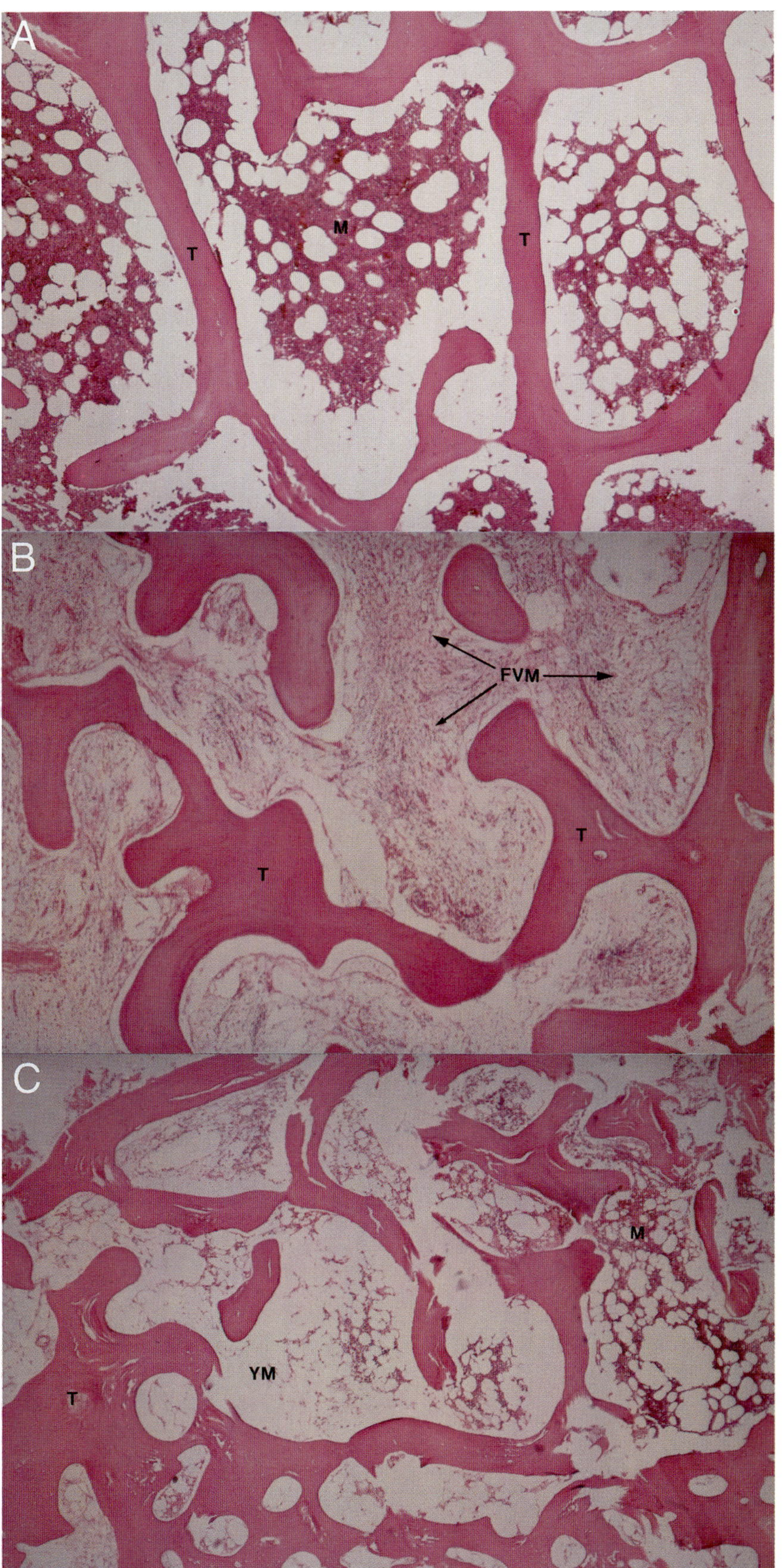

FIG 3–5.
Histology of a normal, type I and type II subcortical vertebral body marrow adjacent to the end plate. **A,** normal marrow is composed of both hematopoietic and lipid elements *(M)*. The bony trabeculae *(T)* are of a normal thickness. **B,** the marrow with type I change shows that fibrovascular tissue has entirely replaced normal marrow *(FVM)* between thickened bony trabeculae *(T)*. **C,** histology of type II marrow change demonstrates an increase in the lipid content *(YM)* of the marrow space when compared to the normal distribution of lipid and hematopoietic elements *(M)*. Thickened, woven bony trabeculae *(T)* are also noted (hematoxylin-eosin).

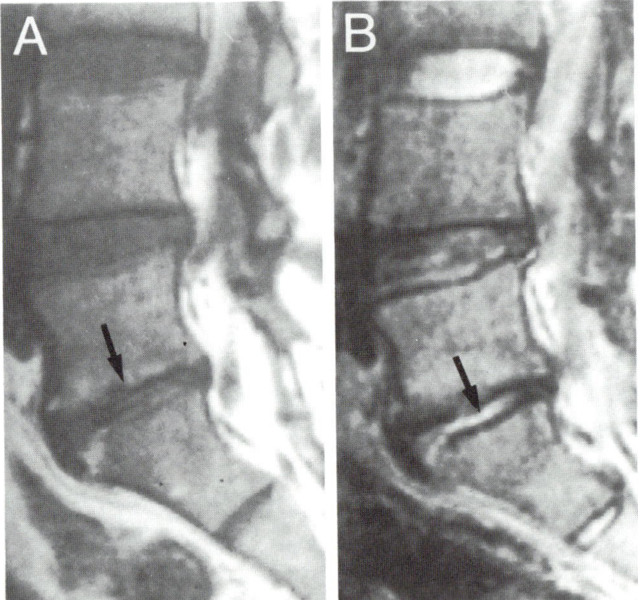

FIG 3–6.
Degenerated L4-5 and L5-S1 disks. **A,** sagittal T_1-weighted SE (500/17). There is narrowing of the L5-S1 disk space *(arrow)* as well as type II change of the anterior margins of the L5 and S1 vertebral bodies. **B,** sagittal T_2-weighted SE (2000/90). There is decreased signal intensity of L4-5 and L5-S1 when compared to L3-4. The high linear increased signal intensity noted at the L5-S1 disk space *(arrow)* is presumably secondary to fluid within a cracked, fissured, degenerated disk.

are represented on spin-echo images as areas of signal void[45] and may not be seen with the same sensitivity as on plain films or computed tomography (CT). Gradient echo images are more sensitive to these changes, apparently related to a magnetic susceptibility effect that allows earlier detection and better characterization (Fig 3–7). However, gradient echo images are not as sensitive to the signal-intensity changes noted on more T_2-weighted images within the disk or T_1 and T_2 changes noted in the adjacent vertebral body with degeneration (see Fig 3–3).

While degeneration may be seen without hernia-

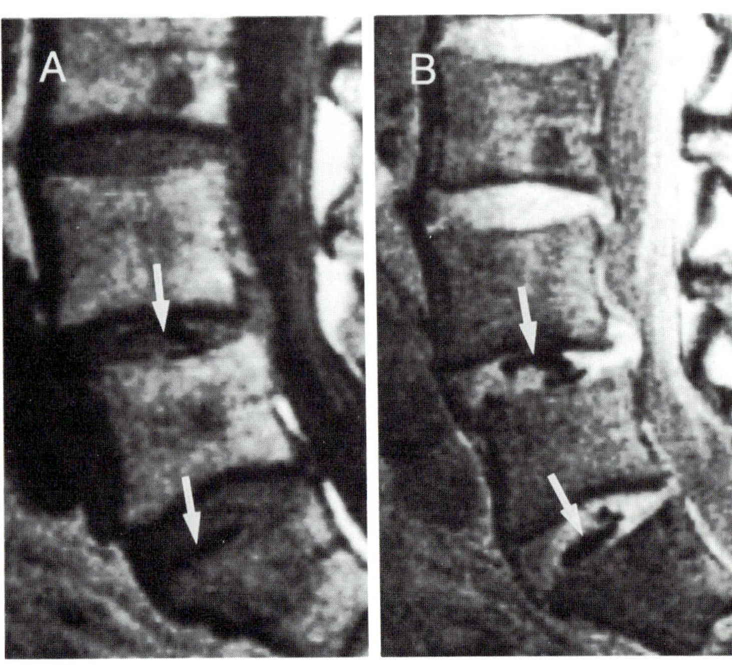

FIG 3–7.
MR of the vacuum phenomenon. **A,** T_1-weighted sagittal SE (500/17) 4-mm midline section. Linear areas of decreased signal are noted in the L4-5 and L5-S1 disks consistent with intradiskal gas or calcification *(arrows).* Incidentally noted is herniation at the L4-5 level. **B,** FLASH sagittal (200/13/50 degrees) 4-mm midline section. The areas of decreased signal (arrows) are now more conspicuous on this gradient echo image when compared to the SE study in **A.**

tion, most herniated disks appear degenerated. Notable exceptions to this are the uncommon juvenile disk herniation and the appearance of an acute disk herniation such as may be noted with spinal trauma.

Sequelae of Disk Degeneration

Disk herniation, especially in the lumbar and thoracic regions, is probably better depicted by MR imaging than by other more conventional modalities.[31–37] Multidimensional imaging allows the direct acquisition of orthogonal views covering long segments of the spine without requiring secondary reconstructions. The outer anulus–posterior longitudinal ligament complex can usually be seen as an area of decreased signal relative to the inner anulus–nucleus pulposus, which helps in characterizing the type of herniation (protrusion, extrusion and/or sequestration).[46] This ability to characterize and differentiate the various subgroups of disk herniation has certain diagnostic and therapeutic ramifications, particularly in the lumbar region.

The distinction between the bulging anulus and herniated disk is important, inasmuch as a bulging disk is considered to be associated less with sciatica than is a herniated disk. The following categories, while not universally accepted, are adapted from the classification scheme utilized by the surgical services at our institution and are similar to those reported by McNab et al.

Abnormal disks can be classified as an anular bulge or herniated (protruded, extruded, or free fragment). An anular bulge is a result of disk degeneration with a grossly intact, albeit lax anulus, usually recognized as a generalized extension of the disk margin beyond the margins of the adjacent vertebral end-plates, regardless of the signal of the interspace. The margin is smooth, symmetric (although occasionally more prominent bilaterally), and without evidence of focal protrusion (Figs 3–8 and 3–9).

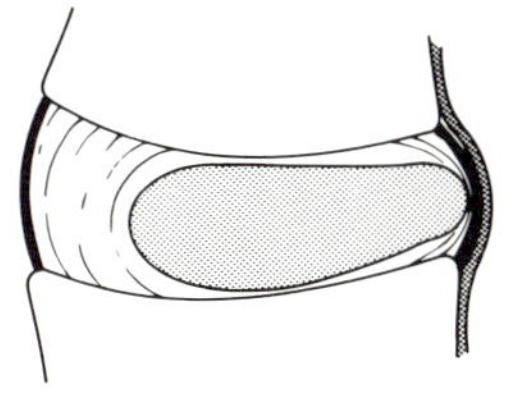

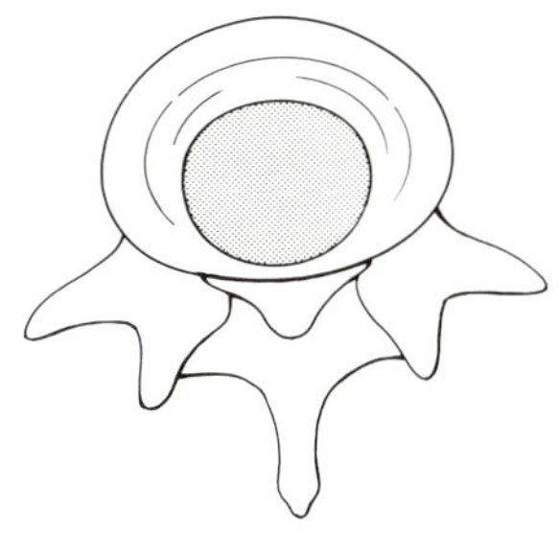

FIG 3–8.
Diagrammatic representation of a bulging intervertebral disk. The bulging anulus fibrosis is recognized as a generalized extension of the disk margin beyond the boundaries of the adjacent vertebral body end plates, regardless of the signal from the interspace on T_2-weighted images.

A protruded disk represents herniation of nuclear material through a defect in the anulus producing a focal extension of the disk margin (Fig 3–10). Orthogonal images are critical for the evaluation of the contour and in separating a bulge from a protrusion, a distinction which may not be as apparent on the sagittal images alone. The signal intensity of the parent nucleus is usually decreased as is the extradural defect particularly on T_2-weighted images. These defects can be central or lateral (Figs 3–11 through 3–13).

An extruded disk represents herniation of nuclear material that results in an anterior extradural mass and remains attached to the nucleus of origin, often via a high-signal pedicle on the T_2-weighted images (Fig 3–14). The signal intensity of the extruded portion may be increased or decreased on T_2-weighted images. The disk usually appears contained by the posterior longitudinal ligament and remaining contiguous portions of the anulus, which appear as curvilinear areas of decreased signal intensity on the T_2-weighted images (Figs 3–15 through 3–17).

The term "free fragment" or "sequestered disk" refers to disk material external to the anulus fibrosis and no longer contiguous with the parent nucleus (Fig 3–18). Free fragments can lie anterior to the posterior longitudinal ligament, especially if they have migrated behind the vertebral bodies where the posterior longitudinal ligament is not in direct opposition (Figs 3–19 and 3–20), posterior to the ligament (Figs 3–21 and 3–22), and even rarely intradurally. Nevertheless, there is almost invariably penetration through the posterior longitudinal ligament either posteriorly, where it is fused with the anulus, or superiorly or inferiorly, where it fuses with the vertebral body margin. Again, contained portions of the anulus and posterior longitudinal ligament may be seen as curvilinear areas of decreased signal intensity surrounding the disk fragment.

A frequent finding with extruded and free fragments is the presence of a high signal intensity extradural defect often surrounded by a curvilinear area of decreased signal intensity that is distinct from the interspace of origin. This separation is best appreciated on sagittal T_2-weighted images where the contrast between the extradural defect and interspace is greatest. It should again be emphasized that visual integration of orthogonal planes is important in the characterization and localization of herniated disk disease.

These distinctions may be important, especially in the recognition of extruded and sequestered disks as such disks (1) may produce misleading localizing signs and symptoms, (2) are a contraindication to the use of chymopapain and percutaneous diskectomy techniques, (3) are a known cause of postoperative back pain, and

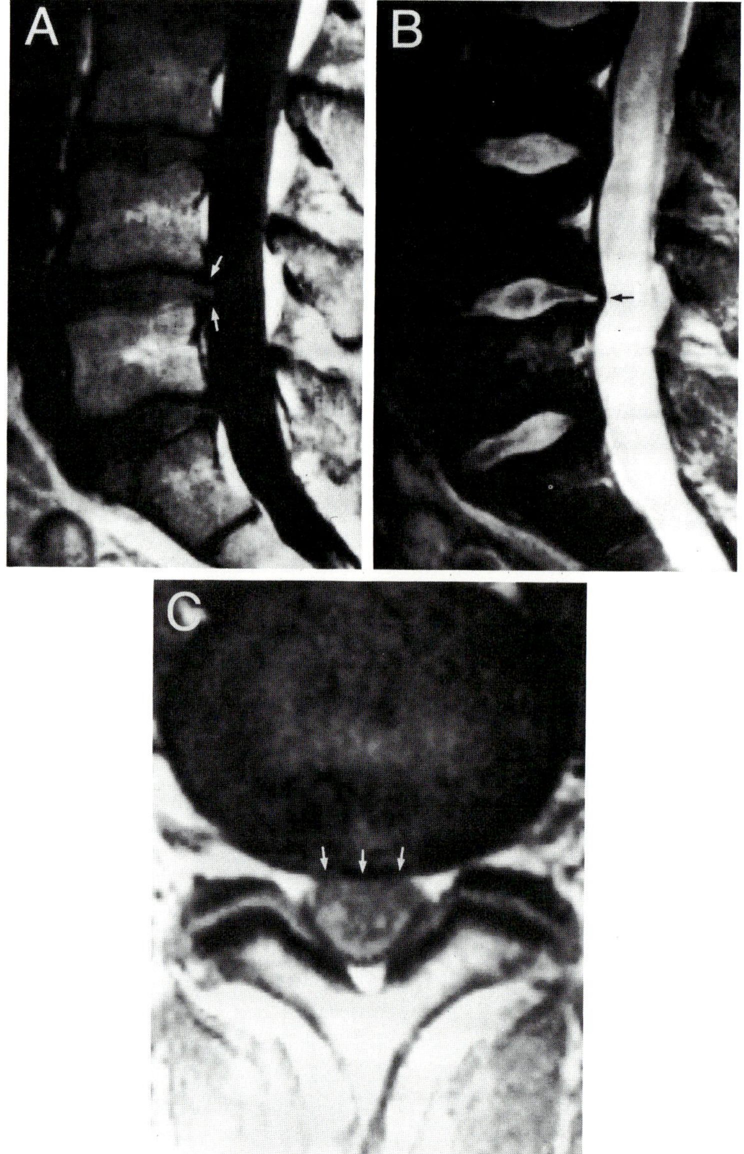

FIG 3–9.
MR of a bulging intervertebral disk. **A,** midline sagittal T_1-weighted SE (500/17) image of the lower lumbar spine demonstrating an extradural defect *(arrow)* at the L4-5 level. **B,** midline sagittal T_2-weighted SE (2000/90) image of the lower lumbar spine again demonstrating a mild anterior extradural defect at the L4-5 level. Notice that there is no focal extension of the high-signal disk material beyond the interspace. However, note the bright signal in a radial tear of the anulus extending back to its confluence with the posterior long ligament *(arrow).* **C,** axial T_1-weighted SE (500/17) image through the L4-5 disk demonstrating smooth symmetric extension of the anulus beyond the margins of the adjacent end plate *(white arrows).*

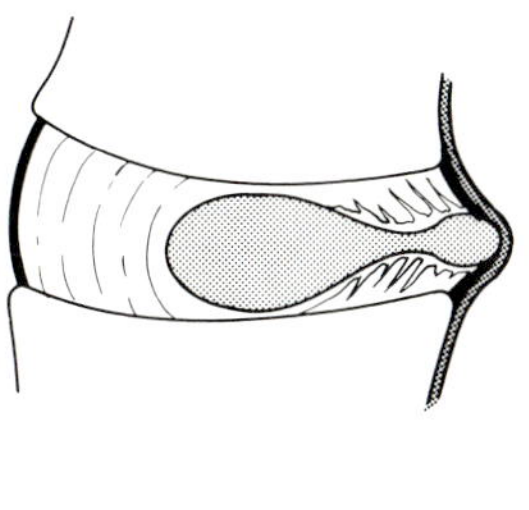
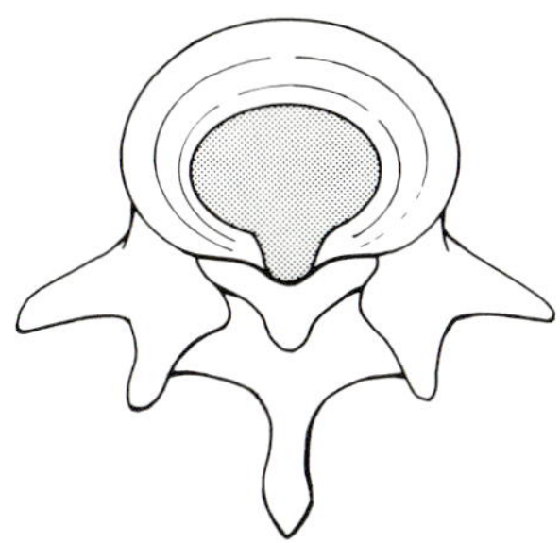

FIG 3–10.
Schematic diagram of disk protrusion. Disk protrusion is recognized as a focal extension of the disk margin in which nuclear material is herniated through a defect in the anulus *(dark, black line).* The anulus, while cracked and/or fissured, remains intact as does the posterior longitudinal ligament. Herniated material is contiguous with the parent nucleus and may or may not have a high signal on T_2-weighted images.

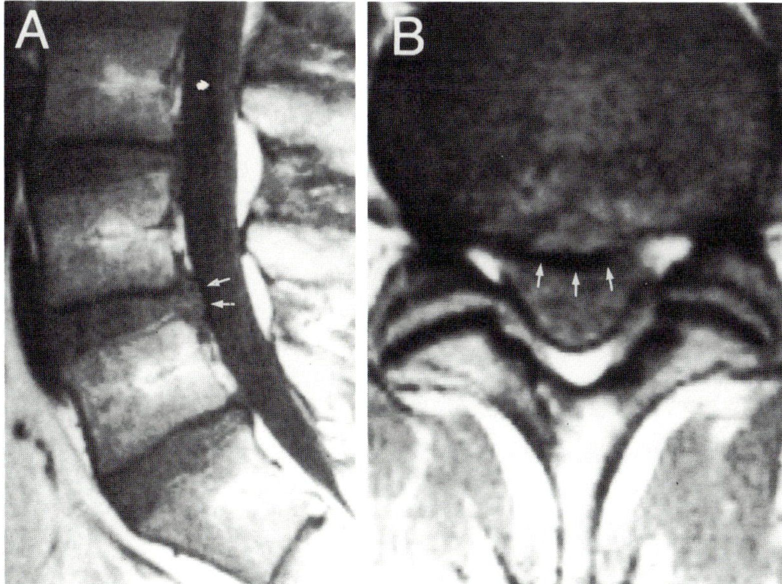

FIG 3–11.
Protrusion of the L4-5 disk. **A,** sagittal midline T_1-weighted SE (500/17) image. *Small white arrows* denote protrusion of disk material beyond the margin of the adjacent vertebral end plates. **B,** axial T_1-weighted SE (500/17) image through the L4-5 disk. There is focal asymmetry of the posterior margin centrally of the L4-5 disk indicative of protrusion *(small white arrows).*

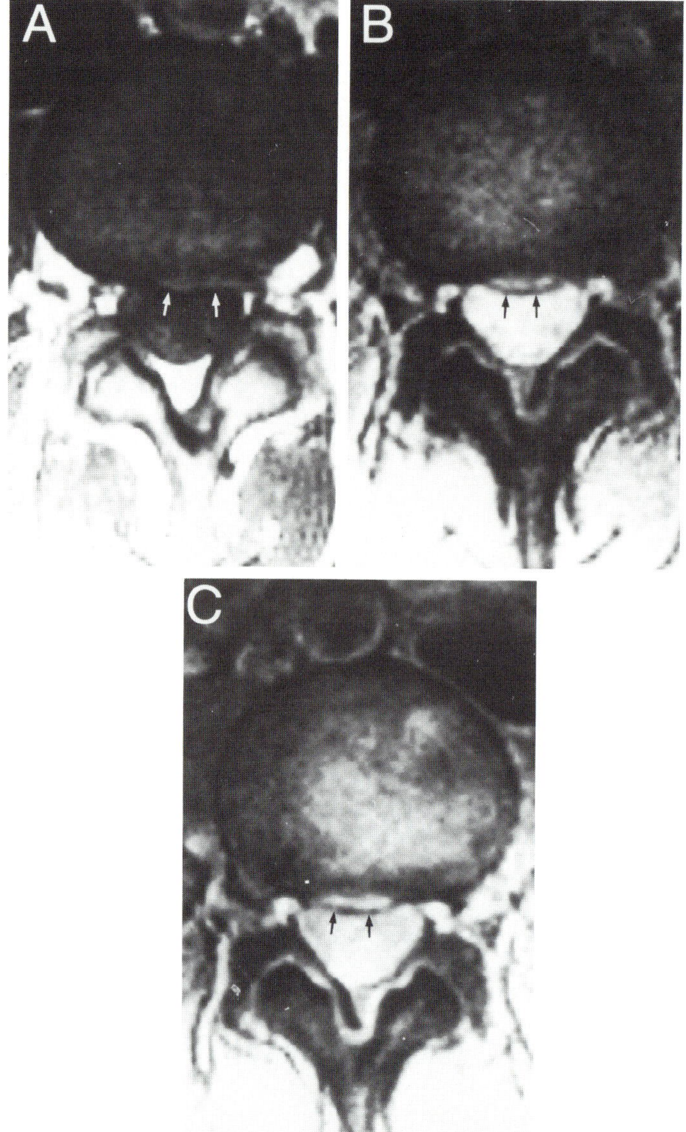

FIG 3–12.
Protrusion of the L3-4 disk. **A,** axial T_1-weighted SE (500/17) image through the L3-4 disk. Note the focal protrusion *(arrow)* of the posterior central portion of the L3-4 disk. **B,** and **C,** axial FLASH (200/13/10 and 40 degree) images through the L3-4 disk. Note the high signal intensity of the protruded segment on these gradient echo studies *(black arrows).*

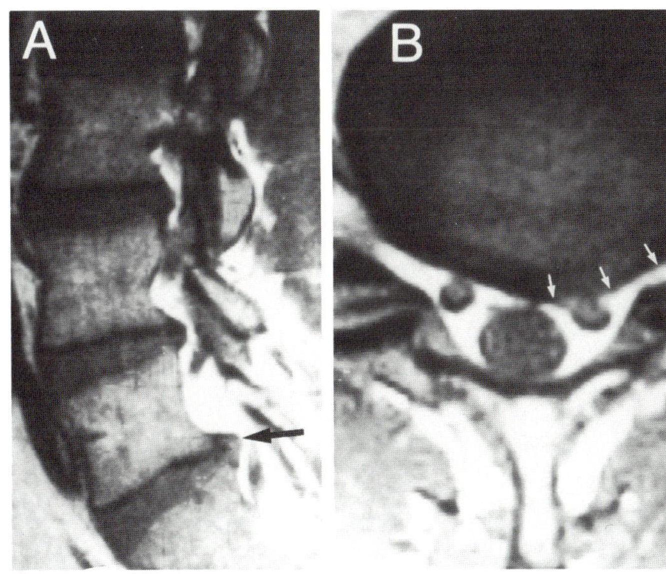

FIG 3–13.
Lateral L5-S1 disk protrusion. **A,** parasagittal T_1-weighted SE (500/17) image through the lumbar spine. *Black arrow* denotes protrusion of the L5-S1 disk. A milder degree of protrusion of the L4-5 disk is also noted. **B,** axial T_1-weighted SE (500/17) image through the L5-S1 disk. Note the asymmetrical protrusion of the L5-S1 disk *(small white arrows)* to the left. There is mild posterior displacement of the S1 nerve root.

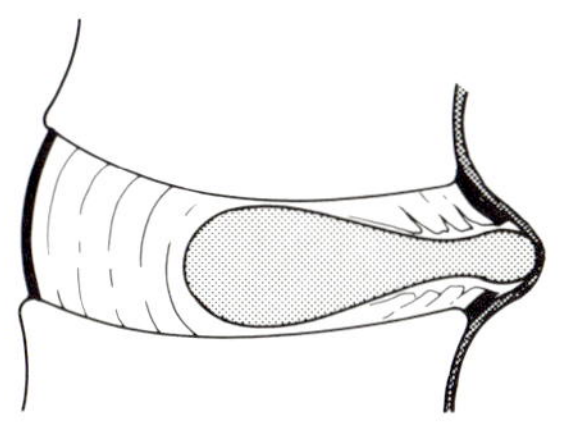

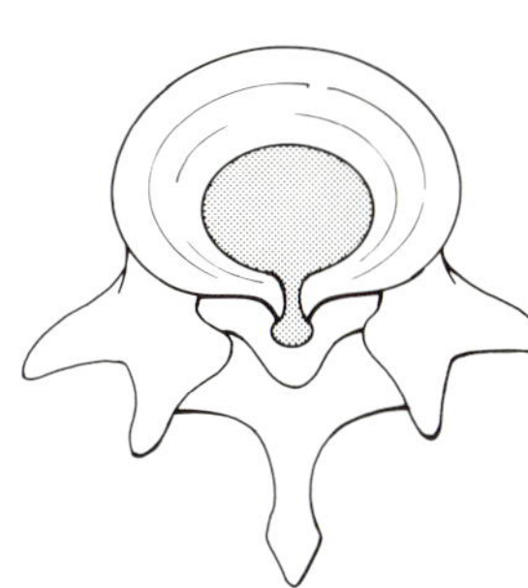

FIG 3–14.
Schematic diagrammatic representation of an extruded lumbar disk. An extruded disk results in a subligamentous mass of nuclear material that remains contiguous with the interspace of origin. The mass may have an increased or decreased signal on T_2-weighted images. Extruded disks have ruptured through the anulus fibrosis *(dark black line)* but are usually contained to some degree by the posterior longitudinal ligament *(dotted gray line).*

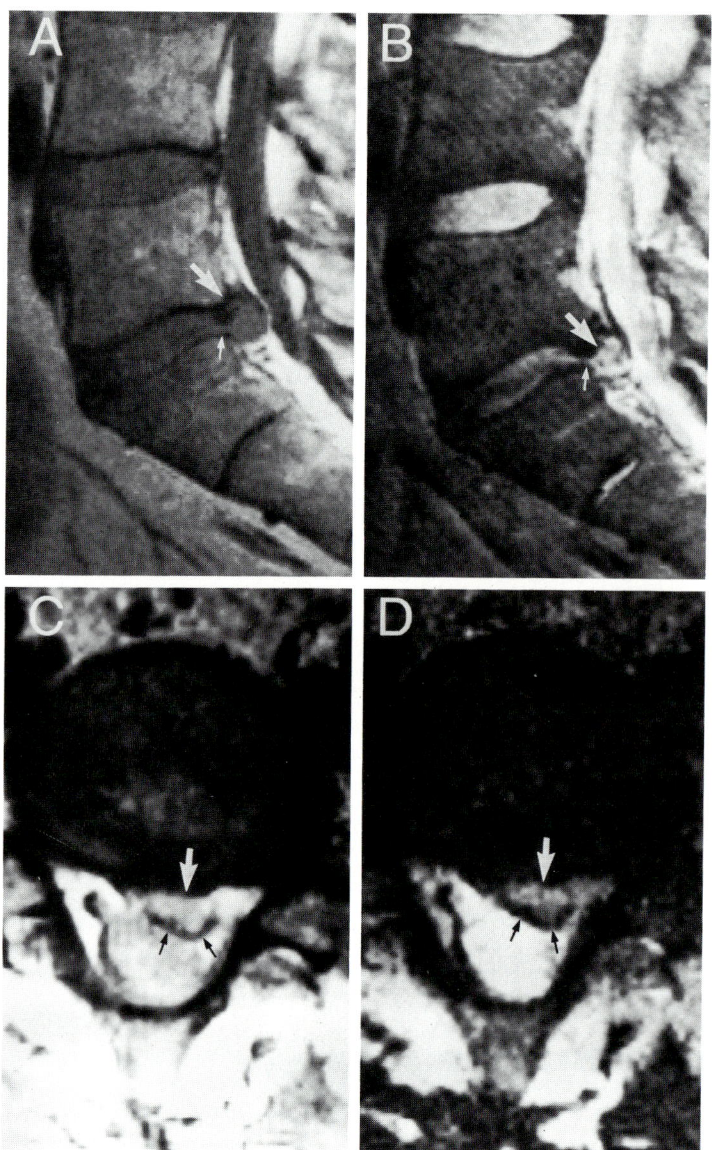

FIG 3–15.
Extruded L5-S1 disk. **A,** sagittal T_1-weighted SE (500/17). There is subligamentous herniation of the L5-S1 disk *(large white arrow).* The disk fragment itself, however, remains connected by a thin pedicle *(small white arrow)* to the parent disk. **B,** sagittal T_2-weighted SE (2000/90). The extruded disk fragment demonstrates a high signal intensity *(large white arrow),* greater than the parent disk. Again a thin pedicle connecting the fragment to the parent disk is noted *(small white arrow).* Intermediate SE (2000/20) (**C**) and T_2-weighted SE (**D**) (2000/90) axial images through the L5-S1 disk herniation. The herniated segment demonstrates a high signal intensity on both sequences *(large white arrow).* Note the curvilinear area of decreased signal intensity outlining the herniated disk segment *(small black arrows)* on both sequences. This area of decreased signal intensity is thought to represent portions of the anulus fibrosis carried with the disk herniation as well as its confluence with the stretched posterior longitudinal ligament.

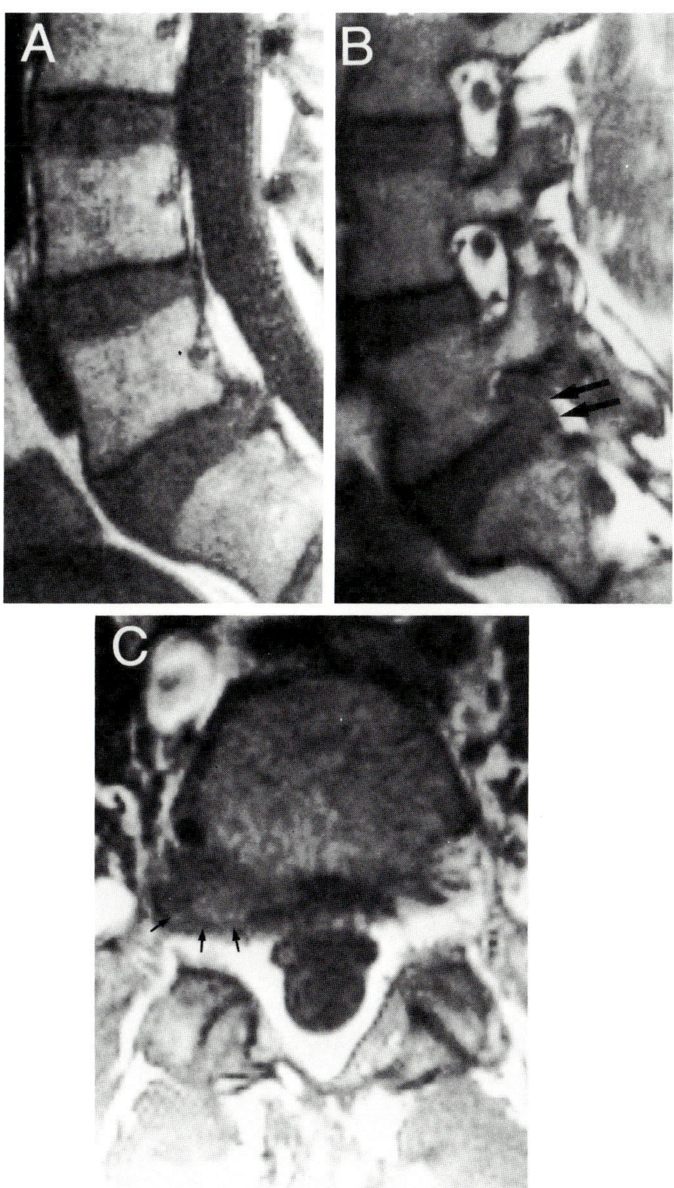

FIG 3–16.
Lateral extruded L5-S1 disk. **A,** sagittal T_1-weighted SE (500/17) image through the lower lumbar spine. Note that there is apparent mild herniation of the posterior aspect of the L5-S1 disk. **B,** parasagittal T_1-weighted SE (500/17) image through the right neural foramina. Note obliteration of the normal epidural fat-signal within the neural foramen and an inability to separate the dorsal nerve root ganglion from the large soft tissue mass contiguous with the L5-S1 disk *(black arrows).* **C,** axial T_1-weighted SE (500/17) image through the L5-S1 neural foramen. Note the soft tissue mass representing a lateral extruded disk *(small black arrows)* within the neural foramen on the right.

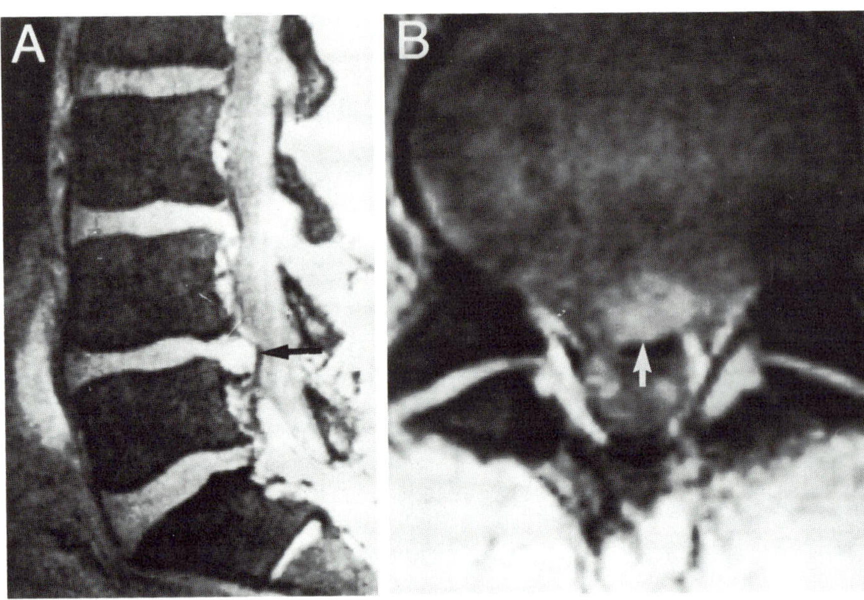

FIG 3–17.
Midline extruded L4-5 disk. **A,** FLASH (200/13/60 degree) image just to the left of midline. *Black arrow* denotes a large central L4-5 disk extrusion. **B,** axial FLASH (200/13/60 degree) image through the L4-5 disk. The *white arrow* denotes the large central disk herniation.

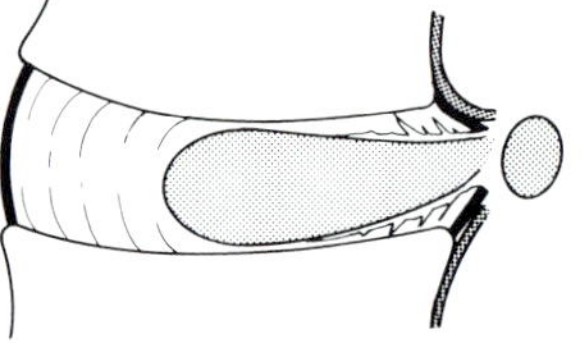

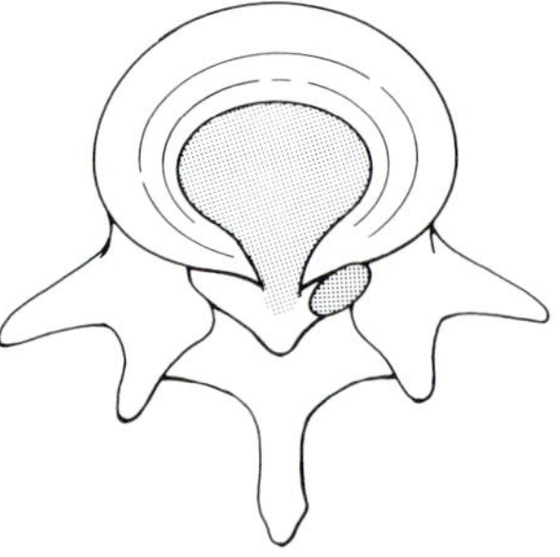

FIG 3–18.
Schematic diagram of a lumbar disk free fragment (sequestered). A sequestered disk is best appreciated on sagittal T_2-weighted images where it can be identified as an isolated fragment of high-signal nuclear material no longer contiguous with the parent disk. They may lie anterior or posterior to the posterior longitudinal ligament and inferior or superior to the adjacent interspace. In this diagram there is disruption of both the anulus *(dark black line)* and posterior longitudinal ligament *(dotted gray line).*

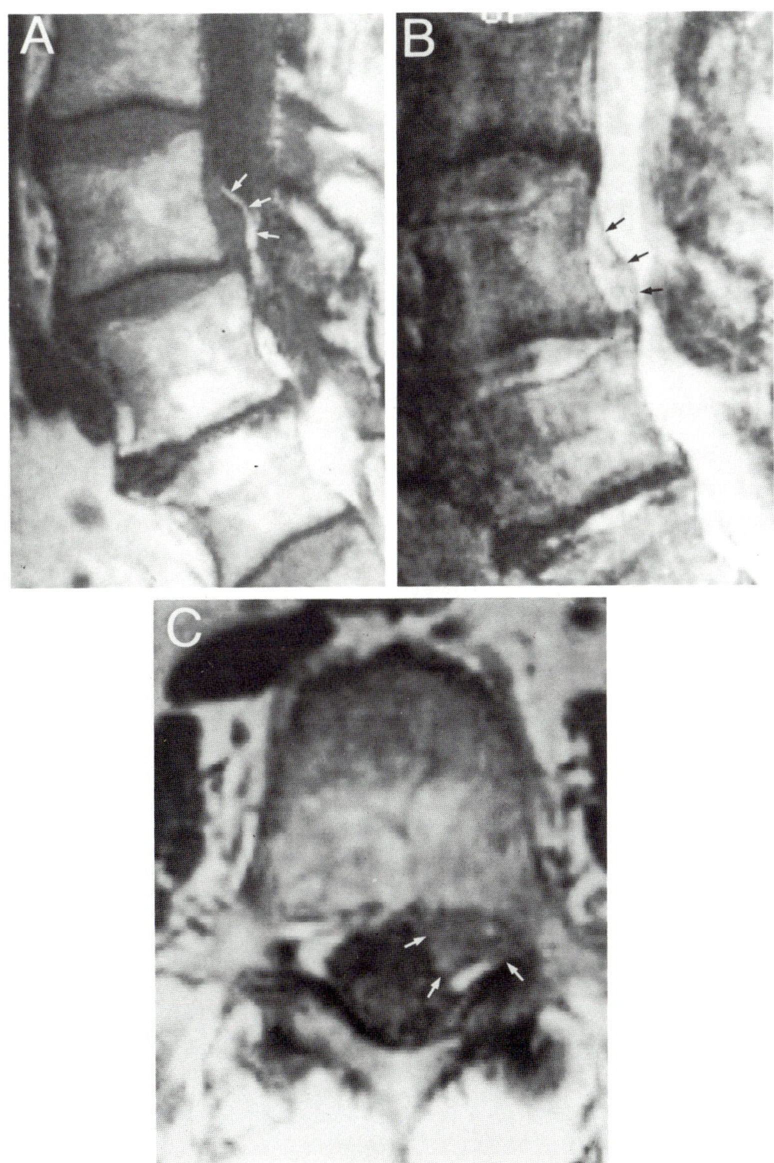

FIG 3–19.

Migrated free fragment, L4-5 disk. **A,** sagittal T_1-weighted SE (500/17) image through the lower lumbar spine. There is narrowing of the L4-5 and L5-S1 disk space with type II vertebral body changes at the later level. There is a soft tissue density identified posterior to the inferior aspect of the L3 vertebral body *(small white arrows).* The high signal intensity surrounding this disk fragment most likely represents epidural fat. This free disk fragment at surgery was found posterior to the vertebral body but anterior to the posterior longitudinal ligament. Sagittal T_2-weighted SE (2000/90) (**B**) and axial T_1-weighted SE (**C**) (500/17) images. The migrated herniated L4-5 disk fragment is again demarcated by the *small arrows.*

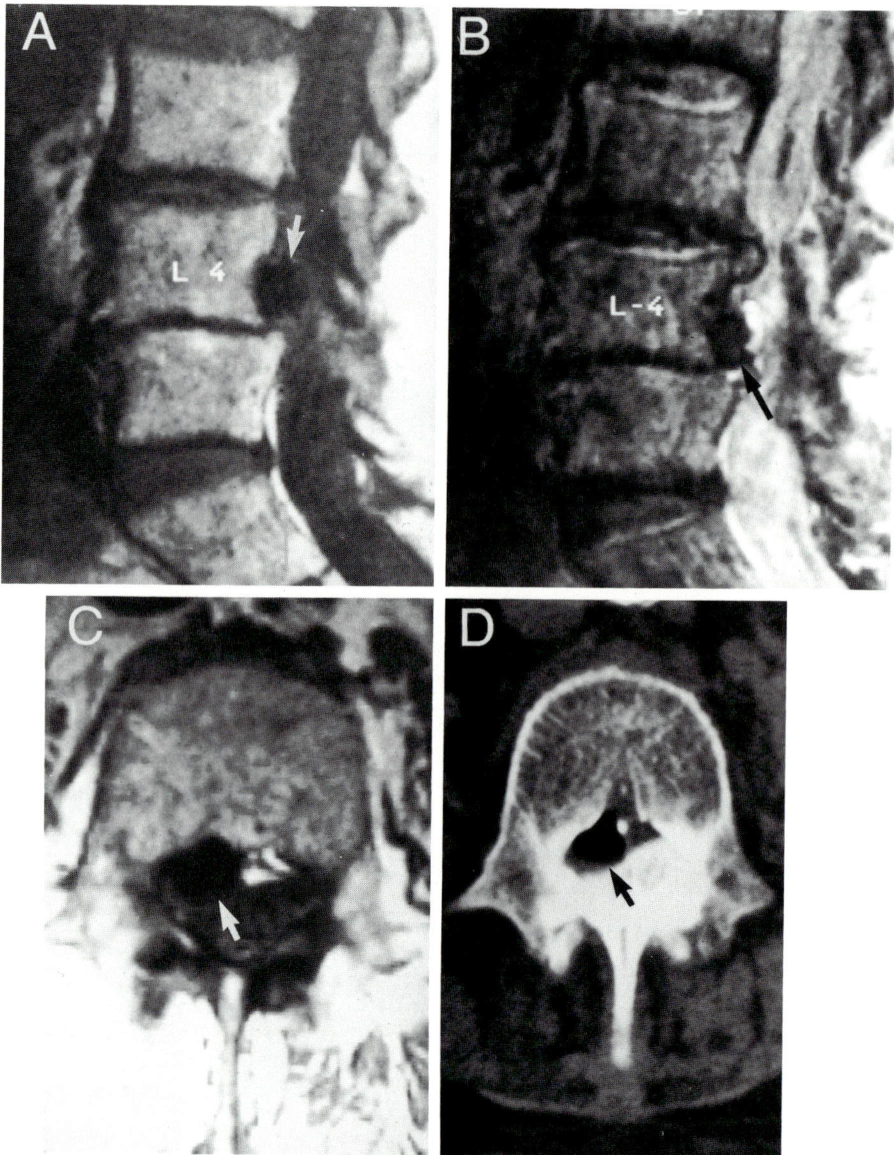

FIG 3–20.

Migrated herniated free fragment, L4-5 disk. Sagittal T_1-weighted SE (500/17) (**A**) and T_2-weighted SE (2000/90) (**B**) images through the lower lumbar spine. There is an ovoid area of decreased signal intensity noted posterior to the inferior aspect of the L4 vertebral body *(white arrow)*. There is moderate to severe narrowing of the L3-4 and severe narrowing of the L4-5 disk. A central disk herniation is noted at the L3-4 level. At surgery this ovoid area of decreased signal intensity represented a large migrated extruded L4-5 disk fragment that contained gas (vacuum phenomenon) *(black arrow)*. Axial T_1-weighted SE (500/17) (**A**) and high-resolution computed tomogram (**D**) (CT) with intrathecal contrast through the inferior aspect of the L4 vertebral body. *Black arrow* denotes the herniated migrated free fragment complete with its own vacuum phenomenon.

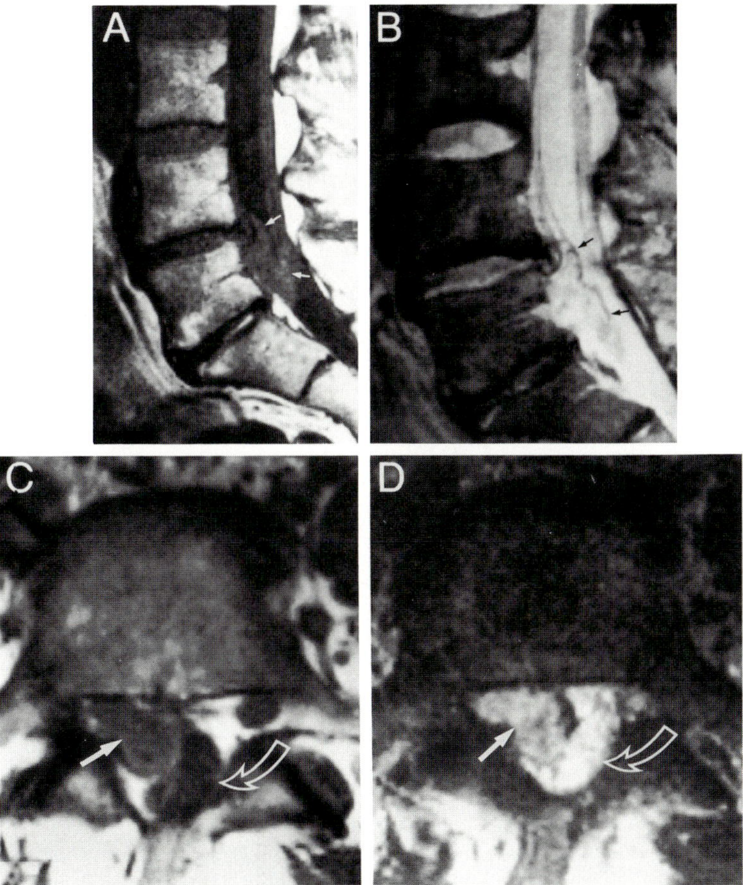

FIG 3–21.
Free fragment, L4-5 disk. Sagittal midline T_1-weighted SE (500/17)(**A**) and T_2-weighted SE (2000/90) (**B**) images. *Arrows* denote a large soft tissue mass that has a high signal intensity on the T_2-weighted sequence occupying a large portion of the spinal canal posterior to the L5 vertebral body. At surgery this was a large free fragment that had ruptured through the posterior longitudinal ligament. Axial T_1-weighted SE (500/17) (**C**) and T_2-weighted SE (2000/90) (**D**) images through the L5 vertebral body level. *Closed white arrow* denotes the large free fragment that is again shown to have a high signal intensity on the T_2-weighted sequence. *Curved open arrow* denotes the markedly displaced and compressed thecal sac at this level.

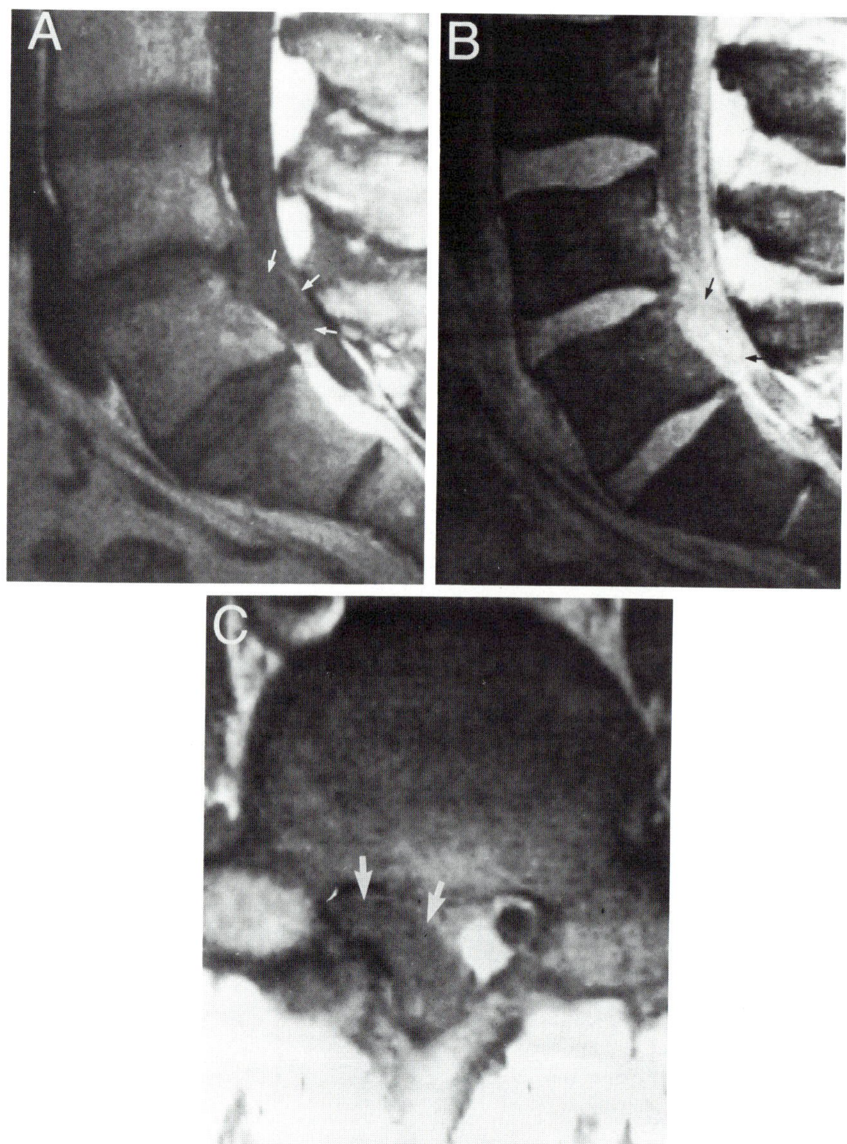

FIG 3–22.
Free fragment, L4-5 disk. **A,** sagittal T_1-weighted SE (500/17) image just to the right of midline. *Small white arrows* denote an ill-defined soft tissue mass lying posterior to the L5 vertebral body. Differentiation of this large free fragment is not as clear on this sequence as on **B,** which is a FLASH (200/13/60 degree) image where the free disk fragment has a high signal intensity relative to the adjacent cerebrospinal fluid (CSF) *(small black arrows).* **C,** axial T_1-weighted SE (500/17) image that demonstrates the large free fragment *(white arrows)* obscuring the region of the S1 nerve root and distorting and displacing the thecal sac posteriorly.

(4) may require a more extensive surgical approach for complete removal.

The reason for the high signal intensity of extruded disks or free fragments is by no means clear. Pech and Haughton[47] have suggested that gross degeneration of intervertebral disks may be present despite their high signal on long TR/TE images. It may be reasonable to assume that such large fragments may be symptomatic early in their clinical course, bringing the patient to seek medical attention (and a diagnostic workup) soon after the onset of symptoms. That is to say, large extruded and sequestered disks that present earlier may have a higher water content than those that present later.

An alternative explanation for the same finding takes into consideration the fact that with rupture and loss of the confined fluid from the disk there is initially a reparative process that leads to a transient gain in water content of the disk.[15,16] Again, assuming an acute

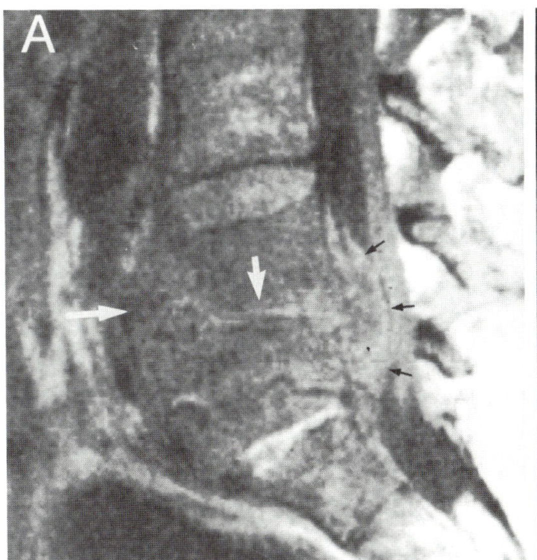

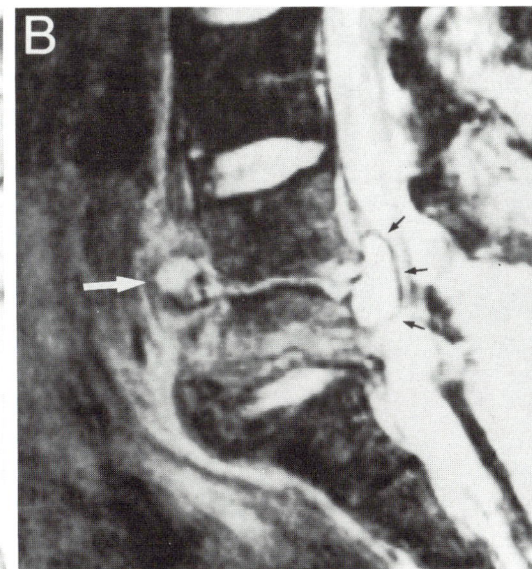

FIG 3–23.
Disk space infection with an epidural abscess formation. **A,** classic appearance of vertebral osteomyelitis is depicted by decreased signal intensity of the adjacent L4 and L5 vertebral bodies and an indiscernible L4-5 interspace. Large ventral and dorsal soft tissue masses *(long white arrow* and *small black arrows)* adjacent to the L4-5 interspace *(short white arrow).* **B,** sagittal T_2-weighted SE (2000/90) image through the lower lumbar spine. There is a linear high nonanatomical signal in the region of the L4-5 interspace that appears to communicate directly with large ventral and dorsal high signal intensity masses *(white and black arrows).* At surgery these represented areas of epidural abscess. Note the mottled high signal intensity of the L5 vertebral body.

clinical presentation, this may present as a high signal intensity on more T_2-weighted images. There are also vascular correlations between disk changes and the number and location of vessels surrounding penetrating areas of disk pathology.

While herniated disks appear more common laterally, presumably because of the absence of fibers of the posterior longitudinal ligament and a thinner portion of the anulus, they can appear both centrally and far laterally in the neural foramina, where they can be confused with neurogenic tumors. When the fragment is adjacent to the interspace, it may have a somewhat rounded configuration, but if it migrates superiorly or inferiorly to the interspace, it frequently appears oval or oblong.

The differential diagnosis for the MR findings of sequestered lumbar disks includes epidural abscesses, extradural neoplasms (such as neurofibroma), and postoperative epidural fibrosis or fluid collections. Epidural abscesses are frequently associated with disk space infection and can be distinguished from free fragments by the characteristic signal changes seen at the infected interspace and adjacent end-plates (Fig 3–23). Extradural or intradural tumor may be more difficult to exclude, although multiplicity of lesions and/or the presence of bone marrow changes would likewise help to narrow the differential diagnosis (Fig 3–24). While postoperative scar in the lumbar spine is typically identified as a loss of signal intensity from the epidural fat on T_1-weighted images, it often demonstrates a high signal intensity on T_2-weighted images, particularly anteriorly and laterally, and may be difficult to separate from a disk fragment (Fig 3–25). The presence or absence of mass effect on the thecal sac may help to distinguish the two. In any event, the utilization of gadolinium diethylenetriamine penta-acetic acid (Gd-DTPA) has proved to be a highly efficient means to differentiate between epidural fibrosis alone and recurrent disk herniation. Postoperative changes may also mimic high signal intensity extradural defects such as free fragments on T_2-weighted images, but they usually resolve within 4 to 6 weeks following surgery.

In a prospective evaluation of surface coil MR, CT, and myelography in lumbar herniated disk disease and canal stenosis, there was an 82.6% agreement between MR and surgical findings for both type and location of disease, 83% agreement between CT and surgical findings, and 71.8% agreement between myelography and surgical findings. There was a 92.5% agreement when MR and CT were used jointly and an 89.4% agreement when CT and myelography were used jointly.[34]

Subsequent improvements in technology such as better optimized surface coils, fast gradient echo scans, oblique images, refocussing sequences, saturated pulses, volume studies, and Gd-DTPA have resulted in im-

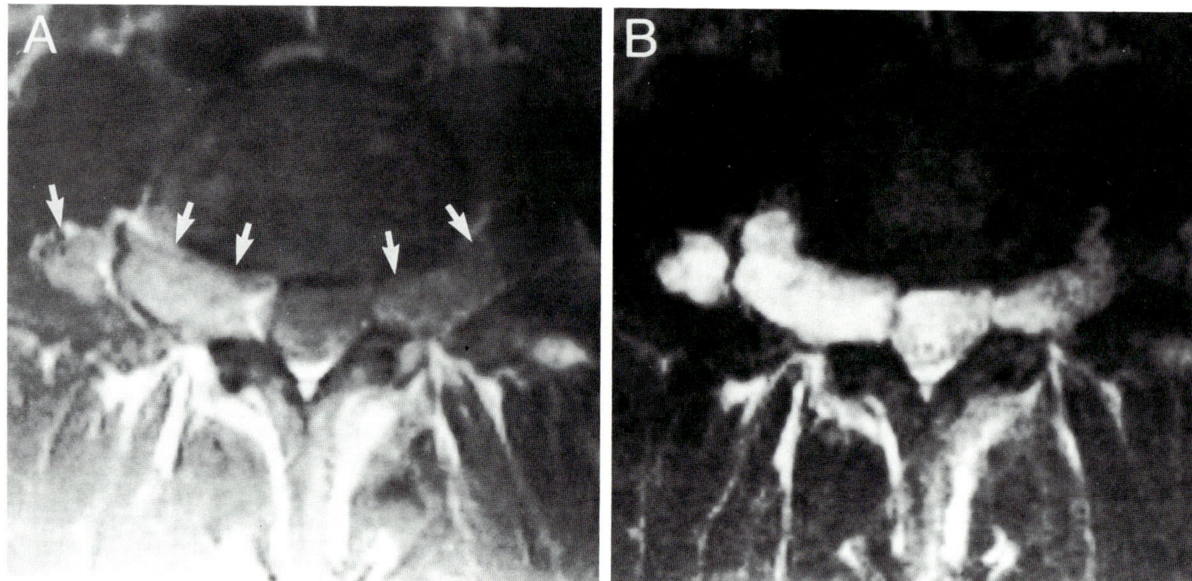

FIG 3–24.
Bilateral neurofibromas, L3-4 level. Axial intermediate SE (2000/20) (**A**) and T_2-weighted SE (2000/90) (**B**) images through the L3-4 neural foramen. *Arrows* denote ovoid masses of high signal intensity occupying the neural foramen bilaterally. At surgery these were documented to represent neurofibromas.

proved image quality, which suggests that the accuracy of MR at this point is even higher.

Thoracic disk herniations, although less common than lumbar cervical herniations, have been noted with a greater frequency with the advancement of imaging techniques[37] (Figs 3–26 and 3–27). The lowermost thoracic interspaces are most frequently involved. Paresthesias below the level of the lesion; loss of sensation, both deep and superficial; and paraparesis or paraplegia are the usual clinical manifestations. The symptom complex,

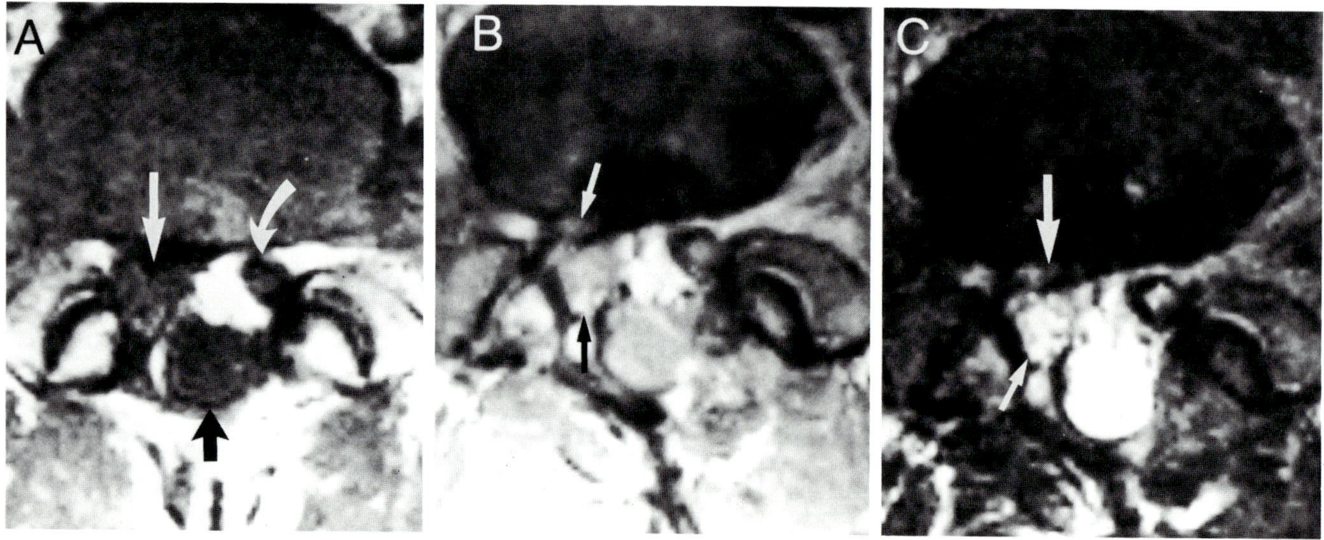

FIG 3–25.
Epidural fibrosis. Axial T_1-weighted SE (500/17) (**A**), intermediate SE (2000/30) (**B**), and T_2-weighted SE (2000/90) (**C**) images through the L5-S1 disk level. A large soft tissue mass is noted on **A** surrounding the region of the S1 nerve root on the right *(large white arrow). Curved white arrow* represents the S1 nerve root on the left. *Black arrow* denotes the thecal sac. Note the laminectomy defect posteriorly on the left. This soft tissue mass surrounding the S1 nerve root is seen on **B** and **C** to have a high signal intensity *(small black and white arrows,* respectively). Anteriorly a small herniated disk (*white arrow,* **B** and *large white arrow,* **C**) is seen. At surgery a large mass of epidural fibrosis was documented, but the region anteriorly where the herniated disk is noted on MR was not surgically visualized.

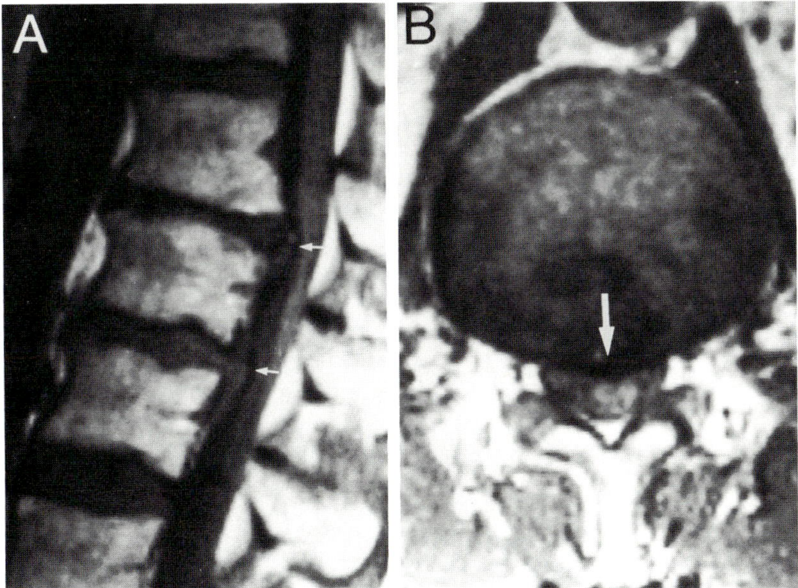

FIG 3–26.
Thoracic disk herniations. **A,** sagittal midline T_1-weighted SE (500/17) images of the lower thoracic spine. Anterior extradural soft tissue masses are noted at the T9-10 and T10-11 levels *(small white arrows).* **B,** axial T_1-weighted SE (500/17) image through the T9-10 disk demonstrating central protrusion *(arrow).* The normal CSF space within the thecal sac anterior to the spinal cord has been obliterated and the posterior margin of the disk is in direct contact with the spinal cord.

however, may be difficult to interpret. Retrospective studies with surface coil MR have shown that it is highly accurate. Over a two-year period, 63 patients who had thoracic examinations with symptoms, where thoracic disk herniation was part of the initial differential, were studied. Magnetic resonance identified 20 thoracic disk herniations in 17 of these patients. Sixteen suspected herniations in 13 patients had a confirmatory imaging study (plain film myelography–computed tomography with metrizamide [PFM-CTM]) and/or surgical verification (8 patients with surgery at 10 levels, including 6 patients with PFM-CTM at 8 levels and 5 patients with PFM-CTM at 6 levels without surgery). The result with CTM-PFM was positive at all 8 surgical levels and at 6 levels without surgery (14/14). When considered alone, PFM showed extradural defects at 9/14 levels. If sagittal and axial images on MR were considered together, then MR defined 16/16 abnormal thoracic levels (surgical verification at 10). Thin slices are critical for adequate evaluation. The configuration of the herniation is similar to that seen in the lumbar and cervical regions, although the extradural defect is usually not as large. Indentation and rotation of the cord are ancillary signs that can be utilized. Caution must be taken, however, in the evaluation of thoracic disk herniations when the usual orientation of the phase-encoded and frequency direction has

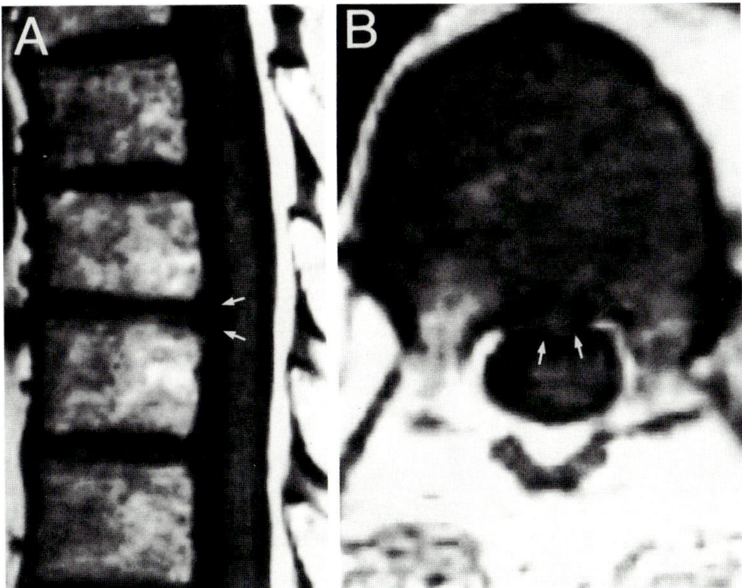

FIG 3–27.
Thoracic disk herniation. **A,** sagittal midline T_1-weighted SE (500/17) image that demonstrates an extruded disk at the T8-9 level *(small white arrows).* **B,** axial T_1-weighted SE (500/17) image through the T8-9 disk. *Small white arrows* demarcate the herniated segment.

been reversed to compensate for cardiac and respiratory ghosting. In these situations, the chemical shift artifact will now appear in an anterior to posterior direction and can obscure disk herniation on the sagittal view.[48]

Cervical disk herniation, especially when central or large, is well appreciated on routine sagittal and axial MR images (Figs 3–28 and 3–29). Again, thin slices (3 mm or less) are critical for accurate diagnosis (Figs 3–30 and 3–31). The signal intensity of the intervertebral disk on T_2-weighted images is not as helpful as it is in the lumbar region for identifying the presence or absence of degeneration. Cervical disk herniation is usually identified on the sagittal images as an anterior or anterior lateral extradural defect that may indent or compress the cervical cord. In a prospective study to compare the accuracy of surface coil MR with metrizamide myelography (MM) and computed tomography with metrizamide (CTM), there was surgical agreement in 74% of patients with surface coil MR, 85% with CTM, and 67% with MM.[35] There was 90% agreement with surgical findings when surface coil MR and CTM were used jointly and 92% agreement when CTM and MM were used jointly. In general, surface coil MR was as sensitive as CTM for identification of disease level but not as specific for type of disease. Metrizamide myelography was a modality least specific for disease type. The major advantage of CTM was its ability to distinguish bone from soft tissue, for which contrast material may be unnecessary. A follow-up study utilizing oblique MR images of the lateral neural canal and foramen improved[36] the accuracy of MR by providing an additional orthogonal view of the foramen (Fig 3–32). Because the routine parasagittal images fail to adequately depict the ventral, inferior, and lateral anatomical courses of the neural foramen in the cervical region, an additional view is often required. Thus if routine sagittal and axial images fail to identify a definite extradural defect in the presence of well-defined radiculopathy, oblique images may be indicated. This problem underscores a long-held radiologic maxim that at least two orthogonal views of an area are frequently necessary for complete characterization of an abnormality. The major advantages of surface coil MR imaging are the capacity to display the foramen magnum and cervical region in their entirety, the characterization of cord contour and delineation of signal alterations within the cord substance, the high quality of the imaging that allows easy evaluation of regions proximal or distal to severe stenosis or block, the easy acquisition of multiple orthogonal planar images in the depiction of the neural foramina, and the ability to obtain images without the use of contrast material. Nevertheless, preliminary work

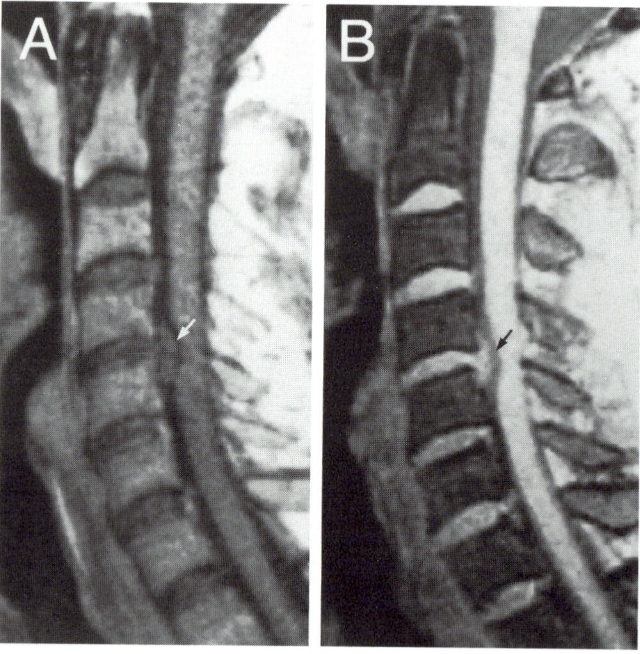

FIG 3–28.
C4-5 disk herniation. **A,** sagittal midline T_1-weighted SE (500/17) image through the cervical spine. There is a moderately large soft tissue mass extending posteriorly from the C4-5 disk space indenting the anterior aspect of the cervical cord *(small white arrow).* **B,** sagittal midline FLASH (200/13/60 degree) image through the cervical spine. Note that the herniated disk is well demarcated from the cervical cord and surrounding CSF *(small black arrow).*

with Gd-DTPA demonstrates that it also may play a role in the evaluation of cervical extradural disease. As has been shown with intravenous CT by Russell et al.,[49] enhancement of the epidural plexus and/or peridiskal scar may prove an aid in increasing the conspicuity of extradural defects (Fig 3–33).

Occasional difficulty in distinguishing bone from soft tissue on surface coil MR imaging is probably due to variable signal intensities encountered in the herniated disk, ligamentous hypertrophy, and osteophytes as well as to partial volume averaging of adjacent structures. The reason for the variable signal from the osteophytes is, we presume, related to the variable presence and composition of bone marrow within them. Osteophyte signal can vary from markedly decreased signal intensity when the bone is dense to an iso- or hyperintensity relative to the disk or the adjacent vertebral body when fatty marrow is more abundant. Hypertrophic bony changes that produce no discernible signal on surface coil MR imaging may be indiscernible from adjacent cerebral spinal fluid without careful T_2-weighted images or fast gradient echo scans with a small flip angle (Fig 3–34).

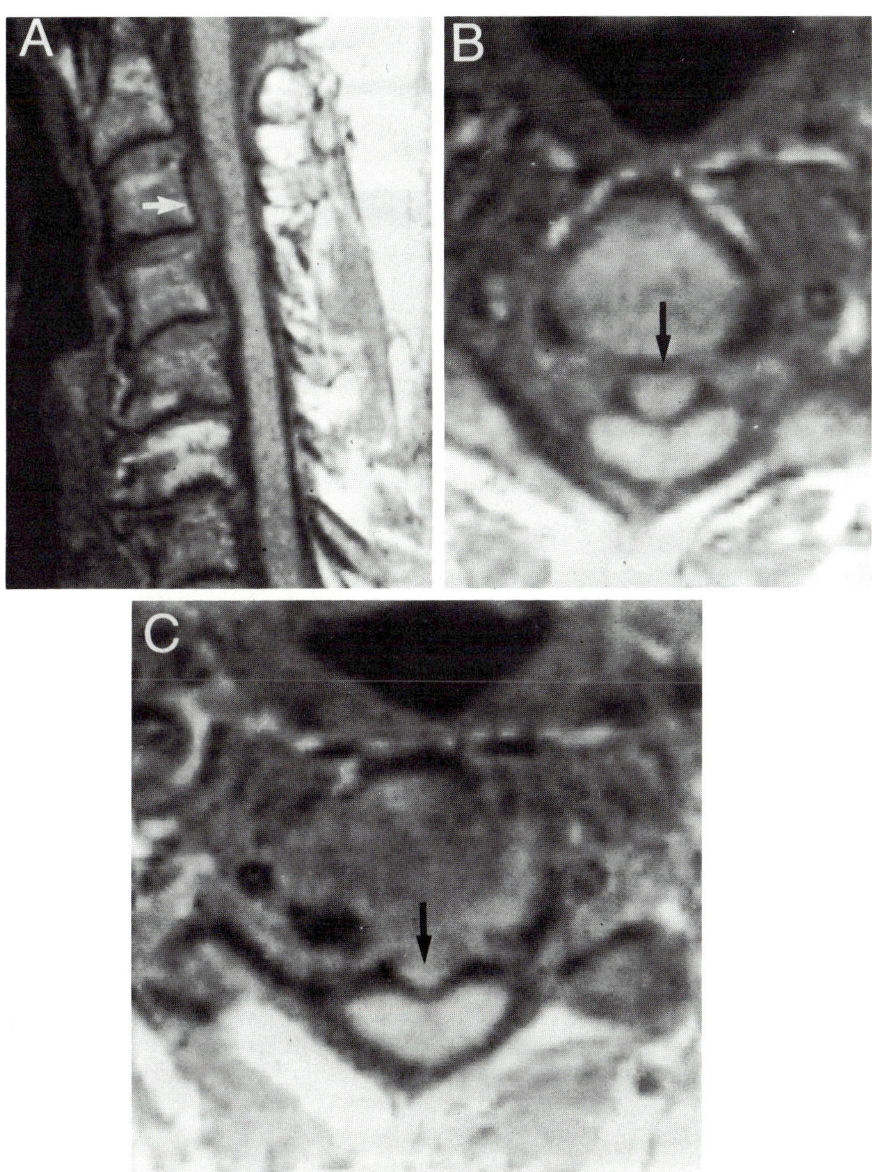

FIG 3–29.
Cervical free disk fragment. **A,** sagittal midline T_1-weighted SE (500/17) image through the cervical spine. There is a large soft tissue mass located posterior to the C3 vertebral body with the inferior extent at the C3-4 disk level *(white arrow).* There is indentation on the anterior aspect of the cervical cord. A smaller disk herniation is noted at the C4-5 level again with indentation on the cervical cord. High signal intensity noted in the C6 vertebral body is thought to represent type II degenerative change. **B** and **C,** axial T_1-weighted SE (500/17) images through the level of the C3 vertebral body and C3-4 disk, respectively. Note the ovoid soft tissue mass anterior to the cord at the C3 vertebral body level *(black arrow)* in **B,** which represents a free disk fragment that has migrated superiorly behind the posterior longitudinal ligament.

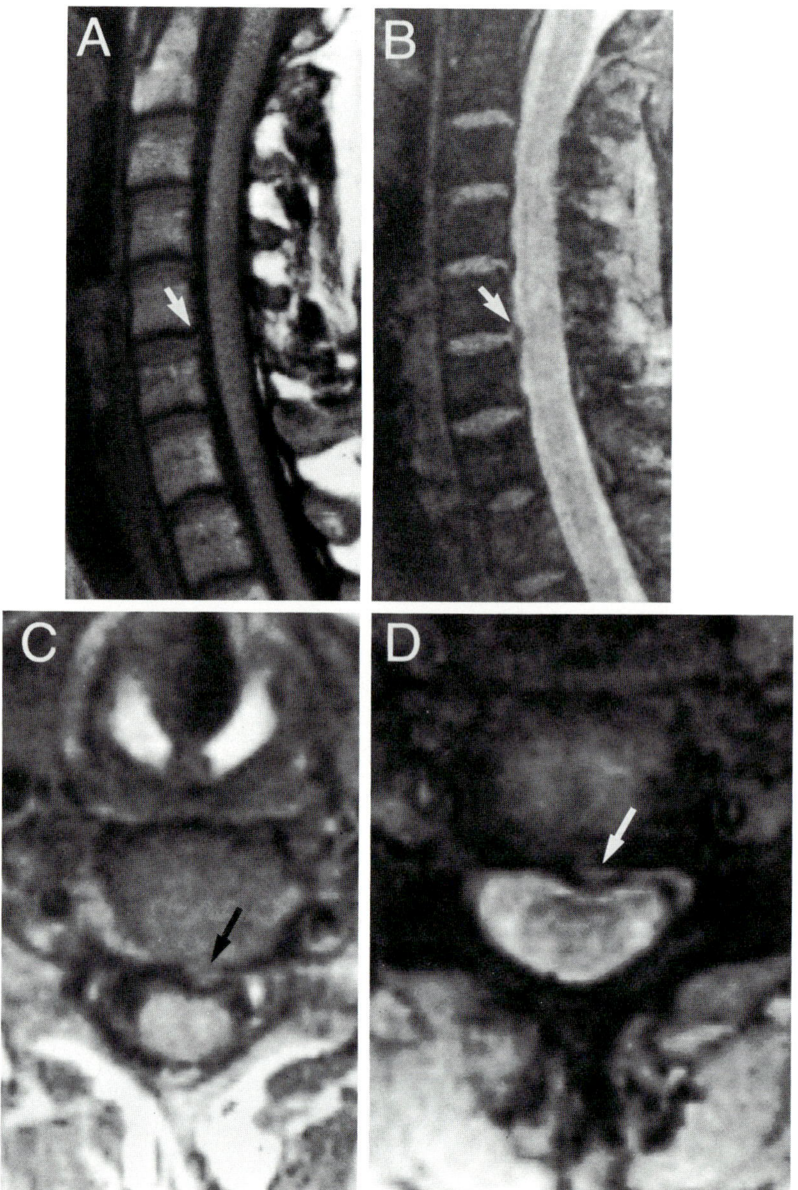

FIG 3–30.

C5-6 disk herniation. **A,** sagittal midline SE (500/17) image through the cervical spine. A small anterior extradural defect is noted at the C5-6 level *(white arrow).* **B,** sagittal midline FLASH (200/13/10 degrees) image through the cervical spine. The small anterior extradural defect is again noted *(white arrow)* outlined by the high signal intensity of the adjacent CSF. **C,** T_1-weighted SE (500/17) axial image through the C5-6 disk. The central left disk herniation is demarcated by the *black arrow.* **D,** FLASH (200/13/10 degree) axial image through the C5-6 disk. The *white arrow* demarcates the high signal intensity in the herniated disk at this level. Note the high signal intensity of the CSF relative to the cord, which is characteristic of this low flip-angle gradient echo scan producing the so-called CSF myelogram effect.

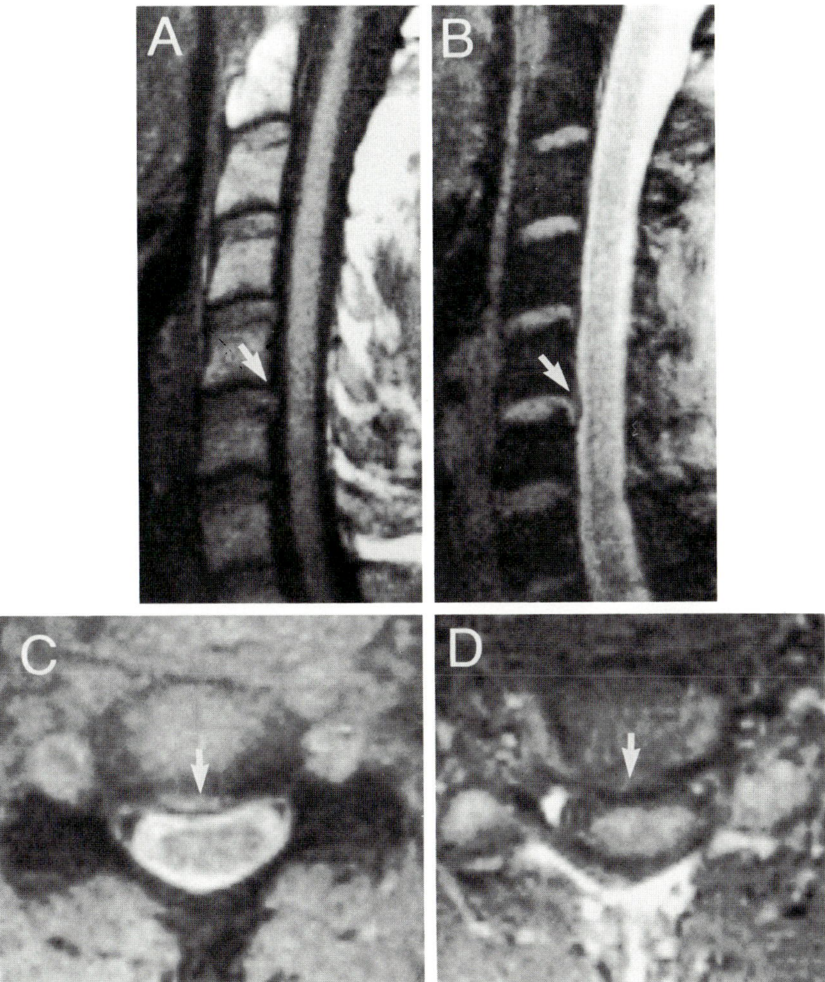

FIG 3–31.
C5-6 disk herniation. **A,** sagittal T_1-weighted SE (500/17) image through the cervical spine. There is an anterior extradural defect at the C5-6 level *(white arrow).* **B,** sagittal FLASH (200/13/10 degree) image through the cervical spine. The *white arrow* denotes the disk herniation. T_1-weighted SE (500/17) (**C**) and FLASH (200/13/10 degrees) (**D**) axial images through the C5-6 disk. A soft tissue mass similar in signal intensity to the adjacent intervertebral disk is noted on both sequences projecting posteriorly *(white arrow).* The conspicuity of the extradural defect is better appreciated on **D** secondary to the high signal intensity of the adjacent CSF.

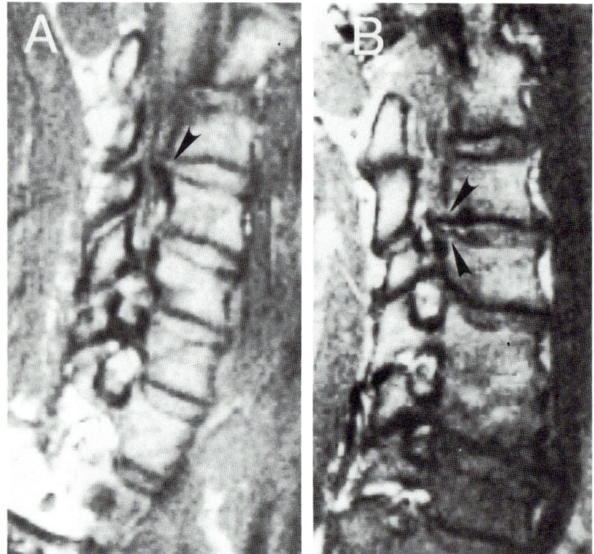

FIG 3–32.
Cervical oblique images. **A** and **B,** 45-degree oblique T_1-weighted SE (500/17) images through the cervical neural foramen. In **A,** the *black arrow* denotes lateral disk herniation at the C3-4 disk level. **B** demonstrates hypertrophic degenerative changes of the inferior posterior aspect of the C3 vertebral body and the uncinate process of the C4 vertebral body producing bony foraminal stenosis. This additional orthogonal plane oriented to the true course of the neural foramen can be useful for better characterization of bone vs. soft tissue abnormalities.

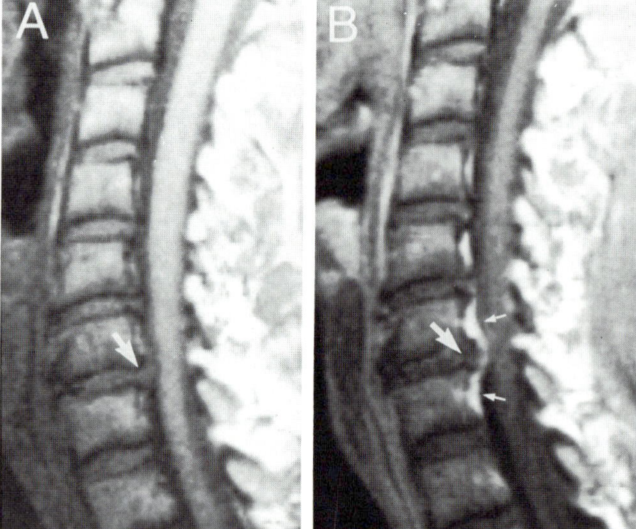

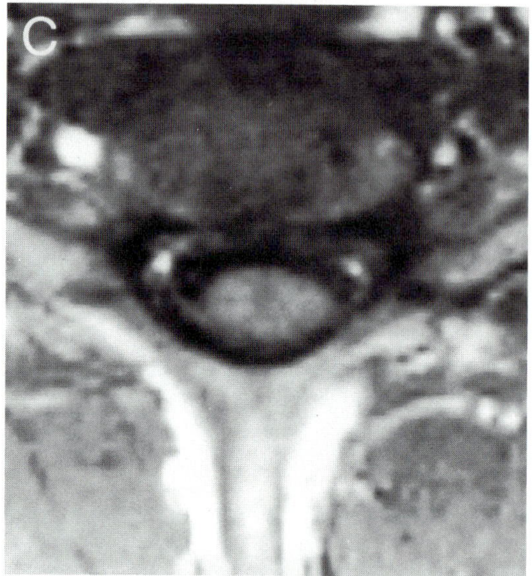

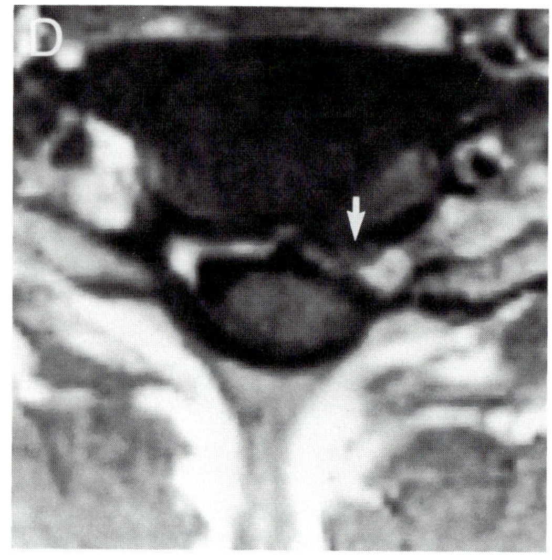

FIG 3–33.
C6-7 disk herniation with and without Gd-DTPA. **A** and **B** represent sagittal T_1-weighted SE (500/17) images through the cervical spine before and after the administration of 0.1 mmole/kg of Gd-DTPA, respectively. The anterior extradural defect at C6-7 on **A** is denoted by the *white arrow.* Following the administration of Gd-DTPA (**B**), there is enhancement of the epidural venous plexus lateral to the midline, which more clearly outlines the anterior extradural defect caused by the cervical disk herniation *(white arrows).* **C** and **D** represent axial T_1-weighted SE (500/17) images through the C6-7 disk before and after the administration of Gd-DTPA, respectively. The lateral disk herniation is not as well appreciated on the precontrast study (**C**) as on the postcontrast study (**D**) because of adjacent enhancement of epidural venous plexus in the latter. The enhancement of the venous plexus appears to increase the conspicuity of extradural defects following the administration of Gd-DTPA. Enhancement of the peripheral margin of the disk may also represent some granulation tissue in addition to the adjacent epidural venous plexus.

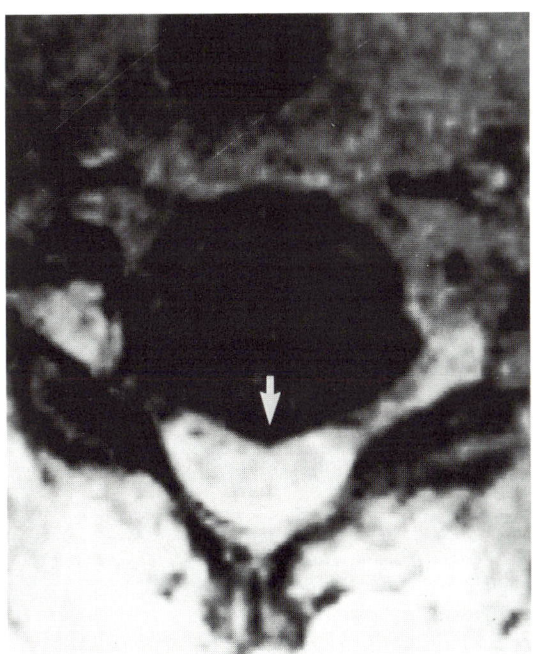

FIG 3–34.
Cervical osteophyte. Axial FLASH (200/13/10 degree) image through the C5 vertebral body. The *arrow* denotes posterior osteophyte formation that indents both the thecal sac and anterior aspect of the cervical cord. The high signal intensity of the CSF on this gradient echo sequence with a low flip angle outlines the decreased signal intensity of the posterior bony osteophyte formation.

While we would maintain that most evaluations of the cervical spine for extradural disease can be done in an adequate fashion with spin-echo T_1-weighted sagittal and axial images, the introduction of fast gradient echo images with small flip angles (less than 15 degrees) has improved the accuracy of the examination by increasing the conspicuity of extradural defects, and recent work has confirmed its value (see Figs 3–28 through 3–31 and 3–34).[50, 51] Gradient echo scans with low flip angles provide a high signal intensity of the cerebrospinal fluid (CSF) relative to the extradural structures providing the so-called CSF myelogram effect in a shorter period of time than can usually be accomplished with T_2-weighted spin-echo images. The major advantages are most apparent in the axial plane. There are sharp delineation of bone and disk margins, excellent contrast between the spinal cord and surrounding subarachnoid space, and clear visualization of the neural foramina and exiting nerve roots. Degenerative bony ridging tends to be of a lower signal intensity than herniated disk material (see Fig 3–34).

This capability, coupled with the potential of utilizing very short TRs (50 msec or less), has stimulated the use of volume imaging for the evaluation of extradural disease in hopes of shortening examination time and decreasing slice thickness. Typically, an anisotropic volume acquired in the sagittal plane with a slab thickness of 10 cm or less can be obtained in less than 10 minutes with partitions producing a contiguous slice thickness of 3 mm or less. When the sagittal plane is used for acquisition, subsequent reconstructions in any plane can be obtained that will produce contiguous sections 2-mm thick or less through the entire field of view. Thus the entire length of the cervical or lumbar spine can be imaged in a multiplanar fashion with one acquisition (Fig 3–35).

The disadvantages of gradient echo imaging relate to problems with field inhomogeneity and contrast detectability of pathologic processes within the cord itself. Thus, if patients present with radiculopathy and myelopathy, or intrinsic cord symptoms alone, additional sagittal multislice multiecho refocussed long TR/TE images (with or without gating) are needed.[50, 52]

An additional adjunct to conventional MR in the evaluation of degenerative disk disease is the utilization of Gd-DTPA. Gadolinium-DTPA is a paramagnetic contrast agent that will show variable degrees of transit from the intravascular space depending on the tissue type. Studies with virgin and postoperative disk herniation indicate that it is the most accurate means of separating epidural fibrosis and disk tissue.[29] There is consistent enhancement of peridiskal fibrosis early (less than 15 minutes postinjection) and variable enhancement of the herniated or degenerated parent disk late (30 minutes postinjection). Enhancement of intervertebral disk does not appear to occur in the normal state and is likely a sequela of the degenerative process[29–53] (Fig 3–36).

Recently, investigators have demonstrated anular tears on MR with T_2-weighted spin-echo that formerly were demonstrated only by diskography or postmortem anatomical studies.[5, 53a] The degenerative changes in the anulus fibrosis in both cadavers and experimental models include several different types of radial tear or rupture. The radial tears have been considered by some to be the most frequent causes of symptomatology. These tears have several stages, including one in which abundant capillaries, precapillaries, and connective tissue enter the tear.[5] Similarly, other studies have noted reactive granulation tissue surrounding herniated disk from nonoperative spines that is similar to that seen postoperatively and appears to reflect scar tissue without evidence of an inflammatory exudate.[12, 21] It makes sense that degenerative disk disease with or without herniation that involves the anulus, posterior longitudinal ligaments, and other associated support structures will result in an attemptive reparative process. Why some but not all de-

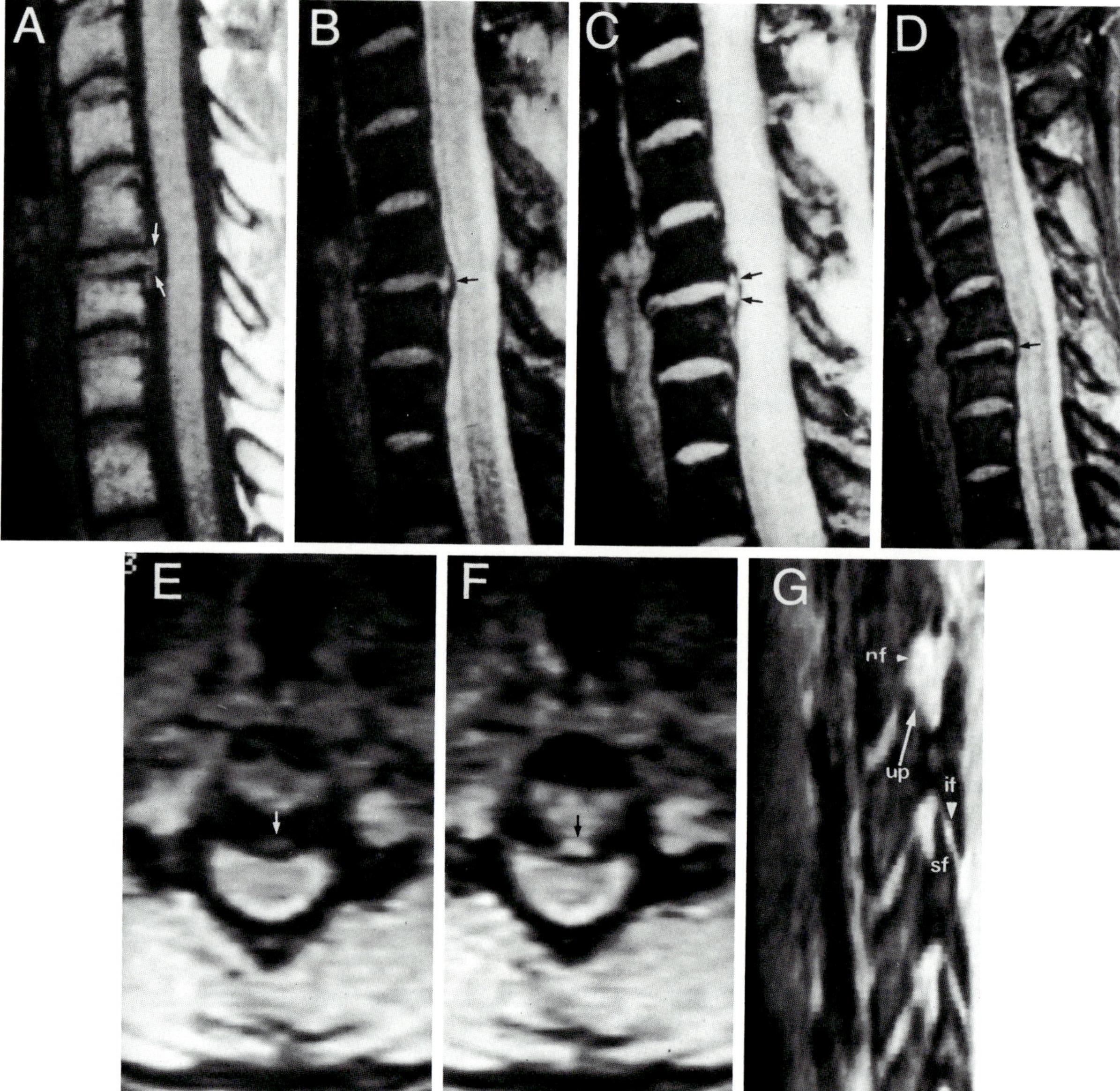

FIG 3–35.
C5-6 disk herniation. **A–C** represent 2D T_1-weighted (500/17), FLASH (200/13/10 degree) and FLASH (200/13/20 degree) images, repectively, through the cervical spine. A cervical disk herniation at the C5-6 level *(arrows)* is noted on all three studies. Note the difference in contrast of the CSF surrounding the cord on the 10- and 20-degree FLASH images. At 10 degrees, the signal intensity of the CSF on 2D imaging is high relative to the adjacent neural structures. There is an isointense zone from approximately 15 to 25 degrees. **D,** a 3-mm FLASH (50/10/10 degree) image that is part of a set of 16 contiguous 3-mm slices obtained in an anisotropic volume mode. The C5-6 disk herniation *(black arrow)* is well seen. **E** and **F,** contiguous 1-mm reconstructions off the anisotropic volume set (**D**) through the C5-6 disk. *Arrows* denote the disk herniation. **G,** 1-mm oblique reconstruction through the neural foramen off this same set. *nf* = neural foramen; *up* = uncinate process; *if* = inferior facet; *sf* = superior facet. The value of volume imaging is that thin contiguous sections can be obtained in a reasonable period of time that can then be reconstructed in any plane without additional acquisitions. This allows 1-mm reconstructions where, for reasons of pathology, spatial resolution is critical.

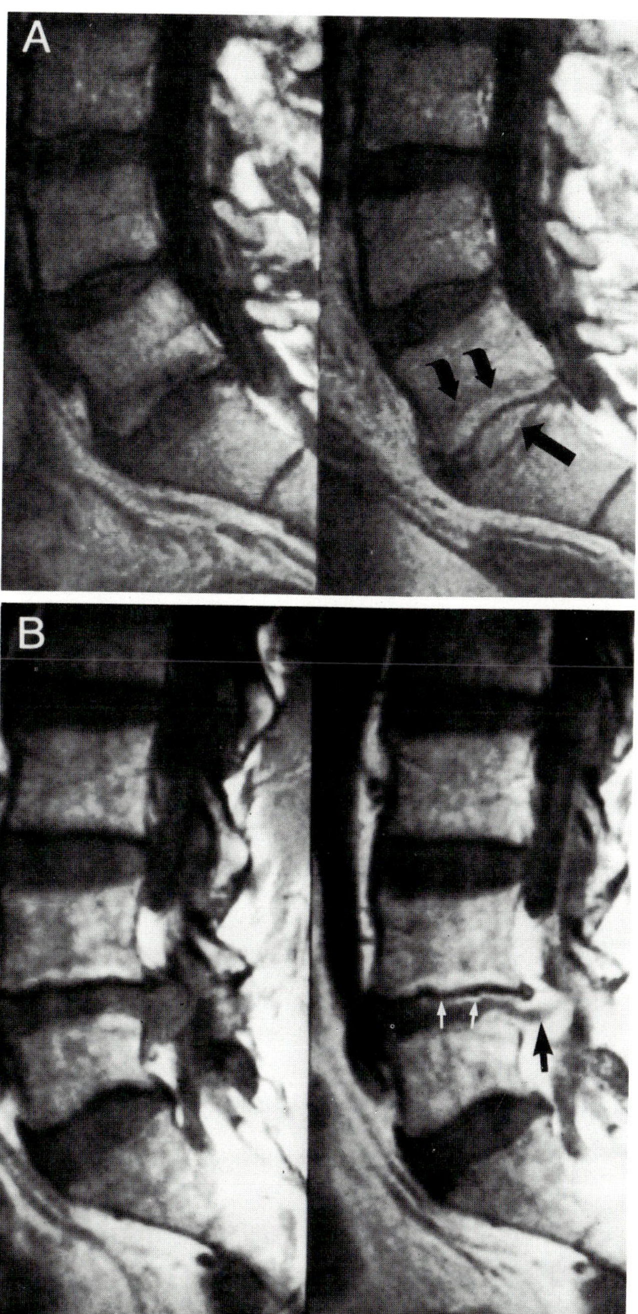

FIG 3–36.
Enhancement of degenerative disks. **A,** T_1-weighted sagittal (500/17) midline section before and 30 minutes after injection of Gd-DTPA. Type I vertebral body changes are noted in the inferior aspect of the L5 vertebral body and contiguous portion of S1. Following injection there is enhancement of these regions *(curved black arrows)* as well as of the entire L5-S1 disk *(straight black arrow).* The enhancement of the disk itself is presumably secondary to diffusion of contrast via fibrovascular granulation tissue within both the vertebral body and/or end plate into the central portion of the disk. **B,** recurrent disk and epidural fibrosis with linear enhancement of the parent degenerated disk. These are T_1-weighted sagittal (500/17) sections before and 8 minutes after injection of Gd-DTPA, respectively. The preinjection scan demonstrates herniation of the L4-5 disk as a soft tissue mass extending posterior and laterally. Following injection there is enhancement of soft tissue surrounding this herniated disk *(black arrow).* Histology revealed granulation tissue in this location. A thin line of enhancement just beneath the inferior cortical margin of the L4 vertebral bodies is noted on the postinjection study and is thought to represent enhancement of granulation tissue within a disrupted end-plate and/or peripheral disk margin *(small white arrows).*

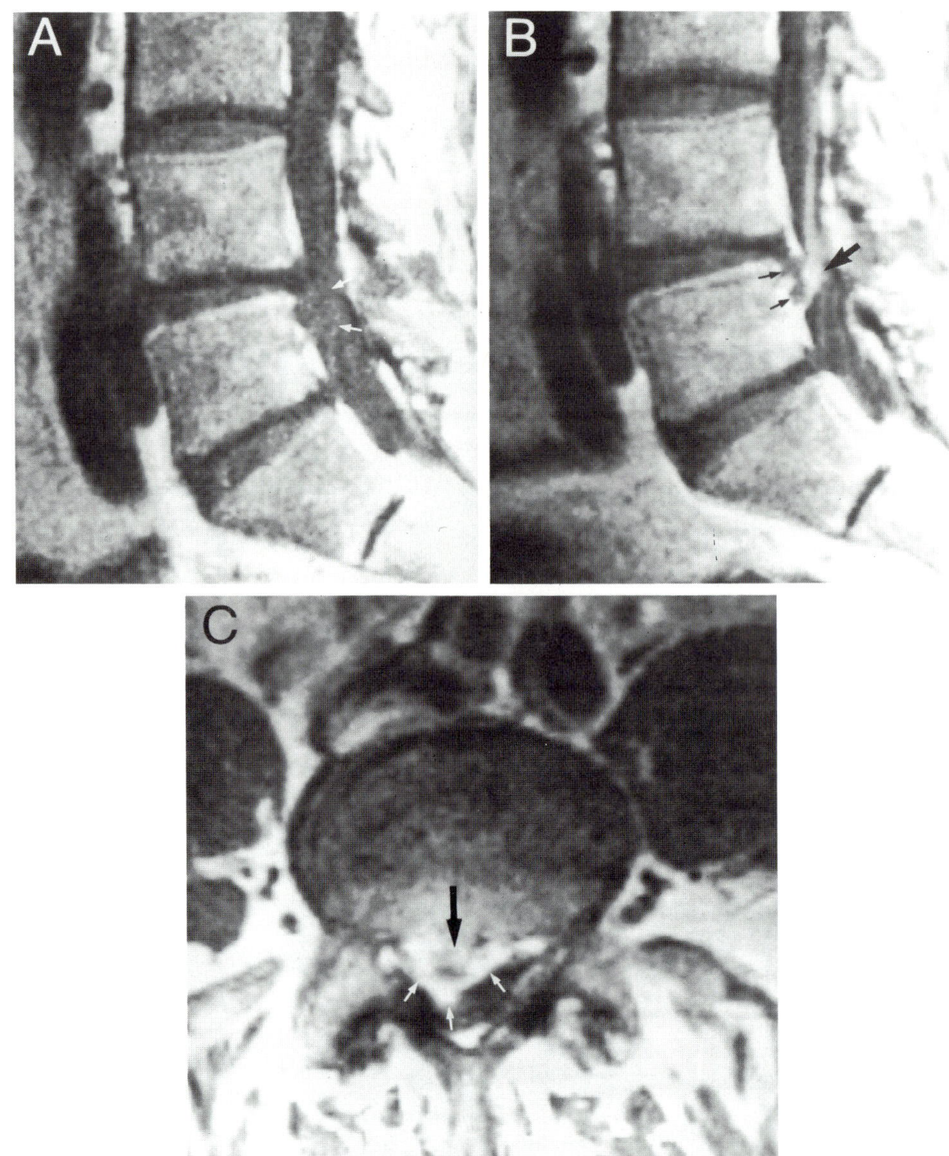

FIG 3–37.
Virgin herniated L4-5 disk before and after administration of Gd-DTPA. **A,** sagittal midline T_1-weighted SE (500/17) sequence through the lumbar spine. *White arrows* demonstrate a poorly defined soft tissue mass posterior to the superior aspect of the L5 vertebral body. **B,** following the administration of Gd-DPTA, there is enhancement surrounding this soft tissue mass. **C,** axial T_1-weighted SE (500/17) image through the inferior aspect of the L4-5 disk and superior L5 vertebral body. There is a large enhancing mass with a central area of decreased signal intensity denoted by the *arrows.* There is posterior displacement and compression of the thecal sac. At surgery the central portion of this mass represented herniated disk surrounded by the peripheral portion (that enhanced on MR) and proved to be granulation tissue. This case demonstrates that in addition to enhancement of the epidural venous plexus by Gd-DTPA for increased conspicuity of extradural defects, there is also enhancement of granulation tissue that is associated with virgin disks as well as the postoperative state.

generated and/or herniated disks exhibit this response and its relationship to the patients' clinical symptomatology remains unclear.

Thus it seems likely that Gd-DTPA may play a role in identifying the sequelae of degenerative disk disease by enhancing the reactive granulation tissue that forms secondary to disruption of the disk and associated structures. This enhancement results in increased conspicuity of extradural defects on T_1-weighted images (Figs 3–37 and 3–38). This result has been confirmed in part by the observation that even herniated virgin disks can be partially outlined by enhancement on MR.

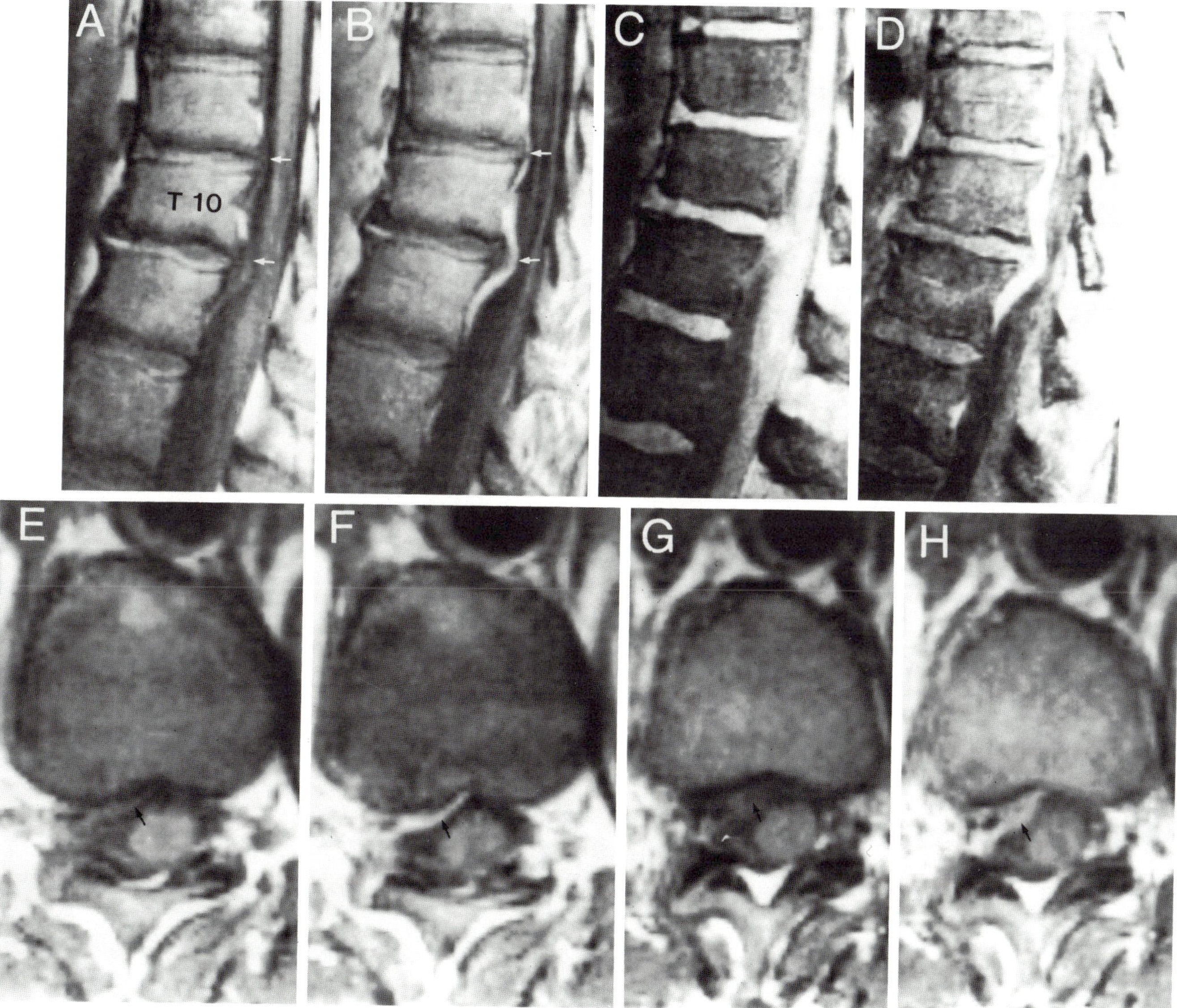

FIG 3–38.

T9-10 and T10-11 disk herniations. **A** and **B** represent sagittal T_1-weighted (500/17) images before and after administration of Gd-DPTA, respectively, and **C** and **D** represent FLASH (200/13/60 degree) images before and after administration of Gd-DTPA, respectively. Note the anterior extradural defects (arrows) at the T9-10 and T10-11 levels that are more clearly outlined following the administration of Gd-DTPA by linear areas of enhancement. **E** and **F** represent axial T_1-weighted (500/17) images before and after administration of Gd-DTPA, respectively, at the T9-10 level and **G** and **H** like images before and after administration of Gd-DPTA, respectively, at the T10-11 levels. The pregadolinium studies show soft tissue signal intensity disk herniations (arrow) to the right of midline (larger at T10-11) that demonstrate peripheral enhancement at the T9-10 level and both peripheral and more diffuse enhancement at the T10-11 level. At surgery these were both noted to represent lateral thoracic disk herniations in association with peridiskal granulation tissue. The enhancement in these cases is a combination of both venous plexus and peridiskal granulation tissue.

Gadolinium-DTPA may be useful in degenerative disk disease for a second reason. Following the intravenous injection of Gd-DPTA, there is consistent, persistent enhancement of the epidural venous plexus following injection for up to 30 to 40 minutes. This again produces increased contrast in the epidural venous structure surrounding the disk space and can result in increased conspicuity of extradural disease when it impacts on the adjacent venous structures (see Fig 3–38). Future applications of Gd-DTPA will be its utilization with fast gradient echo volume scans to produce contrast that may not be inherently apparent.

In addition to the changes within the disk, including herniation, secondary changes are noted both in animal models and humans following disk degeneration. The stability of a motion segment depends on the integrity of all of its components. Diseases occurring in this area are circumferential, one joint affecting the other. Degeneration of the disk leads to a loss of disk height and forces the facet joints into malalignment, so-called "rostrocaudal subluxation." This results in an increase in the biomechanical forces experienced at the facet joint with increasing joint relaxation and instability, secondary facet and arthritic changes, and potentially fractures. Similarly, abnormal movements allowed by disk degeneration and facet changes add stress to the posterior ligaments and can result in hypertrophy. A vicious degenerative cycle is established that includes degenerative disk disease, facet arthrosis, ligamentous and capsular hypertrophy, spine instability, and lumbar stenosis.[54]

SPINAL STENOSIS

Spinal stenosis results from an overall diminution of the spinal canal, lateral recess, or neuroforamen. It occurs more commonly in the lumbar and cervical regions. The symptoms of spinal stenosis are usually a reflection of the compressive pathology. In the cervical region, the most frequently observed manifestations are multiple unilateral or bilateral radiculopathy and/or myelopathy. Neck or shoulder pain are frequent complaints but are not specific and may only reflect general myotomal innervation. Myelopathic syndromes usually present with some degree of spasticity and weakness. This is usually secondary to involvement of the cortical spinal tracks, spinal thalamic tracks, and/or posterior columns below the level(s) of involvement.[55] In the lumbar region, canal stenosis can cause compression of the cauda equina and/or individual nerve roots. The classical description of the neurogenic claudication from spinal stenosis is bilateral radicular pain, disorders of sensory function, and motor deficits that develop when the patient is standing or walking, and absent when the patient is recumbent. Interestingly, this claudication, unlike vascular claudication, may actually be more severe when the subject is standing still. More frequently, arthritic symptoms such as back pain and the subjective symptoms of coldness, tingling, burning, and sciatica are noted. As a rule, the symptoms and signs of spinal stenosis do not appear until the fifth or sixth decade but can occur much earlier for acquired disease superimposed on a developmental form.

Etiologically, stenosis can be divided into two main types. The first is developmental or congenital stenosis, which includes idiopathic, achondroplasia, Morquio's disease, and various bony dysplasias. Congenital stenosis may be associated with thick pedicles and a reduced interpedicular distance.

This form is often further complicated by the second type, acquired stenosis, which can be seen after trauma and with degenerative disease, spondylolisthesis, postoperative changes, and various miscellaneous disorders including ankylosing spondylitis, ossification of the posterior longitudinal ligament or ligamentum flavum, Paget's disease, acromegaly, and fluorosis.

Three factors, either alone or in combination, are felt to be responsible for the development of symptoms in most cases. The first is some degree of developmental narrowing of the neural canal. The second is tethering of involved nerve roots secondary to hypertrophic vertebral body or facet joint disease that may interfere with the normal vascular supply. The last is rotary or lateral instability secondary to disk and facet degeneration.[55] Regrdless of the etiology, the common denominator of spinal stenosis is narrowing of the canal that may be central, peripheral, or both. From the therapeutic standpoint, it seems more practical to describe the changes of spinal stenosis in relationship to the regions and anatomical structures involved.

The first is central, which refers to the portion of the bony spinal canal bounded by the pedicles laterally and facet joints, laminae, and spinous process posteriorly, with the disk anterior. The second is subarticular, which refers to the subarticular segment of the nerve root canal including the lateral recess. The third is the intervertebral canal (intervertebral foramina), which refers to the infrapedicular segment of the nerve root canal and intervertebral foramen. Involvement of these last two regions is often referred to as peripheral stenosis. Central and peripheral stenosis often coexist.

Lumbar Spine

Central stenosis tends to occur at multiple levels but is most frequent and usually most severe at the L4-5 level where it may occur alone (Figs 3–39 through 3–41). Central stenosis tends to produce complicated radicular signs and symptoms with or without claudication. This region is particularly susceptible to impingement by osteophytes from the vertebral bodies or facet joints, thickening of the ligaments, and bulging of the intervertebral disks. Ligamentous stenosis can occur even when the dimensions of the central bony canal are normal. This includes reduction in the overall dimensions by hypertrophy of the ligamentum flavum as well as by calcification of the posterior longitudinal ligament. While this reduction is more common in the cervical

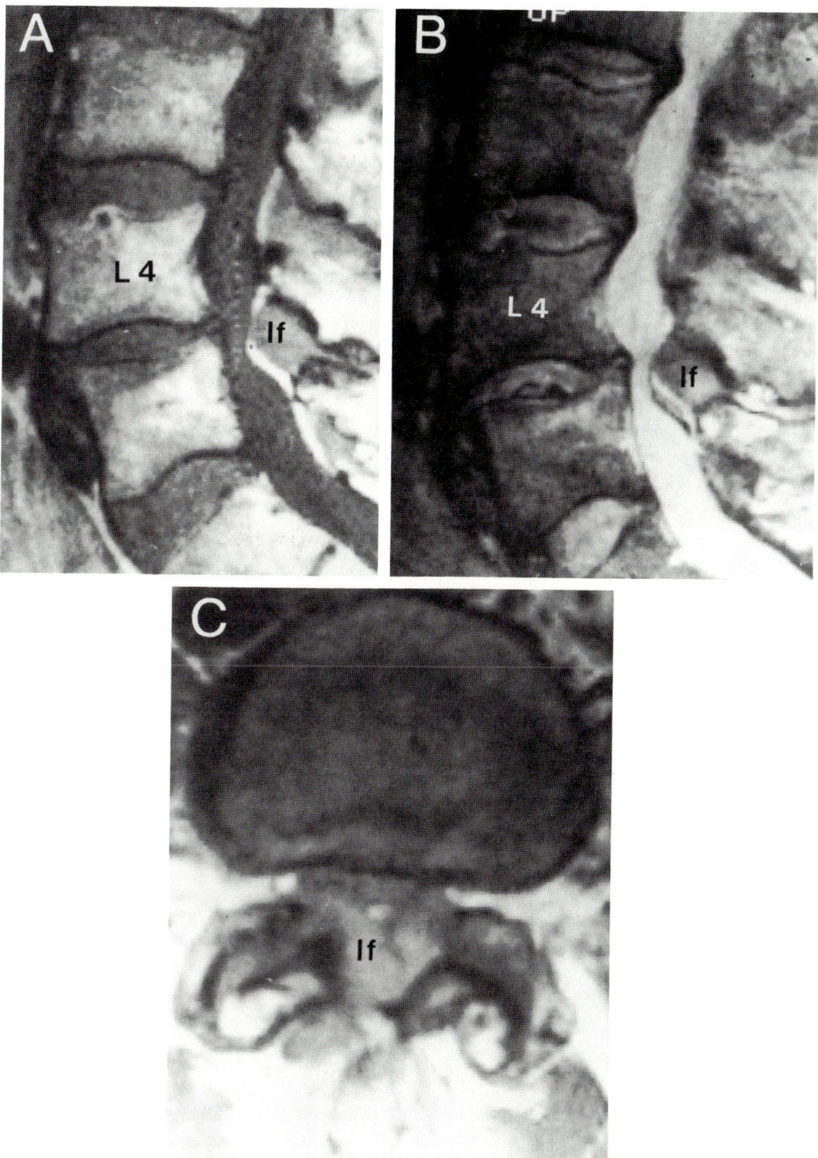

FIG 3–39.
Central lumbar canal stenosis, L4-5 level. **A,** sagittal midline T_1-weighted SE (500/17) image. There is marked narrowing of the central lumbar canal at the L4-5 interspace primarily secondary to enlargement of the ligamentum flavum *(LF)*. **B,** sagittal T_2-weighted SE (2000/90) image through the same level as **A.** Again marked canal stenosis is noted at the L4-5 interspace. **C,** axial T_1-weighted SE (500/17) image through the L4-5 disk. Markedly enlarged ligamenta flava are noted *(LF)*. The thecal sac is markedly reduced in size. The facet joints are enlarged and show evidence of hypertrophic degenerative change.

region, it can also occur in the thoracic or lumbar region. This latter finding is seen in up to 25% of patients with diffuse idiopathic skeletal hyperostosis. Paget's disease may also cause spinal canal narrowing secondary to diffuse bony overgrowth. Following surgery, secondary stenosis of the spinal canal may occur secondary to hypertrophy of bone grafts, overgrowth of bone, or spondylolisthesis.

The transverse and sagittal dimensions of the central neural canal are best depicted by integrating orthogonal planes, e.g., axial and sagittal images. Gradient echo images with low flip angles or more T_2-weighted SE sequences provide the best depiction of the overall dimensions of the thecal sac by providing a relative gray-scale inversion of the CSF and extradural elements.[50, 51] Besides an overall reduction of the size of the neural canal, several ancillary signs may be noted that often are a cause for confusion. First, especially in the lumbar re-

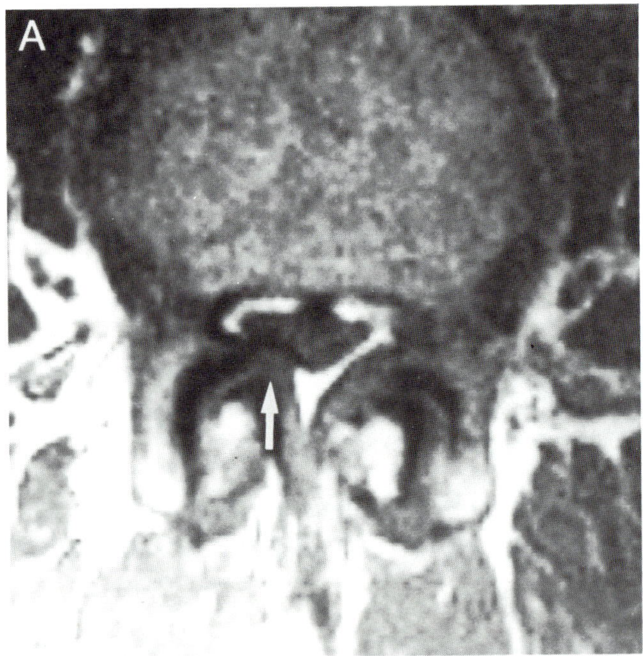

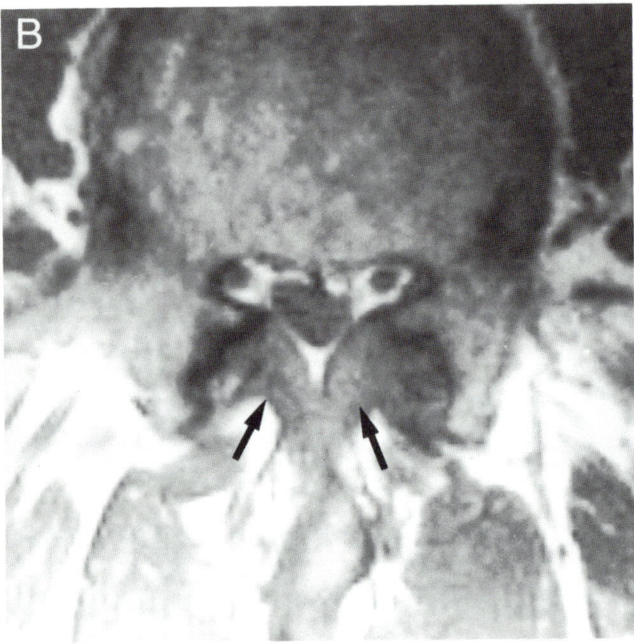

FIG 3–40.
Central canal stenosis at the mid-L3 vertebral body level. **A** and **B,** T_1-weighted axial SE (500/17) images at the mid-L3 level. There is canal stenosis produced by hypertrophic changes in the facets *(white arrow)* as well as posterolateral indentation of the thecal sac from the enlarged facet capsule complex. Note thickening enlargement of the ligamentum flavum posteriorly *(black arrows).*

gions, central canal stenosis can cause central consolidation of the nerve roots, resulting in an intermediate signal intensity within the thecal sac on T_1-weighted images. This can be confused with clumping secondary to arachnoiditis or an intradural mass. Second, canal stenosis can dampen the CSF pulsations, resulting in a higher signal intensity distally that can be diffuse or focal on both sagittal and axial images, again not to be confused with arachnoiditis or an intradural mass. There is often a reduction of ghosting, and the signal intensity of the CSF is often well preserved on T_2-weighted sequences for similar reasons.

Peripheral stenosis may occur alone or in combination with central stenosis (Fig 3–42). The height of the lateral recess is defined as the distance between the most anterior portion of the superior articular facet and the posterior portion of the vertebral body in the same plane. The height of 4 mm or less is usually associated with symptoms. More laterally, neural foraminal stenosis can occur from bony overgrowth, spondylolisthesis, and/or degenerative bulging or herniation of the intervertebral disk. Postoperative fibrosis can also cause symptoms identical to bony stenosis. It must be remembered that severe morphological changes can occur without symptomatology because the nerve root only occupies a small portion of the superior neural foramen. Narrowing of the inferior portion is a relatively common finding in the aging population and is less likely to cause symptoms.

Peripheral stenosis is best appreciated on T_1-weighted images where the separation between neural structures and epidural fat is well maintained. The signal intensity between neural elements and fat is less well seen on more T_2-weighted and gradient echo images, although bony overgrowth can be identified. In the lumbar region, the parasagittal and axial images together allow accurate identification of the lateral recess and neural foramina and their corresponding relationship to the vertebral body, disk, and facets. In this fashion, accurate description of the various anatomical zones where stenosis can occur can be obtained. It should be noted that lateral disk bulging into the inferior aspect of the foramen is common in the aging population. This is, by itself, rarely a cause of symptoms as the neural elements pass laterally in a more superior plane underneath the pedicle. In the cervical region, oblique images are more useful than the parasagittal images as they provide a more accurate second orthogonal plane in conjunction with the axial images.

The malalignment concomitant with spondylolisthesis produces anatomical derangement of the neural foramina that causes stenosis. Associated true disk herniation is uncommon at the level of a pars defect but

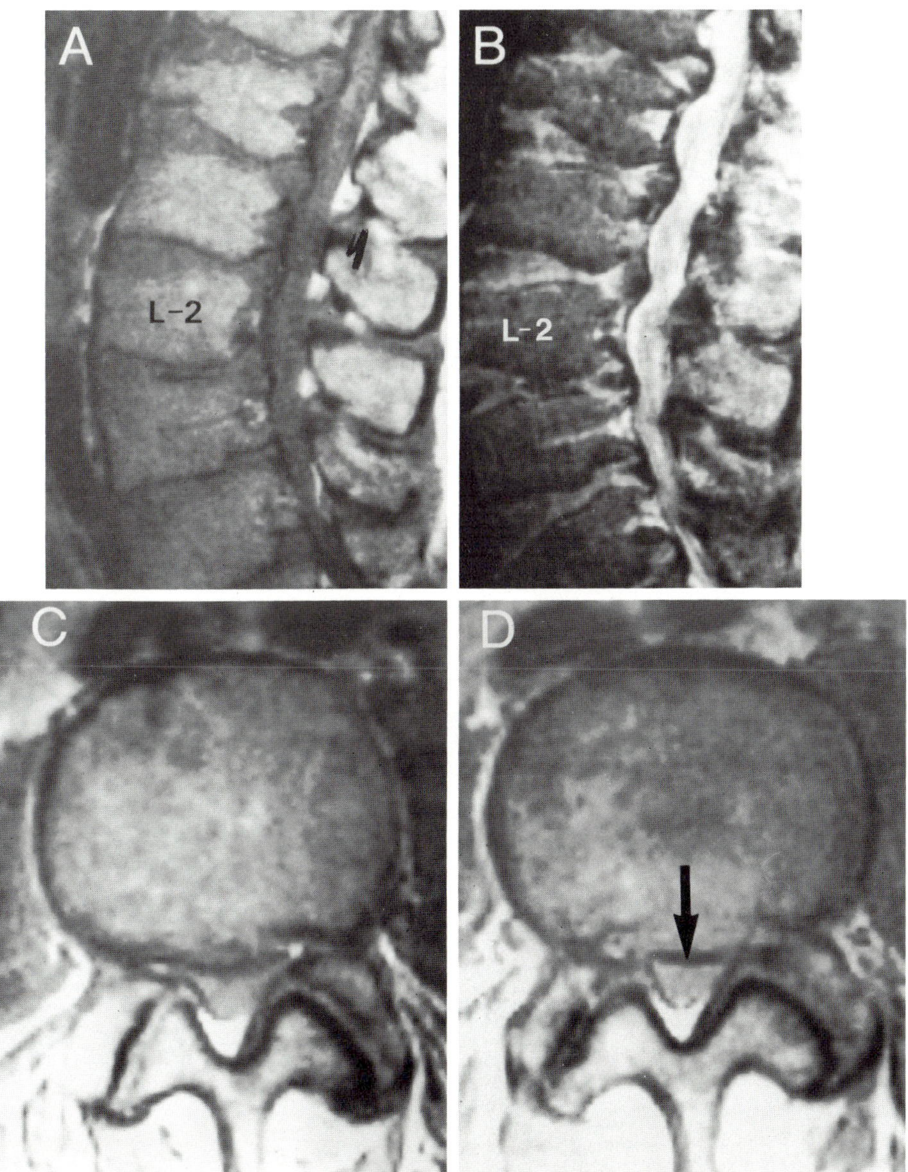

FIG 3–41.
Lumbar canal stenosis. **A,** sagittal midline T_1-weighted SE (500/17) image. Sagittal midline T_2-weighted SE (2000/90) image (**B**) and axial T_1-weighted SE (500/17) images (**C** and **D**) through the L4 neural foramina demonstrate diffuse central and peripheral stenosis in this 36-year-old female. There is complete obliteration of the normal neural foramina from hypertrophic degenerative changes of both the facet joints and vertebral bodies at all levels. The signal intensity of the CSF is higher than one would anticipate on the T_1-weighted images. This is secondary to both the decreased pulsations of the thoracic CSF and the clumping centrally of the nerve roots in the cauda equina *(black arrow,* **D**).

may be seen at the inner space above. Compression of the nerve root in spondylolisthesis may occur secondary to the buildup of fibrocartilage rather than to the pars defect and malalignment itself. The height of the neural foramina becomes reduced at the level of segment involved by the pedicle, which forms the roof as it becomes positioned more inferiorly. Encroachment of the central spinal canal also occurs secondary to forward displacement.

Thoracic Spine

Symptomatic spinal stenosis in the thoracic region is much less common than in the cervical and lumbar regions unless it is associated with metabolic disease or spinal trauma. This is, to a large degree, secondary to the relatively large size of the thoracic canal relative to the cord. Thus there must be a marked decrease in the overall dimensions of the thoracic canal to produce

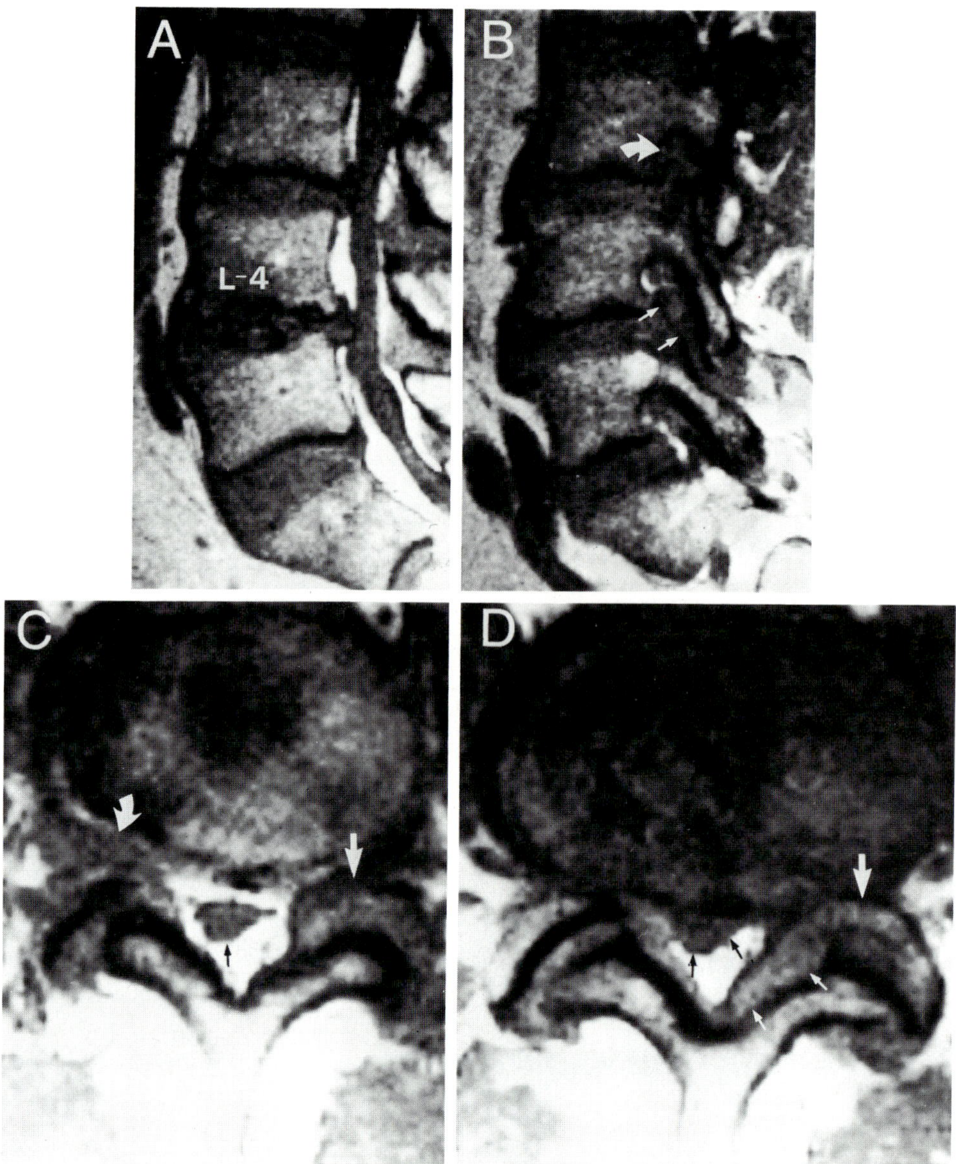

FIG 3–42.
Lumbar canal stenosis. Midline (**A**) and parasagittal (**B**) T_1-weighted SE (500/17) images. **C** and **D,** axial T_1-weighted SE (500/17) images through the level of the neural foramen at L4. There is diffuse central and peripheral lumbar canal stenosis. Note obliteration of the normal epidural fat signal and the inability to discern the dorsal root ganglion beneath the pedicles in **B** *(curved and small white arrows).* The axial images demonstrate marked hypertrophy of the ligamentum flavum, facet joints, and capsule totally obliterating the neural foramen *(white arrows).* The thecal sac is small *(black arrows),* and despite the severe stenosis, there is still abundant epidural fat centrally. The L4-5 disk is diffusely herniated both centrally and laterally.

compressive symptomatology. The symptoms of thoracic spinal stenosis are varied and may consist of myelopathy, sensory changes, radiculopathy, and a syndrome of claudication with low back pain similar to that seen with lumbar disease but without leg pain. The pathology noted is usually hypertrophy of the posterior spinal bony and/or ligamentous elements.[56]

Cervical Spine

In the cervical spine, degenerative changes affect all major spinal articulations, including the intervertebral disk, apophyseal joints, ligamentous connection between vertebral bodies, and the vertebral bodies themselves. The term spondylosis is used to refer to changes

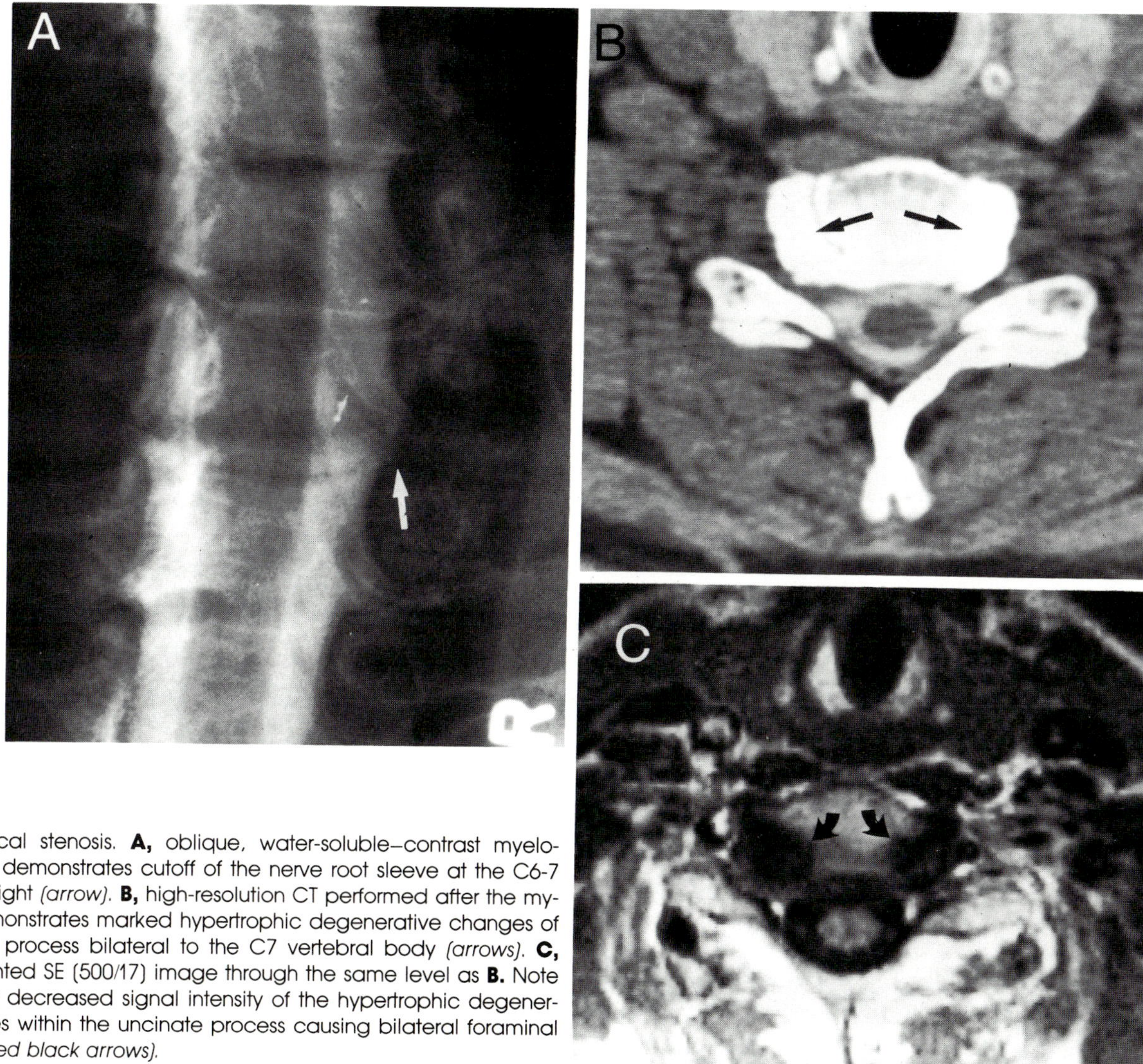

FIG 3–43.
Lateral cervical stenosis. **A,** oblique, water-soluble–contrast myelogram image demonstrates cutoff of the nerve root sleeve at the C6-7 level on the right *(arrow)*. **B,** high-resolution CT performed after the myelogram demonstrates marked hypertrophic degenerative changes of the uncinate process bilateral to the C7 vertebral body *(arrows)*. **C,** axial T_1-weighted SE (500/17) image through the same level as **B.** Note the markedly decreased signal intensity of the hypertrophic degenerative changes within the uncinate process causing bilateral foraminal stenosis *(curved black arrows)*.

involving the intervertebral disk and vertebral bodies, in contrast to degenerative changes of the apophyseal joints, which are more often classified as osteoarthritis. A common factor in both spondylosis and osteoarthritis is concomitant degenerative disease of the intervertebral disk that results in the loss of elasticity of the disk and surrounding ligaments. Bulging of the disk margin tends to produce traction in the longitudinal ligaments of the vertebral bodies, producing an irritative reaction resulting in the formation of osteophytes. Ironically, the formation of osteophytes may have a stabilizing effect on the spine. This mechanism is more important in the formation of anterior rather than posterior or posterolateral osteophytes, which are usually the most important clinically.

With degenerative collapse of the intervertebral disk space and/or posterior intervertebral joints, there is narrowing of the intervertebral foramina that tends to compress the individual nerve roots. The development of uncovertebral spurs that lie medially and laterally in the spinal canal usually occurs concomitantly (Fig 3–43). Thus the major cause of cervical spinal stenosis results from osteophytic overgrowth at the posterolateral margins of the body, posterior protrusion of the disk material, hypertrophy of the ligamentum flavum, and dorsal intrusions into the canal by osteophytes secondary to apophyseal arthritic changes (Figs 3–44 and 3–45). Not all individuals with evidence of cervical spondylosis and osteoarthritis have cord compression, and those that do tend to have small spinal canals irrespective of the sec-

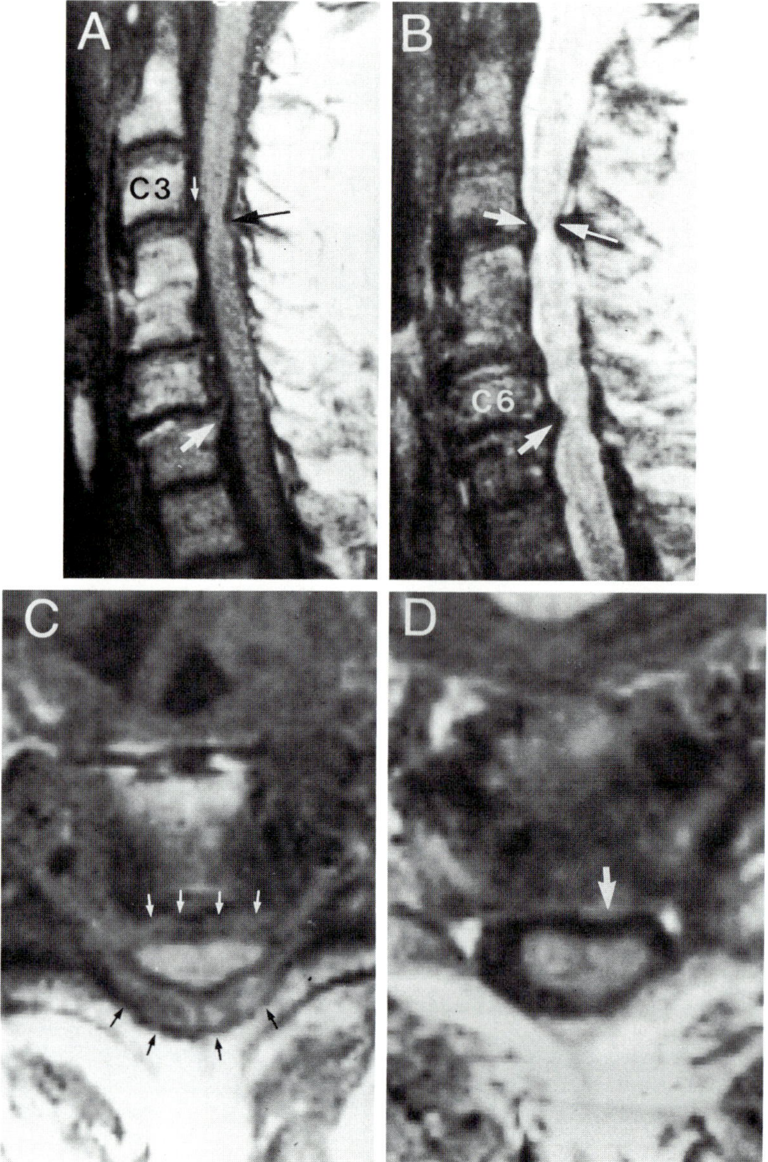

FIG 3–44.
Cervical stenosis. Sagittal T_1-weighted SE (500/17) (**A**) and T_2-weighted SE (2000/90) (**B**) images through the cervical spine. There is stenosis at the C3-4 level both anteriorly *(small white arrow)* and posteriorly *(large black arrow)* as well as evidence of hypertrophic degenerative changes and canal narrowing at the C6-7 level anteriorly *(large white arrow).* Axial T_1-weighted SE (500/17) images through the C3-4 (**C**) and C6-7 (**D**) levels. Note that at C3-4, the small *white and black arrows* demonstrate marked ligamentous and soft tissue cervical canal stenosis with compression of the spinal cord. **D** demonstrates an intermediate signal intensity of the hypertrophic degenerative bone from the superior aspect of the C7 vertebral body *(white arrow)* causing an anterior extradural defect and cervical stenosis.

ondary changes. This is exacerbated in extension, as the maximal canal size is achieved in slight flexion. Relaxation of bulge in the ligamentum flavum into the canal and hyperextension may also be a cause of stenosis. (One of the reasons stenosis may appear more severe on myelography than with MR is because of the difference in positions, i.e., hyperextensional with myelography and neutral with MR.) Degenerative changes of the posterior articulations may allow mild retrolisthesis of the superior vertebra on the inferior partner, which also results in a decrease in the sagittal diameter.

A less common cause of cervical spinal stenosis is ossification of the posterior longitudinal ligament (OPLL) (Fig 3–46). The basic pathophysiologic process of OPLL is similar to heterotopic bone formation elsewhere secondary to mechanical stress. With time, the

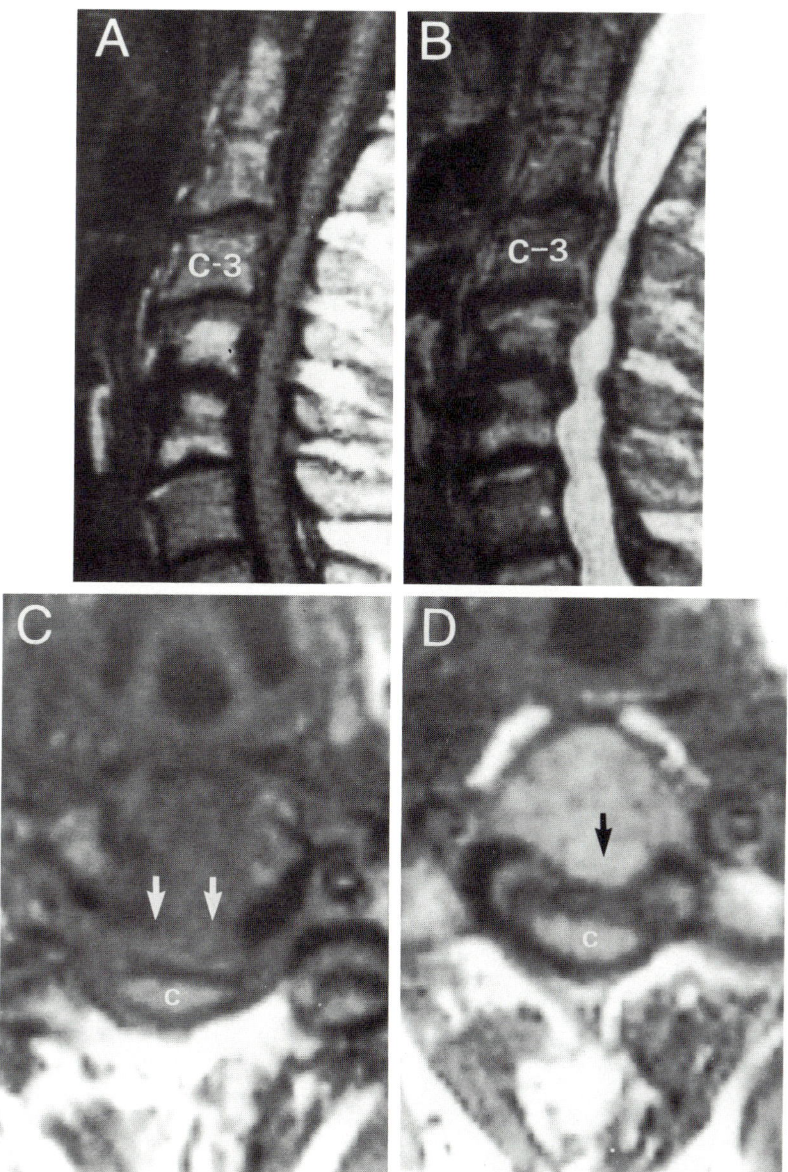

FIG 3–45.
Cervical stenosis. Sagittal T_1-weighted SE (500/17) (**A**) and T_2-weighted SE (2000/90) (**B**) images through the cervical spine. There is severe cervical canal stenosis from the C2-3 through the C4-5 levels. **C,** axial T_1-weighted SE (500/17) image through the C2-3 level that demonstrates herniation of the intervertebral disk *(white arrows)* and marked cervical cord compression. **D,** axial T_1-weighted SE (500/17) image through the C5 vertebral body. Note the large osteophyte anteriorly *(black arrow)* and cord compression.

OPLL mass progressively enlarges in thickness, width, and length. Again, OPLL is more likely to produce symptomatic cord compression in a canal already compromised by congenital stenosis, spondylosis, or hypertrophy of the ligamentum flavum than in a canal with normal dimensions.[57]

On MR, the following features are important for analysis: facet joint size and contour; osteophyte formation of the facet joints or vertebral bodies; hypertrophy and/or calcification of ligamentous structures; and transverse and sagittal dimensions of the neural canal, lateral recess, and neural foramina.

Bony osteophytes can present as either decreased, intermediate, or high signal intensity relative to the adjacent vertebral body and facet joints.[35] Signal differences presumably reflect variable amounts of yellow marrow. While usually appreciated on T_1-weighted images, they are reportedly easier to see and distinguish

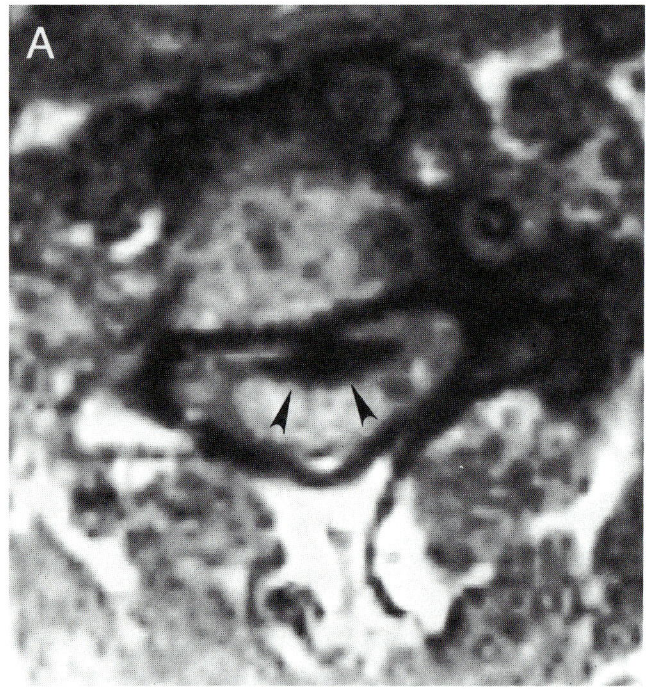

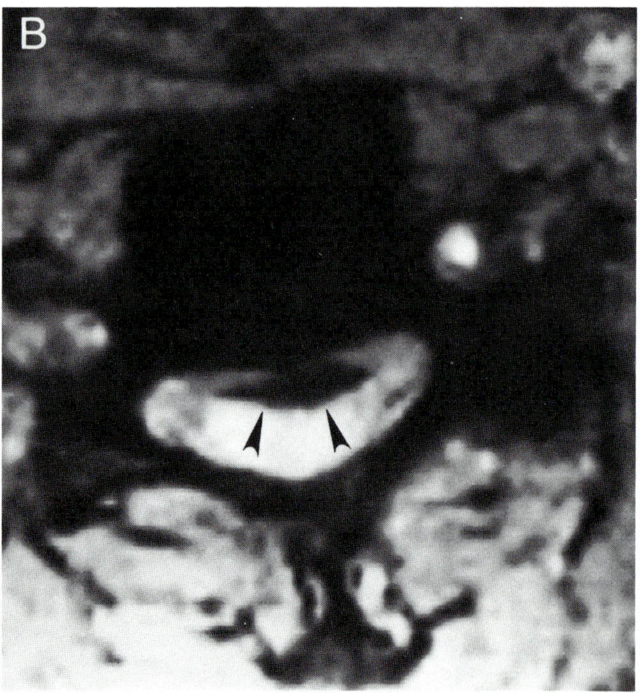

FIG 3–46.
Ossification of the posterior longitudinal ligament. Axial T_1-weighted SE (500/17) (**A**) and FLASH (200/13/60 degree) (**B**) images through the C6 vertebral body level. A mass of decreased signal intensity is identified anterior to the cord *(black arrowheads)* on both the T_1-weighted SE and gradient echo images. Although equally well seen in this example, gradient echo images tend to depict ossification of the posterior longitudinal ligament better than SE images secondary to a presumed susceptibility effect of the heterotopic bone formation within the posterior longitudinal ligament.

from soft tissue on long TR/short TE images. On T_1-weighted images, those with a higher content of lipid marrow are easier to identify than the sclerotic osteophytes, which usually have a low signal intensity that may blend with adjacent ligamentous structures or CSF. Gradient echo images, especially with low flip angles, depict hypertrophic changes as decreased signal in contrast to the CSF or adjacent paraspinal fat.

Thickening of the ligamentum flavum can be identified on both the axial and sagittal planes.[58] In the axial plane in normal persons, its mean thickness is 5.5 ± 1.3 mm. Hypertrophy can be unilateral or asymmetric (see Fig 3–39). In the cervical region it measures from 1 to 3 mm and approximately 2 mm in the thoracic region. Thickening is identified with degeneration, aging, or buckling, and it is usually seen concomitantly with facet and degenerative disk disease. The high signal intensity of the ligamentum flavum relative to the posterior longitudinal ligaments, especially on T_1-weighted or gradient echo images, has been reported to be related to its high elastin (80%) and low type I collagen (20%) content.[58] Calcification of the ligamentous structures may be difficult to appreciate on T_1-weighted spin-echo images as the decreased signal intensity may blend with signal from the adjacent CSF within the thecal sac. This is particularly true in ossification of the posterior longitudinal ligaments. Its decreased signal intensity can be identified in sharp contrast to the CSF on more T_2-weighted images. Alternatively, gradient echo scans appear more sensitive to the presence of calcification secondary to susceptibility effect, which allows their identification with greater sensitivity and accuracy than on T_1-weighted SE sequences (see Fig 3–46).

Facet Joint Disease

While facet arthrosis constitutes an important cause of acquired lumbar stenosis, degenerative change can occur independently and may be one of the most common causes of low back pain and radiculopathy.[54, 59] Like any diarthrodial synovium-lined joint, the facet joints are predisposed to arthropathies. This may result in alterations of the articular cartilage leading to osteochondral fragments that can act as joint mice. With advancing disease and progressive evolution of articular cartilage, subchondral bony sclerosis and degenerative cysts develop. Synovial villi can be entrapped, and joint effusions may be produced. Osteophytes may develop in areas of bone stress, which may in addition lead to hypertrophy of the entire facet joints or parts thereof, usually the superior articular facet. Herniation of synovium through the facet joint capsule may result in a synovial cyst that can act as a mass lesion.

Back pain can be caused by two mechanisms of facet joint disease. The first is direct compression of nerve roots secondary to facet hypertrophies, osteophytes, or rostrocaudal subluxation and expansion of the facet joint capsule caused by joint effusions. Secondly, and perhaps more competently, the synovial linings and joint capsule of the facet joint are richly innervated,[54] and pain may be produced by local internal derangements resulting in direct irritation of local pain fibers that can produce muscle spasm, focal or diffuse back pain, and sciatica.

As mentioned previously, degenerative changes of the facet joints most commonly involve the superior articular facet that with hypertrophy and focal osteophyte formation can produce both central or lateral stenosis. Enlargement of the superior articular facet can cause stenosis in the region of the lateral recess and with rostrocaudal subluxation can produce narrowing in the upper portion of the neural canal. Posterolateral protrusion of the facet joint into the central canal can also be noted. It must be emphasized that undiagnosed facet disease has been implicated as one of the causes of the failed back surgery syndrome and thus must be looked for carefully in all preoperative evaluations. Postoperative changes may also be seen with a development of contralateral facet joint disease following foraminotomies and diskectomy. This procedure may lead to additional stress on the facet joints, most often manifested on the contralateral side since the ipsilateral side is usually sufficiently decompressed.[54]

On MR the facet joints are best evaluated by visually integrating the sagittal and axial images. Again, osteophytes are easier to identify on gradient echo images or spin-echo images with long TRs. Those that contain marrow are also better demarcated than those that are sclerotic, which can be confused with the adjacent capsular ligamentous structures, particularly at the posterior inferior aspect of the joint where the capsule always demonstrates low signal intensity. Altered signal intensity in bone marrow consistent with fatty replacement has also been reported to be commonly associated.[58] Although both facet joints can be involved, the superior is more common. The articular cartilage can be directly visualized on both T_1- or T_2-weighted spin-echo images, but thinning is difficult to measure accurately because of variable axial obliquity and chemical shift artifact from the adjacent facet. Nevertheless, notable changes appear to correlate well with those identified on CT. More recently, gradient echo examinations have demonstrated that they provide better conspicuity of the articular cartilage itself as distinct from adjacent osseous structures. Preliminary data suggest that their appraisal is better with this technique. This potentially could allow direct visualization of thinning and irregularities of the cartilage itself, which is not possible with other modalities. Changes in the underlying bone such as facet erosions or cyst formation can also be noted.

References

1. Kelsey JL, White AA III, Pastides H, et al: The impact of musculoskeletal disorders in the population of the United States. *J Bone Joint Surg* [*Am*] 1979; 61:959–964.
2. Dillane JB, Frye J, Colton G: Acute back syndrome—a study from general practice. *Br Med J* 1966; 2:82–84.
3. Rowe ML: Low back pain in industry: A position paper. *J Occup Med* 1969; 11:161–169.
4. Resnick D: Degenerative diseases of the vertebral column. *Radiology* 1985; 156:3–14.
5. Haughton VM: MR imaging of the spine. *Radiology* 1988; 166:297–301.
6. Penning L, Wilmink JT, Woerden HH, et al: CT myelographic findings in degenerative disorders of the cervical spine: Clinical significance. *AJNR* 1986; 7:119–127.
7. Teresi LM, Lufkin RB, Reicher MA, et al: Asymptomatic degenerative disk disease and spondylosis of the cervical spine: MR imaging. *Radiology* 1987; 164:83–88.
8. Rothman SL, Glenn WV: Spondylosis and spondylolisthesis, in Newton TH, Potts DG (eds): *Computed Tomography of the Spine and Spinal Cord*. San Anselmo, Calif, Clavadel Press, 1983, pp 267–280.
9. Pritzer KPH: Aging and degeneration in the lumbar intervertebral disc. *Orthop Clin North Am* 1977; 8:65–67.
10. White AA, Gordon SL: Synopsis: Workshop on idiopathic low-back pain. *Spine* 1982; 7:141–149.
11. Quinet RJ, Hadler NM: Diagnosis and treatment of backache. *Semin Arthritis Rheum* 1979; 8:261–287.
12. Coventry MB: Anatomy of the intervertebral disk. *Clin Orthop* 1969; 67:9–15.
13. Adams P, Eyre DR, Muir H: Biochemical aspects of development and ageing of human lumbar intervertebral discs. *Rheumatol Rehabil* 1977; 16:22–29.
14. Brown MD: The pathophysiology of disc disease, symposium on disease of the intervertebral disc. *Orthop Clin North Am* 1971; 2:359–370.
15. Lipson SJ, Muir H: Experimental intervertebral disc degeneration. Morphological and proteoglycan changes over time. *Arthritis Rheum* 1981; 24:12–21.
16. Lipson SJ, Muir H: Proteoglycans in experimental intervertebral disc degeneration. *Spine* 1984; 6:194–210.
17. Naylor A: Intervertebral disk prolapse and degeneration: The biochemical and biophysical approach. *Spine* 1976; 1:108–114.
18. Bisla RS, Marchisello PJ, Lockshin MD, et al: Auto-immunological basis of disk degeneration. *Clin Orthop* 1976; 121:205–211.
19. Bobechko WP, Hirsch C: Auto-immune response to nucleus pulposus in the rabbit. *J Bone Joint Surg* [*Br*] 1965; 47:574–580.

20. Moskowitz RW, Adler H: Spondylosis in sand rats: A model of intervertebral disk degeneration. *Arthritis Rheum* 1986; 29:S17.
21. Lindblom K, Hultqvist G: Absorption of protruded disk tissue. *J Bone Joint Surg* 1950; 22:557–560.
22. Brown T, Hansen RJ, Yorra AJ: Some mechanical tests on the lumbosacral spine with particular reference to the intervertebral discs: A preliminary report. *J Bone Joint Surg [Am]* 1957; 39:1135.
23. Evans FG, Lissner HR: Strength of intervertebral discs (abstract). *J Bone Joint Surg [Am]* 1954; 36:195.
24. Nachemson A: The load on lumbar disks in different positions of the body. *Clin Orthop* 1966; 45:107–122.
25. Roaf R: A study of the mechanics of spinal injuries. *J Bone Joint Surg [Br]* 1960; 42:810.
26. Axel LL: Surface coil magnetic resonance imaging. *J Comput Assist Tomogr* 1984; 8:381–384.
27. Enzmann DR, Rubin JB, Wright A: Use of cerebral spinal fluid gating to improve T_2 weighted images: I: The spinal cord. *Radiology* 1987; 162:763–767.
28. Haacke EM, Lenz G: Improving MR image quality in the presence of motion by using rephasing gradients. *AJR* 1987; 148:1251–1258.
29. Hueftle M, Modic MT, Ross JS, et al: Lumbar spine: Postoperative MR imaging with Gd-DPTA. *Radiology* 1988, 167:817–824.
30. Edelman RR, Atkinson DJ, Silver MS, et al: FRODO pulse sequences: A new means of eliminating motion, flow and wrap around artifacts. *Radiology* 1986; 166:231–236.
31. Chafetz NI, Genant HK, Moon KL, et al: Recognition of lumbar disk herniation with NMR. *AJR* 1983; 141:1153–1156.
32. Edelman RR, Shoukimas GM, Stark ED, et al: High resolution surface coil imaging in lumbar disk disease. *AJR* 1985; 144:1123–1129.
33. Maravilla KR, Lash HP, Weinreb JC, et al: Magnetic resonance imaging of the lumbar spine with CT correlation. *AJNR* 1985; 6:237–245.
34. Modic MT, Masaryk TJ, Boumphrey F, et al: Lumbar herniated disc disease and canal stenosis: Prospective evaluation by surface coil MR, CT and myelography. *AJNR* 1986; 7:709–717.
35. Modic MT, Masaryk TJ, Mulopulos GP, et al: Cervical radiculopathy: Prospective evaluations with surface coil MR imaging, CT with metrizamide and metrizamide myelography. *Radiology* 1986; 161:753–759.
36. Modic MT, Masaryk TJ, Ross JS, et al: Cervical radiculopathy: Value of oblique MR imaging. *Radiology* 1987; 163:227–231.
37. Ross JS, Perez-Reyes N, Masaryk TJ, et al: Thoracic disk herniation: MR imaging. *Radiology* 1987; 165:511–515.
38. Modic MT, Pavlicek W, Weinstein MA, et al: Magnetic resonance imaging of intervertebral disk disease: Clinical and pulse sequence considerations. *Radiology* 1984; 152:103–111.
39. deRoos A, Kressel H, Spritzer C, et al: MR imaging of marrow changes adjacent to end plates in degenerative lumbar disk disease. *AJR* 1987; 149:531–534.
40. Modic MT, Steinberg PM, Ross JS, et al: Degenerative disk disease: Assessment of changes in vertebral body marrow with MR imaging. *Radiology* 1988; 166:193–199.
41. Aoki J, Yamamoto I, Kitamura N, et al: End plate of the discovertebral joint: Degenerative change in the elderly adult. *Radiology* 1987; 164:411–414.
42. Masaryk TJ, Boumphrey F, Modic MT, et al: Effects of chemonucleolysis demonstrated by MR imaging. *J Comput Assist Tomogr* 1986; 10:917–923.
43. Modic MT, Feiglin DH, Piraino DW, et al: Vertebral osteomyelitis: Assessment using MR. *Radiology* 1985; 157:157–166.
44. Yu S, Ho PS, Sether LM, et al: Nucleus pulposus degeneration: MR imaging, presented at the 73rd Scientific Assembly of the Radiological Society of North America, Chicago, 1987.
45. Grenier N, Gorssman RI, Schiebler ML, et al: Degenerative lumbar disk disease: Pitfalls and usefulness of MR imaging in detection of vacuum phenomenon. *Radiology* 1987; 164:861–865.
46. Masaryk TJ, Ross JS, Modic MT, et al: High-resolution MR imaging of sequestered lumbar intervertebral disks. *AJNR* 1988; 9:351–358.
47. Pech P, Haughton VM: Lumbar intervertebral disk: Correlative MR and anatomic study. *Radiology* 1985; 156:699–701.
48. Enzmann DR, Griffin L, Rubin J: Potential false-negative MR images of the thoracic spine in disk disease with switching of phase and frequency-encoding gradients. *Radiology* 1987; 165:635–637.
49. Russell EJ, D'Angelo CM, Zimmerman RD, et al: Cervical disk herniation: CT demonstration after contrast enhancement. *Radiology* 1984; 152:703–712.
50. Hedberg MC, Drayer BP, Flom RA, et al: Gradient echo (GRASS) MR imaging and cervical radiculopathy. *AJNR* 1988; 9:145–151.
51. Enzmann DR, Rubin JB: Cervical spine: MR imaging with a partial flip angle, gradient refocussed pulse sequence: I. General considerations and disk disease. *Radiology* 1988; 166:467–472.
52. Enzmann DR, Rubin JB: Cervical spine: MR imaging with a partial flip angle, gradient refocussed pulse sequence: II. Spinal cord disease. *Radiology* 1988; 166:473–478.
53. Ross JS, Delamarter R, Hueftle MG, et al: Gadolinium DTPA enhanced postoperative lumbar spine MRI: Time course and mechanism of enhancement. *AJNR* (in press).
53a. Yu S, Sether LA, Ho PS, et al: Tears of the anulus fibrosus: Correlation between MR and pathologic findings in cadavers. *AJNR* 1988, 9:367–370.
54. Schellinger D, Wener L, Ragsdale BD: Facet joint disorders and their role in the production of back pain and sciatica. *RadioGraphics* 1987; 7:923–944.
55. Dorwart RH, Vogler JB III, Helms CA: Spinal stenosis—symposium on CT of the lumbar spine. *Radiol Clin North Am* 1983; 21:301–323.
56. Yamamoto I, Matsumae M, Ikeda A, et al: Thoracic spinal stenosis: Experience with 7 cases. *J Neurosurg* 1988; 68:37–40.

57. Harsh GR III, Sypert GW, Weinstein PR, et al: Cervical spine stenosis secondary to ossification of the posterior longitudinal ligament. *J Neurosurg* 1987; 67:349–357.
58. Grenier N, Kressel HY, Schiebler ML, et al: Normal and degenerative posterior spinal structures: MR imaging. *Radiology* 1987; 165:517–525.
59. Harris RI, McNab I: Structural changes in the lumbar intervertebral disks: Their relationship to low back pain and sciatica. *J Bone Joint Surg [Br]* 1954; 36:304–322.

4

Postoperative Spine

Jeffrey S. Ross, M.D.

Mark G. Hueftle, M.D.

POSTOPERATIVE LUMBAR SPINE

A difficult diagnostic problem from the clinical and radiographic viewpoints is the evaluation of patients with symptoms following spinal surgery. This failed back surgery syndrome is a spectrum of diseases characterized by pain and functional incapacitation. From 10% to 40% of patients may fall into this category following spinal surgery. The causative factors accounting for the failed back surgery syndrome include recurrent disk herniation (12% to 16%), lateral (58%) or central (7% to 14%) spinal stenosis, arachnoiditis (6% to 16%), and epidural fibrosis (6% to 8%).[1] Less frequent causes include meningocele formation, mechanical instability (including facet subluxations and pseudoarthroses), nerve injury, and wrong-level surgery. In evaluating the postoperative patient, plain radiographs are generally unrewarding since they reveal only the usual postoperative bony changes such as laminectomy site, fusion masses, and degenerative disk-space narrowing. Myelography may show arachnoiditis or a focal extradural defect at the surgical site. However, the myelographic distinction between scar and herniated disk is considered by many to be impossible.[2–4] High-resolution computed tomographic (CT) scanning of the lumbar spine was a major inroad to understanding the causes of failed back surgery syndrome, and the CT findings in the postoperative spine have been described.[5] More recently, magnetic resonance (MR) has been applied to the postoperative spine patient, with encouraging results towards the diagnosis of a wide variety of disease entities.[6]

Sequences

If paramagnetic contrast agents are not available, then a routine MR examination of the postoperative patient consists of T_1-weighted spin-echo sagittal as well as T_1- and T_2-weighted spin-echo axial images. The use of surface coils will provide the optimum signal-to-noise ratio (S/N). The T_1-weighted spin-echo images provide good spatial resolution and S/N. The T_2-weighted images are not an absolute necessity but will occasionally better define the extradural tissues (scar vs. disk), extradural interface, and nerve roots than is possible with only a T_1-weighted sequence. We have also used gradient echo fast scans with variable flip angles (usually 40 to 60 degrees for the lumbar spine) to better define the extradural interface.

Unenhanced Magnetic Resonance Imaging

Before images of abnormalities in postoperative patients can be interpreted, knowledge of the normal postoperative sequence of events that is demonstrable by MR is a necessity. The following findings are based on 15 patients who underwent MR imaging prior to, 1 to 10 days after, and 2 to 6 months after a variety of lumbar spine surgeries. The majority of surgeries were laminectomy and diskectomies (Fig 4–1).

Laminectomy sites are quite apparent due to the bone removal involved (Figs 4–2,B and 4–3,B). The regions of the missing lamina are identified on axial and sagittal images as a loss of the normal low-signal cortical bone and high-signal marrow on T_1-weighted images. In

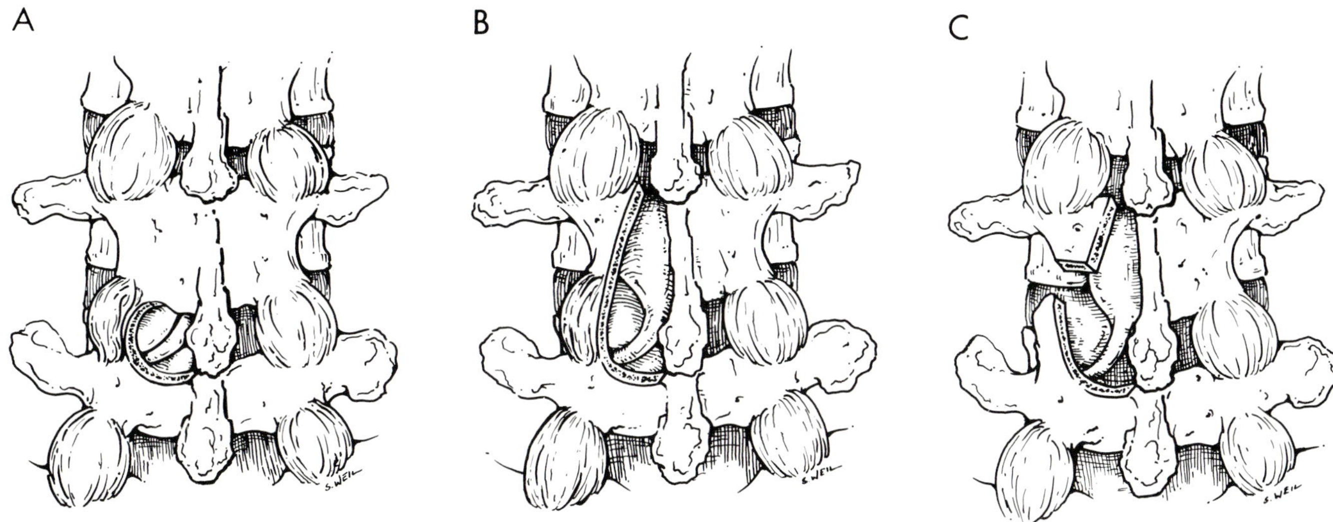

FIG 4–1.
A, laminotomy. Only a small amount of bone is removed from the inferior and superior laminae both above and below the herniated nucleus pulposus (HNP) level, respectively. **B,** laminectomy. The length of the laminae is removed to improve exposure of the HNP. **C,** laminectomy and facetectomy. The exposure is widened by removal of a variable amount of facet joint, not only to better visualize the HNP, but also to relieve lateral recess or foraminal stenosis.

the immediate postoperative period, this is replaced by a variable amount of postoperative soft tissue edema exhibiting slightly heterogeneous intermediate signal on T_1-weighted images and hyperintense signal on T_2-weighted images (see Figs 4–2 and 4–3). This soft tissue signal obliterates the normal muscle-fat planes of the paraspinal musculature along the operative tract. Mass effect is not usually present on the dural tube from this posterior edema. Midline sagittal images also well define the portions of the spinous processes remaining due to their high-signal fatty marrow. The minimal soft-tissue disruption caused by microsurgical techniques may be difficult or impossible to localize. With a laminotomy, only the absence of the ligamentum flavum will denote the site of previous surgical intervention. Studies obtained 2 to 6 months postoperatively show persistence of these posterior soft tissue changes (i.e., scar) that have become more homogeneous in appearance. The disruption of the normal muscle-fat planes continues. Following laminectomy, the thecal sac will maintain a smooth rounded contour, although it may be slightly posteriorly displaced or protruding into the soft tissues. Expansion of the thecal sac to normal contour will occur quite rapidly in the immediate postoperative period, even if there was severe canal stenosis preoperatively (Fig 4–4).

Diskectomy produces unique changes on MR. Sagittal and axial T_1-weighted images immediately following diskectomy will show intermediate soft tissue signal anterior to the thecal sac at the original site of disk herniation and operation. This soft tissue signal will blend smoothly with the posterior portion of the disk, especially at the site of diskectomy on T_1-weighted images and show increased signal on T_2-weighted images. This soft tissue can be as large as the original disk herniation and produce mass effect on the anterior dural tube (see Fig 4–2,B). Of the 13 patients we studied who underwent diskectomy, mass effect mimicking preoperative findings was present in 9. The amount of this anterior extradural soft tissue usually decreases by 2 to 6 months postoperatively. Specifically, these anterior extradural changes were seen to improve in appearance by the late postoperative study in 8/9 cases where initial mass effect was present (see Figs 4–2,C and 4–3,C).

Sagittal T_2-weighted images are excellent for showing the distribution of the normally low signal of the outer fibers of the posterior anulus fibrosis/posterior longitudinal ligament at the site of diskectomy. The high signal of the nucleus pulposus may be seen on T_2-weighted images extending posteriorly to where the anulus was disrupted by surgery (Fig 4–5). This area will merge with the high cerebrospinal fluid (CFS) signal in this region. Axial T_2-weighted images can show similar findings with a tract of increased signal extending laterally from the diskectomy site into the central portion of the nucleus pulposus where curettage took place. This disruption of the posterior aspect of the anulus fibrosis is generally not visible on T_1-weighted images. However, on T_2-weighted images, this anulus disruption or "anular rent" was seen in 11/13 cases in the immediate

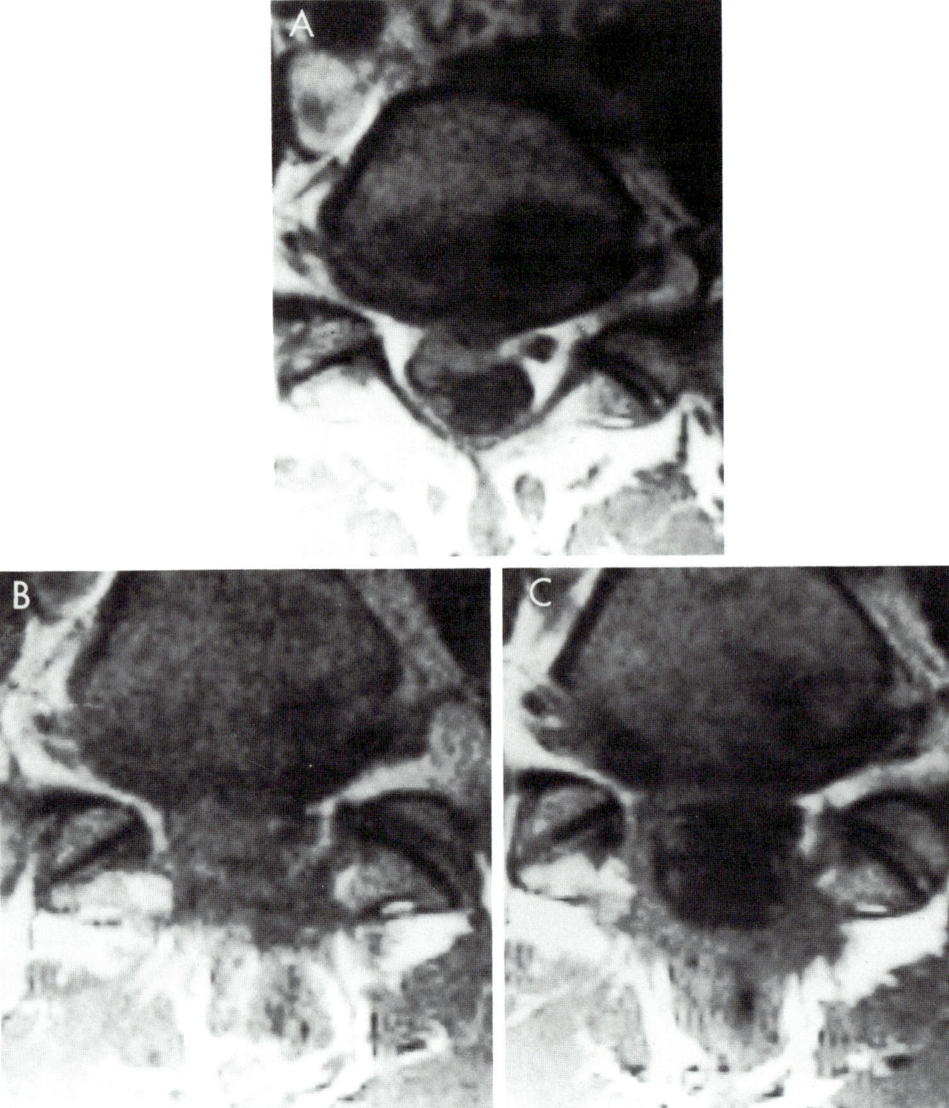

FIG 4–2.
Normal sequence of events following laminectomy and diskectomy. **A,** preoperative axial T_1-weighted MR shows a large central disk herniation at L5-S1 compressing the thecal sac. **B,** immediate postoperative axial T_1-weighted MR shows disruption of the epidural soft tissues and indistinct thecal sac margin. **C,** late postoperative (6 months) axial T_1-weighted MR shows restoration of the thecal sac margin, which is now surrounded by epidural fibrosis.

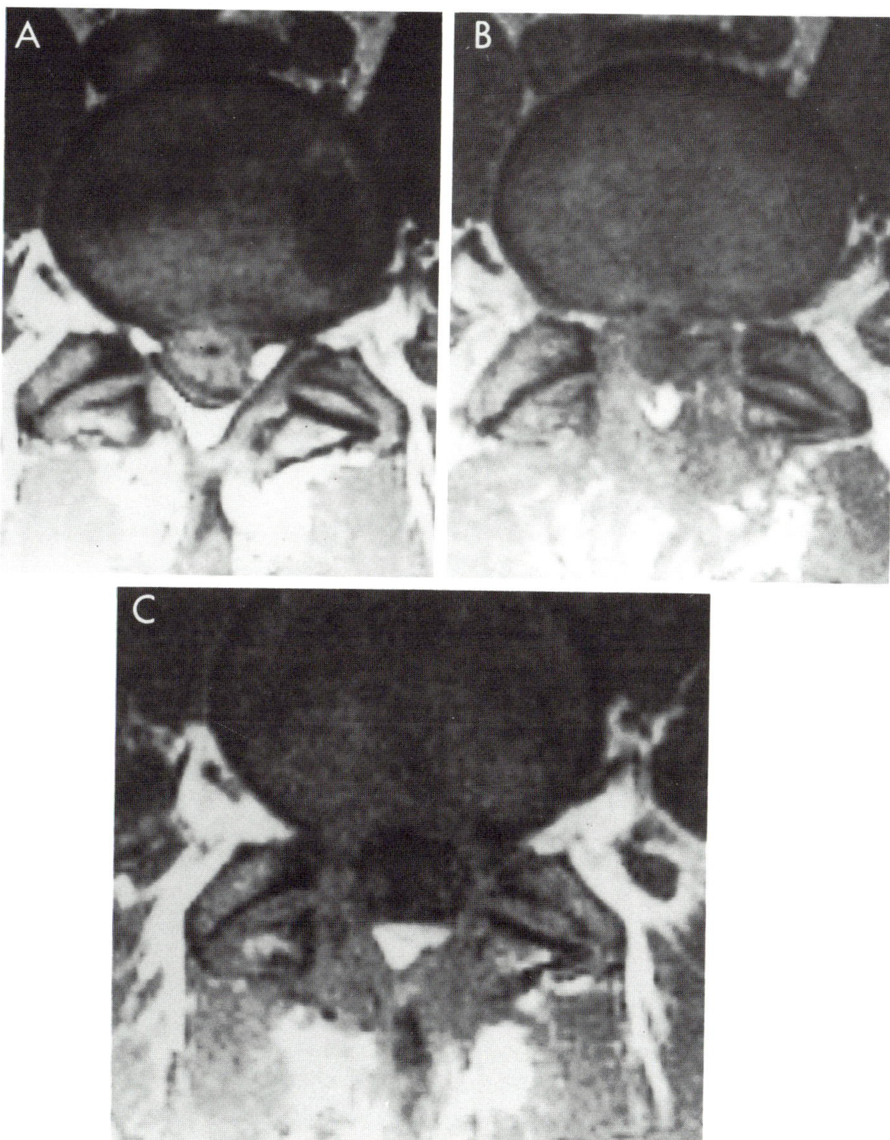

FIG 4–3.
Normal sequence of events following laminectomy and diskectomy. **A,** axial T_1-weighted image shows an enormous central disk herniation. **B,** immediate postoperative T_1-weighted axial image shows disruption of the epidural tissues and an indistinct thecal sac. The herniation appears to have been removed. **C,** late postoperative axial T_1-weighted image shows a normal thecal sac contour but extensive epidural fibrosis.

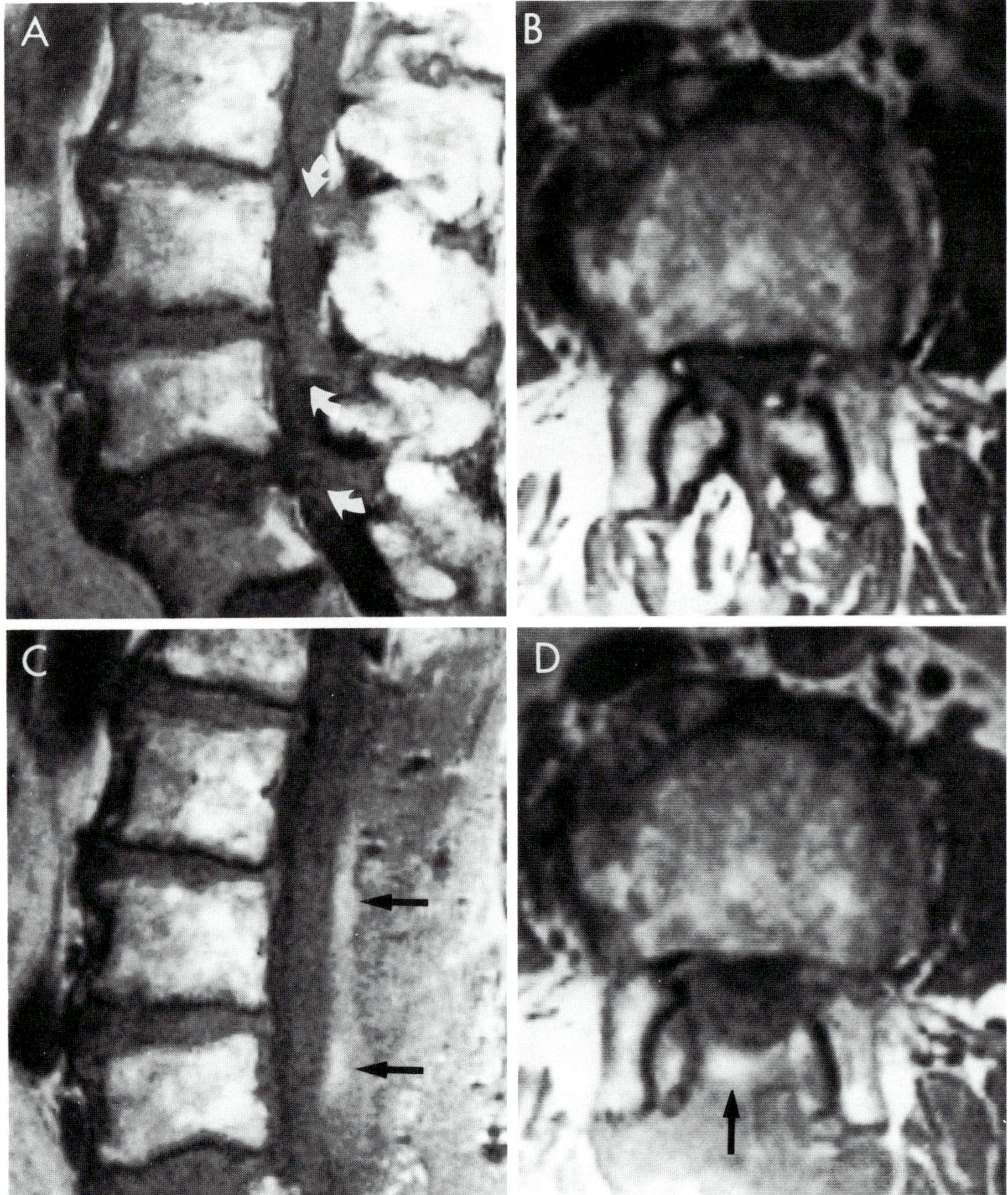

FIG 4–4.
Preoperative sagittal (**A**) and axial (**B**) T_1-weighted images demonstrate severe canal stenosis at several levels. The hypertrophied ligaments are seen as indistinct masses encroaching on the thecal sac on the sagittal view *(arrows)*. Increased signal is present from the cerebrospinal fluid (CSF) in the lumbar spine due to dampened CSF pulsations secondary to the stenosis. Postoperative sagittal (**C**) and axial (**D**) T_1-weighted images demonstrate a more normal contour to the thecal sac following an extensive laminectomy. High signal intensity posterior to the sac *(arrows)* is presumed to be blood (methemoglobin). (From Ross JS, Masaryk TJ, Modic MT, et al: Lumbar spine: Postoperative assessment with surface-coil MR imaging. *Radiology* 1987; 164:851–860. Used by permission.)

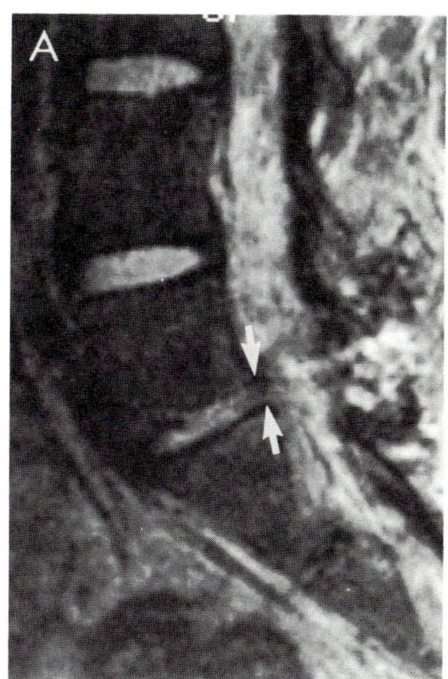

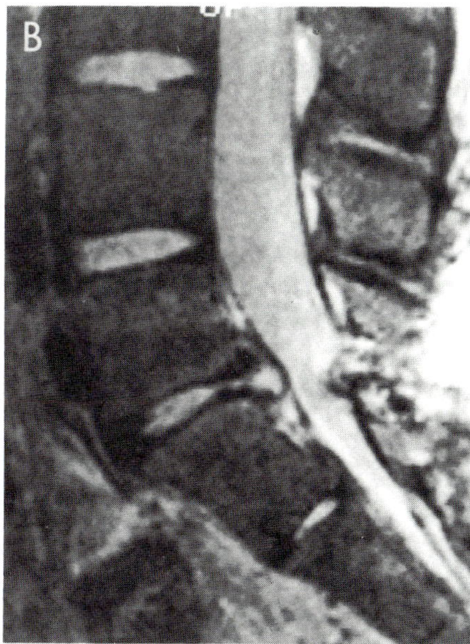

FIG 4–5.
A, immediate postoperative T_2-weighted image following laminectomy and diskectomy shows the site of disruption of the posterior annulus fibrosis/posterior longitudinal ligament due to disk curettage *(arrows)* **B,** image lateral to **A** shows an apparent continued disk herniation. These generally decrease in size with time. From Ross JS, Masaryk TJ, Modic MT, et al: Lumbar spine: Postoperative assessment with surface-coil MR imaging. *Radiology* 1987; 164:851–860. Used by permission.

postoperative period. It is important to realize that the anulus lateral to the site of diskectomy can retain its preoperative appearance, (whether normal in configuration, bulging, or even protruded) if imaged soon enough following surgery.

Late follow-up studies 2 to 6 months postoperatively will show that the rent in the anulus at the diskectomy site is less, or no longer apparent. In the 10 patients where comparison could be made on last postoperative studies, the anular rent resolved in 8/10. With "healing," the original high signal on T_2-weighted images from the rent is replaced with linear vertical decreased signal on T_2-weighted sagittal images similar to the appearance of the preoperative anulus fibrosis. While the configuration of the anulus away from this site of diskectomy can remain unchanged, more commonly the disk bulge or protrusion will become less apparent with a concomitant decrease in disk-space height as further degeneration occurs. This lack of change in the appearance of the disk herniation, combined with the epidural surgical disruption makes an unenhanced MR examination within the first 8 weeks following surgery nearly useless in defining residual disk material.

Changes in the adjacent lumbar vertebral bodies are uncommon with simple diskectomy. Only 1 of our 15 patients showed a rectangular area of hypodensity in the posterior superior end-plate of the L5 vertebral body following L5–S1 diskectomy (Fig 4–6). This is presumably due to curettage of the end-plate during diskectomy. In an additional three patients, type I vertebral body marrow changes occurred adjacent to the site of diskectomy on the late postoperative study.[7]

In the immediate postoperative period, soft tissue changes following foraminotomy are confined to the level where foraminal exploration and operation were performed. These are seen on T_1-weighted images as an increased amount of soft tissue signal material sur-

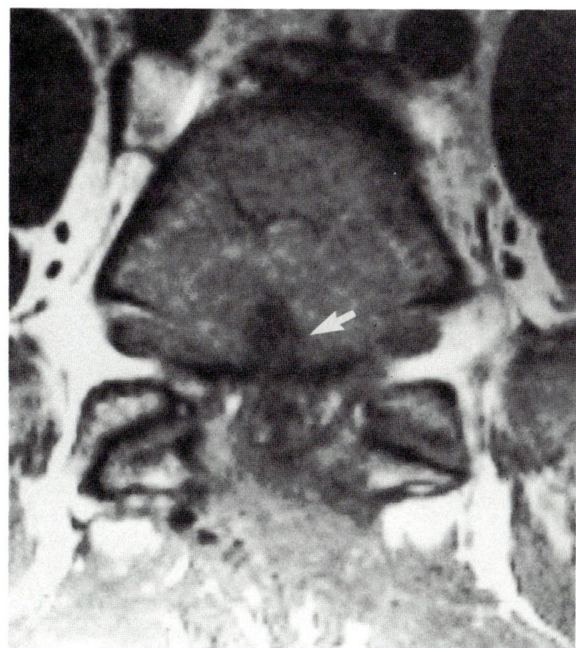

FIG 4–6.
Area of decreased signal within the superior S1 end-plate *(arrow)* due to inadvertent curettage during surgery. (From Ross JS, Masaryk TJ, Modic MT, et al: Lumbar spine: Postoperative assessment with surface-coil MR imaging. *Radiology* 1987; 164:851–860. Used by permission.)

rounding the nerve roots that obliterates the usual foraminal fat. This soft tissue commonly will show increased signal on T_2-weighted images.

Increased soft tissue lateral to the dural tube can be seen immediately after a variety of surgeries and is not limited to foraminotomy or facetectomy. Lateral epidural soft tissue signal changes are present in virtually all patients following laminectomy and diskectomy. This lateral soft tissue can merge with the soft tissue edema anterior and posterior to the thecal sac in a circumferential pattern. Increased signal on T_2-weighted images is also seen with lateral epidural edema. Initially, mass effect can displace the dural tube away from the operative site. Two to 3 months postoperatively, these lateral epidural soft tissue changes become smaller and more homogeneous in appearance with a loss of the initial mass effect. These areas of epidural fibrosis continue to show increased signal on T_2-weighted images (Fig 4–7).

In the immediate postoperative period, posterior and posterolateral fusions appear as large areas of soft tissue signal intensity on T_1-weighted images containing scattered pieces of graft bone in the region of the trans-

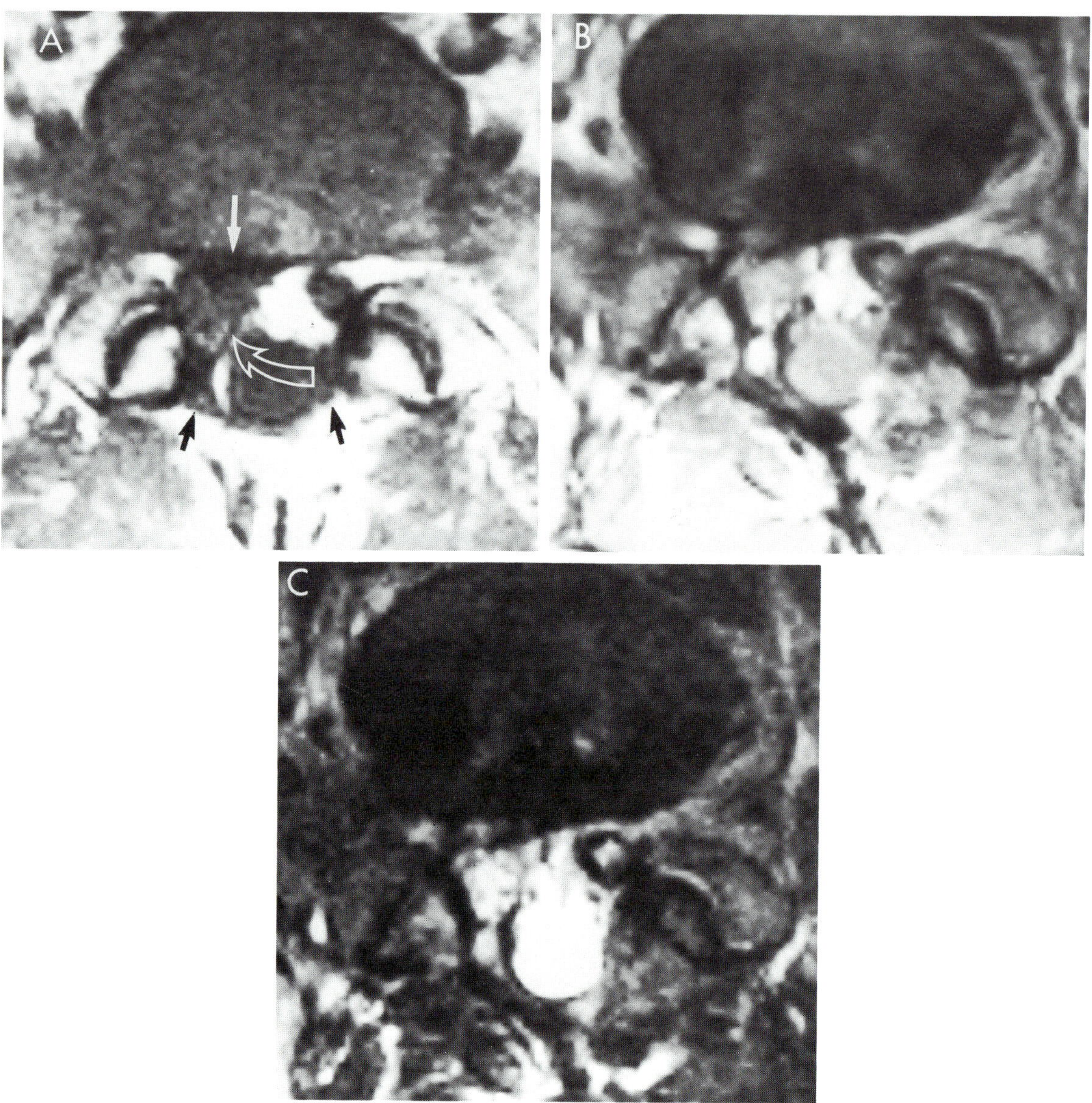

FIG 4–7.
Axial T_1-(**A**), spin-density (**B**), and (**C**) T_2-weighted images show epidural scar anterior to and laterally to the right of the thecal sac following laminectomy. The anterior scar encases the right S1 roots and demonstrates increased signal on the T_2-weighted images *(open arrow)*. Small disk herniation anterior to scar *(white arrow)* remains low in signal intensity on all three sequences. Posterior laminectomy scar *(black arrows)* shows no increase in signal with T_2-weighting.

verse processes and facet joints. The involved regions show loss of a normal fat signal and muscle-fat planes. The appearance of the bone grafts is quite variable and depends on its type. Allografts will tend to show decreased signal on T_1- and T_2-weighted images. Autografts tend to show higher signal on T_1-weighted images due to their presence of marrow. However, decreased signal on T_1-weighted images and increased signal on T_2-weighted images may also be seen with autografts. The thecal sac contour is not disrupted by the posterior soft tissue signal. This soft tissue signal will merge imperceptibly with the posterior and lateral epidural scar from the operation.

Solid bony fusion masses are outlined by the low signal intensity of cortical bone on T_1- and T_2-weighted images. Solid fusions show increased signal on T_1-weighted images due to the marrow content (Fig 4–8). Fibrous portions of the fusions are generally decreased signal on T_1- and T_2-weighted images. However, low signal-intensity areas may be either fibrous or bony if fatty marrow is not present. The continuity of fusion masses is generally quite difficult to determine by MR, due to the variable signal of graft marrow. Computed tomography or tomography is generally more helpful in defining areas of nonunion or pseudoarthrosis.

Subacute soft tissue hemorrhage has a characteristic appearance by MR showing increased signal on T_1- and T_2-weighted images (see Fig 4–4). In several patients, we have observed moderately well-defined, homogeneous areas of increased signal on T_1- and T_2-weighted images around the dural tube. While pathologic confirmation is not available in these asymptomatic patients, we feel these areas are compatible with postoperative hematomas.[8–10] Significant mass effect on the thecal sac was not observed in our cases. One patient who was imaged 2 months postoperatively showed complete resolution of these areas of increased signal on T_1- and T_2-weighted images, and these areas were replaced with homogeneous scar formation. Patients imaged within 24 hours following surgery may show a different hematoma appearance. These may be isointense on T_1-weighted images and show strikingly decreased signal on the T_2-weighted images due to deoxyhemoglobin (Fig 4–9).

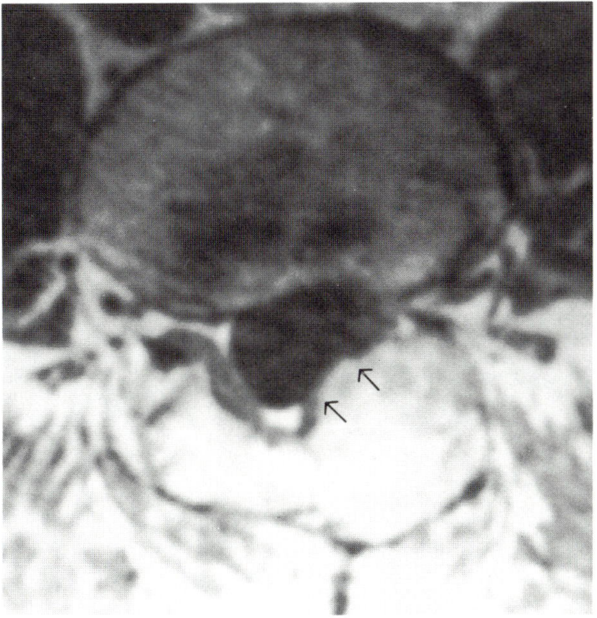

FIG 4–8.
Bony stenosis. Posterior fusion mass compresses the left posterolateral aspect of the thecal sac *(arrows)*. (From Ross JS, Modic MT, Masaryk TJ, et al: The postoperative spine. *Semin Roentgenol* 1988; 13:125–136. Used by permission.)

We have been unable to predict the clinical course of the patient by the appearance of the initial postoperative MR studies. Patients who were pain free may show significant anterior and lateral epidural scar tissue on the late postoperative studies.

Scar vs. Disk

The distinction between epidural fibrosis and recurrent disk herniation is of considerable importance since removal of extradural scar often leads to further scar formation, while removal of disk herniation is generally beneficial. Intravenous contrast-enhanced CT is felt by some investigators to be a reliable means of separating disk from scar but has not gained widespread usage in the routine workup of the postoperative patient.[11, 12] A prospective study[13] on 27 patients to evaluate MR and secondarily intravenous contrast-enhanced CT in the differentiation of epidural scar from herniated disk material showed that MR agreed with surgical findings in 83%. Protruded disks exhibited decreased signal intensity relative to epidural fibrosis on T_2-weighted sequences. Free fragments can demonstrate slightly increased signal on T_1-weighted images relative to the epidural fibrosis but a hyperintense signal intensity on T_2-weighted images similar to scar.

The intensity characteristics of epidural scar differ according to their location. Anterior epidural scars were hypointense to isointense relative to the adjacent disk material on T_1-weighted images. Anterior epidural scars were hyperintense on both spin-density and T_2-weighted sequences (see Fig 4–7). In general, the lateral scars exhibited similar characteristics, but not as consistently. As one moves posteriorly towards the site of laminectomy, the signal intensity of the scar becomes more variable. However, increased signal intensity is generally seen in the paraspinal musculature at the operative site with the T_2-weighted sequences. This study shows that

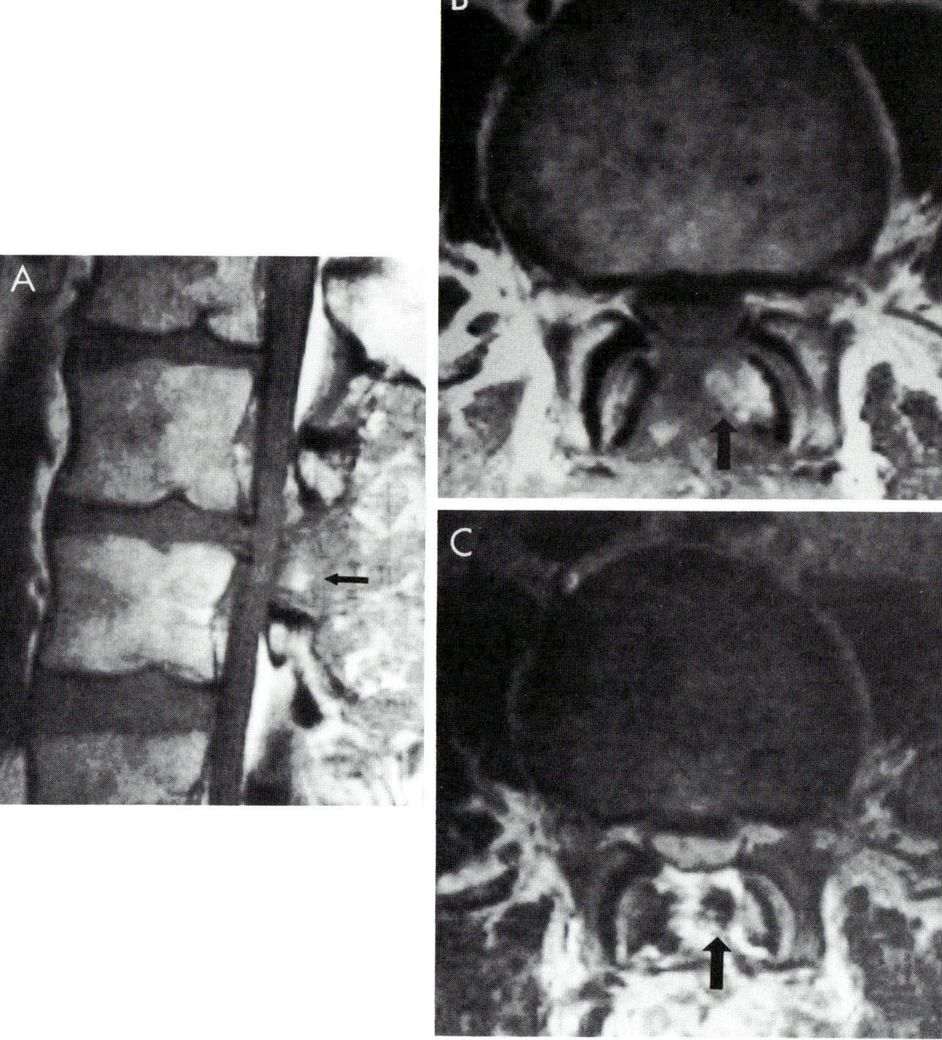

FIG 4–9.
Postoperative hematoma. Sagittal (**A**) and axial (**B**) T_1-weighted images following laminectomy show areas of intermediate and increased signal intensity in the posterior epidural tissue *(arrows)*. These areas show decreased signal on the axial T_2-weighted image (**C**) consistent with intracellular deoxyhemoglobin and methemoglobin *(arrow)*. (From Ross JS, Modic MT, Masaryk TJ, et al: The postoperative spine. *Semin Roentgenol* 1988; 13:125–136. Used by permission.)

when the criteria of morphology, epidural location, and mass effect are used, scar and disk may be differentiated on unenhanced MRI with an accuracy comparable to that of intravenous contrast-enhanced CT. Herniated disks will show continuity with the intervertebral disk space (except free fragments) and mass effect. Scarring will generally show increased signal on T_2-weighted images without mass effect. Large protruded or extruded disks may show decreased signal along their periphery on T_2-weighted images, while the central portion shows increased signal (similar to nucleus pulposus) (Fig 4–10).

Signal intensity of severely extruded or free fragments can be increased relative to the apparent disk or adjacent vertebral bodies on the T_2-weighted sequences. Similar signal intensity changes are also observed with epidural scar. In this small study, half the surgically proved free disk fragments showed hyperintensity on the T_1-weighted sequences relative to epidural fibrosis. No surgically demonstrated free fragments appeared hypointense relative to the desiccated postoperative disk or adjacent bone. However, scar appeared slightly hypointense or isointense on T_1-weighted images where it could easily be separated from fat. Both epidural scar and fat conform to the available space, while herniated

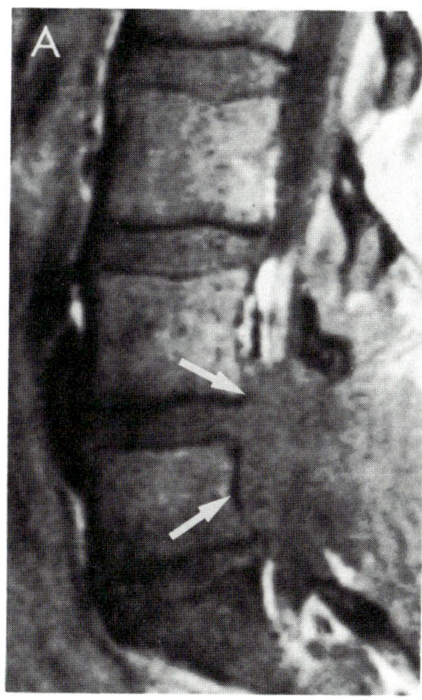

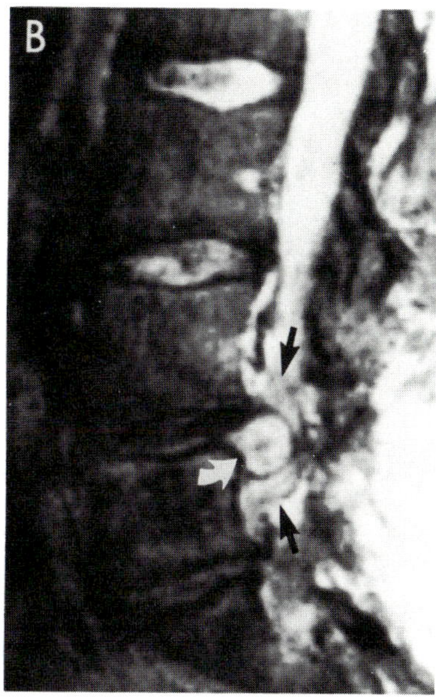

FIG 4–10.
Postoperative recurrent disk herniation. **A,** sagittal T_1-weighted image shows a large area of intermediate signal intensity at the L4-5 level and extending inferiorly over the L5 body *(arrows)*. **B,** sagittal T_2-weighted image shows a large high signal intensity mass extending into the canal from the L4-5 interspace, representing recurrent disk material *(curved arrow)*. Epidural scar surrounds the disk herniation and is also of increased intensity *(black arrows)*. No abnormal increased signal is seen in the central portion of the L4-5 intervertebral disk nor of the adjacent vertebral end-plates to suggest disk space infection despite the rather ominous T_1-weighted images appearance.

disk compresses and distorts it. Mass effect may be the only finding that will aid in the discrimination of free fragments from anterior or lateral recess scar.

Besides the differentiation of scar from disk, which is usually the primary concern in these postoperative patients, MR is also capable of defining a wide variety of additional postoperative findings.

Postoperative Fluid Collections

A pseudomeningocele results from a dural tear during surgery.[14] The fluid collection may be formed as the arachnoid herniates through the tear and proliferates into an arachnoid pouch, or the CSF may extravasate into the soft tissues that develop a fibrous capsule. Magnetic resonance will show a rounded area of CSF intensity immediately posterior to the thecal sac at the site of previous laminectomy (Fig 4–11). If the fluid contains blood products, then the T_1-weighted images may show slightly increased signal. This was present in one patient who had a large fluid collection of the right and posterior to the thecal sac following resection of an extradural component of a dumbbell-shaped neurofibroma. This collection demonstrated increased signal on the T_1- and T_2-weighted images. At reoperation, the presence of a pseudomeningocele containing xanthochromic fluid was verified.

Not uncommonly, well-defined areas of decreased signal on T_1-weighted and of increased signal on T_2-weighted images will be seen in the midline posteriorly along the incision site (Fig 4–12). Out of five patients we have examined with these small collections, no clinical symptoms were referable to the areas. These are presumed to be small postoperative serous fluid collections. A similar-appearing fluid collection that may also lie posteriorly along the incision site is a wound abscess. This also shows low signal on T_1-weighted images, and increased signal on T_2-weighted images. The MR changes are nonspecific for these fluid collections, and MR is unable to differentiate by signal characteristics or morphology the appearance of benign postoperative fluid collection, pseudomeningoceles, or wound abscesses. A pseudomeningocele should not be mistaken for the normal posteriorly placed thecal sac that occurs with simple laminectomy.

Stenosis

In a recent series of 73 postoperative patients, recurrent disk herniation was present in only 67% of cases. On the other hand, lateral bony stenosis is implicated as a cause of failed back surgery syndrome in up to 60% of cases.[1] An additional cause of stenosis is the upward migration of the superior facet (with concomitant narrowing of the foramen) secondary to disk degeneration and loss of height after diskectomy. Bony stenosis may have a wide variety of appearances on MR. This is due to the variability of the marrow content of the vertebral body and bony fusion masses as well as to various degrees of bony sclerosis. Osteophytes of compact or sclerotic bone will have low signal intensity on T_1- and T_2-weighted images (Fig 4–13). These may be apparent only by the displacement of the epidural fat or mass effect on the thecal sac and nerve roots. At the

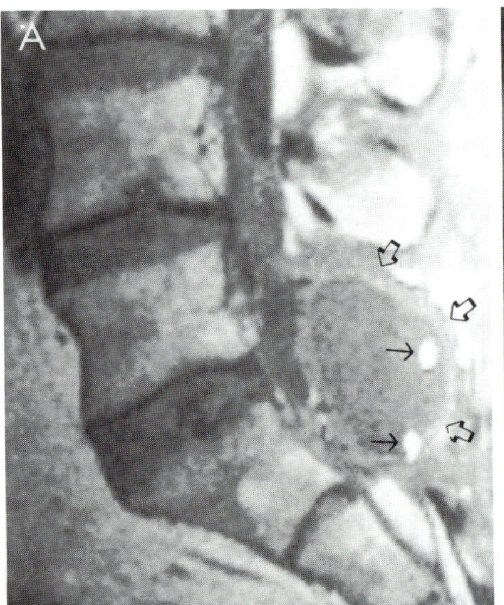

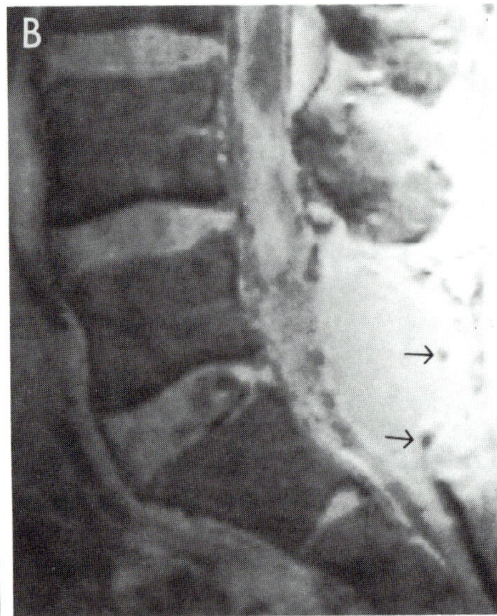

FIG 4–11.
Pseudomeningocele. Sagittal T_1-weighted image (**A**) shows a posterior CSF collection *(open arrows)* with a well-defined capsule. Small droplets of iophendylate (Pantopaque) *(arrow)* lie in the dependent portion of the pseudomeningocele. Note the clumped nerve roots at the L4 level indicating arachnoiditis. **B,** gradient echo FISP image (α = 60 degrees) shows similar findings with the iophendylate now low in signal.

other extreme, spurs containing fatty marrow are easily recognized by their high signal intensity on T_1-weighted images (see Fig 4–8). We have seen postoperative bony stenosis in 10/62 patients in our series. In 5 of these, the narrowing was generalized secondary to disk degeneration. In our series with MR, as well as in the series of Teplick and Haskins[5] using CT, epidural fibrosis is a much more common finding than severe bony stenosis.

One method used in an attempt to decrease epidural fibrosis is the placement of free fat or pedicle fat grafts over the laminectomy site.[15] Posterior fat grafts are easily recognized as globular collections of increased signal on T_1-weighted images posterior to the dural tube (Fig 4–14). The fat grafts may be associated with minimal epidural scarring or be included in extensive scarring that appears to stop just where the graft is present. A small amount of posterior epidural scar is often interposed between the dural tube and the graft.

Arachnoiditis is covered more fully in the chapter on inflammation. Magnetic resonance is capable of vi-

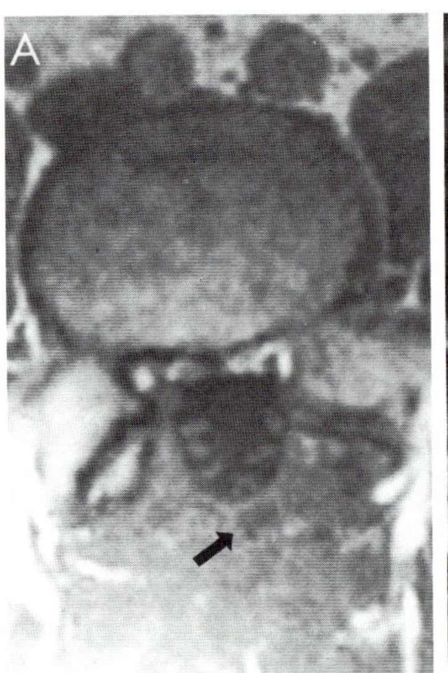

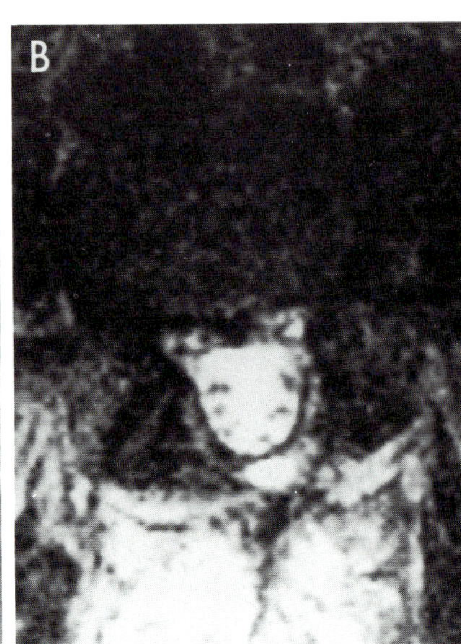

FIG 4–12.
Small round area of decreased signal *(arrow)* on the axial T_1-weighted image (**A**) and increased signal on T_2-weighted image (**B**) in the posterior epidural tissue is consistent with a small serous fluid collection. Note the abnormal high signal intensity from the paraspinal muscles along the operative tract. (From Ross JS, Masaryk JJ, Modic MT, et al: Lumbar spine: Postoperative assessment with surface-coil MR imaging. *Radiology* 1987; 164:851–860. Used by permission.)

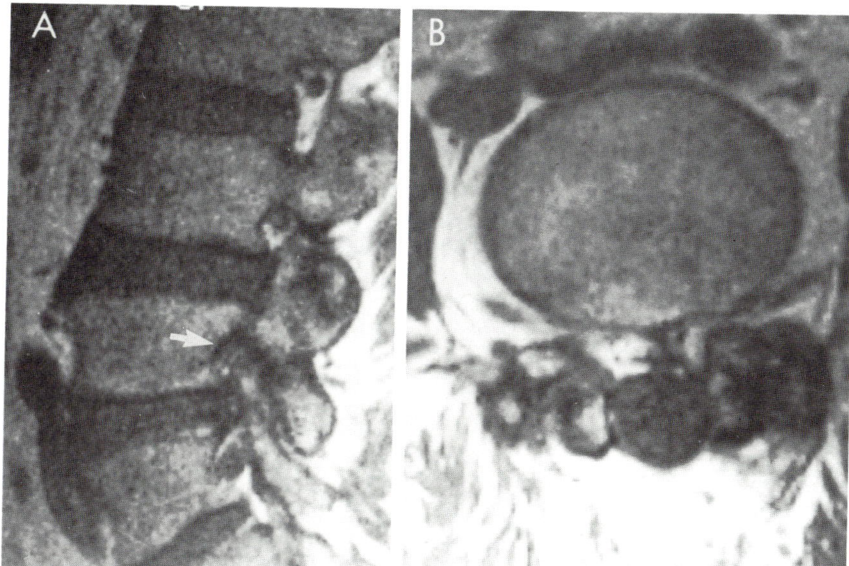

FIG 4–13.
Foraminal stenosis. Sagittal (**A**) and axial (**B**) T_1-weighted images show severe bilateral foraminal stenosis in this patient who is status post laminectomy. The superior articular facets compress the exiting nerve roots *(arrow)*. (From Ross JS, Modic MT, Masaryk TJ, et al: The postoperative spine. *Semin Roentgenol* 1988; 13:125–136. Used by permission.)

sualizing central adhesions of nerve roots as increased soft tissue within the central portion of the thecal sac on T_1- and T_2-weighted images. Peripheral adhesions of roots to the meninges may also occur, giving rise to an apparently "empty thecal sac," seen as homogeneous CSF signal within the dural tube on both T_1- and T_2-weighted images (Fig 4–15). With more severe arachnoiditis, increased soft tissue signal may be seen in the thecal sac obliterating the normal CSF signal. This finding correlates with marked irregularity of the thecal sac or a myelographic block.[16]

Field distortion due to changes in magnetic susceptibility are frequently observed in postoperative spine patients due to minute metallic particles from surgical instruments. During surgery, small metallic fragments that are not visible on plain x-rays or CT can be sheared off the instruments either by contact with other metal instruments or when dense sclerotic bone is drilled (see Fig 4–15). In the lumbar spine, these artifacts are commonly seen in the regions of the foramina and lateral recesses. These artifacts consist of either field distortion, loss of signal, or a halo of increased signal. Occasionally the field distortions are great enough to impede diagnosis.[17]

Gelfoam is an absorbable gelatin sponge primarily used for hemostasis during surgery, since it acts as a matrix for thrombus formation.[18] Gelfoam appears to have a characteristic appearance by MR, that is, decreased signal on T_1- and T_2-weighted images. In two patients, we have seen linear well-defined areas of decreased signal on both T_1- and T_2-weighted images posterior to the dural tube where Gelfoam had been placed at surgery (Fig 4–16). Follow-up study 60 days later in one patient showed apparent reabsorption of the Gelfoam with loss of the areas of decreased signal intensity.

Methyl methacrylate is commonly used in orthopedic procedures to distribute the mechanical forces imposed by metal hardware on endosteal or cancellous bony surfaces. Methyl methacrylate shows decreased signal on T_1- and T_2-weighted images.[17] Occasionally, the appearance of the methacrylate may be rather unusual depending on its area of placement. One patient who had removal of fusion hardware placed through the pedicles and into the vertebral bodies showed linear areas of low signal intensity representing residual methyl methacrylate within the pedicles. These appeared as "ghost shadows" of the spiral configuration of the screws.

Lumbar interbody fusions often utilize bank bone grafts. These demonstrate a uniform decreased signal intensity on T_1- and T_2-weighted images within the graft. The margins of the graft are well defined and linear. Axial images will show the graft as a square-shaped area of low signal intensity on T_1-weighted images at the level of the intervertebral disk (Fig 4–17). We have not observed adjacent vertebral body marrow signal changes with these grafts.

Fibular grafts may be utilized for posterior interbody fusions of the lumbar spine for severe spondylolisthesis. The fibular grafts demonstrate a rim of decreased signal on T_1- and T_2-weighted images representing cortical bone, with the marrow spaces showing more variable appearance (Fig 4–18). Commonly, the graft marrow space will show decreased signal on T_1-weighted and increased signal on T_2-weighted images compared to the normal fibular marrow signal. This change in the central marrow signal can be seen in the immediate postoperative period and may persist over at least a 6 month period. Other grafts will show only the

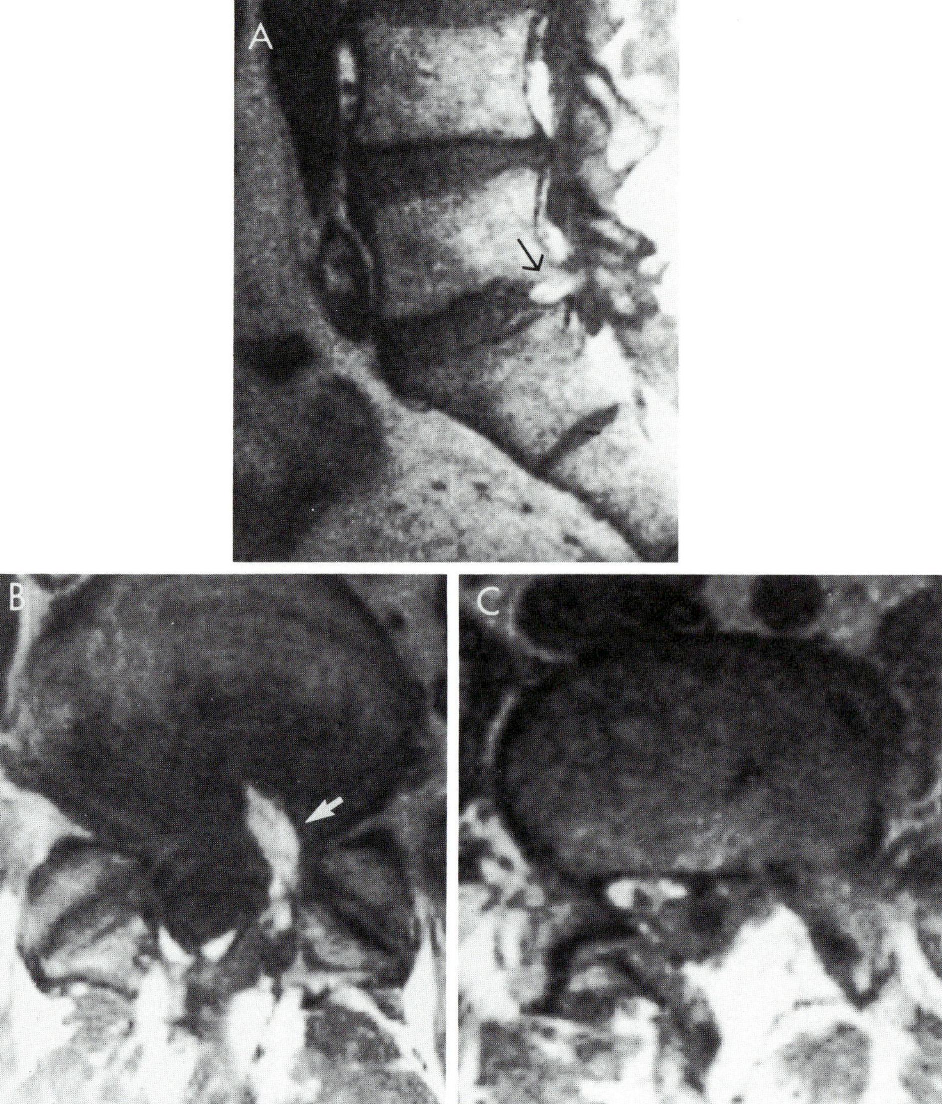

FIG 4–14.
Fat grafts. Sagittal (**A**) and axial (**B**) T_1-weighted images show a graft extending from the left epidural space into the disk at the site of previous curettage *(arrow)*. **C,** more typical appearing fat graft fills in the left hemilaminectomy site precluding significant epidural fibrosis.

high signal on T_1-weighted images from normal appearing marrow. Whether these signal changes on MR relate to graft revascularization is presently unknown.

Conclusion

Early postoperative changes demonstrated by MR are dramatic and affect every portion of the neural canal. In the immediate postoperative period following diskectomy, the anular rent where diskectomy and curettage has taken place is easily demonstrated. Increased soft tissue signal (edema) is commonly seen anterior and lateral to the dural tube that obliterates the normal epidural fat signal. These changes also greatly distort the dural tube contour. The intervertebral disk may continue to show a herniation in the immediate postoperative period. This lack of intervertebral disk change, coupled with extensive epidural disruption, precludes a useful unenhanced MR study in the immediate postoperative period for continuing symptomatology except for excluding a postoperative hemorrhage. The high signal intensity of hemorrhage on T_1- and T_2-weighted im-

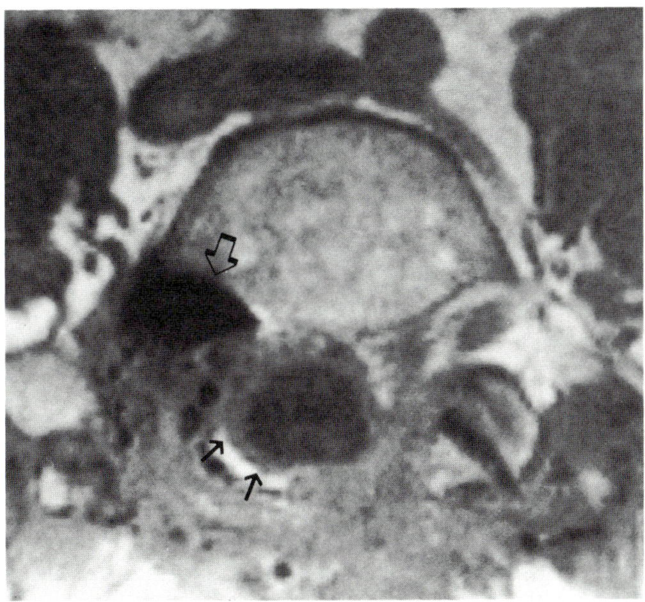

FIG 4–15.
Metal artifact. Ovoid area of decreased signal overlying the right foramen *(large arrow)* is secondary to minute metallic fragments sheared off instruments during surgery. The CT scan showed no metallic density. Additionally, the nerve roots are adhered to the meninges, giving an "empty thecal sac" appearance of arachnoiditis *(arrows)*. The small posterior protrusion of the thecal sac *(arrows)* is normal following laminectomy.

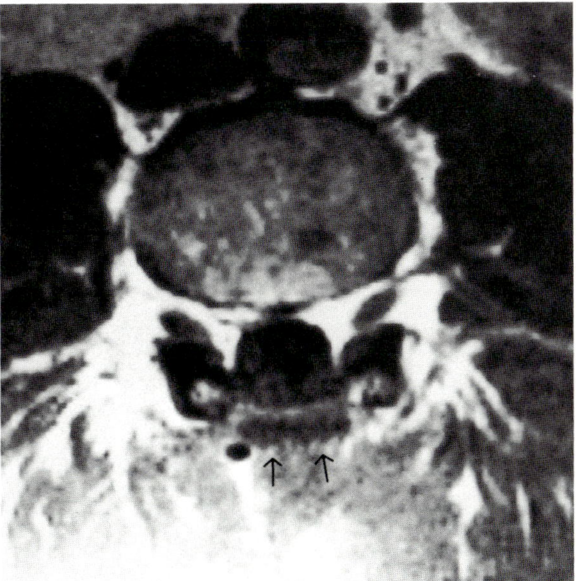

FIG 4–16.
Gelfoam. Axial T_1-weighted image demonstrates a linear band of decreased signal posterior to the thecal sac immediately following laminectomy *(arrows)*. This most likely represents gelfoam placed at surgery. Small dot of decreased signal posterolateral to the Gelfoam is a gas bubble.

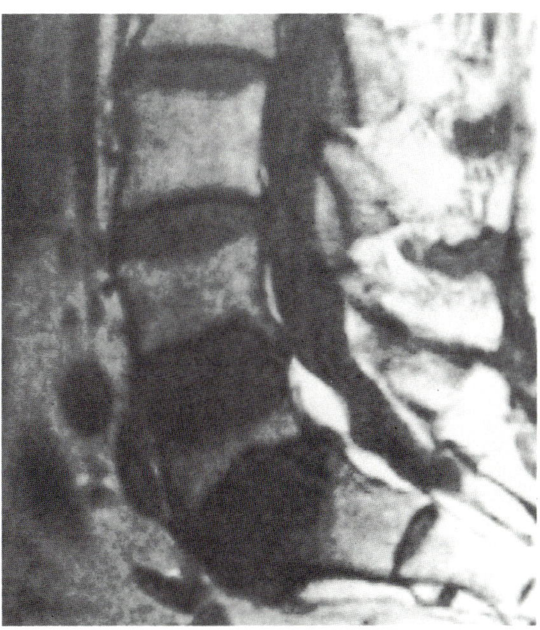

FIG 4–17.
Lumbar anterior fusion (total disk replacement). Disk replacements have been performed at L4-5 and L5-S1. These are seen as well-defined areas of decreased signal on this sagittal T_1-weighted image.

ages allows tissue contrast with the intermediate intensity of epidural edema.

T_2-weighted sagittal images appear to be the most helpful in discriminating in the site of anulus disruption and the morphology of the remaining disk. T_1-weighted images in this immediate postoperative period are less helpful, generally showing ill-defined increased soft tissue signal involving the anulus, nucleus, and anterior and lateral epidural tissues. Later in the postoperative course, the anular rent will heal and become inapparent with a concomitant disk degeneration and resolution of any remaining disk protrusion away from the diskectomy site. Epidural changes will improve in appearance and become more homogeneous and lose any initial mass effect. Scar formation tends to be ubiquitous in lumbar surgery except for a simple laminectomy or laminectomy and fusion. Epidural fibrosis conforms to the dural tube outline and usually does not demonstrate mass effect. Scarring anterior and lateral to the dural tube will generally show increased signal on T_2-weighted images. The changes present in the immediate postoperative period are consequence of the surgical intervention and should not be confused with pathology. These changes instead reflect a dynamic course of the normal process of repair.

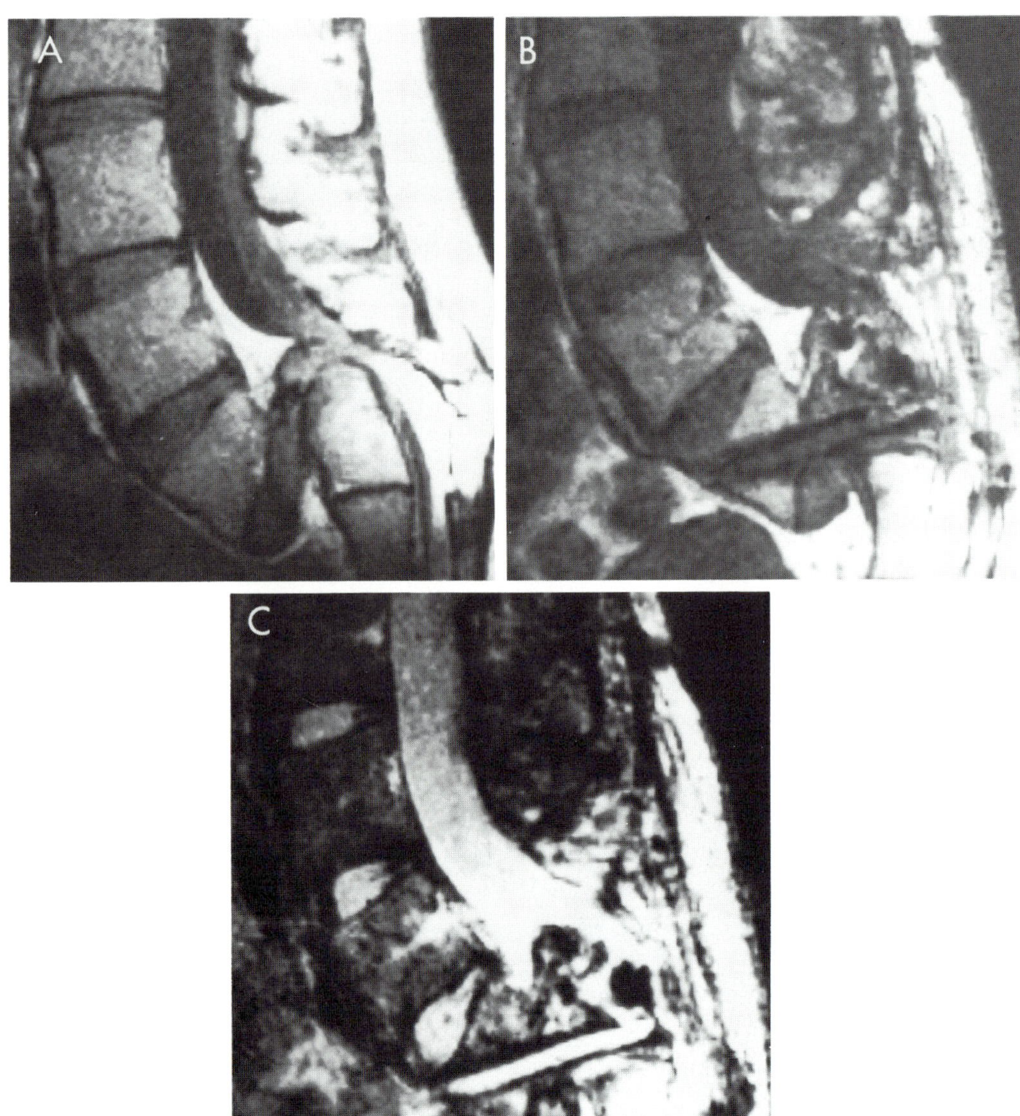

FIG 4–18.
Interbody fusion. Preoperative sagittal T_1-weighted image (**A**) demonstrates a grade IV spondylolisthesis of L5 on S1. Postoperative sagittal T_1-weighted (**B**) and T_2-weighted (**C**) images show placement of a fibular strut through L5 and S1 to stablilize the spine. The strut is outlined by low-signal cortical bone. The marrow signal is increased on the T_2-weighted image that could reflect edema due to the operative procedure. (From Ross JS, Masaryk TJ, Modic MT, et al: Lumbar spine: Postoperative assessment with surface-coil MR imaging. *Radiology* 1987; 164:851–860. Used by permission.)

Gd-DTPA Enhanced Magnetic Resonance Imaging

Gadolinium diethylenetriamine penta-acetic acid (Gd-DTPA) is a paramagnetic contrast agent used in MR imaging. It has been shown in humans and animal models to enhance the MR intensity of various tissues following intravenous administration.[19–23] Gadolinium DTPA has a biodistribution compatible with an extracellular fluid compartment and is rapidly excreted by the kidneys. Gadolinium DTPA has a high degree of paramagnetism, has strong complex formation, and appears well tolerated.[24, 25] It is useful as a contrast agent for evaluating inflammatory or tumorous lesions as well as for denoting any disruption within the blood-brain barrier. Gadolinium DTPA has a short half-life in blood of approximately 20 minutes and a relatively high LD_{50} in rats (18 mmole/kg).[21]

As previously indicated in this chapter, the differentiation of epidural fibrosis from recurrent or persistent disk herniation is of prime importance in imaging patients with the failed back surgery syndrome. A large amount of time and effort has been expended in trying to identify an imaging modality and/or diagnostic criteria that will allow this distinction. Myelography has not proved useful in this regard.[3, 4] In the series of Firooznia et al.,[26] unenhanced CT scanning was diagnostic in 60% of cases. The accuracy of intravenously enhanced computed tomography (IVCT) has been variously reported in the literature between 67% to 100%.[27–31]

Unenhanced MR has recently been addressed by Bundschuh et al.[13] who have found a similar accuracy to that of IVCT. More recently, Gd-DTPA–enhanced MR has been used to evaluate scar and disk herniations. Based on our initial experience with 30 cases (14 reoperated), we feel that Gd-DTPA–enhanced MR has tremendous potential toward accurate differentiation of scar from disk.[32]

All patients selected for this initial study were suffering from the failed back surgery syndrome with complaints referable to previously operated disk levels. To prevent any confusion during the immediate postoperative period, all selected patients had had surgery more than 6 months before the study. All the patients were studied before and after intravenous (IV) gadolinium administration with T_1-weighted sagittal and axial spin-echo sequences, T_2-weighted sagittal and axial spin-echo sequences, and gradient echo low flip-angle images.

Of the 14 operated patients (17 disk levels) there were 6 levels with scar, 7 combinations of scar and disk herniation, and 2 with only disk herniation. The final 2 levels had no aberrant soft tissue in the epidural space. Magnetic resonance was accurate in each of the cases, all of which had had a histologic diagnosis.

Epidural fibrosis was consistently enhanced (Fig 4–19). Enhancement of scar was seen to be diffuse but rather inhomogeneous on the early T_1-weighted spin-echo studies. By the delayed scans, (greater than 30 minutes after injection) this enhancement became homogeneous. In the operated group, half of the cases of scar demonstrated mass effect on the thecal sac. Additionally, 4/7 scars were located in a position contiguous with the disk space, an additional point of confusion with disk herniation.

Of the 9 levels where disk material was found at reoperation, 7 revealed peripheral enhancement following Gd-DTPA administration. Peridiskal scar was found in all of these cases at surgery and on histologic study (Figs 4–20 and 4–21). The 2 remaining cases were disk herniations at levels other than that previously operated and consisted solely of disk material as predicted by MR. One herniation did demonstrate peripheral enhancement following Gd-DTPA injection that was felt to represent epidural venous plexus. Of considerable significance, delayed enhancement of disk material was present in 7/9 reoperated cases. Four of these cases had initial peripheral enhancement that became more extensive and appeared to involve the periphery of the disk on the later scans. Three of these cases revealed diffuse enhancement of the disk material by the delayed study.

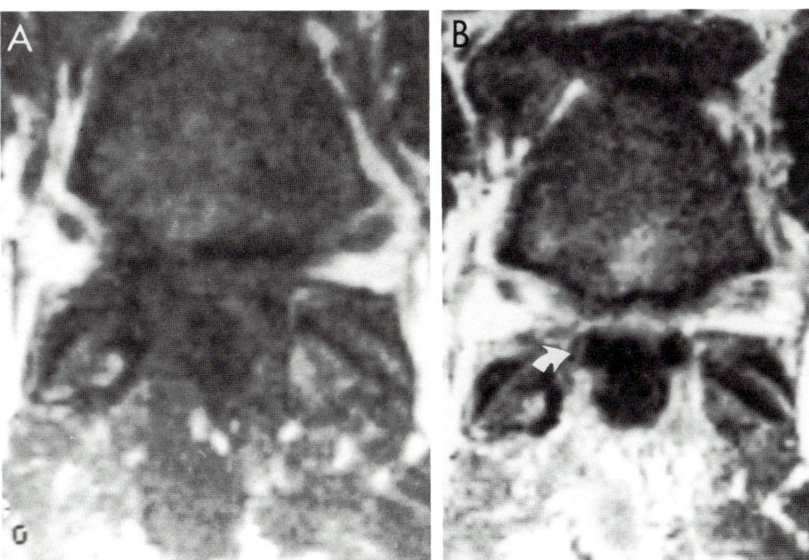

FIG 4–19.
Gd-DTPA enhancement of epidural fibrosis. Precontrast axial T_1-weighted image (**A**) shows circumferential soft tissue signal about the thecal sac. The differentiation of a recurrent disk from scar is not possible. Following Gd-DTPA (0.1 mmole/kg IV) the epidural scar is enhanced (**B**), allowing definition of the thecal sac and nerve roots *(arrow)*. No disk herniation is seen. (From Ross JS, Modic MT, Masaryk TJ, et al: The postoperative spine. *Semin Roentgenol* 1988; 13:125–136. Used by permission.)

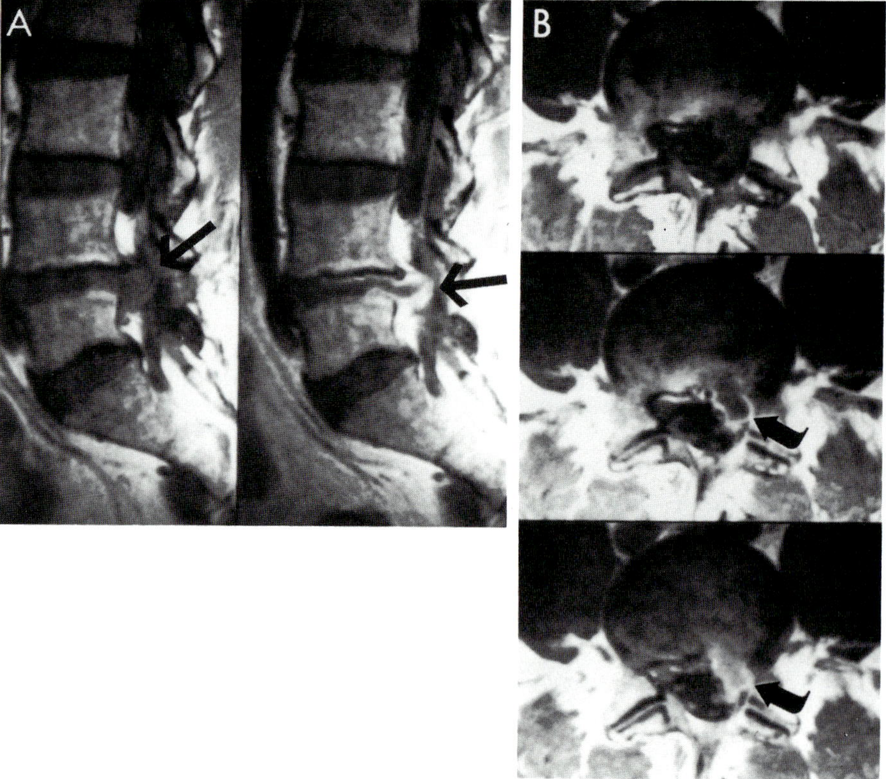

FIG 4–20.
Scar and disk herniation. **A,** precontrast T_1-weighted sagittal MR. The image on the *left* shows a large mass of aberrant soft tissue anterior to the thecal sac at the L4-5 level *(arrow)* in this patient with previous L4-5 diskectomy. Postcontrast sagittal image *(right)* shows marked enhancement of the peridiskal fibrosis *(arrow)* with nonenhancing disk present centrally. **B,** precontrast axial image *(top)* shows aberrant tissue anterior and to the left of the dural tube. Immediate postcontrast axial image *(middle)* shows enhancement of peripheral scar *(tailed arrow)* but no enhancement of disk herniation. Late postcontrast axial image *(bottom)* (greater than 30 minutes after injection) now shows enhancement of disk herniation and scar *(tailed arrow).* (From Hueftle MG, Modic MT, Ross JS, et al: Lumbar spine: Postoperative imaging with Gd-DTPA. *Radiology* 1988; 167:817–824. Used with permission.)

A similar finding has been noted by DeSantis et al.[33] with IVCT delayed scans. This finding can be quite helpful in differentiating small disk fragments from nerve roots. If enhancement is seen on delayed images, but not on the early study, then the diagnosis should be disk material. If no enhancement is identified, then the tissue could still be either herniated disk material or nerve root. Assessment of the contiguous images will help define the expected course of the nerve roots and can help in the distinction between disk fragments.

Venous plexus enhancement was seen in all 30 cases and was felt to be helpful in delineating the etiology of the aberrant soft tissue. The most dramatic enhancement of the venous plexus was seen in cases with large herniated disk causing dilatation of the venous plexus above and below the herniation. This finding can be used in a manner similar to that of Russell et al.[34] in their evaluation of cervical herniated disks. Enhancement of the anular rent was noted in 4/14 operated cases as well as in 4 of the remaining cases (Fig 4–22). In those patients who were reoperated at this same level, the thecal sac was noted to be adherent to the rent secondary to scar formation. Parent disk enhancement was seen in 4/14 operated cases and 7 cases total. This had a variable appearance with 5 being linear near one or both end-plates, with one case demonstrating diffuse homogeneous enhancement, and a final case showing a mottled pattern of enhancement. This enhancement may relate to scar formation in the disk space that has previously been curettaged. An additional hypothesis for this would be ingrowth of vascularity as has been described by Coventry et al.[35]

A real advantage of MR is its ability to directly image in the sagittal plane, in contrast to CT. This point is especially important in evaluating enhancement and in preventing partial volume averaging. The continuity of abnormal soft tissue extending from the parent disk space can be evaluated exquisitely with sagittal MR in a

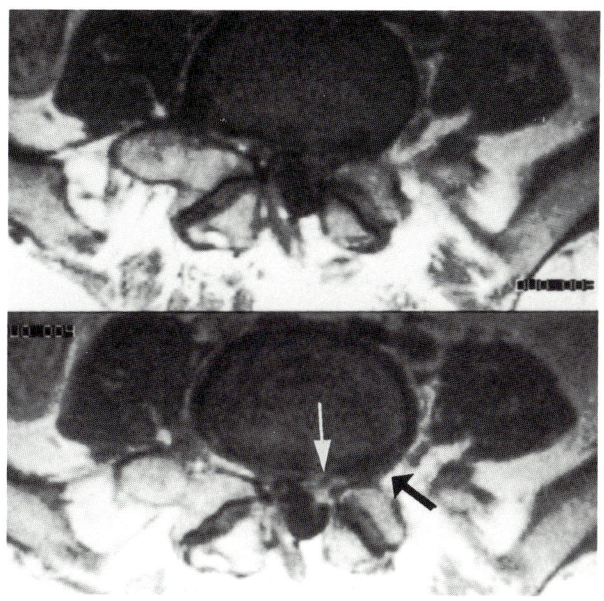

FIG 4–21.
Scar and recurrent disk herniation. **A,** axial precontrast image *(top)* shows aberrant soft tissue anterior and to the left of the dural tube. **B,** axial postcontrast image *(bottom)* shows enhancement of medial scar *(white arrow)* with good definition of the lateral disk herniation *(black arrow)*. (From Hueftle MG, Modic MT, Ross JS, et al: Lumbar spine: Postoperative imaging with Gd-DTPA. *Radiology* 1988; 167:817–824. Used by permission.)

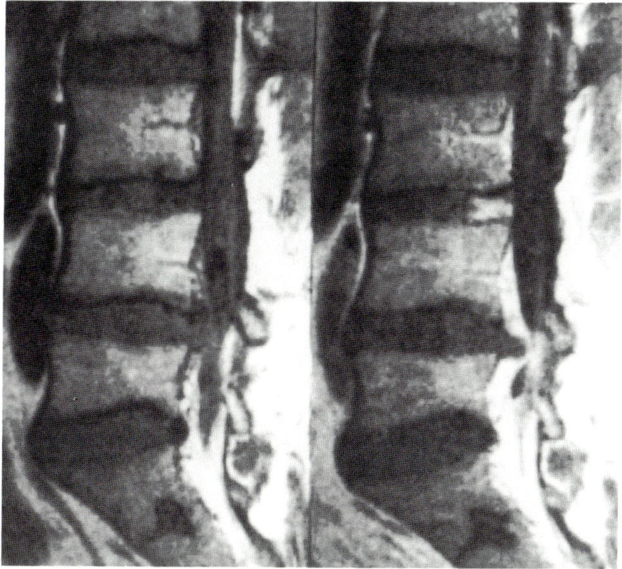

FIG 4–22.
Anular rent enhancement following laminectomy and diskectomy at L3-4. Precontrast sagittal T_1-weighted image *(left)* shows a large anterior extradural defect at L4-5. Postcontrast sagittal T_1-weighted image *(right)* shows a rectangular-shaped area of enhancement involving the L3-4 disk that abuts the anterior thecal sac. This likely represents scar tissue within the disk at the site of previous curettage. The dura can be adherent to this scar tissue. The disk herniation is outlined by enhancing epidural plexus at L4-5. (From Hueftle MG, Modic MT, Ross JS, et al: Lumbar spine: Postoperative imaging with Gd-DTPA. *Radiology* 1988; 167:817–824. Used by permission.)

manner unobtainable with other imaging modalities. In addition, the multislice capabilities of MR allows numerous levels to be studied at one time.

Our initial study suggests that Gd-DTPA–enhanced MR is the most accurate means for identifying and characterizing aberrant soft tissue in the postoperative lumbar spine. If there is a discrepancy in the diagnosis, then enhancement should supersede any other diagnostic criteria. In other words, if it is enhanced on the early T_1-weighted studies, then it is epidural fibrosis. Sagittal and axial scans are needed to prevent partial volume averaging and to optimally evaluate the enhancement characteristics. Early T_1-weighted sagittal and axial images are the best sequence for evaluating tissue morphology and contrast enhancement.

POSTOPERATIVE CERVICAL SPINE

A multiplicity of surgical procedures has been developed for cervical disk disease and spondylosis. The initial surgical approach for treating spondylosis was posterior. The problem with this approach is the difficulty in removing anteriorly compressive structures. This approach has generally fallen out of favor in lieu of the anterior approach, popularized in the 1950s by Bailey and Badgley, Cloward, and Robinson and Smith.[36–38] Partial vertebrectomies with radical anterior decompression over multiple levels may be used for severe spondylotic myelopathy or in cases of cervical trauma with cord compression. Iliac or fibular grafts may be used for multilevel stabilization.

Anterior cervical spine fusion may be roughly grouped into three types: Smith-Robinson, Cloward, and the strut graft. These fusions involve removing the offending intervertebral disk and a portion of the vertebral bodies, including osteophytes, and insertion of a bone graft (Fig 4–23). The bone graft functions for fusion, as well as for maintaining the proper disk space height and alignment. Anterior fusion can be applied to a variety of cervical spine disorders, including disk disease with radiculopathy, spondylosis, instability, dislocations and fractures, tumors, and infection.

The Smith-Robinson technique involves removing the disk material and cartilaginous end-plates from an anterior approach.[38] The bony osteophytes are generally not removed with this technique. A rectangular iliac bone graft is then cut to fit the curetted disk space. Trac-

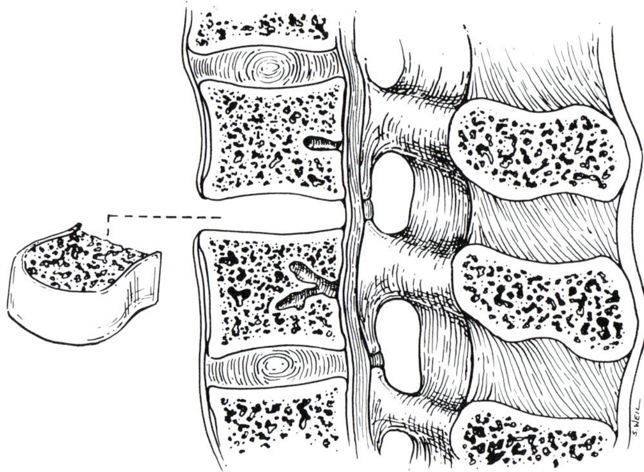

FIG 4–23.
Appearance of iliac crest bone graft and positioning for a Smith-Robinson anterior diskectomy and fusion.

tion is applied to widen the space, and the graft is inserted and counter sunk.

The Cloward technique involves drilling a round hole in the disk space and adjacent end-plates with a specialized tool.[37] Into this drilled space is then inserted a prefit dowel of bone. Prior to graft insertion, the posterior and posterolateral osteophytes are removed. The graft material may be iliac, autograft, or allograft.

Strut grafts are larger segments of bone used to obtain stabilization following multilevel diskectomy or corpectomy. This graft material may be iliac, rib, tibial, or fibular bone. The anterior aspects of the uppermost and lowermost receptor vertebral bodies must be carefully preserved so the graft ends will lock in place and not become dislodged.

Some immediate surgical complications of the anterior approach include pneumothorax, perforation of the esophagus, permanent cord damage, infection, graft extrusion, and damage to the recurrent laryngeal nerve.[39] Of these, only infection and graft extrusion will be considered in this chapter. Late complications that will be considered include bony stenosis, degenerative disease, (including disk herniations above and below the fusion site) bony deformity, and intrinsic cord abnormalities.

Anterior Diskectomy and Fusion

Patients imaged within the first few days following anterior diskectomy and fusion (ADF) will demonstrate a fairly characteristic appearance (Fig 4–24).[40] The bone grafts are visible as discrete rectangular areas of altered signal intensity within the central portion of the disk space. The signal intensities of the grafts themselves may be quite variable. Hyperintense, hypointense, and isointense signals from cervical graft material have been seen when compared with adjacent normal marrow signal (Fig 4–25). These signal changes most likely reflect the state of the graft marrow, whether cellular or fatty. The adjacent vertebral body end-plates and subchondral bony signal may be normal, or just as commonly, may show decreased signal on T_1-weighted images. If decreased signal on T_1-weighted images is present within the bony end-plates, then these areas will show increased signal on T_2-weighted images. These changes are presumed to represent marrow edema from the operative trauma.

Patients imaged months to 1 to 2 years following ADF will show a wide variety of graft and adjacent ver-

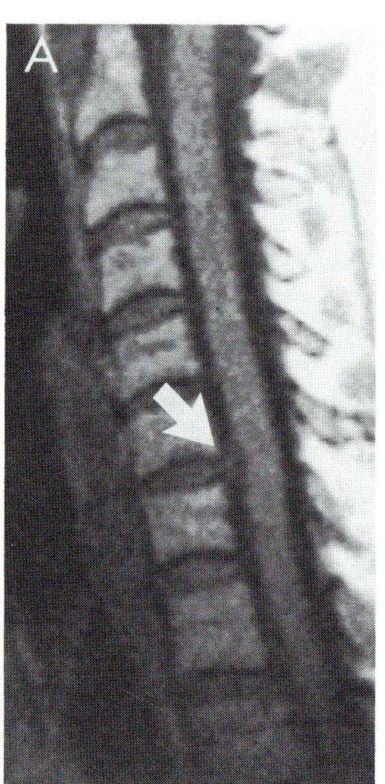

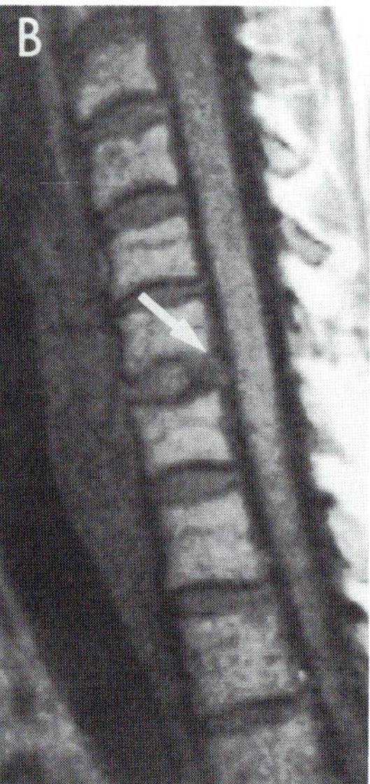

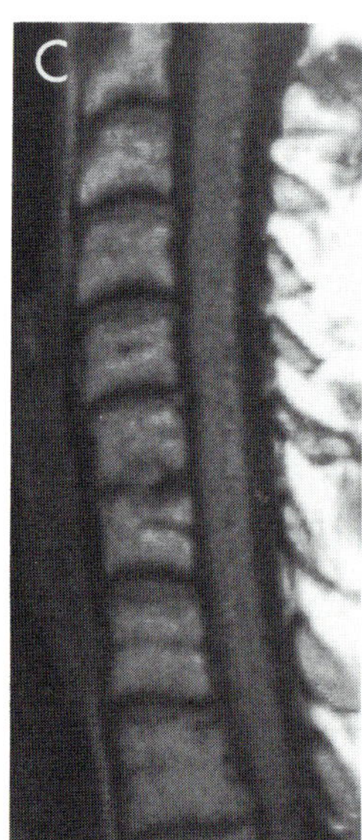

FIG 4–24.
Normal postoperative changes following anterior diskectomy and fusion. **A,** preoperative T_1-weighted image demonstrates a large disk herniation *(arrow)* at C6-7. **B,** immediate postoperative study shows graft as intermediate signal within the disk space causing an "apparent" anterior extradural defect. **C,** T_1-weighted image 9 months following surgery shows incorporation of the graft that now has indistinct margins. The anterior extradural defect is no longer apparent. (From Ross JS, Masaryk TJ, Modic MT: Postoperative cervical spine: MR assessment. *J Comput Assist Tomogr* 1987; 11:955–962. Used by permission.)

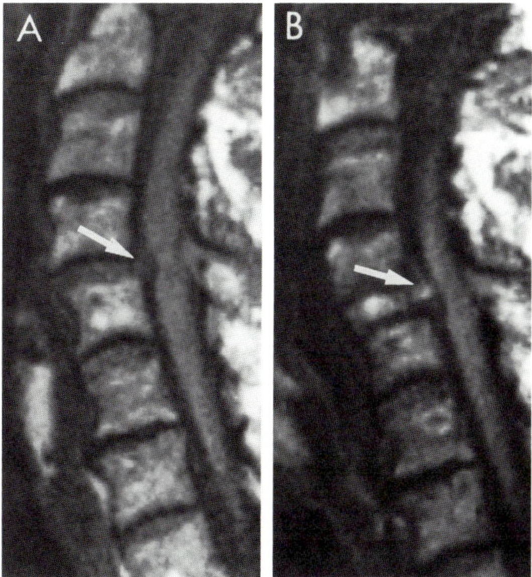

FIG 4–25.
Complication of anterior diskectomy. **A,** preoperative T_1-weighted image shows a large disk herniation at C4-5 compressing the cord *(arrow).* **B,** immediate postoperative T_1-weighted image shows the graft extending posteriorly to continue compressing the cord *(arrow).* The high signal within the graft is presumably due to yellow marrow. (From Ross JS, Masaryk TJ, Modic MT: Postoperative cervical spine. MR assessment. *J Comput Assist Tomogr* 1987; 11:955–962. Used by permission.)

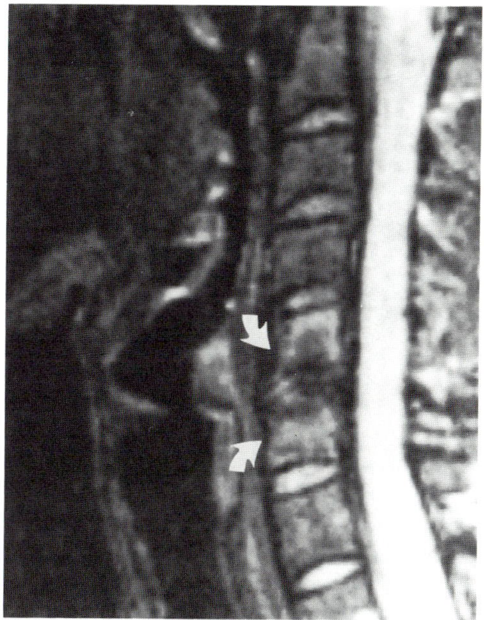

FIG 4–26.
Postoperative vertebral body changes. Immediate postoperative T_1-weighted image following anterior diskectomy and fusion (ADF) at C5-6 shows increased signal from the adjacent vertebral body *(curved arrows)* thought to represent marrow edema. (From Ross JS, Masaryk TJ, Modic MT: Postoperative cervical spine: MR assessment. *J Comput Assist Tomogr* 1987; 11:955–962. Used by permission.)

tebral body signal changes. In general, the grafts continue to be visible as horizontal, linear areas of decreased signal on T_1- and T_2-weighted images. The adjacent vertebral body signal changes will vary from isointense or hypointense on T_1-weighted images to isointense or hyperintense on T_2-weighted images. The etiology of these varied grafts and vertebral body signal changes in the postoperative spine is unknown. It probably represents a combination of (1) the initial status of the vertebral body and graft marrow, (2) the amount of trauma received by the end-plate vertebral body and graft during the operative procedure, (3) the postoperative stress placed on the fusion mass, and (4) the amount of revascularization that is present (Fig 4–26). In addition, a series of vertebral body signal changes occur in the spine in association with acute and chronic disk degeneration. Acute disk degeneration as seen with chymopapain injection in the lumbar spine shows decreased signal on T_1-weighted images and increased signal on T_2-weighted images from the vertebral end-plates.[41] Changes within the vertebral end-plates associated with chronic disk degeneration typically show increased signal on T_1-weighted images and isointense to slightly increased signal on T_2-weighted images. This is secondary to fatty marrow conversion.[7] Similar changes have been seen within the cervical spine. The traumatic effects on the vertebral body and graft marrow would reflect marrow edema showing decreased signal on T_1-weighted and increased signal on T_2-weighted images, or perhaps even the varied signal intensities of hemorrhage.

Solid bony fusions are more consistent in their appearance. They are seen as continuous marrow signal without evidence of an original intervertebral disk space or definable bone graft. The marrow of the fusion mass may be isointense to the adjacent normal marrow (approximately 50% of the time) or can demonstrate a more patchy or spotty increased signal on T_1-weighted images (Fig 4–27).

Corpectomy

Areas of vertebral body resection appear as homogeneous areas of decreased signal on T_1-weighted images with respect to the normal marrow signal. These areas may be isointense or, more commonly, may show increased signal on T_2-weighted images. Disk material is not visible within the midportion of the disk spaces where corpectomy has been performed. However, away from the corpectomy site at the lateral aspects of the vertebral bodies, the intervertebral disk space again will be-

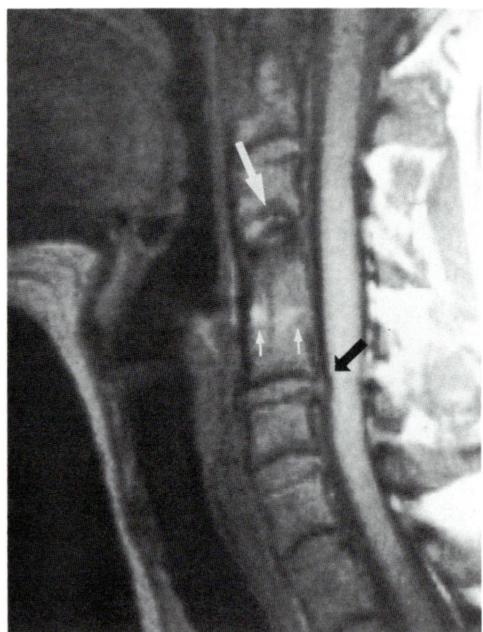

FIG. 4–27.
Late appearance of cervical fusions. Sagittal T_1-weighted image shows typical appearance of a solid fusion at C4-5 9 years following surgery. Linear area of high signal *(small arrows)* presumably represents focal increased yellow marrow. A mixed-intensity graft is present at C3-4 9 months following surgery *(white arrow)*. A new disk herniation is present below the fusion mass *(black arrow)*. (From Ross JS, Masaryk TJ, Modic MT: Postoperative cervical spine: MR assessment. *J Comput Assist Tomogr* 1987; 11:955–962. Used by permission.)

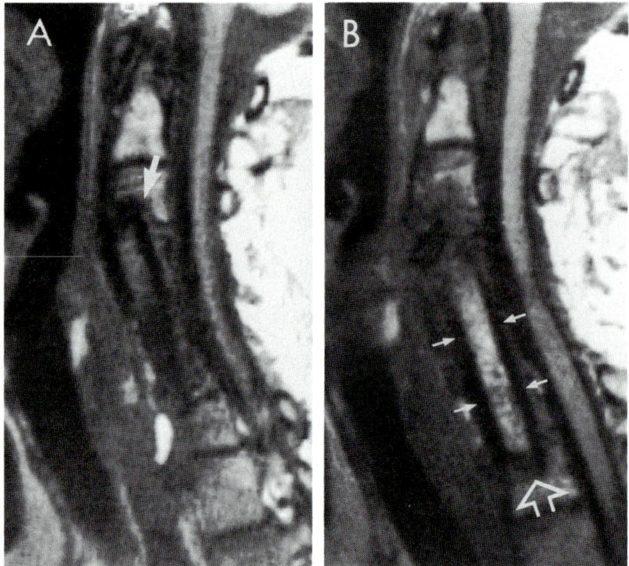

FIG 4–28.
Cervical strut graft. (a-b) Immediate postoperative sagittal T_1-weighted images show a fibular strut graft placed from C3 to C7. The sequential 4-mm images allow good definition of the superior *(white arrow,* **A***)* and inferior *(open arrow,* **B***)* extent of the graft. The anterior-posterior dimensions of the graft are also visualized due to the cortical bone *(small white arrows,* **B***)*. A focal area of cord atrophy is present at the C5 level. The patient has previously undergone a C3-5 laminectomy. (From Ross JS, Masaryk TJ, Modic MT: Postoperative cervical spine: MR assessment. *J Comput Assist Tomogr* 1987; 11:955–967. Used by permission.)

come well defined and retain its normal signal intensity.

The outlines of the strut graft material itself is well defined by the low-signal cortical bone (Fig 4–28). Strut graft marrow signal may be isointense or may demonstrate increased signal on T_1-weighted images when compared to the adjacent normal vertebral body signal. The precise positioning of the ends of the strut grafts are visible as very low signal graft cortical bone contrasted with the variable signal intensity (slightly hypointense or isointense) of the corpectomy site. Portions of strut graft marrow commonly show increased signal on T_2-weighted images. These high signal areas will correspond to the areas of decreased signal on the T_1-weighted images and most likely reflect graft marrow edema or revascularization.

Bony Stenosis

The most significant postoperative changes that we have identified by MR in the postoperative cervical spine are bony stenosis and new disk herniations. We have identified bony stenosis at the fusion sites in up to 26% of our patients. This stenosis is most often secondary to hypertrophic bone from the anterior fusion mass that encroaches on the cord or neural foramen (Fig 4–29). The hypertrophic bone can be visualized as an anterior extradural defect that is isointense with the vertebral body on T_1-weighted images, shows increased signal, or shows very low signal. These latter osteophytes may be visible only by the mass effect they exert on the cord. In these cases where the osteophytes are very low signal, T_2-weighted or gradient echo low flip-angle images are necessary to confirm the presence of the extradural defects. The sensitivity of MR for extradural disease but its lack of specificity regarding differentiating disk vs. bone has been previously noted.[42] However, at least in the cervical spine, this nonspecific appearance may be of less importance since recurrent disk herniations are uncommon due to their total removal under direct vision.

An additional type of bony stenosis seen immediately following ADF is anterior or posterior graft extrusion. We have seen two cases of graft extrusion where MR defined the extruded graft when patients were imaged within the first few days following ADF. In one case, no new symptomatology was present following a Smith-Robinson ADF at C4–5. The postoperative images showed the graft in close approximation to the cord,

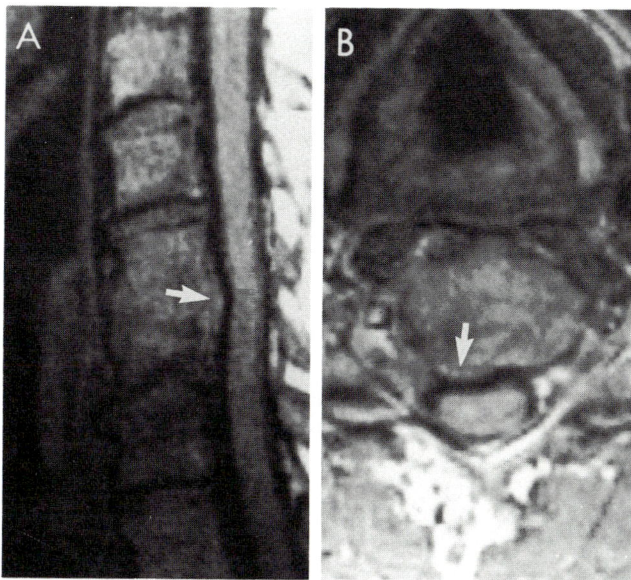

FIG 4–29.
Bony stenosis. **A,** sagittal T_1-weighted image shows a solid fusion mass at C5-6. An area of bony hypertrophy compresses the cord *(arrow)*. **B,** axial T_1-weighted image confirms the bony compression on the cord *(arrow)*.

which mimicked the preoperative appearance of the disk herniation (see Fig 4–25). One other patient underwent a C5–6, C6–7 ADF with postoperative quadriparesis. The MR examination performed five days postoperatively showed a large anterior extradural defect at C4–5 that compressed the cervical cord. Additional cord compression was produced by a large anterior extradural defect at C5–6, at the site of the bone graft (Fig 4–30). All of these findings were confirmed at reoperation.

Disk Herniation

Following anterior diskectomy and fusion, instability and disk degeneration or herniation can develop above or below the fusion site due to excess stress placed on these joints. This is especially true when multiple levels have been fused. Disk degeneration at levels adjacent to the fusion may occur in as many as 81% of cases.[43] We have observed disk herniations in up to 29% of our cases. These herniations were fairly evenly distributed above and below the fusion site. These herniations have the typical appearance of intermediate soft tissue signal on the T_1-weighted images and low signal anterior extradural defects on gradient echo images (see Figs 4–27 and 4–30,C). The vast majority of the herniations were seen in patients following ADF. Occasionally, multiple herniations may be seen in patients who have undergone wide cervical laminectomies since they were the cause for the initial operation.

Soft Tissues

Areas of high signal intensity may be present within the prevertebral region on T_2-weighted images immediately following anterior diskectomy and fusion. These regions are isointense with muscle on T_1-weighted images and most likely represent edema along the operative tract (see Fig 4–30,B). With time, the size and signal intensity of the prevertebral space will return to normal. Any high signal intensity within the prevertebral space on T_1-weighted images should be considered suspicious for a hematoma.

Bony Deformity

Midline sagittal images allow excellent definition of bony deformities such as kyphosis and subluxations. We observed cervical kyphosis in 6/73 postoperative patients, all of whom had undergone anterior diskectomy and fusions. Of significance, all of these patients had evidence of bony encroachment on the canal and cervical cord from the fusion sites.

Metal Artifacts/Posterior Approaches

Cervical laminectomies are easily recognized by the absence of the bony posterior elements. Axial images commonly show loss of the normal muscle-fat interfaces at the surgical site. This can be replaced by relatively homogeneous intermediate signal on T_1-weighted images representing scar or simply be replaced with high signal intensity fat.

Posterior cervical fusions involving sublaminar or intraspinous process wiring are defined by the local metal artifacts they produce. The metal artifacts are usually confined to the posterior soft tissues or perhaps to the posterior margin of the subarachnoid space when spin-echo images are used (Fig 4–31). Gradient echo images are more susceptible to metal artifacts that commonly extend to involve the cervical canal. Occasional patients will have metal artifacts anteriorly at the site of anterior diskectomy and fusion produced by a shearing off of small metal drill particles during the diskectomy or corpectomy. The artifacts vary in size from small, which mimics a small anterior extradural defect, to large, which obscures the fusion mass and cervical cord.[44]

Pseudomeningocele

Pseudomeningoceles are defined as sharply marginated areas of decreased signal intensity on T_1-weighted

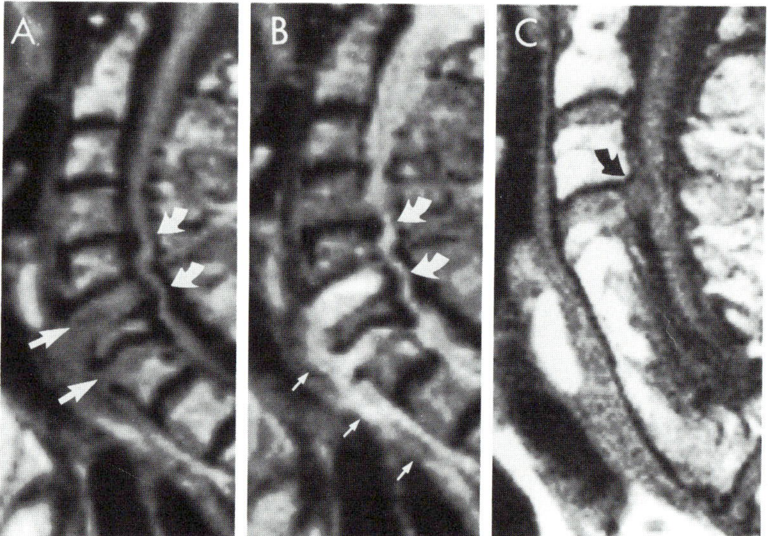

FIG 4–30.
79-year-old woman who underwent anterior diskectomy and fusion at C5-6, C6-7 levels with postoperative quadriparesis. **A,** initial sagittal T_1-weighted image shows homogeneous low signal from the diskectomy sites *(arrows)*. There continues to be large extradural defects at C4-5 and C5-6 with marked cord compression *(curved arrows)*. **B,** sagittal T_2-weighted image also shows large anterior extradural defects at C4-5, C5-6 *(curved arrows)* with a smaller defect at C3-4. The grafts and prevertebral space *(small arrows)* show high signal intensity. (From Ross JS, Masaryk TJ, Modic MT: Postoperative cervical spine: MR assessment. *J Comput Assist Tomogr* 1987; 11:955–962. Used by permission. **C,** follow-up T_1-weighted sagittal image 2 years following fibular graft placement from C4 through C7. The graft appears well incorporated into the bodies. There is now a very large disk herniation at the C3-4 level *(arrow)*.

images and increased signal on T_2-weighted images, similar to that of CSF. These are most commonly seen posterior to the upper cervical thecal sac following suboccipital craniotomy and decompression. Sagittal and axial images are usually necessary to define the full extent of the pseudomeningocele and the site of connection with the subarachnoid space.

Intrinsic Cord Abnormalities

A variety of abnormalities involving the cervical cord can be defined by MR in the postoperative patient. Diffuse cord atrophy can occur from a variety of etiologies including cervical spondylosis, trauma, and tumor surgery.

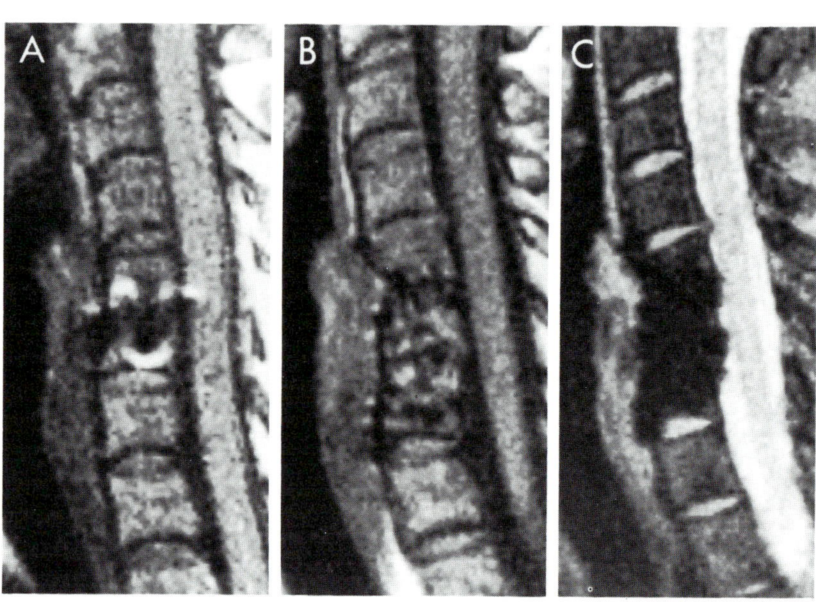

FIG 4–31.
Metal artifacts. **A,** spin-echo T_1-weighted image shows decreased signal with a halo of increased signal at the site of anterior fusion. **B,** spin-echo T_1-weighted image in a different patient shows mottled, diffuse low signal from the C5-6, **C** 6-7 fusions. **C,** gradient echo 10-degree flip-angle image in the same patient as **B** shows extensive area of the low signal due to minute metal fragments within the fusions.

Severe cervical spondylosis can allow repetitive trauma to take place with limited amounts of flexion and extension. This repetitive trauma can cause areas of cord cavitation (Fig 4–32). These are usually seen as well-defined areas of decreased signal intensity on T_1-weighted images within the central portion of the cord.[45–47] If the patient is imaged within a few days following trauma and posterior stabilization, then evidence of cord hematoma may be seen. This is usually seen as an ill-defined area of high signal intensity on T_1-weighted images within the cord secondary to the methemoglobin content.

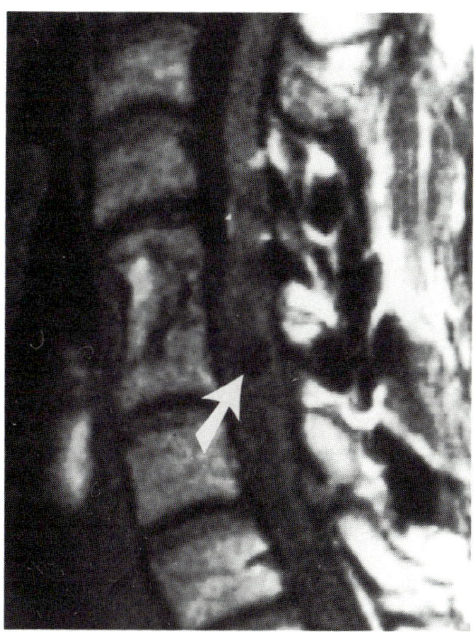

FIG 4–32.
Post-traumatic cord cavitation. Sagittal T_1-weighted MR following fracture/subluxation of C5 and C6, with subsequent fusions anteriorly and posteriorly. The cord is enlarged and contains a small cyst *(arrow)*. Posterior fusion wires give moderate artifact.

Conclusion

A variety of signal changes are present within the postoperative course of graft healing in the cervical spine. These would appear not to, in and of themselves, represent a pathologic process but rather the complex series of graft–vertebral body interactions in the course of healing. Magnetic resonance is also capable of defining a wide variety of postoperative abnormalities, the most common being disk herniation above or below the fusion level and bony stenosis from the fusion mass.

POSTOPERATIVE THORACIC SPINE

Initial surgical assaults on thoracic disk disease and vertebral body fractures with cord compromise were by means of laminectomy, with the intention of decompressing the spinal cord. From this experience, it became quite clear that laminectomy resulted in an unacceptably high incidence of neurologic deterioration and instability. These complications occurred without any attempts to remove the offending anterior bone or disk fragments responsible for cord compression.[48]

Since the first reports of transthoracic (1958) and anterolateral (1960) procedures for thoracic disk disease, it is now agreed that a lateral or anterior approach gives the best neurologic results, without compromising spine stability.[49–50]

There are three general types of anterior or lateral approaches: (1) posterior-lateral (costotransversectomy), (2) extrapleural anterior-lateral (modified costotransversectomy), and (3) transthoracic, transpleural (Fig 4–33).[51]

These procedures allow removal of the pedicle on the side of approach, as well as a variable amount of vertebral body above and below the disk space, and the intervertebral disk. The amount of vertebral body removed will depend on the cause for surgery. A thoracic diskectomy may require only removal of a small amount of the posterior-inferior and posterior-superior endplates above and below the herniation, respectively. Correction of kyphosis, burst fracture, or tumor may require radical corpectomy. The surgical procedures requiring removal of larger amounts of vertebral body necessitate graft placement. Bone graft material may be either iliac or rib. The superior and inferior ends of the graft are carefully incorporated into the central recesses of the upper and lower receptor vertebral bodies. Cancellous bone chips may be placed anterior to the graft itself.[52]

Pulse Sequences

The usual postoperative evaluation of the thoracic spine includes sagittal and axial T_1-weighted images, as well as sagittal T_2-weighted images. The T_1-weighted images allow assessment of the vertebral body marrow condition at the operative site, as well as the amount and location of scar. The T_1-weighted images are usually adequate for evaluating presence or absence of extradural mass effect on the cord. However, with more extensive corpectomies, occasionally the interface between the surrounding postoperative soft tissue edema and scar cannot be discerned from the dural tube itself. In these situations, a gradient echo image with higher flip angles (approximately 40 to 60 degrees) is useful. With this degree of flip angle, CSF has a lower signal intensity than does the cord. This usually allows better definition

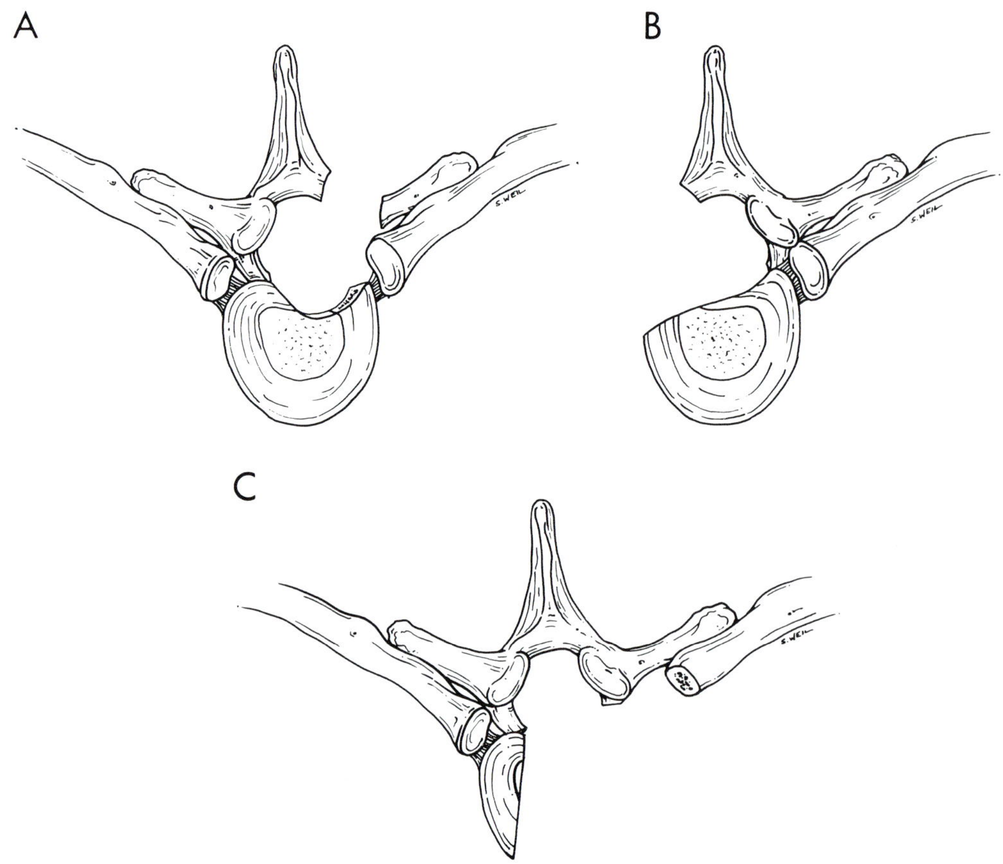

FIG 4–33.
Approaches for thoracic cord decompression. **A,** posterolateral or lateral gutter approach allows more of an anterior decompression than is possible with a conventional posterior exposure. **B,** lateral approach or costotransversectomy allows access to the entire posterior margin of the vertebral body. **C,** anterolateral or transthoracic-transpleural approach allows wide resection of the offending vertebral body.

of the cord than may be possible with a standard spin-echo T_2-weighted image. The disadvantage of using the gradient echo is its increased susceptibility to local magnetic field inhomogeneity. This is often present due to the surgical clips used to ligate vessels in these surgeries.

The appearance of the postoperative thoracic spine might be expected to parallel that of the cervical spine since the approaches, types of surgeries, and grafts are similar. This is indeed the case, up to a certain point.

Posterior lateral approaches for thoracic disk disease show absence of the pedicle below the operated disk level, as well as a portion of the posterior vertebral body adjacent to the dural tube. These areas are replaced by intermediate soft tissue signal material (scar) on T_1-weighted images (Fig 4–34). This can be fairly homogeneous and extend medially to conform to the smooth outer border of the dural tube. The anterior extent of the scar is to the region of the costotransverse articulation, which may also be removed during the operation. Laterally, the scar will be seen to encompass the neural foramen, with obliteration of the normal foraminal fat signal. With a posterolateral approach, the dural tube should continue to be well defined and oval in shape. The epidural and paravertebral scarring show a more variable appearance on T_2-weighted images, being either isointense or hyperintense with respect to normal marrow signal. The margins of the dural tube are graphically defined by the high signal CSF.

We have not as yet observed changes in signal intensity within the vertebral body marrow adjacent to the intervertebral disk space in the thoracic spine following anterior graft placement. This is more commonplace in the cervical and lumbar regions. The thoracic vertebral bodies adjacent to the disk continue to show normal marrow signal on T_1- and T_2-weighted images. A small amount of metal artifact is commonly seen along the lateral aspect of the vertebral body due to clipping of the segmental vessels.

Regions of more extensive corpectomy also show replacement with intermediate soft tissue signal scar on

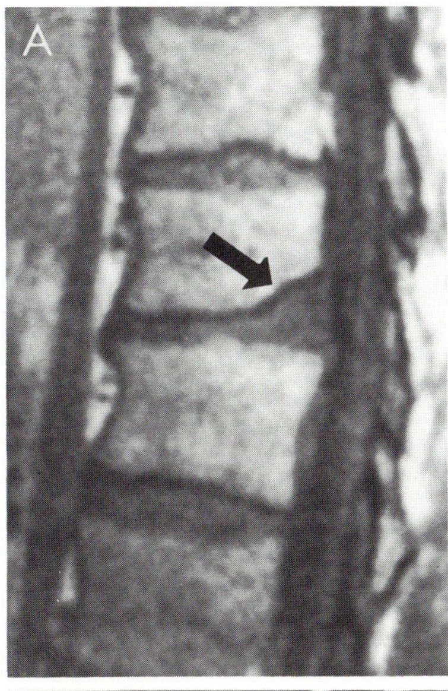

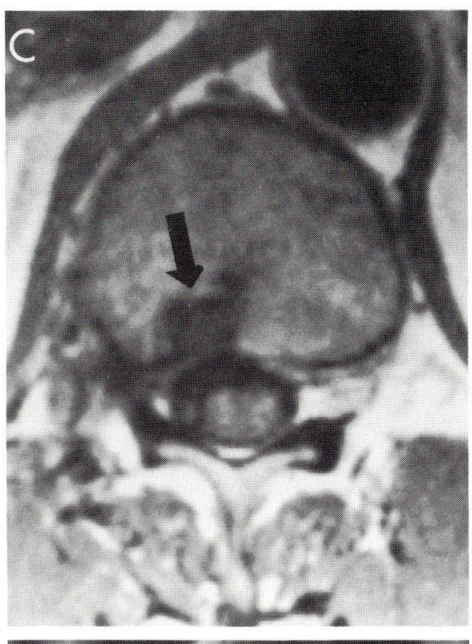

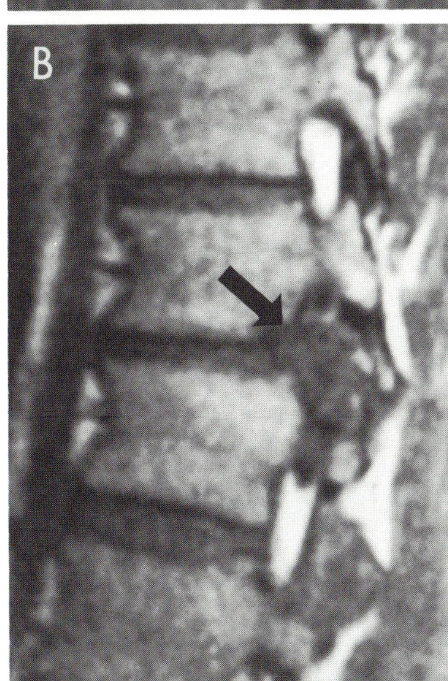

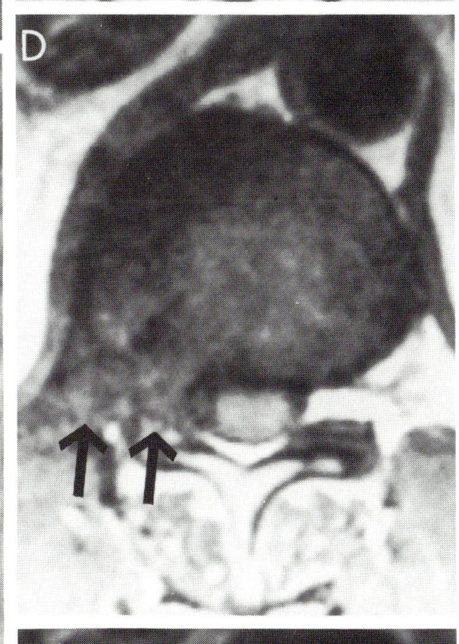

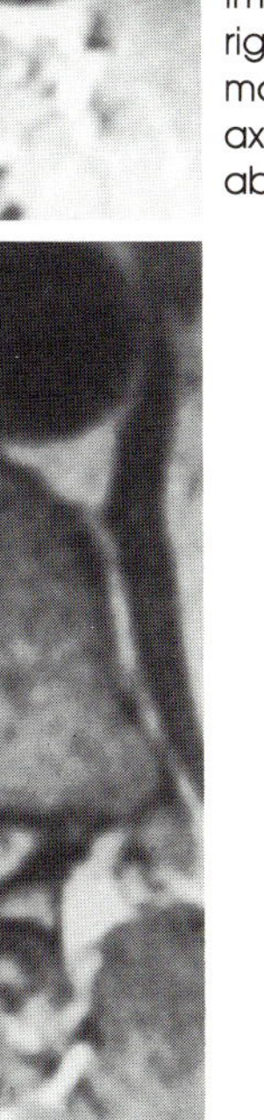

FIG 4–34.
Normal appearance following costotransversectomy for thoracic disk herniation. **A,** sagittal T_1-weighted MR just to the right of midline shows the operative defect in the inferior end-plate *(arrow)*. This allows room for safe curettage of the disk material from an anterior-lateral approach. **B,** sagittal T_1-weighted image through the neural foramina. There is obliteration of the normal foraminal fat signal by scar tissue *(arrow)*. Note the removal of the pedicle below the operative disk level. **C,** axial T_1-weighted image shows the defect in the inferior end-plate *(arrow)* comparable to that in **A. D,** axial T_1-weighted image just inferior to **C** shows the scar within the right neural foramen *(arrows)*. The posterior disk margin is slightly convex, but otherwise normal. **E,** axial T_1-weighted image just inferior to **D** shows the absent pedicle on the right.

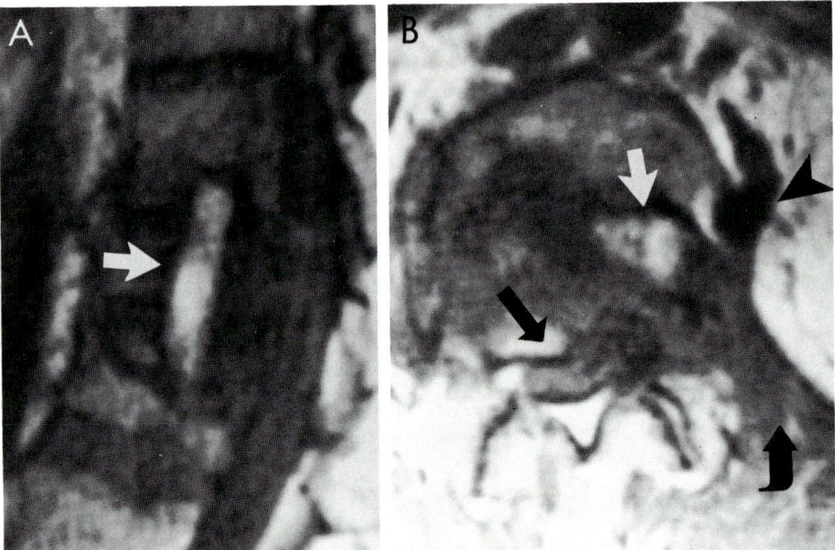

FIG 4–35.
Corpectomy and iliac grafting following burst fracture. **A,** sagittal T_1-weighted image shows a rectangular high signal intensity graft *(arrow)* spanning the corpectomy site that is hypointense. **B,** axial T_1-weighted image shows the graft to the left *(white arrow)*. Circular hypointensity with a hyperintense halo *(arrowhead)* is metal artifact. There continues to be compression of the cord by a retropulsed bone fragment of hyperintense signal *(straight black arrows)*. Note the low signal intensity following the extraperitoneal approach on the left *(tailed arrow)*.

T_1-weighted images. The interface of the scar with the remaining normal vertebral bodies is well defined. Areas of scar can show very high signal on T_2-weighted images, similar to CSF. Of considerable importance is that the normal postoperative soft tissue changes can obscure the dural tube on sagittal and axial images. This soft tissue precludes adequate evaluation of the potential mass effect on the thecal sac postoperatively.

Graft material may have a wide variety of signal intensities as it has within the cervical spine (Figs 4–35

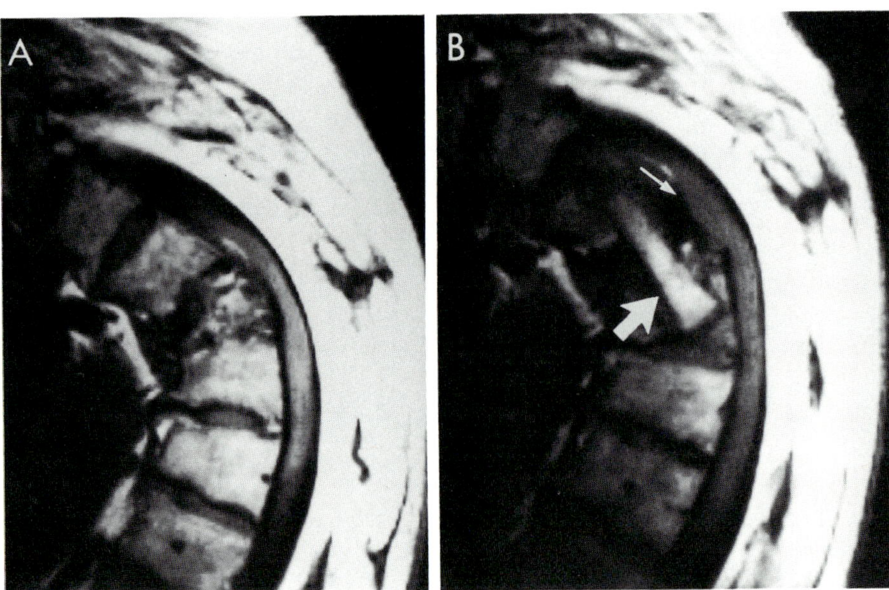

FIG 4–36.
Thoracic osteonecrosis. **A,** sagittal T_1-weighted image preoperatively shows heterogeneous signal from a collapsed vertebral body. There is mild compression of the cord at this level, and a severe kyphosis. **B,** sagittal T_1-weighted image following corpectomy and iliac grafting shows the well-defined graft traversing the corpectomy site *(large arrow)*. The caudal portion of the graft is well defined and is seated within the inferior vertebral body. The cord now follows the concavity of the corpectomy site *(small arrow)*.

and 4–36). On T_1-weighted images, graft marrow signal may be isointense, slightly hyperintense, or quite hyperintense with respect to normal vertebral body marrow. The edges of the grafts are well defined due to the decreased signal of the cortical bone. With more extensive corpectomies, metal artifact may be a more significant impediment to interpretation. This is especially true when gradient echo images are used.

Laminectomies

Thoracic laminectomies are performed for a variety of reasons including resection of tumors, syringes, and cord exploration. The site of laminectomy, as in other areas of the spine, is defined by the lack of posterior elements. A variable amount of scar tissue may be present in the posterior epidural region. This has an intermediate signal intensity on T_1-weighted sequences and is usually isointense to slightly hyperintense on T_2-weighted sequences.

Conclusion

No studies yet exist in the literature documenting the effectiveness of MR in evaluating the postoperative thoracic spine. Until comparisons of MR with more conventional modalities are made, it is prudent to continue to use the latter modalities as the primary investigative tool. Morphology of the thecal sac and spinal cord following anterior or lateral approach is most efficiently imaged by either water-soluble contrast myelography and/or CT myelography.

REFERENCES

1. Burton CV, Kirkaldy-Willis WH, Young-Hing K, et al: Causes of failure of surgery on the lumbar spine. *Clin Orthop* 1981; 157:191–199.
2. Cronqvist S: The postoperative myelogram. *ACTA Radiol [Stockh]* 1959; 52:45–51.
3. Quencer RM, Tenner M, Rothman L: The postoperative myelogram. *Radiology* 1977; 123:667–679.
4. Shapiro R: *Myelography,* ed 3. Chicago, Year Book Medical Publishers, 1975; p 203.
5. Teplick JG, Haskin ME: Computed tomography of the postoperative lumbar spine. *AJR* 1983; 141:865–884.
6. Ross JS, Masaryk TJ, Modic MT, et al: Lumbar spine: Postoperative assessment with surface-coil MR imaging. *Radiology* 1987; 164:851–860.
7. Modic MT, Tyrrell R, Haccke EM, et al: MR imaging assessment of vertebral-body changes in degenerative disc disease, 72nd Scientific Assembly and annual meeting of the RSNA. Chicago, 1986.
8. Ehrman RL, Berquist TH: Magnetic resonance imaging of musculoskeletal trauma. *Radiol Clin North Am* 1986; 2:291–319.
9. Unger EC, Glazer HS, Lee JKT, et al: MRI of extracranial hematomas: Preliminary observations. *AJR* 1986; 146:403–407.
10. Dooms GC, Fisher MR, Hricak H, et al: MR imaging of intramuscular hemorrhage. *J Comput Assist Tomogr* 1985; 9:908–913.
11. Teplick JG, Haskin ME: Intravenous contrast enhanced CT of the postoperative lumbar spine. *AJR* 1984; 143:845–855.
12. Braun IF, Hoffman JC, Davis PC, et al: Contrast enhancement in CT differentiation between recurrent disk herniation and postoperative scar: Prospective study. *AJR* 1985; 145:785–790.
13. Bundschuh CV, Modic MT, Ross JS, et al: Epidural fibrosis and recurrent disk herniation in the lumbar spine: Assessment with MR. *AJNR* 1988; 9:169–178.
14. Teplick JG, Peyster RG, Teplick S, et al: CT identification of post laminectomy pseudomeningocele. *AJNR* 1983; 4:179–182.
15. Gill GG, Scheck M, Kelley ET, et al: Pedicle fat grafts for the prevention of scar in low-back surgery. *Spine* 1985; 10:662–667.
16. Ross JS, Masaryk TJ, Modic MT, et al: Magnetic resonance of lumbar arachnoiditis. *AJNR* 1987; 8:885–892 and *AJR* 1987; 149:1025–1032.
17. Heindel W, Friedman G, Burke J, et al: Artifacts in MR imaging after surgical intervention. *J Comput Assist Tomogr* 1986; 10:596–599.
18. Harrington DP: Particulate embolization materials, in Abrams HL (ed): *Abrams Angiography: Vascular and Interventional Radiology,* ed 3. Boston, Little Brown & Co, 1983, pp 2138–2139.
19. Brasch RC, Weinmann HJ, Wesley GE: Contrast enhanced MR imaging: Animal studies using gadolinium-DTPA complex. *AJR* 1984; 142:625–630.
20. Runge VM, Clanton JA, Herzer WA, et al: Intravascular contrast agents suitable for magnetic resonance imaging. *Radiology* 1984; 153:171–176.
21. Weinmann HJ, Brasch RC, Press WR, et al: Characteristics of gadolinium-DTPA complex: A potential NMR contrast agent. *AJR* 1984; 142:619–624.
22. Carr DH, Brown J, Bidder GM, et al: Gadolinium-DTPA as a contrast agent in MRI: Initial clinical experience in 20 patients. *AJR* 1984; 143:215–224.
23. Felix R, Schoerner W, Laniado M, et al: Brain tumors: MR imaging with gadolinium-DTPA. *Radiology* 1985; 156:681–688.
24. Gadian DG, Payne JA, Bryant DJ, et al: Gadolinium-DTPA as a contrast agent in MR imaging—theoretical projections. *J Comput Assist Tomogr* 1985; 9:242–248.
25. Wolf GL, Fobben ES: The tissue proton T1 and T2 response to Gadolinium-DTPA injection in rabbits. A potential renal contrast agent for NMR imaging. *Invest Radiol* 1984; 19:324–328.
26. Firooznia H, Kricheff II, et al: Lumbar Spine after surgery: Examination with intravenous contrast enhanced CT. *Radiology* 1987; 163:221–226.
27. Yang PJ, Seeger JF, et al: High dose IV contrast in CT

scanning of the postoperative lumbar spine. *AJNR* 1986; 7:703–707.
28. Teplick GJ, Haskin ME: Intravenous contrast enhanced CT of the postoperative lumbar spine: Improved identification of recurrent disc herniation, scar, arachnoiditis and diskitis. *AJNR* 1984; 5:373–383.
29. Braun IF, Hoffman JC, et al: Contrast enhancement in CT differentiation between recurrent disc herniation and postoperative scar: Prospective study. *AJNR* 1985; 6:607–612.
30. Schubiger O, Valabanis A: CT differentiation between recurrent disc herniation and postoperative scar formation: The value of contrast enhancement. *Neuroradiology* 1982; 22:251–254.
31. Weiss T, Treisch J, et al: CT of the postoperative lumbar spine: The value of intravenous contrast. *Neuroradiology* 1986; 28:241–245.
32. Hueftle M, Modic MT, Ross JS, et al: Lumbar spine: Postoperative MR imaging with Gd-DPTA. *Radiology* 1988; 167:817–824.
33. DeSantis M, Crisi G, Folch I, et al: Late contrast enhancement in the CT diagnosis of herniated disc. *Neuroradiology* 1984; 26:303–307.
34. Russell EJ, D'Angelo CM, et al: Cervical disk herniation: CT demonstration after contrast enhancement. *Radiology* 1984; 152:703–712.
35. Coventry MB, Ghormley RK, Kernohan JW: The intervertebral disc: It's microscopic anatomy and pathology: III. Changes in the intervertebral disc concomitant with age. *J Bone Joint Surg* [*Am*] 1945, vol 27.
36. Jacobs B: Anterior cervical spine fusion. *Surg Ann* 1976; 8:413–446.
37. Cloward RB: The anterior approach for removal of ruptured cervical discs. *J Neurosurg* 1958; 15:602–614.
38. Robinson RA, Smith GW: Anterolateral cervical disc removal and interbody fusion for cervical disc syndrome. *Bull Johns Hopkins Hosp* 1955; 96:223.
39. Whitecloud TS: Management of radioculopathy and myelopathy by the anterior approach, in the Cervical Spine Research Society: *The Cervical Spine*. Philadelphia, JB Lippincott Co, 1983, pp 411–424.
40. Ross JS, Masaryk TJ, Modic MT: Postoperative cervical spine: MR assessment. *J Comput Assist Tomogr* 1987; 11:955–962.
41. Masaryk TJ, Boumphrey F, Modic MT, et al: Effects of chemonucleolysis demonstrated by MR imaging. *J Comput Assist Tomogr* 1986; 10:917–923.
42. Modic MT, Masaryk TJ, Mulopulous GP, et al: Cervical radiculopathy: Prospective evaluation with surface coil MR imaging, CT with metrizamide and metrizamide myelography. *Radiology* 1986; 161:753–759.
43. Simone FA, Rothman RH: Cervical disc disease, in Rothman RH, Simeone FA (eds): *The Spine*. Philadelphia, WB Sanders Co, 1982, p 491.
44. Heindel W, Friedmann G, Burke J, et al: Artifacts in MR imaging after surgical intervention. *J Comput Assist Tomogr* 1986; 10:596–599.
45. Regenbogen VS, Rogers LF, Atlas SW, et al: Cervical spinal cord injuries in patients with cervical spondylosis. *AJR* 1986; 146:277–284.
46. Jinkins JR, Baskir R, Al-Mefty O, et al: Cystic necrosis of the spinal cord in compressive cervical myelopathy: Demonstration by Iopamidol CT-myelography. *AJR* 1986; 147:767–775.
47. Sherman JL, Barkovich AJ, Citrin CM: The MR appearance of syringomyelia: New observations. *AJR* 1987; 148:381–391.
48. Benjamin V: Diagnosis and management of thoracic disk disease. *Clin Neurosurg* 1983; 30:577–605.
49. Crafoord C, Hiertonn T, Lindblom K, et al: Spinal cord compression caused by a protruded thoracic disc. Report of a case treated with antero-lateral fenestration of the disc. *Acta Orthop Scand* 1958; 28:103–107.
50. Hulme A: The surgical approach to thoracic intervertebral disc protrusion. *J Neurol Neurosurg Psychiatry* 1960; 23:133–137.
51. Dohn DF: Thoracic spinal cord decompression: Alternative surgical approaches and basis of choice. *Clin Neurosurg* 1980; 27:611–623.
52. Bohlman HH, Eismont FJ: Surgical techniques of anterior decompression and fusion for spinal cord injuries. *Clin Orthop Rel Res* 1981; 154:57–67.

5

Cervicomedullary and Craniovertebral Junction

Jeffrey S. Ross, M.D.

Benjamin Kaufman, M.D.

Magnetic resonance imaging (MRI) has opened vistas in diagnosing disorders of the brain stem, medulla, upper cervical cord, cervicomedullary junction (CMJ), and the encompassing bony and ligamentous structures of the craniovertebral junction (CVJ). The neurologic symptoms produced from the diverse disorders of this region relate to compression or distortion of the neurovascular structures of the CMJ either from intrinsic diseases or from alterations (acquired and congenital) of the CVJ. These abnormalities may be congenital, osseous, neoplastic, inflammatory, or traumatic.

Magnetic resonance imaging has proven extremely useful in evaluating this region because of its ability to directly image in the sagittal and coronal planes.[1] While the lack of signal from cortical bone may cause some initial trepidation in determining bony outlines, this is not as large a problem as once feared. The lack of signal from cortical bone is, in fact, a diagnostic asset when compared to computed tomography (CT) of the posterior fossae. The role of conventional evaluation of the complex anatomy of this region is undergoing revision with the result that MR has assumed the place of a primary imaging modality.

SEQUENCES AND TECHNIQUES

Sagittal images provide the best views of the brain stem, fourth ventricle, and upper cervical spine. Short echo time (TE) repetition time (TR) spin-echo (SE) sequences are optimal for defining the gross anatomy of the cervicomedullary junction, while keeping the cerebrospinal fluid (CSF) signal intensity low. However, the precise imaging planes are determined by the need to image particular anatomical structures, e.g., the cerebellar tonsils may be evaluated best by a combination of coronal and sagittal planes. The key to diagnosing a large part of the CVJ pathology lies in precise definition of the anatomy, which is best done with high signal-to-noise T_1-weighted images. Parenchymal lesions (tumors, multiple sclerosis) may be better identified with long TR/TE sequences. In particular, refocussed and/or gated T_2-weighted images allow high signal from CSF and pathology while minimizing CSF pulsation artifact. Additional rephasing gradients may also be added to improve spatial misregistration and dephasing from CSF flow. Gradient echo techniques with low flip angles (10 degrees) are also capable of giving a "CSF-myelogram"–like effect with the advantage of short imaging times. The gradient echo examination appears excellent for extradural disease but fairly unreliable for defining intramedullary disease. An extremely useful technique is obtaining sagittal T_1-weighted images of the patient in neutral, flexed, and extended positions to assess the atlantodental interval (ADI), basion-dental interval (BDI), and effects of the dens and ligaments on the cervicomedullary junction. Our routine examination for the CMJ consists of sagittal and axial T_1-weighted images (4-mm slice thickness, 50% gap, 256 matrix), and a sagittal low flip-angle (10 degrees) gradient echo examination. If there is a question of instability, then flexion and extension sagittal T_1-weighted images are obtained.

NORMAL ANATOMY

Figures 5–1 through 5–4 show normal anatomy of the CMJ and CVJ at various planes. The occipitoatlan-

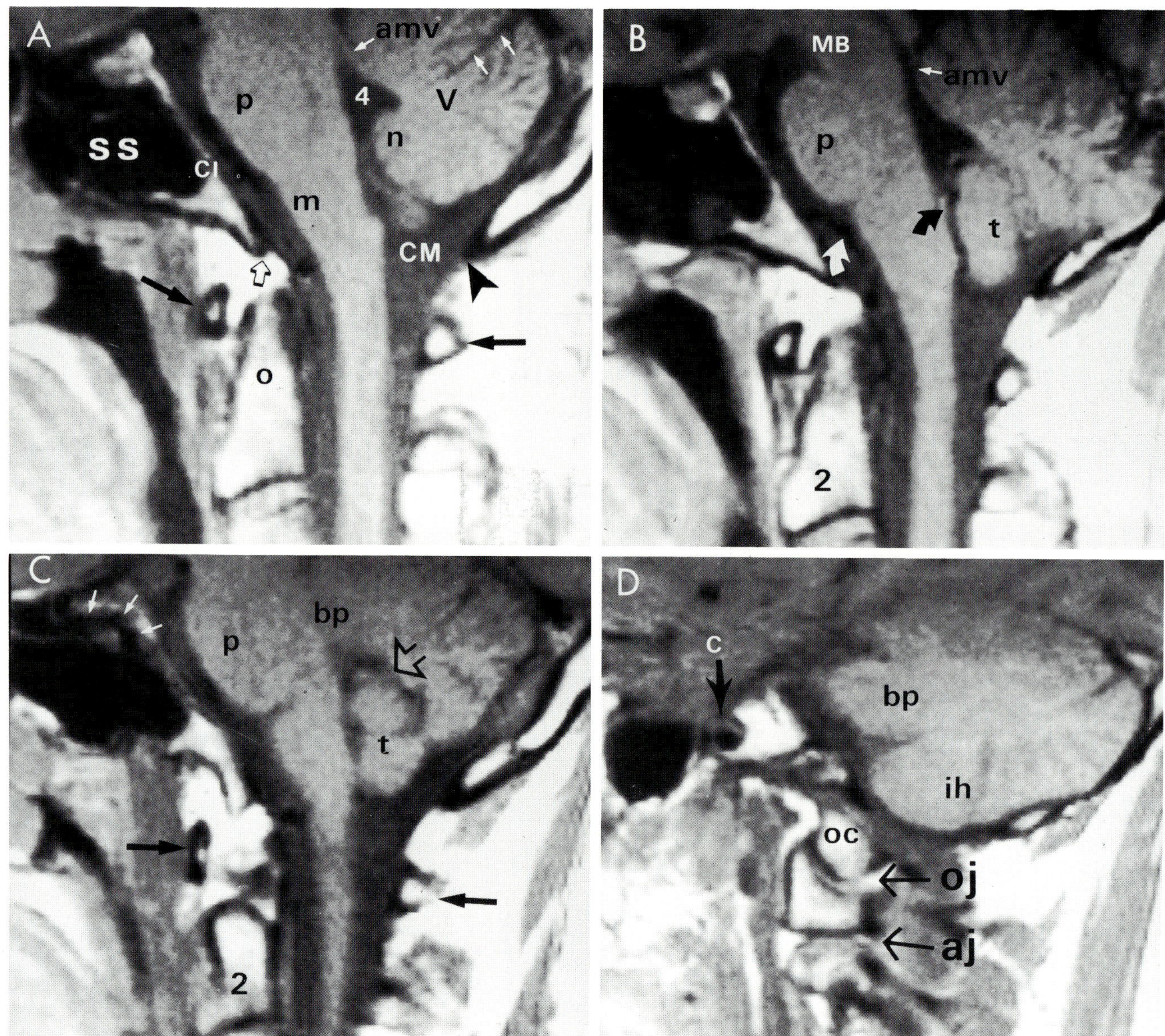

FIG 5–1.
A–D, normal anatomy: sagittal. (For explanation of abbreviations and symbols, see p. 151.) *(Continued)*

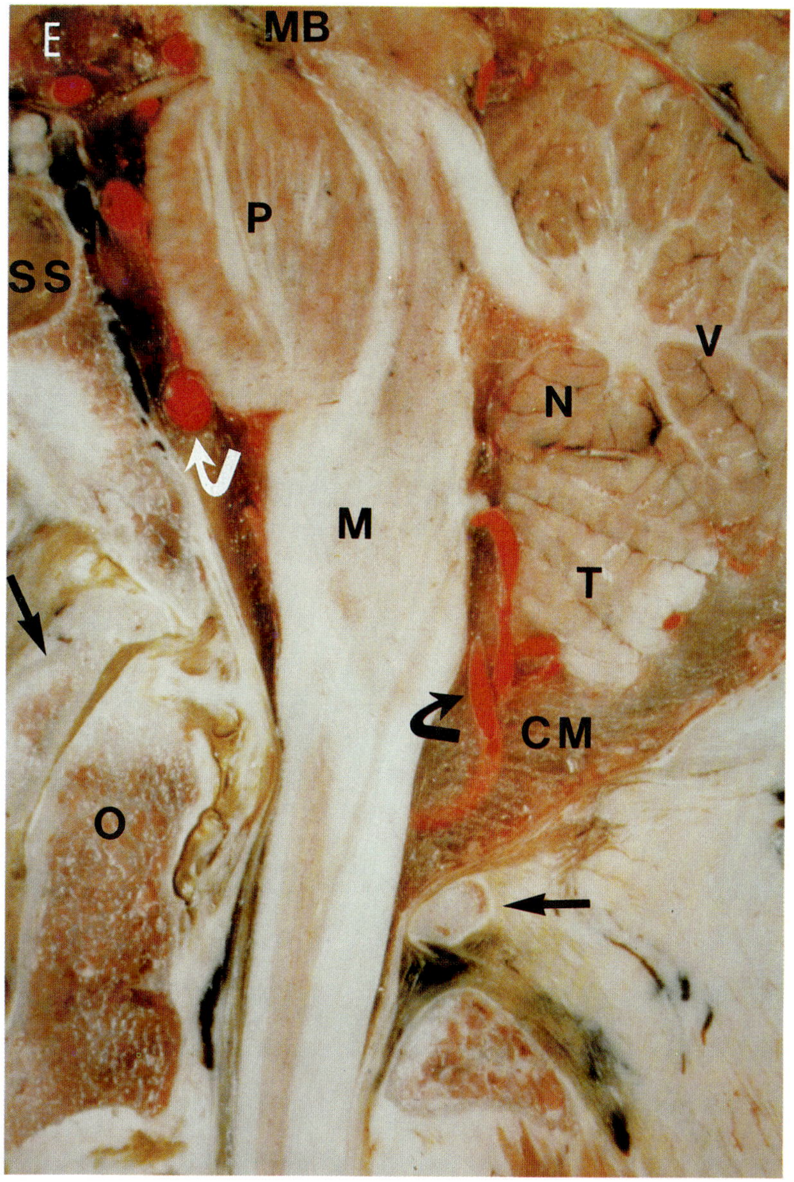

FIG 5–1 (cont.)
E, normal anatomy: sagittal. *aj* = atlantoaxial joint; *amv* = anterior medullary velum; *bp* = brachium pontis; *c* = carotid artery; *Cl* = clivus; *CM* = cisterna magna; *ih* = inferior hemisphere of cerebellum; *m* = medulla; *MB* = midbrain; *N* = nodulus; *O* = odontoid; *oc* = occipital condyle; *oj* = occipitoatlantal joint; *p* = pons; *ss* = sphenoidal sinus; *t* = cerebellar tonsil; *V* = vermis; *2* = C2 body; *4* = fourth ventricle. C1 *(black arrows);* opisthion *(arrowhead);* basion *(small open arrow);* carotid siphon *(three white arrows);* primary cerebellar fissure *(two white arrows);* basilar artery *(curved white arrow);* posterior inferior cerebellar artery (PICA) *(curved black arrow);* lateral recess of fourth ventricle; obex *(asterisk).*

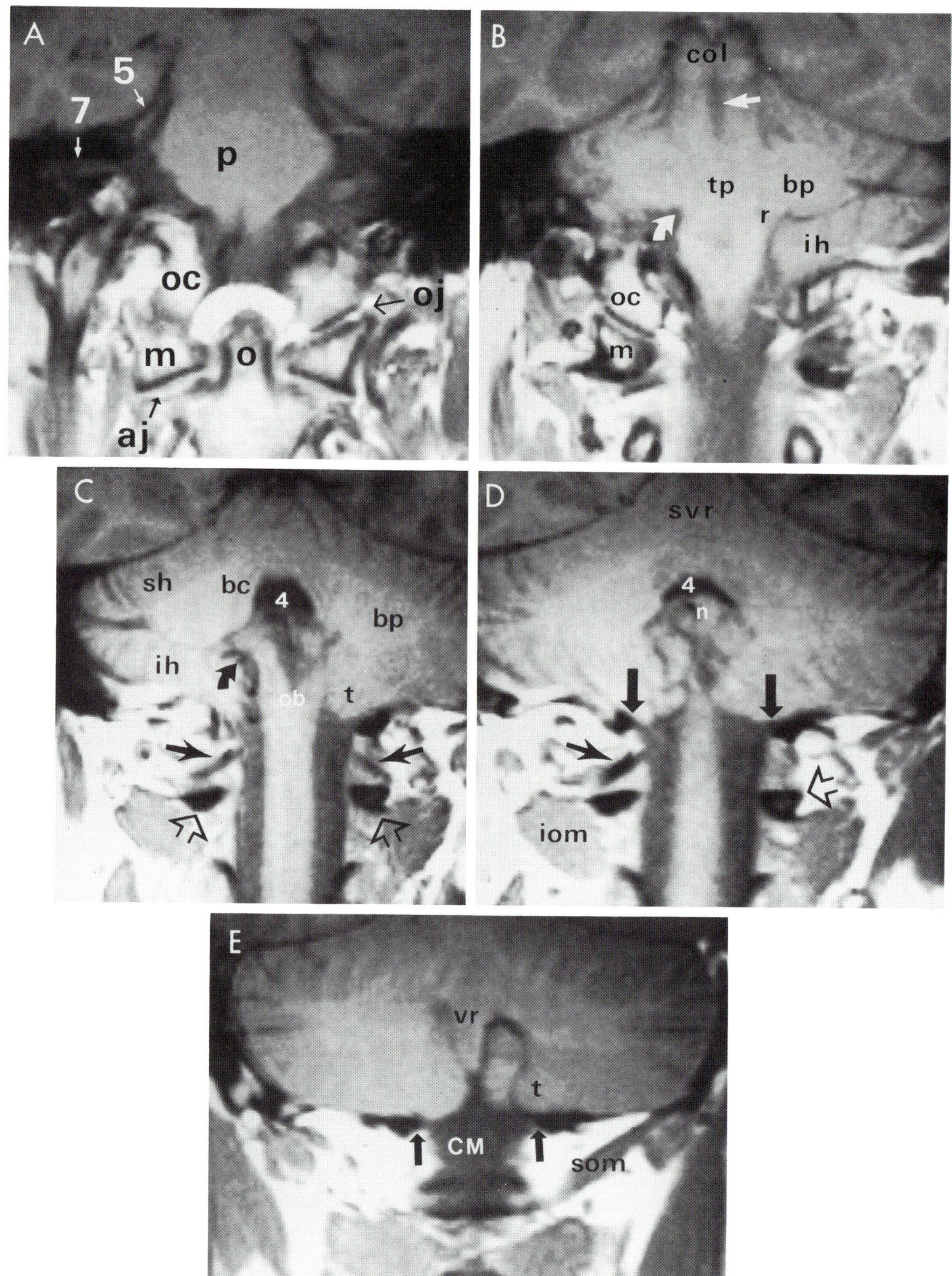

FIG 5–2.

A–E, normal anatomy: coronal. *aj* = atlantoaxial joint; *bc* = brachium conjunctivum (superior cerebellar peduncle); *bp* = brachium pontis (middle cerebellar peduncle); *CM* = cisterna magna; col = colliculi; *ih* = inferior hemisphere of cerebellum; *iom* = inferior oblique muscle; *m* = lateral mass C2; *n* = nodulus; *ob* = obex; *o* = odontoid; *oc* = occipital condyle; *oj* = occipitoatlantal joint; *p* = pons; *r* = restiform body (inferior cerebellar peduncle); *sh* = superior hemisphere cerebellum; *som* = superior oblique muscle; *svr* = superior vermis; *tp* = tegmentum of pons; *t* = tonsil; *vr* = vermis; *7* = cranial nerves VII and VIII in internal auditory canal; *5* = cranial nerve V; *4* = fourth ventricle; aqueduct of Sylvius *(white arrow);* lateral recess of fourth ventricle *(curved white arrow);* posterior inferior cerebellar artery (PICA) *(curved black arrow);* vertebral arteries *(black arrows);* foramen magnum margin *(vertical black arrows);* posterior arch of C1 *(open arrows).*

toaxial joints consist of two occipitoatlantal articulations and three atlantoaxial joints. Each of the atlanto-occipital joints involves the superior facet of the lateral mass of the atlas and an occipital condyle. The atlantal facets are concave and tilted medially, articulating with the ellipsoid surface of the occipital condyle. There is intercommunication of the synovial joints of the lateral masses of C1 and C2, as well as of the joint between the dens and atlas arch anteriorly, and the transverse ligament posteriorly. The unique combination of stability and complex motion of the CVJ is provided by the complex ligaments of the region. The anterior ligaments consist of (1) the anterior atlanto-occipital membrane, which is the superior extension of the anterior longitudinal ligament and connects the anterior margin of the foramen magnum to the anterior arch of the atlas; (2) the transverse ligament, which consists of a broad ligamentous band that crosses the ring of the atlas and secures the dens in contact with the anterior arch of C1. A small upper band connects the basilar part of the occipital bone, while a lower band attaches to the posterior surface of the body of the axis. This whole ligament thus forms a cross and is referred to as the cruciform ligament; (3) the alar ligaments, which are strong bands that connect the dens to the medial aspect of the occipital condyles; (4) the apical ligament, which connects the tip of the odontoid to the anterior margin of the foramen magnum; and (5) the tectorial membrane, which is a cephalad extension of the posterior longitudinal ligament and attaches to the upper surface of the basilar occipital bone in front of the foramen magnum (see Fig 5–4).

The posterior structures that are responsible for stability are the ligamentum nuchae, interspinous ligament, posterior atlanto-occipital membrane, ligamentum flavum, and cervical musculature.

Since cortical bone does not produce signal on MR, care must be taken when the bony margins are identified, as with the foramen magnum. Nevertheless, the low signal from the cortical bone of the anterior foramen magnum margin (basion) and the posterior margin (opisthion) usually provides enough contrast against the surrounding soft tissue and CSF to allow fairly precise measurements. The high-signal yellow marrow in the skull base is quite variable and should not be used as an indicator of bony margins. The signal intensity of the dens is also quite variable depending on the marrow content (e.g., red or yellow) and pathologic alterations such as edema, erosions, and bony sclerosis. The odontoid often has decreased signal on parasagittal images due to partial-volume averaging of the cortical bone and periodontoid soft tissue. A variable amount of fat is routinely seen between the tip of the dens and the basion. Absence of fat should signify CVJ pathology.

Certain measurements of the CVJ relationships were first applied to plain films and are identifiable and applicable with MR. Some of the more classical ones are briefly described below:

1. Platybasia: An increase in the basal angle of the skull. This may be defined by the angle between lines drawn along the plane of the sphenoid bone and another line along the clivus. Platybasia exists if the angle is greater than 143 degrees (normal range, 125 to 143).[2]
2. Basilar impression
   a. Chamberlain's line: A line drawn between the hard palate and the opisthion. Projection of up to one third of the top of the dens above this line has been considered normal.[2]
   b. McGregor's line: A line drawn between the hard palate to the caudal point of the occipital curve.[3] It has the same significance as Chamberlain's line.
   c. Fischgold's digastric line: A line drawn tangent to the diagastric grooves. This line in Fischgold's article relates to the location of the skull base, e.g., if the skull base is above the line, basilar invagination is present.[4] Other publications have related this line to the location of the odontoid tip.[5]
   d. Wachenheim's line: A line drawn along the posterior surface of the clivus. The dens should lay inferior to this line, and any intersection is considered abnormal.[6]
3. Foramen magnum margin
   a. McRae's line: A line drawn between the basion and opisthion. This is normal if it measures approximately 35 mm in diameter.[7]

CONGENITAL ANOMALIES

Chiari I Malformation

The Chiari I malformation consists of tonsilar displacement through the foramen magnum into the cervical spinal canal. The fourth ventricle retains its normal position. Common reported associations are syringomyelia and bony CVJ anomalies. Symptomatic populations tend to be older children and adults. A variety of symptoms can be present including brain-stem and cranial nerve findings such as facial pain, deafness, and vertigo. Cerebellar signs and paresthesias can also occur. Multiple sclerosis is a common mimicking diagnosis.

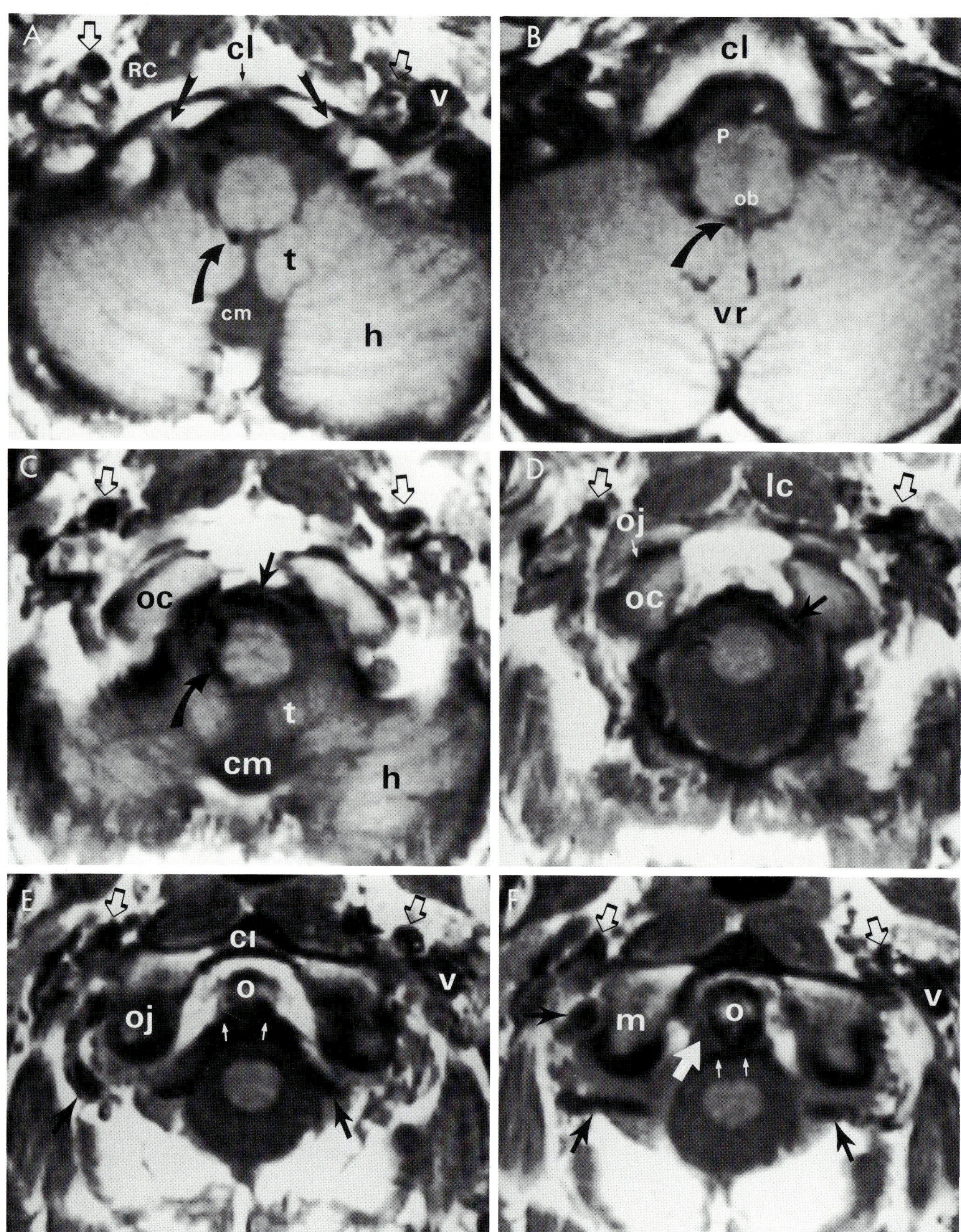

FIG 5–3.

A–I, normal anatomy: axial. *aj* = atlantoaxial joint; *C1* = anterior arch of C1; *cl* = clivus; *cm* = cisterna magna; *C2* = body of C2; *h* = hemisphere; *lc* = longus colli; *m* = lateral mass C1; *o* = odontoid; *ob* = obex; *oc* = occipital condyle; *oj* = atlanto-occipital joint; *P* = pyramid; *pcl* = posterior arch C1; *RC* = rectus capitis; *s* = cervical cord; *t* = tonsil; *v* = jugular vein; *vr* = vermis. Vertebral arteries *(straight black arrows);* posterior inferior cerebellar artery (PICA) *(curved black arrow);* hypoglossal canal *(tailed arrows);* carotid arteries *(open arrows);* tectorial membrane *(small white arrows);* alar ligament *(large white arrow);* transverse ligament *(curved black arrow).*

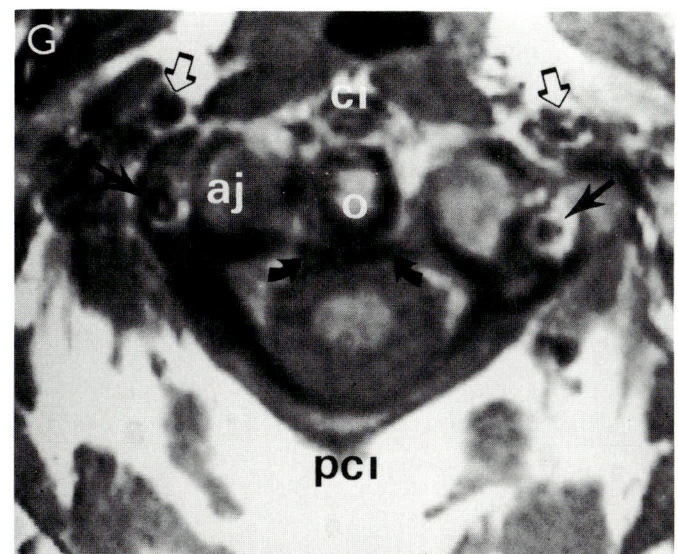
G
C1
aj
O
pC1

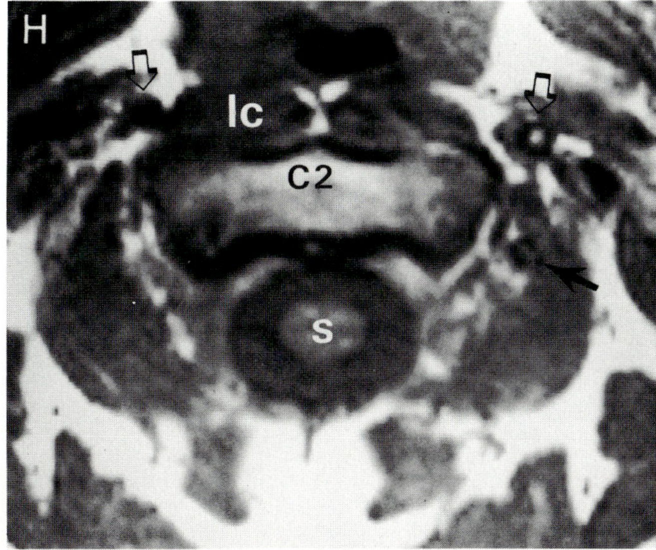
H
lc
C2
S

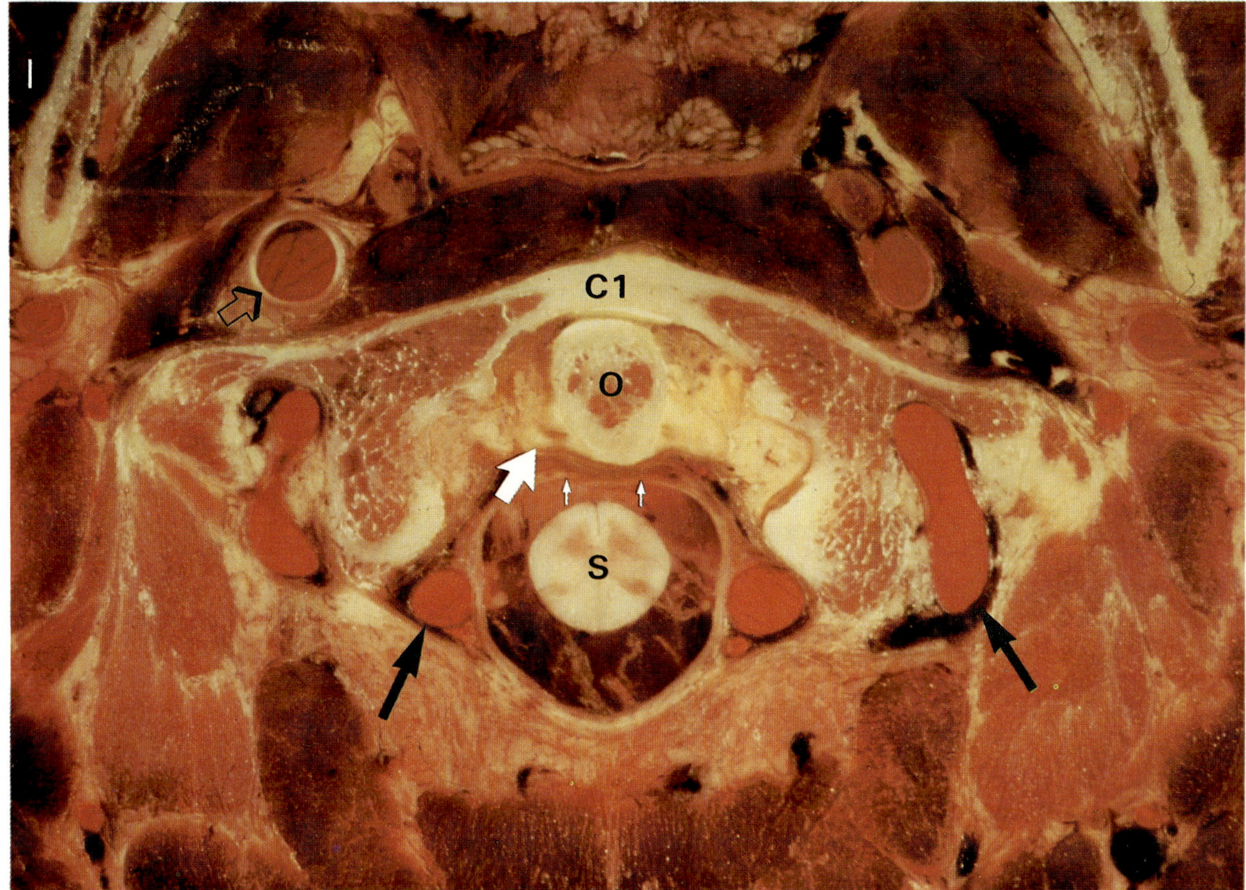
I
C1
O
S

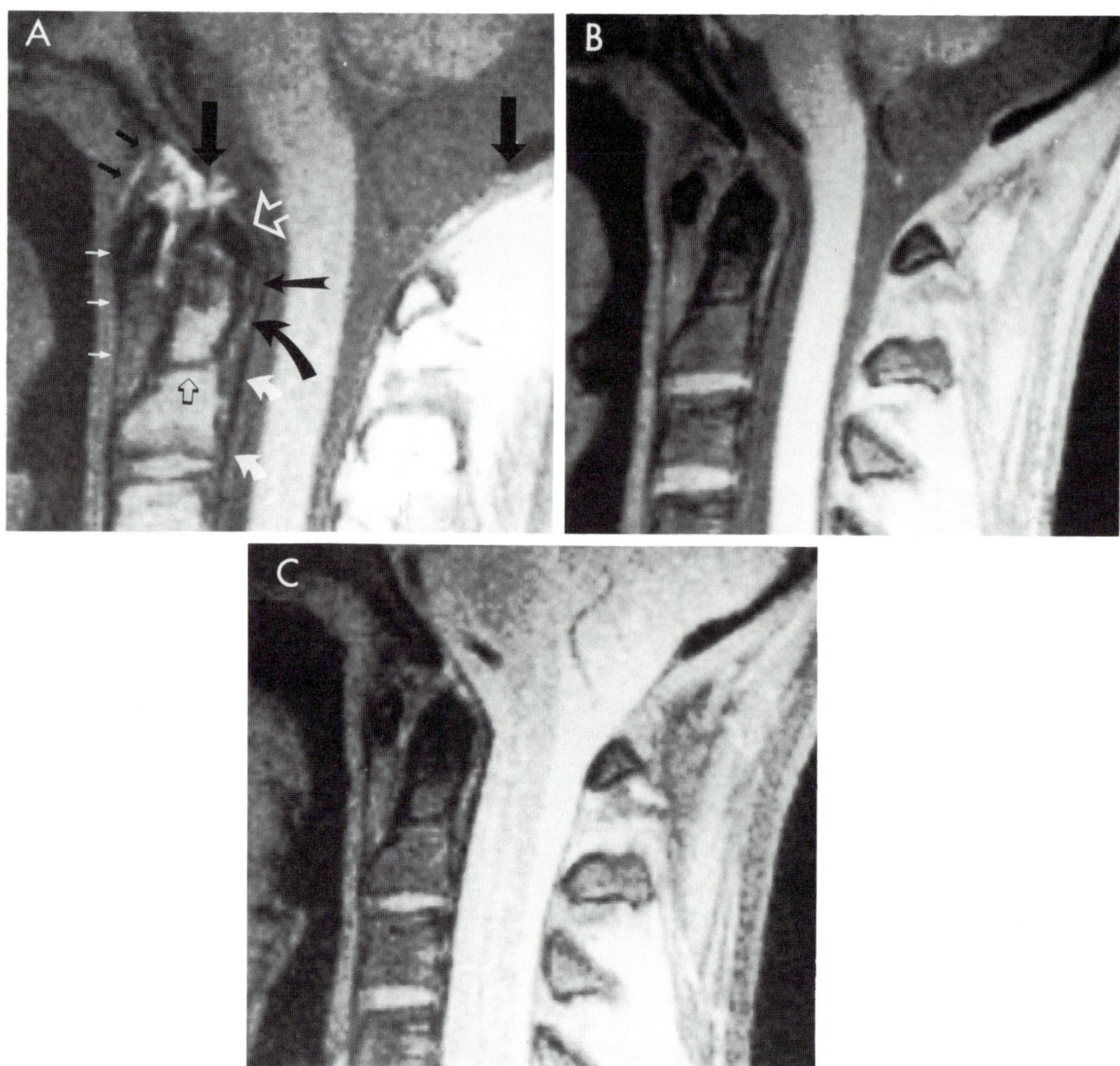

FIG 5–4.
Normal anatomy: midline sagittal. **A,** SE T_1-weighted image; **B,** gradient echo scan, $\alpha = 60$ degrees; **C,** gradient echo scan, $\alpha = 10$ degrees. Anterior longitudinal ligament *(small white arrows);* posterior longitudinal ligament *(curved white arrows);* subdental synchondrosis *(small open arrow);* anterior atlanto-occipital membrane *(small black arrows);* inferior fascicle of cruciate ligament *(curved black arrow);* tectorial membrane and superior fascicle cruciate ligament *(open white arrow);* transverse ligament *(tailed back arrow);* foramen magnum margin *(vertical black arrows).*

Magnetic Resonance Findings

Minor downward displacement of the tonsils ("tonsillar ectopia") and Chiari I malformation tend to form a spectrum of abnormalities. In tonsillar ectopia, the cerebellar tonsils project slightly below the foramen magnum but retain their normal globular configuration. The brain stem and fourth ventricle are usually normal, and there is no syrinx. Various minor degrees of caudal displacement have been described.[8] A reasonable upper limit of normal by sagittal MR is that the tonsils may project 2 mm below a line drawn from the inferior margin of the basion to the opisthion[9] (Fig 5–5). The tonsils should have a smooth rounded configuration in both the coronal and sagittal planes.

A Chiari I malformation will have tonsillar herniation anywhere from 3 mm to several centimeters below the foramen magnum margin. The tonsils assume an abnormal "peg-like" configuration. Arachnoiditis can mat the tonsils, medulla, and cord together. Occasionally the tonsils may be so adherent that they are difficult to separate from the dorsal cord surface (Fig 5–6). An additional clue to the diagnosis would be the presence of a

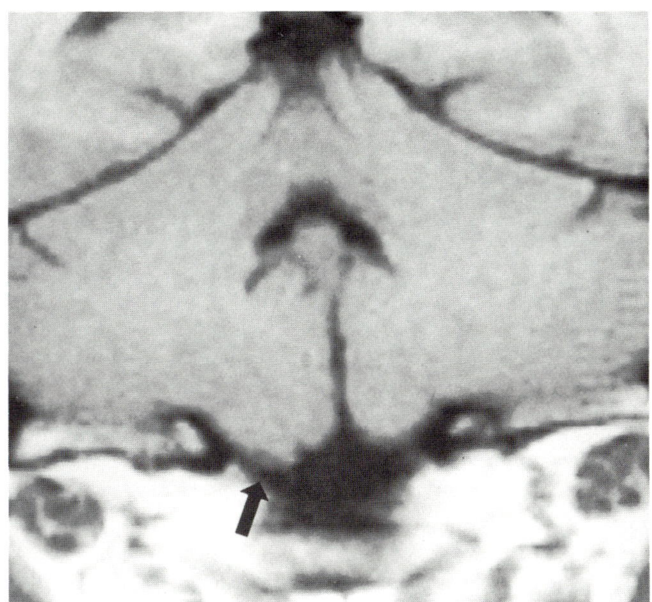

FIG 5–5.
Tonsillar ectopia. Coronal T_1-weighted image shows slight inferior displacement of the right tonsil *(arrow)*. The tonsil maintains a normal globular configuration.

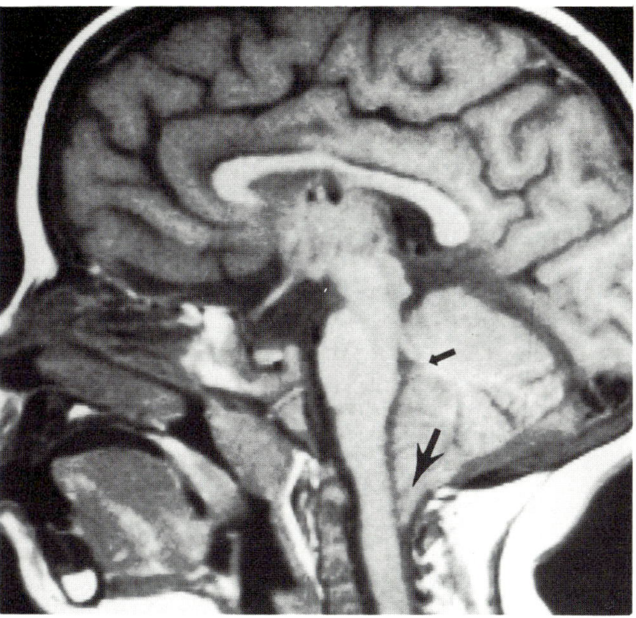

FIG 5–6.
Chiari I malformation. There is downward displacement of the cerebellar tonsils that has an abnormal "peg"-like configuration *(large arrow)*. The fourth ventricle maintains a normal position *(small arrow)*.

syrinx cavity. Basilar invagination has been reported in up to 50% of Chiari I patients. The cisterna magna is usually small in these patients. The incidence of hydrocephalus varies greatly from 0% to 44%.[10–12]

Chiari II Malformation

The Chiari II (Arnold-Chiari) malformation is defined by downward displacement of the brain stem and inferior cerebellum into the cervical spinal canal (Fig 5–7). The fourth ventricle is a long sagittally flattened cavity with no obvious lateral recesses. The fourth ventricle also extends into the cervical spinal canal. The medulla may characteristically buckle in on itself (the cervicomedullary kink or spur) as it descends behind and below the upper cervical cord. This kink usually occurs between C2 and C4. The bony posterior fossa is quite small and the foramen magnum symmetrically enlarged. A sagittal diameter of the C1 ring is less than that of the foramen magnum, so C1 may appear to be displaced upward into the foramen magnum. The lower vertebral column invariably demonstrates a myelocele or myelomeningocele. A syrinx is present in 40% to 95% of cases. Approximately 6% of cases will demonstrate diastematomyelia below C3.[13–17]

Depending on the source consulted, basilar impression and/or assimilation of C1 to the occiput may or may not be associated with Chiari I and/or Chiari II malformations. With the superb anatomical fidelity of MR, determining this association becomes simply a matter of defining the parenchymal pathology and/or the bony CVJ anomalies present.

Dandy-Walker Malformation

The Dandy-Walker malformation is a well-defined entity consisting of three features:

1. Hydrocephalus
2. Incomplete fusion of the cerebellar vermis
3. Retrovermian cyst that is contiguous with the fourth ventricle[18, 19] (Fig 5–8).

The size of the cyst and whether or not it communicates with the subarachnoid space has no bearing on the diagnosis. The term "Dandy-Walker variant," (which has been applied to cases with a narrow slit between the cerebellar hemispheres) may be inappropriate since these cases do have the three necessary conditions to be simply "Dandy-Walker." Other associated congenital anomalies include agenesis of the corpus callosum, holoprosencephaly, heterotopic gray matter, and occipital encephalocele (Fig 5–9). Sagittal and axial T_1-weighted images are usually all that is required for identification of the malformation. Sagittal images are especially useful in defining the dysplastic vermis and the connection of the cyst to the fourth ventricle. Look-a-likes include a

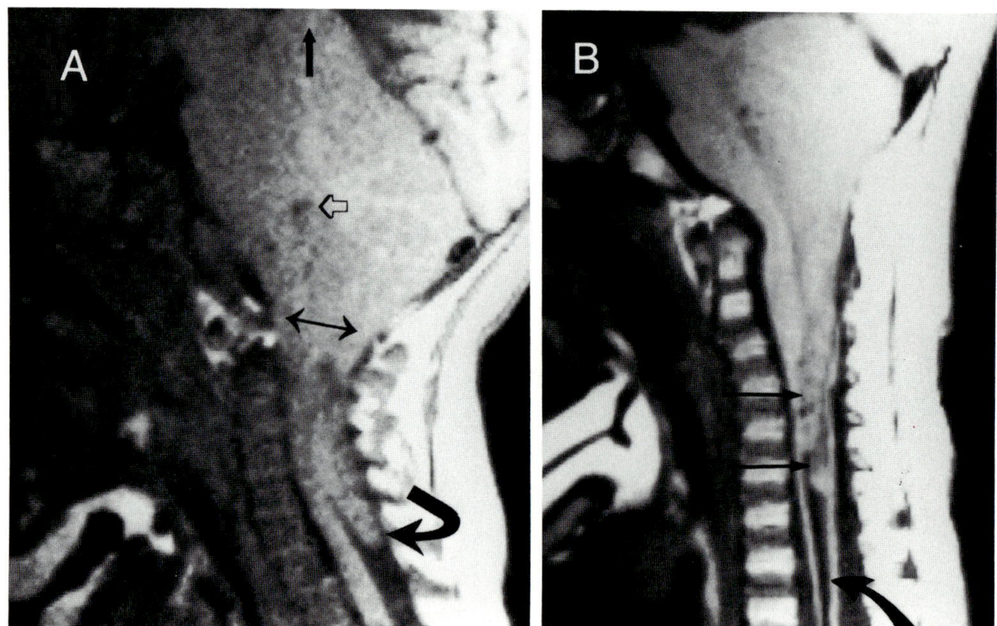

FIG 5–7.
Chiari II malformation. **A,** there is marked caudal displacement of the cerebellar tonsils *(curved arrow)* below the foramen magnum margin *(double-headed arrow)*. The fourth ventricle is attenuated and barely visible *(open arrow)*. Note the superior projection of the vermis *(arrow)*, also called the cerebellar "pseudomass." **B,** Chiari II malformation where the choroid plexus *(arrows)* lies entirely within the cystic prolongation of the fourth ventricle, contiguous with the cervical syrinx cavity *(curved arrow)*.

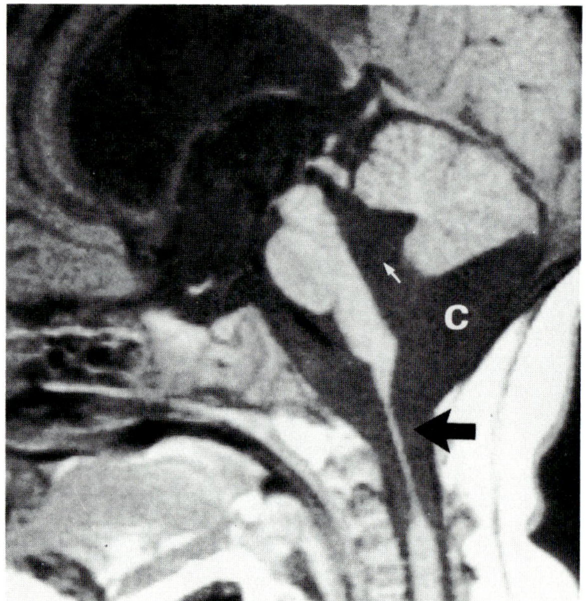

FIG 5–8.
Dandy-Walker malformation. The three components of the malformation are demonstrated in this case: (1) hydrocephalus, (2) inferior vermian dysplasia, and (3) a retrovermian cyst (**C**) that communicates with the fourth ventricle *(white arrow)*. There is marked atrophy of the cervicomedullary junction *(black arrow)* due to birth trauma.

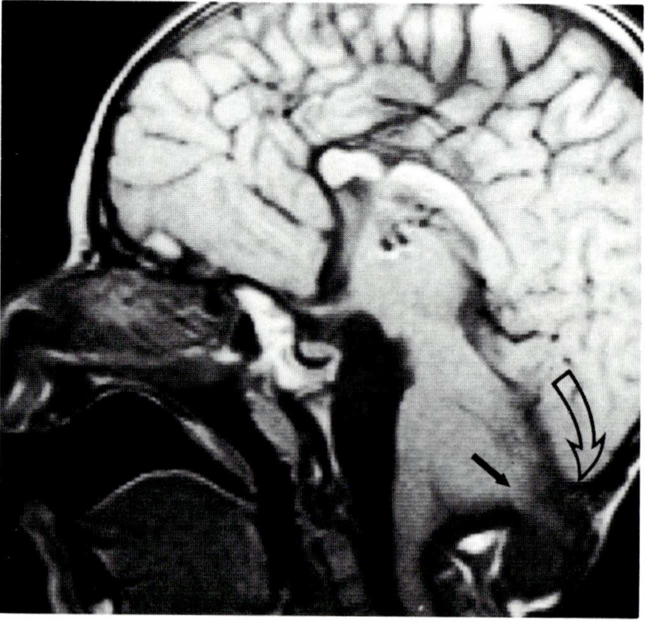

FIG 5–9.
Occipital encephalocele. The brain stem is tethered posteriorly by the cerebellum *(arrow)* herniating through the occipital-bone defect *(curved arrow)*. (Courtesy of Dr. Allison Smith.)

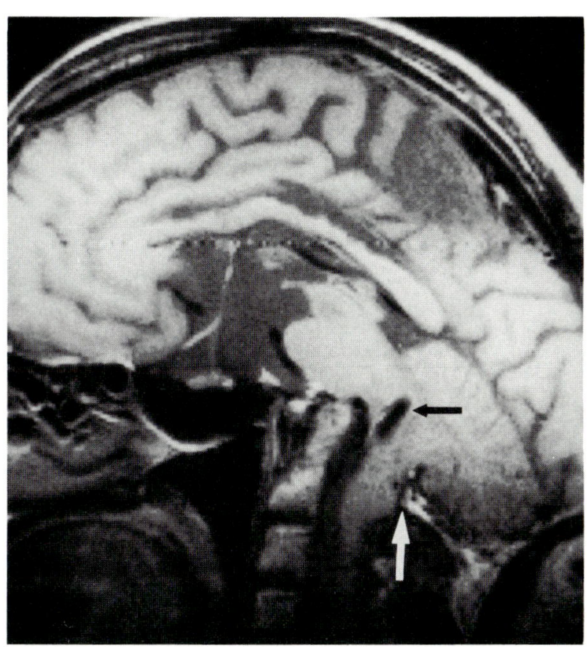

FIG 5–10.
Osteogenesis imperfecta. There is basilar invagination with the odontoid compressing the pontomedullary junction. The opisthion is also superiorly displaced with mass effect on the posterior medulla *(white arrow)*. There is extreme platybasia (*arrow* indicates tortuous vertebral artery).

large cisterna magna and posterior fossae arachnoid cyst. However, neither of these will show the dysplasia and connection to the fourth ventricle of a true Dandy-Walker malformation.

Basilar Invagination

Basilar impression (or invagination) is a common congenital anomaly in the atlanto-occipital region. It involves upward migration of the skull base around the foramen magnum and may be associated with intracranial extension of the dens. A primary congenital cause is occipitalization of the atlas. There are several secondary causes related to malacic or abnormal bone structures such as osteogenesis imperfecta, Paget's disease, rickets, osteomalacia, and hyperparathyroidism (Fig 5–10). Midline T_1-weighted MR images are ideal for defining the position of the odontoid bone with respect to the foramen magnum but more importantly for defining the effect the odontoid bone has in neutral/flexion/extension on the cervicomedullary junction.

Achondroplasia

Achondroplasia is a congenital abnormality transmitted as an autosomal dominant. The features of achondroplasia of the lumbar spine, such as small spinal canal with progressively narrowing interpediculate spaces is well known. More of a problem in the pediatric population is a small foramen magnum, or foramen magnum coarctation (Fig 5–11). This may be a cause of respiratory problems, quadriparesis, and communicating hydrocephalus.[20] The hydrocephalus may be secondary to outlet obstruction from the small foramen magnum, or perhaps to venous outflow obstruction.[21] The foramen magnum may be extremely small and narrowed in the transverse plane. Coronal imaging may be necessary to reveal the precise degree of cord impingement laterally. Basilar impression is seen in up to 50% of cases.[22]

Morquio's Syndrome

Morquio's syndrome is a lysosomal storage disease thought to be secondary to an enzyme defect (galactosamine-6-sulfate–sulfatase or β-galactosidase) and is transmitted as an autosomal recessive. Atlantoaxial subluxation is a regular feature of Morquio's syndrome, secondary to ligamentous laxity. The foramen magnum may also be quite small and narrow in the transverse plane similar to that seen in achondroplasia.[20] Patients with mucopolysaccharidosis may have leptomeningeal thickening, dural involvement, as well as spinal stenosis and subluxation. Cord compression may be caused by atlantoaxial subluxation or by deposits of mucopolysaccharide in the anterior soft tissues. Water-soluble contrast myelography has been recommended for evaluating the cervical spine in these patients to precisely define the spinal soft tissues. Magnetic resonance imaging may also define CVJ abnormalities, including the deposits of mucopolysaccharide.[23, 24]

Osseous Abnormalities

The CVJ osseous abnormalities may be quite complex, consisting of a variety of segmentation errors and subluxations. Polytomography or CT scanning with bone algorithms may be necessary to precisely define the bony anatomy. Magnetic resonance is capable of roughly defining the bony anatomy using the combination of signal void produced by cortical bone and high signal from yellow marrow (e.g., clivus, anterior and posterior arches of C1, and the dens). Magnetic resonance excels in defining any distortion of the brain stem or cervical cord by the osseous abnormalities on T_1-weighted sagittal images. Flexion and extension views add the element of motion and can detect C1–2 subluxations and basilar invagination, as well as determine whether or not they are reducible.

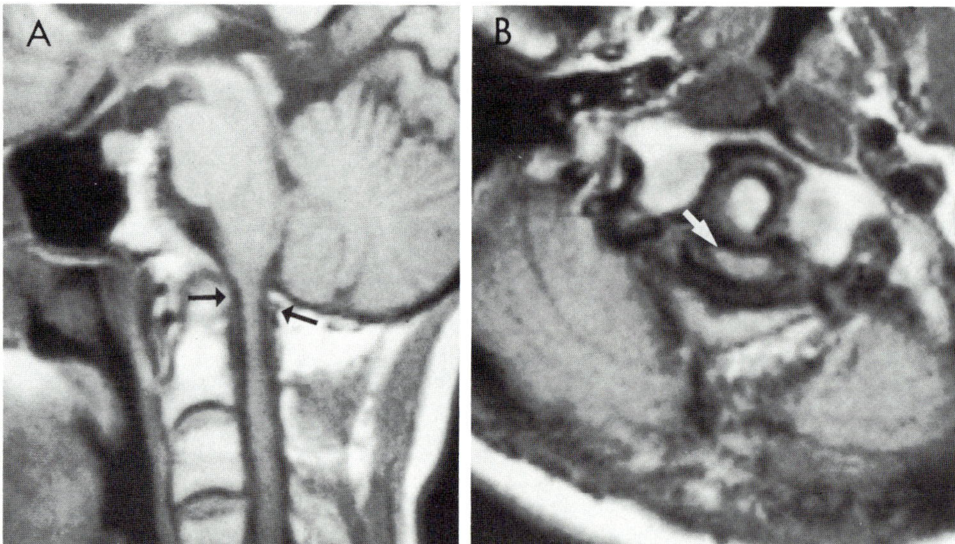

FIG 5–11.
Achrondroplasia. **A,** there is marked narrowing of the foramen magnum with compression of the cervicomedullary junction *(arrows).* **B,** axial image confirms the significant anterior compression of the cord *(arrow).*

Atlantoaxial Subluxations

In children, the ADI should be no larger than 4 mm, while the upper limit of normal in adults is 2.5 to 3 mm. It must be kept in mind that these measurements are based on the ossified portions of the C1 anterior arch by plain radiographs. Care is needed in applying these measurements to MR images in children where cartilage and synovial joints may be readily visualized. Congenital causes of atlantoaxial instability include Down's syndrome, spondyloepiphyseal dysplasia, osteogenesis imperfecta, and neurofibromatosis. However, with these congenital causes, the presence of an increased ADI in flexion may not signal the need for stabilization, nor are the patients necessarily symptomatic. Of a more physiologic importance is the space available for the cord (SAC), measured from the dens to the nearest posterior bony structure (such as the opisthion or the posterior arch of C1). Cord impression always occurs if the SAC is 14 mm or less.[25]

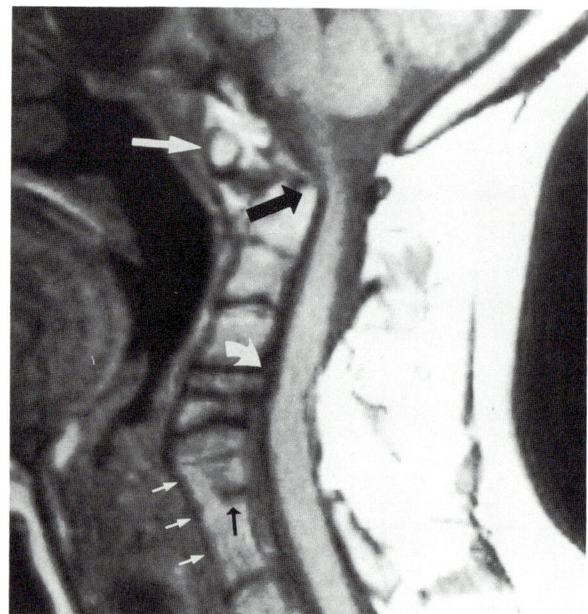

FIG 5–12.
Klippel-Feil syndrome. There are segmentation anomalies involving C2–3 and C6–7. Level C6–7 has a "wasp-waist" configuration *(small white arrows)* with only a small remnant of the disk space *(small black arrow).* There is reverse atlantoaxial subluxation with compression of the cervicomedullary junction *(black arrow).* Additionally there is a disk herniation at C4–5 *(curved arrow).* Anterior arch of C1 *(white arrow).*

Klippel-Feil Syndrome

Klippel-Feil syndrome refers to a condition in patients with congenital fusion of the cervical vertebra (Fig 5–12). The classic clinical triad consists of low posterior hairline, limited range of motion, and a short neck. While occipitalization of the atlas, hemivertebra, and basilar impression occur more frequently in this syndrome, as isolated entities they are not designated as Klippel-Feil syndrome.[26] Sagittal T_1-weighted sequences define the levels of congenital fusion by the thinner, "wasp-waste" appearance of the fused segments. The segments demonstrate normal marrow signal. Frequently, a thin horizontal line of decreased signal intensity is present in a central portion of the fusion representing the rudimentary disk space. Flexion and extension views are useful in determining any atlantoaxial instability. Due to the changes in stress on the spine secondary to the fusions, disk herniations are common above and below the fusion levels.

Os Odontoideum

A true os odontoideum is a relatively rare manifestation of a segmentation error and is manifested as a separate bone between the basion and the normal odontoid tip. Many cases described as os odontoideum are the result of an unrecognized fracture through the base of the odontoid, which subsequently becomes distracted by the traction of the alar ligaments towards the basion[27] (Fig 5–13). When there is complete resorption of the fractured dens, the mistake is to consider this congenital absence of the dens.

TUMORS

Brain stem gliomas are a fairly common tumor representing 10% to 15% of childhood neoplasms or 20%

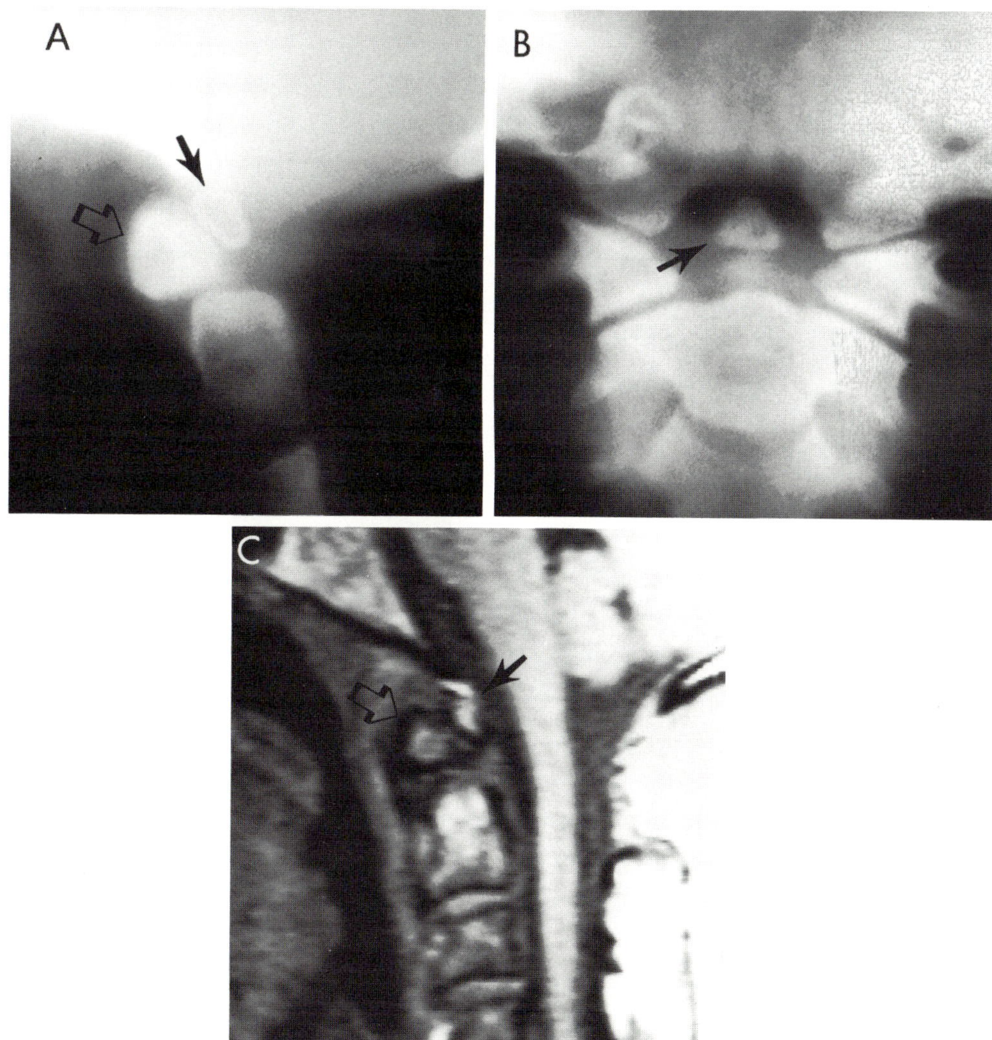

FIG 5–13.
Old odontoid fracture. **A,** sagittal tomogram shows a hyperplastic anterior arch of C1 *(open arrow)* and a small remnant of the odontoid *(arrow)*. **B,** coronal tomogram demonstrates the smoothly corticated odontoid fragment *(arrow)*. **C,** sagittal MR also demonstrates the fragment *(arrow)* in relation to the anterior C1 arch *(open arrow)*. Odontoid fracture status after posterior fusion.

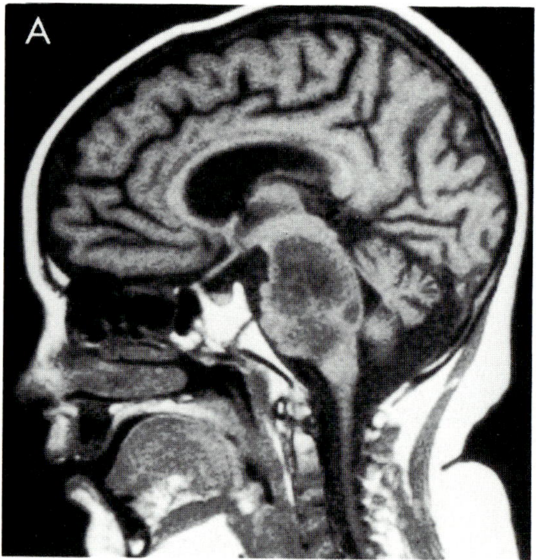

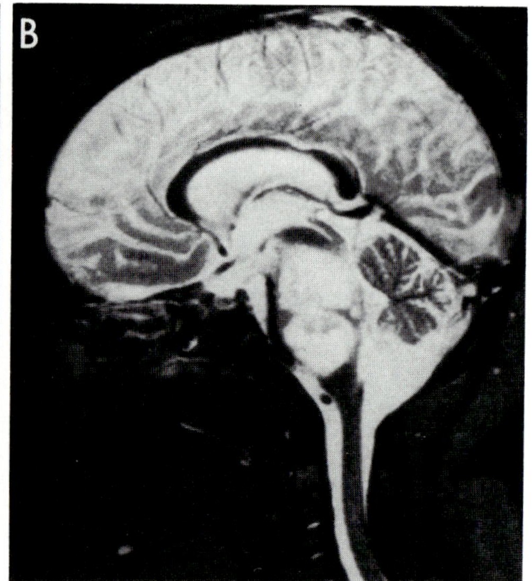

FIG 5–14.
Brain stem glioma. T_1-weighted (**A**) and cardiac-gated T_2-weighted (**B**) images show a large exophytic brain stem mass showing prolonged T_1 and T_2 relaxation times. The caudal and cephalad edges of the tumor are well defined.

of infratentorial childhood tumors. Histologic evidence of malignancy is common. Sagittal and axial T_1- and T_2-weighted images are superb for defining areas of pathology, as well as compression of adjacent structures such as the fourth ventricle or midbrain (Fig 5–14). Brain stem gliomas usually show marked expansion of the brain stem, which will appear hypointense on T_1-weighted and hyperintense on T_2-weighted images. The exophytic components and their relationship to the basilar artery (seen well due to flow void) are also easily defined. A large expansile mass in the brain stem with these signal characteristics is pathognomonic for a brain stem glioma in a child.[28] In adults, metastatic disease must be a prime consideration. Other intraparenchymal lesions of the posterior fossae that must be included in the differential are cerebellar hemispheric or tonsillar gliomas, infection, and infarction. Tumors and infection distort architecture and produce mass effect. Infarcts generally preserve the gross morphology of the gray and white matter (albeit abnormal in signal intensity) and produce less mass effect for the overall lesion size.

The most common extra-axial lesions occuring at the CVJ are meningiomas and neurinomas (Figs 5–15 through 5–17). The posterior fossa accounts for approximately 10% of intracranial meningiomas. These are usually smooth, well defined tumors that displace the cervicomedullary junction, causing symptoms by pressure or vascular compromise rather than parenchymal destruction. Meningiomas are commonly isointense on T_1- and T_2-weighted images to brain parenchyma, so the gross anatomical picture must be carefully evaluated. Neurinomas may closely resemble the appearance of meningiomas, being well-defined extramedullary lesions. They are usually isointense on T_1-weighted sequences but may be isointense to hyperintense on T_2-weighted sequences. Both meningiomas and neurinomas show marked enhancement with paramagnetic contrast agents on T_1-weighted sequences. However, not all

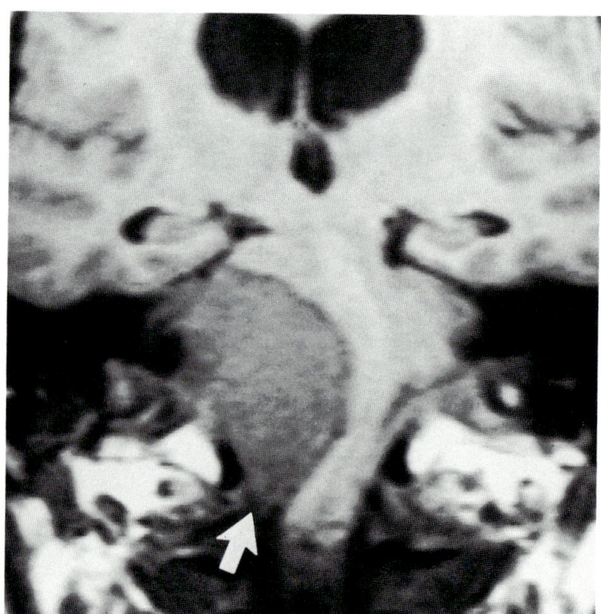

FIG 5–15.
Meningioma. The large extra-axial mass compresses the brain stem and causes hydrocephalus. The tumor extends below the level of the foramen magnum *(arrow)*.

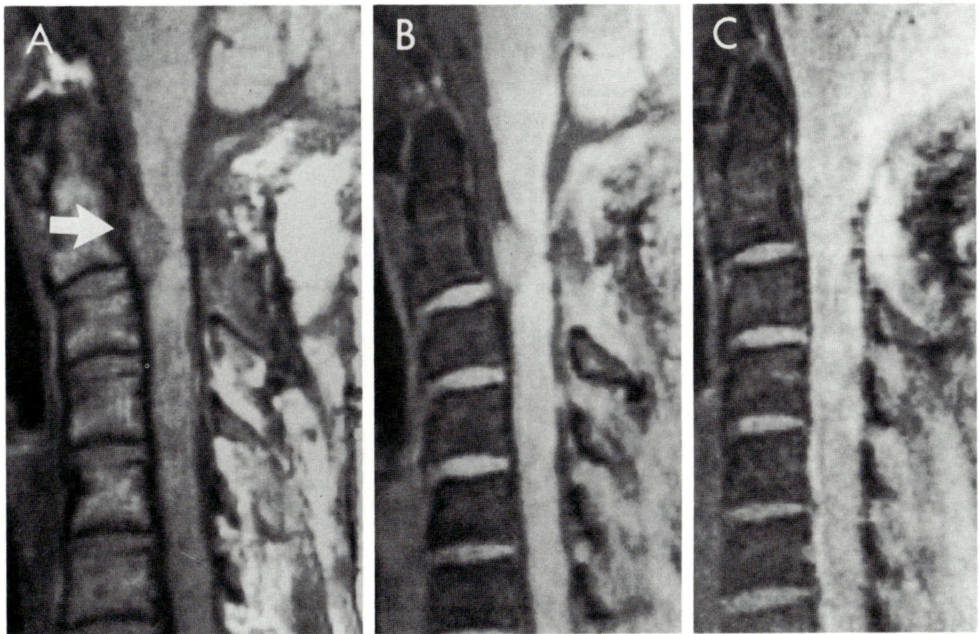

FIG 5–16.
Neurofibroma. **A,** sagittal T_1-weighted SE image shows the extramedullary mass arising anteriorly at the C2 level *(arrow).* **B,** gradient echo fast low-angle shot (FLASH) with a 60-degree flip angle. The tumor is still well visualized as a extramedullary lesion. **C,** gradient echo (FLASH) with a 10-degree flip angle causes the CSF to increase in signal relative to parenchyma, thus obscuring the pathology.

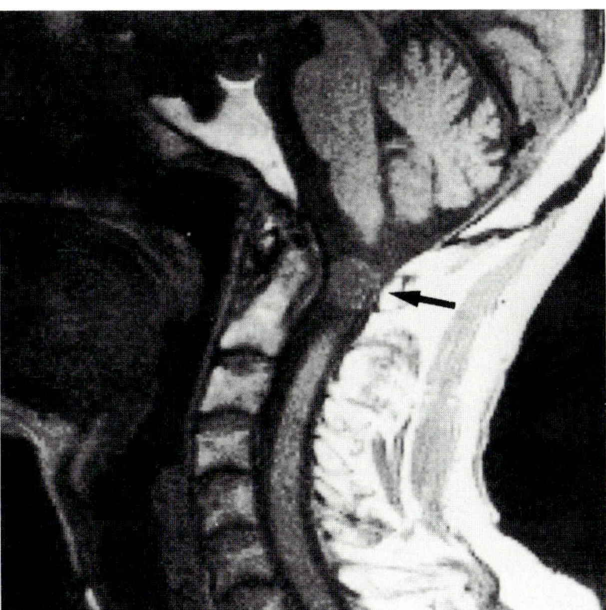

FIG 5–17.
Neurofibroma. Sagittal T_1-weighted image shows a large soft tissue mass at the C1 level displacing the cord out of the midline *(arrow).*

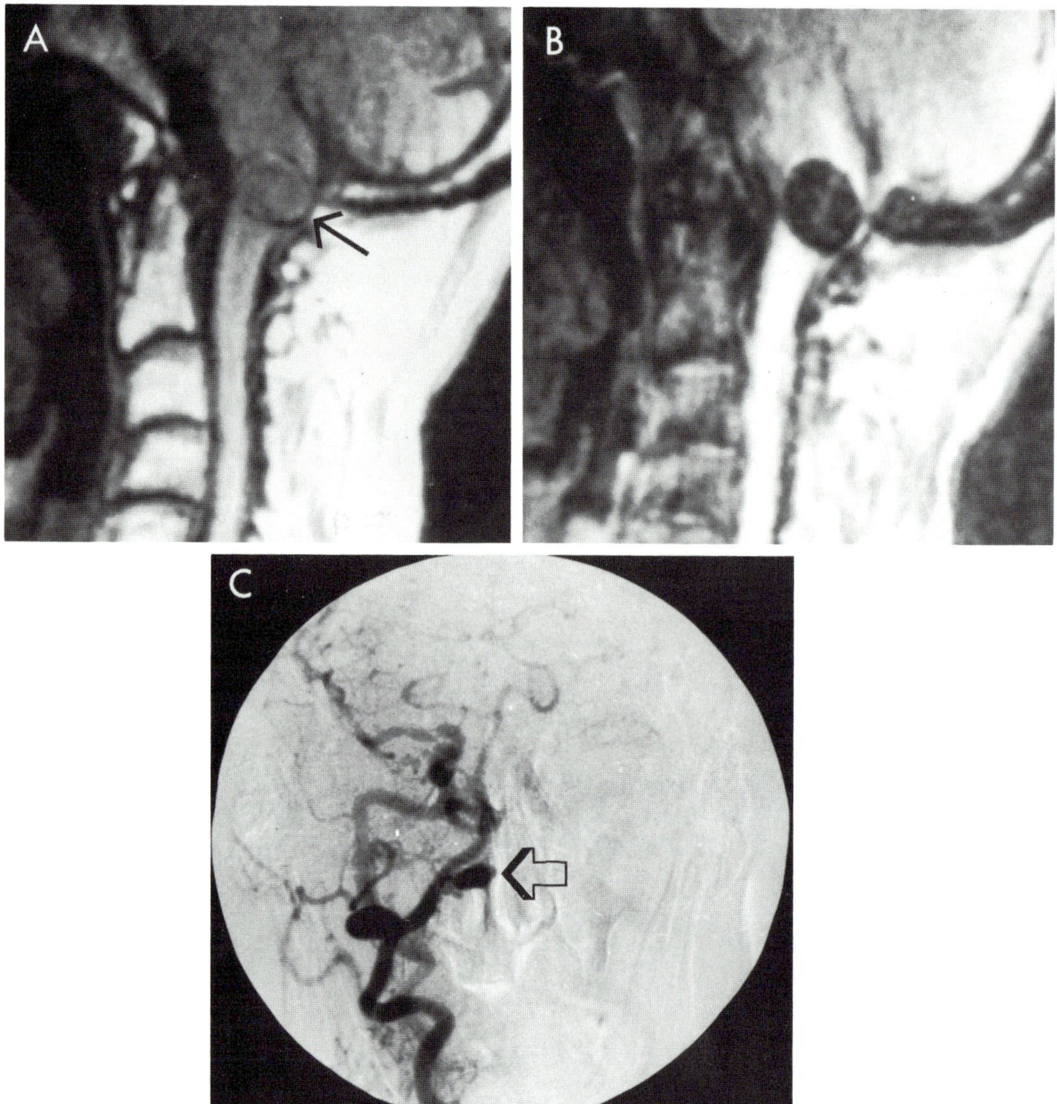

FIG 5–18.
Partially thrombosed posterior inferior cerebellar arterial (PICA) aneurysm. **A,** sagittal T_1W image shows a well-defined circular mass *(arrow)* of peripheral low signal intensity at the foramen magnum level. **B,** T_2-weighted image shows markedly decreased signal from the aneurysm due to preferential T_2 relaxation from the thrombus. **C,** anteroposterior digital subtraction angiogram (DSA) shows the aneurysm arising off the origin of the right PICA *(arrow).*

extramedullary tumoral masses of the CVJ are meningiomas or neurofibromas. We have seen one case of a posterior inferior cerebellar arterial (PICA) aneurysm that was initially interpreted as a meningioma due to its low signal on T_1- and T_2-weighted images, which in retrospect was secondary to organized thrombus within the aneurysm (Fig 5–18). Other extra axial prepontine tumors that must be considered include chordomas, nasopharyngeal carcinomas, metastases, and multiple myeloma, chondroma, osteochondroma, and osteoma (Figs 5–19 and 5–20). All of these may present as a soft tissue mass destroying the clivus.

Chordomas are uncommon tumors derived from notochord remnants. These tumors tend to be locally aggressive and infrequently metastasize. Plain films and CT will show calcification (20% to 70%) and bone destruction.

Because they arise from notochordal remnants, chordomas may be found throughout the spinal column, with a preponderance in the sacrococcygeal (50% to 70%) and clival (15% to 25%) regions. In the spine, the cervical (especially C2) region is the most common location. The MR findings are nonspecific and show intermediate signal on T_1-weighted images destroying or in-

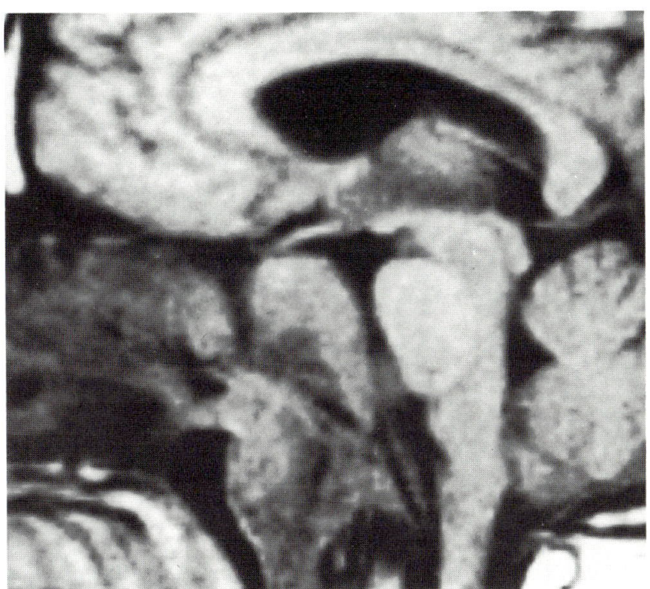

FIG 5–19.
Nasopharyngeal carcinoma. Sagittal T_1-weighted image shows soft tissue replacing the nasopharynx, clivus, and prevertebral space. The pituitary is not distinctly seen. (Courtesy of Dr. Frederick Dengel.)

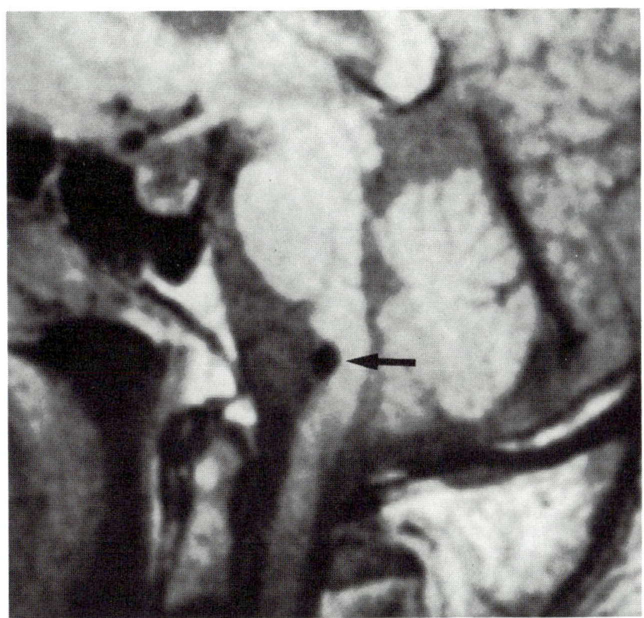

FIG 5–21.
Dolichoectasia of the vertebrobasilar system. A tortuous vertebral artery *(arrow)* indents the anterior medulla.

volving bone. Like other tumors, they will show increased signal on T_2-weighted images.

DOLICHOECTASIA OF THE BASILAR ARTERY AND VERTEBRAL ARTERIES

The most common correctable reason for trigeminal neuralgia and hemifacial spasm is vascular compression of the fifth and seventh cranial nerves. This may be caused by a tortuous or dolichoectatic vertebral basilar system. A loop of the superior cerebellar artery usually is responsible for fifth-nerve symptoms, while a loop of the anterior-inferior cerebellar artery compresses the seventh nerve exit zone.[29]

The course of the vascular system is usually well defined on T_1-weighted sagittal and axial images, as is the mass effect on the brain stem (Fig 5–21). Long TR/TE odd-echo images will provide excellent contrast be-

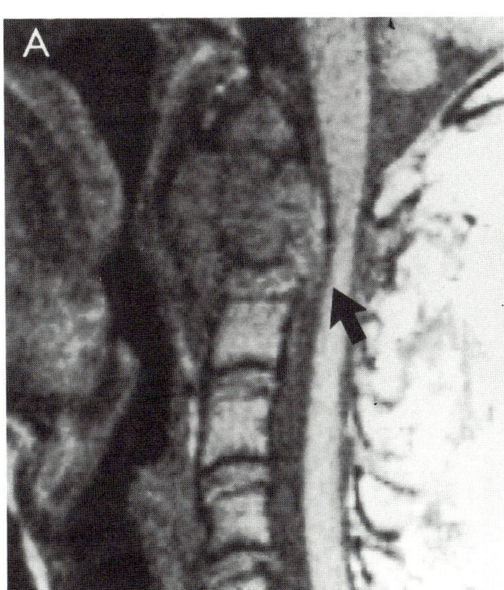

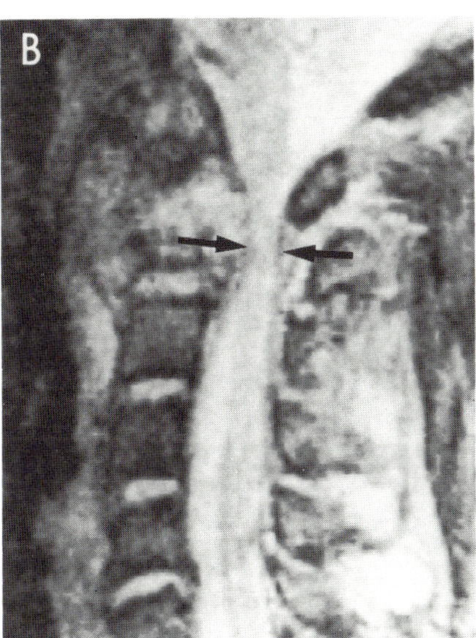

FIG 5–20.
Metastatic paraganglioma. **A,** sagittal T_2-weighted image shows a large soft tissue mass destroying the C2 body and compressing the cervical cord *(arrow)*. **B,** gradient echo (FLASH) with 10-degree flip angle. The destruction of C2 and the cord compression *(arrows)* are well visualized.

tween the increased signal CSF and the flow void within the vessels. Even-echo T_2-weighted images may rephase enough flow to decrease the conspicuity of the vessels. Slow flow may demonstrate increased signal on T_1-weighted images. However, a significant degree of compression by MR may or may not correlate with a patients symptomatology.

REFERENCES

1. Lee BC, Kneeland JB, Deck MDF, et al: Posterior fossae lesions: Magnetic resonance imaging. *Radiology* 1984; 153:137–143.
2. Taveras JM, Wood EH: *Diagnostic Neuroradiology*. Baltimore, Williams & Wilkins, 1976, pp 51–60.
3. McGregor M: The significance of certain measurements of the skull in diagnosis of basilar impression. *Br J Radiol* 1948; 21:171.
4. Fischgold H, David M, Bregeat P: *La Tomographie de la Base du Crane en Neurochirurgie et Neuro-ophthalmologie*. Paris, Masson and Cie, 1952.
5. Hinck VC, Hopkins CE: Measurement of the atlanto-dental interval in the adult. *AJR* 1960; 84:945–951.
6. VanGilder JC, Meneges AH: Craniovertebral junction abnormalities. *Clin Neurosurg* 1983; 30:514–530.
7. McRae DL, Barnum AS: Occipitalization of the atlas. *AJR* 1953; 70:23–46.
8. Baker H: Myelographic examination of the posterior fossa with positive contrast medium. *Radiology* 1963; 81:791–801.
9. Barkovich AJ, Wippold FJ, Sherman JL, et al: Significance of cerebellar tonsillar position on MR. *AJR* 1986; 97:795–799.
10. DuBoulay G, Shah SH, Currie JC, et al: The mechanism of hydromyelia in Chiari type I malformations. *Br J Radiol* 1974; 47:579–587.
11. Rhoton AL: Microsurgery of Arnold-Chiari malformations in adults with and without hydromyelia. *J Neurosurg* 1976; 45:473–487.
12. Forbes WS, Isherwood I: Computed tomography in syringomyelia and the associated Arnold-Chiari type I malformation. *Neuroradiology* 1978; 15:73–78.
13. Naidich TP, Pudlowski RM, Naidich JB, et al: Computed tomographic signs of the Chiari II malformation: I. Skull and dural partitions. *Radiology* 1980; 134:65–71.
14. Naidich TP, Pudlowski RM, Naidich JB: Computed tomographic signs of Chiari II malformation: II. Midbrain and cerebellum. *Radiology* 1980; 134:391–398.
15. Naidich TP, Pudlowski RM, Naidich JB: Computed tomographic signs of the Chiari II malformation: III. Ventricles and cisterns. *Radiology* 1980; 134:657–663.
16. Naidich TP, McLane DG, Fulling KH: The Chiari II malformation: IV. The midbrain deformity. *Neuroradiology* 1983; 25:179–197.
17. Wolpert SM, Anderson M, Scott RM, et al: Chiari II malformation: MR imaging evaluation. *AJNR* 1987; 8:783–792.
18. Harwood-Nash DC, Fritz CR: Congenital malformations of the brain, in Harwood-Nash DC, Fritz CR (eds): *Neuroradiology in Infants and Children*. St Louis, CV Mosby Co, 1976, vol 3, pp 998–1053.
19. Masdeu JC, Dobben GD, Azar-Kia B: Dandy-Walker syndrome studied by computed tomography and pneumoencephalography. *Radiology* 1983; 147:109–114.
20. Naidich TP, McLane DG, Harwood-Nash DC: Systemic malformations in Newton TH, Potts DG (eds): *Computed Tomography of the Spine and Spinal Cord*. San Anselmo, Calif, Clavadel Press, 1983.
21. Yamada H, Nakamura S, Tajima M, et al: Neurological manifestations of pediatric achondroplasia. *J Neurosurg* 1981; 54:49–57.
22. Luyendijk W: *J Neurol Neurosurg Psychiatry* 1978; 41:1053.
23. Edwards MK, Harwood-Nash DC, Fitz CR, et al: CT metrizamide myelography of the cervical spine in Morquio syndrome. *AJNR* 1982; 3:666–669.
24. Kulkarni MV, Williams JC, Yeakley JW, et al: Magnetic resonance imaging in the diagnosis of the cranio-cervical manifestations of the mucopolysaccharidoses. *Magn Reson Imaging* 1987; 5:317–323.
25. Greenberg AD: Atlanto-axial dislocations. *Brain* 1968; 91:655.
26. Pizzutillo PD: Klippel-Feil, in the Cervical Spine Research Society: *The Cervical Spine*. Philadelphia, JB Lippincott Co, 1983, pp 174–188.
27. Fielding JW, Hensinger RN, Hawkins RJ: Os odontoideum. *J Bone Joint Surg* [*Am*] 1980; 62:376.
28. Hueftle MG, Han JS, Kaufman B, et al: MR imaging of brainstem gliomas. *J Comput Assist Tomogr* 1985; 9:263–267.
29. Sobel D, Norman D, Yorke CH, et al: Radiography of trigeminal neuralgia and hemifacial spasm. *AJNR* 1980; 1:251–253.

6

Inflammatory Disease

Jeffrey S. Ross, M.D.

Inflammatory disorders of the spine that will be covered in this chapter include arachnoiditis, disk space infection (DSI), and rheumatoid arthritis. These diverse processes have equally diverse presenting symptomatology that are often nonspecific. Imaging plays a key role in defining the abnormalities and guiding clinicians toward proper management. Magnetic resonance imaging (MRI) has replaced the more conventional imaging modalities (myelography for arachnoiditis, scintigraphy for DSI) and is capable of specific and early diagnosis.

ARACHNOIDITIS

In 6% to 16% of patients who have had spinal surgery, spinal arachnoiditis is the cause of persistent symptoms.[1] Its clinical diagnosis is often difficult since it has no distinct symptom complex. The pathogenesis of spinal arachnoiditis is very similar to the repair process of serous membranes, such as the peritoneum, which demonstrate little inflammatory cellular exudate and predominance of fibrinous exudate. The fibrin-covered roots stick to themselves and to the thecal sac. With time, dense collagenous adhesions are formed by the proliferating fibrocytes during the repair phase.[2]

Previously, the diagnosis of arachnoiditis was confirmed by myelography, and less commonly by computed tomography (CT) and surgery. Myelography in spinal arachnoiditis may show a variety of patterns. These include prominent cauda equina nerve roots, a homogeneous contrast pattern without nerve root shadows, and subarachnoid filling defects with concomitant narrowing and shortening of the thecal sac. Jorgensen et al.[3] divided the myelographic patterns into a type I group that is due to adhesions of the roots inside the meninges giving a root "sleeveless" appearance and a type II pattern that demonstrates filling defects, narrowing, shortening, and occlusion of the thecal sac. Type I is seen with mild disease, while type II is the picture of more extensive adhesions.[4] By CT myelography, the early adhesions are seen in the distal thecal sac as a loss of nerve root sleeve filling. Roots will become adherent to each other and to the meninges, which leads to the appearance of an "empty sac."[5] As this transmeningeal fibrosis continues, clumping becomes more prominent until the thecal sac and roots become one confluent soft tissue mass. This produces a myelographic block and has been considered the "end stage" of arachnoiditis.[6] Surface coil MR utilizing slice thickness less than 5 mm can also define abnormal patterns of nerve roots within the thecal sac.

Sequences

Both T_1- and T_2-weighted sequences are useful for the optimum definition of arachnoiditis. The single most efficient sequence for visualization of arachnoiditis is probably the axial T_1-weighted sequence. It allows moderate confidence in defining all types of arachnoiditis. A recent report has stated the inability of heavily T_2-weighted sequence to distinguish inflammatory tissue (such as arachnoiditis) within the thecal sac by using body coil MR.[7] In our experience with surface coil MR, the T_2-weighted axial study is helpful in defining the distribution of roots within the thecal sac with greater contrast sensitivity than provided by the T_1-weighted images, at least in the less severely affected groups. However, the pathology in the type II group of Jorgensen et al.[3] with a large soft tissue mass within the thecal sac could potentially be masked due to the high signal from the fibrosis and adhesions mimicking normal cerebrospinal fluid (CSF) signal on the T_2-weighted study.

Normal Variations

Since the pattern and positioning of new roots within the thecal sac is critical for defining arachnoiditis, the normal variations must first be considered. We examined 20 patients referred for an MR study for back pain and with no previous history of myelography or spinal surgery as a control group for nerve root distribution. Ten of these 20 patients had plain film myelograms or CT myelograms within 1 week of the MR study. We examined a total of 54 vertebral body levels. At the L2 level, the roots are seen as a mass of intermediate soft tissue signal on T_1-weighted images in the dependent portion of the thecal sac. The roots form a smooth crescent following the curvature of the posterior thecal sac. At the L3 level, the roots are often amassed posteriorly (the dependent position). These may be globular and irregular in appearance or crescentic and smooth. The roots about to exit the dural tube are placed anterolaterally in a symmetric pattern. At the L4 level, the roots have dispersed so that they are seen as separate delicate entities arranged in a symmetric pattern within the CSF. By the L5 level, the few roots present are equally spaced from each other within the thecal sac. Central conglomeration within the thecal sac is conspicuously lacking at the L5 level. Midline sagittal images show the roots as a single band of intermediate signal intensity on T_1-weighted images following the posterior thecal sac. This band of roots gradually tapers from the conus to the L4 level. Parasagittal images nicely demonstrate the roots dispersing from the conus in a fan-shaped manner as they travel from the posterior-superior position of the conus to the anterior-inferior L5 level.

Pathology

The MR morphological changes may be divided into three groups.[8] In a group I arachnoiditis, the predominant MR findings are large conglomerations of nerve roots that reside centrally within the thecal sac (Fig 6–1). The nerve roots are seen on T_1-weighted images as well-defined rounded areas of intermediate soft tissue signal. Some improvement in definition of the clumped roots can be seen with the high contrast provided by the CSF signal on T_2-weighted images. The CT myelographic appearance in this group is similar to that of the T_2-weighted MR images, showing central thickening of the nerve roots. Myelograms in this group may vary in appearance from loss of definition of the root sleeves with thickened roots present intrathecally to moderate narrowing and irregularity of the contrast column.

In group II, MR demonstrates clumped nerve roots attached peripherally to the meninges (Fig 6–2). This appears as areas of focal thickening of the meninges, with few or no nerve roots visible within the subarachnoid space. T_2-weighted images provide the best definition of the peripheral nerve roots and the central homogeneous CSF signal. The appearance is essentially one of an "empty thecal sac." Computed tomographic myelograms also will show the focal thickening of the soft tissue attenuation nerve roots peripherally along the meninges. The central portion of the subarachnoid space will show homogeneous intrathecal contrast with no nerve roots appreciated. Myelograms in this group will show a capacious thecal sac with a smooth outer border, amputation of the root sleeves, and no nerve roots within the caudal thecal sac.

In group III, T_1-weighted MR images will demonstrate increased soft tissue signal within the thecal sac below the conus, obliterating the majority of the subarachnoid space (Fig 6–3). T_2-weighted images will show increased signal diffusely from the thecal sac without definition of individual nerve roots. Computed tomographic myelography will show increased soft tissue attenuation material within the subarachnoid space. Small loculated areas of contrast material may be seen peripherally. Myelography commonly demonstrates a block of the subarachnoid space, with the distally visualized subarachnoid space being irregular and assuming a "candle dripping" appearance. Of course, the variations and combinations of these groups may be seen. One fairly frequently observed combination is that of group I and group II (Fig 6–4). Often, at the L3 or L4 level, the roots are seen to be clumped centrally. As the roots progress caudally, they fan out and are attached peripherally to the meninges giving an empty thecal sac appearance by the L5 level.

These abnormalities of nerve roots are uniformly seen at the L3 level or below. In over 25 patients we have studied with lumbar arachnoiditis, the abnormal configuration of nerve roots has been seen over at least two vertebral body levels.

In one series, we identified the changes of arachnoiditis by MR in 11 of 12 cases that had been demonstrated by CT myelography and plain film myelography. This represented a sensitivity of 92%, specificity of 100%, and accuracy of 99%. Our group I and group II patients appear to fall within the type I category of Jorgensen et al.,[3] the main difference being the distinction between central and peripheral clumping of nerve roots. More severe disease categorized by Jorgensen type II is reflected in our group III. These latter groups show a soft tissue replacing the subarachnoid space on CT and MR, which gives rise to the myelographic block.

False negative and false positive MR studies are inevitable. Both may be caused by suboptimal MR scans

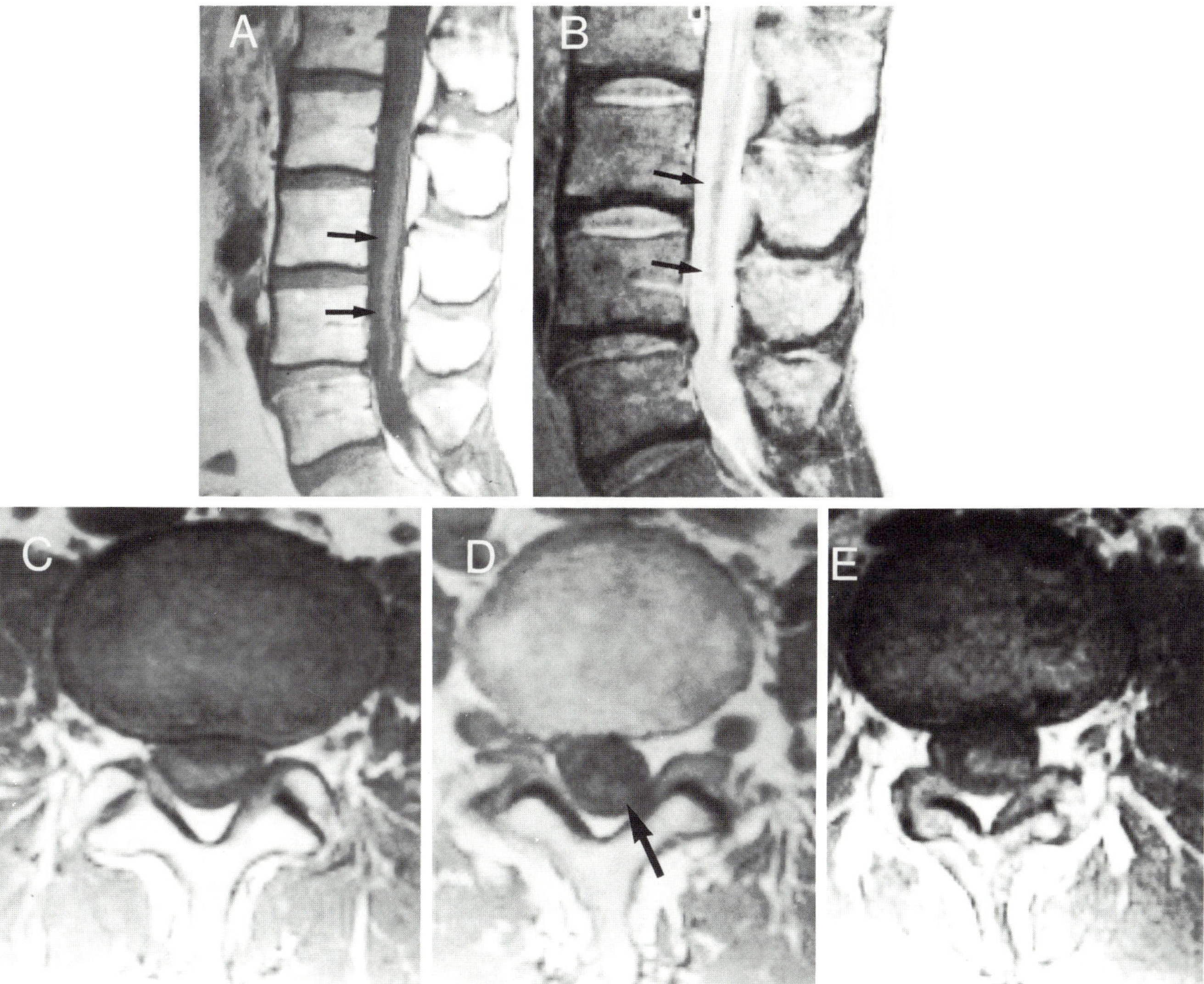

FIG 6–1.
Group I arachnoiditis. Sagittal T_1-weighted (**A**) and T_2-weighted (**B**) images show nerve roots to be adhered centrally into one linear mass of soft tissue signal *(arrows)*. Axial T_1-weighted image (**C**) at the L3–4 level also demonstrates the abnormally clumped roots. At the L5 body level (**D**), the roots continue to be centrally clumped *(arrow)*. Axial T_1-weighted image (**E**) in a different patient shows the typical appearance of centrally clumped nerve roots. (From Ross JS, Masaryk TJ, Modic MT, et al: MR imaging of lumbar arachnoiditis. *AJNR* 1987; 8:885–892. Used by permission.)

where patient motion or poor signal-to-noise can give the appearance of lack of nerve roots within the thecal sac, as well as a false positive appearance of central clumping.

Potentially, the normal appearance of nerve roots at the L2 or L3 level could be mistaken for arachnoiditis. In routine practice, however, this is not a problem since arachnoiditis involves the L3 level and below and also extends over at least two lumbar body levels. It is difficult to diagnose arachnoiditis on a single axial image. A much more confident diagnosis can be made by the visual integration of the appearance of the roots over several levels. Clumping of lumbar nerve roots is very commonly seen with lumbar canal stenosis, which could potentially mimic a group III arachnoiditis. However, the associated findings in bone and ligament will allow a correct diagnosis to be made. The distinction between group III arachnoiditis and an intrathecal tumor may be impossible by MR, except for any secondary findings of previous surgery and/or iophendylate (Pantopaque) myelography. If the tumor has been present long enough, then ancillary findings such as scalloping of the posterior margins of the vertebral bodies may be an additional clue. Neoplastic CSF seeding could produce soft

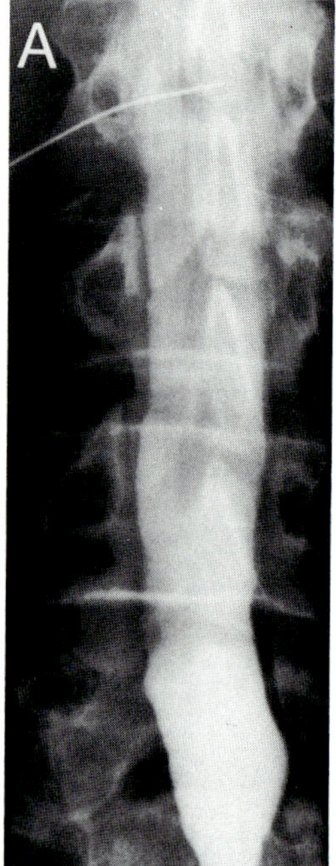

FIG 6–2.
Group II arachnoiditis. **A,** water-soluble contrast myelogram shows an amorphous collection of contrast material in the caudal thecal sac with no visible nerve roots or root sleeves. Computed tomography following the myelogram **B** confirms that the roots are adhered peripherally to the meninges *(arrow).* **C,** axial T_1-weighted MR also shows the "empty thecal sac" and the peripherally clumped roots *(arrow).* **D,** axial T_2-weighted image confirms that no roots are visible within the thecal sac. (From Ross JS, Masaryk TJ, Modic MT, et al: MR imaging of lumbar arachnoiditis. *A JNR* 1987; 8:885–892. Used by permission.)

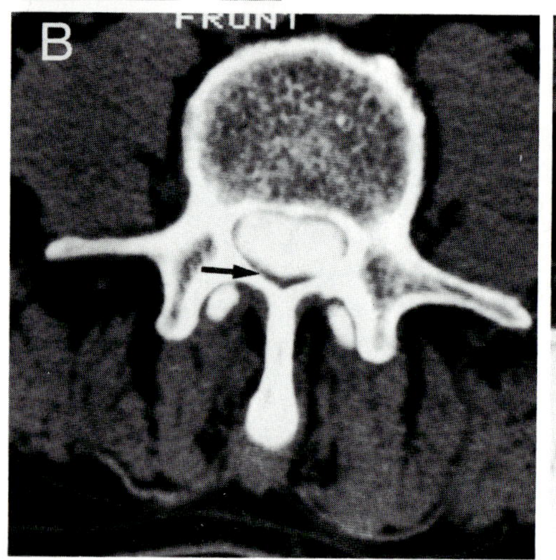

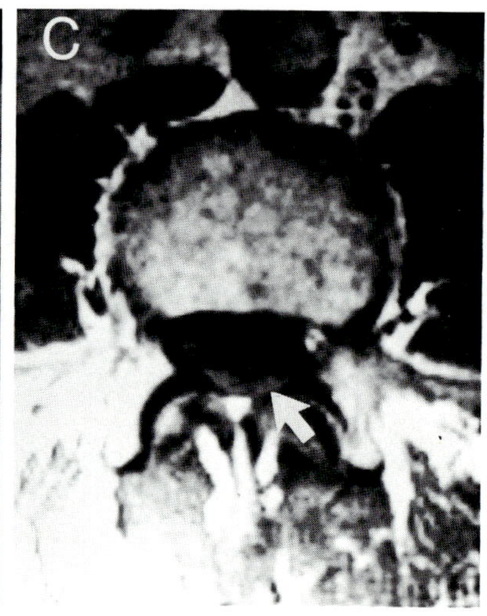

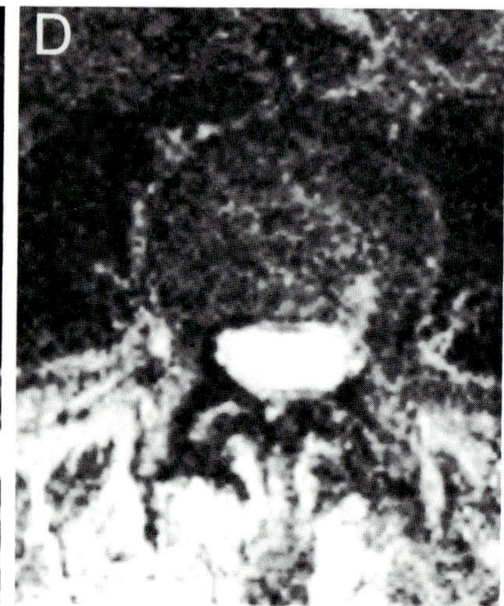

tissue masses within the thecal sac indistinguishable from group I changes. However, more commonly, the roots seen with group I arachnoiditis are smooth and tapered, in contradistinction to the focal, irregular tumor masses seen with CSF seeding.

Thoracic arachnoiditis may be visualized as thickening of the leptomeninges, which is best imaged using axial T_1-weighted spin-echo (SE) sequences. The cord may or may not be involved in the inflammation with subsequent adhesion to the dura. If the cord is adhered, then it will lie eccentrically within the canal. Thoracic arachnoiditis appears to predispose the cord to syringomyelia. The syrinxes have relatively indistinct margins when compared to the archetype syrinx associated with a Chiari I malformation. The syrinxes are formed presumably due to the markedly altered CSF dynamics secondary to the adhesions. Arachnoid cysts are also commonly formed in association with thoracic arachnoiditis.[9]

Causes of spinal arachnoiditis are varied and include infection, intrathecal steroids or anesthetic agents, surgery, trauma, and intrathecal hemorrhage.[10] While surgery is probably the most common cause, retained iophendylate is an additional cause that gives a fairly characteristic appearance on MR. The T_1 value of Pantopaque is approximately 134 msec, which is slightly less than that of subcutaneous fat. Iophendylate will therefore give a very high signal intensity on T_1 value within the thecal sac and continue to show decreased signal intensity on T_2-weighted images.[11–12] The signal intensity

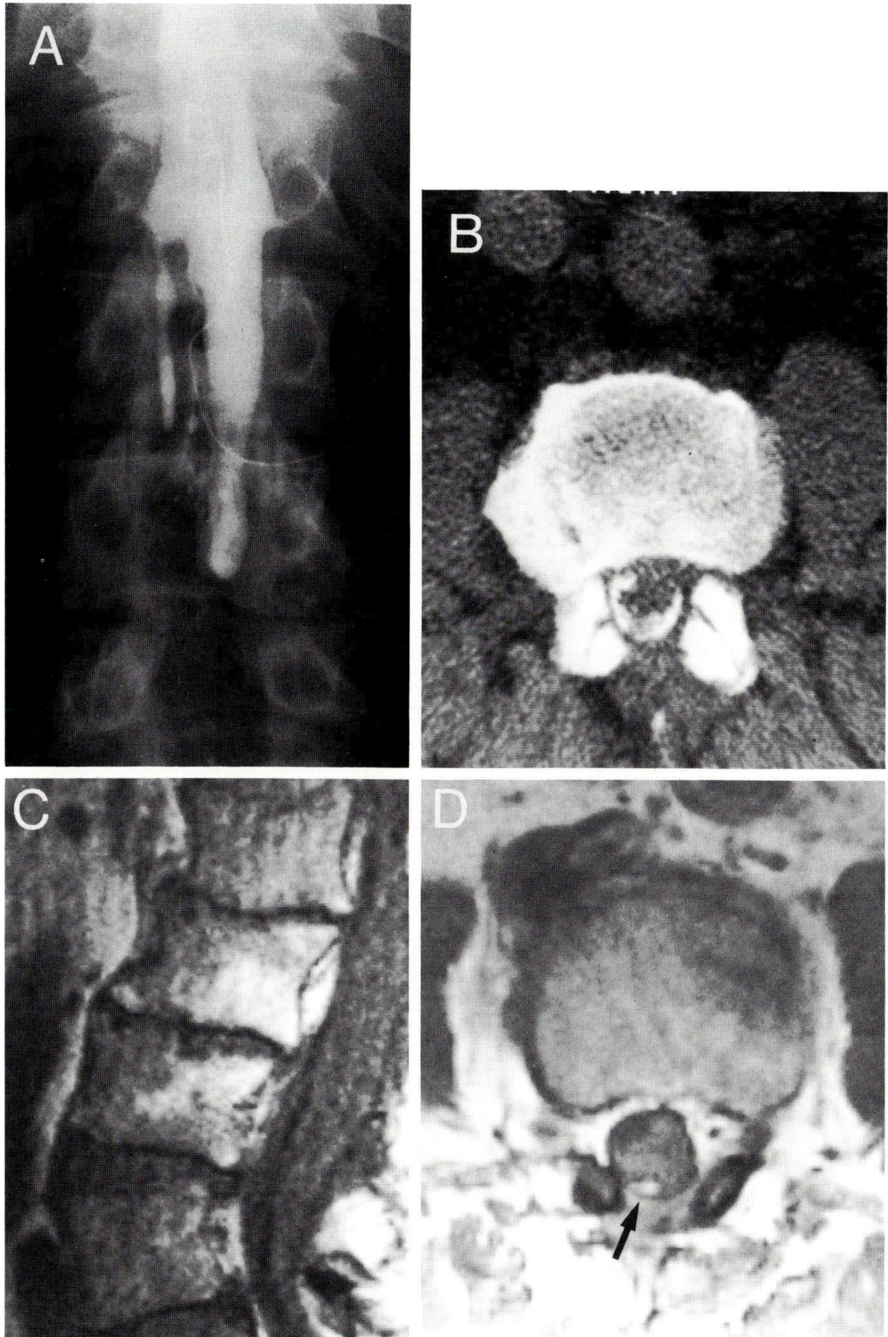

FIG 6–3.
Group III arachnoiditis. Water-soluble contrast myelogram (**A**) shows an irregular block at the L2–3 level with a "candle-dripping" appearance. Thin wire along the midline is a dorsal column simulator for pain control. Computed tomographic scan following myelogram (**B**) shows abnormal soft tissue attenuation material within the thecal sac. **C,** sagittal T_1-weighted MR shows large mass of inflammatory tissue filling the thecal sac. Note the extensive laminectomy. **D,** axial T_1-weighted MR also shows the intrathecal soft tissue mass with a small amount of pantopaque posteriorly *(arrow).* (From Ross JS, Masaryk TJ, Modic MJ, et al: MR imaging of lumbar arachnoiditis. *AJNR* 1987; 8:885–892. Used by permission.)

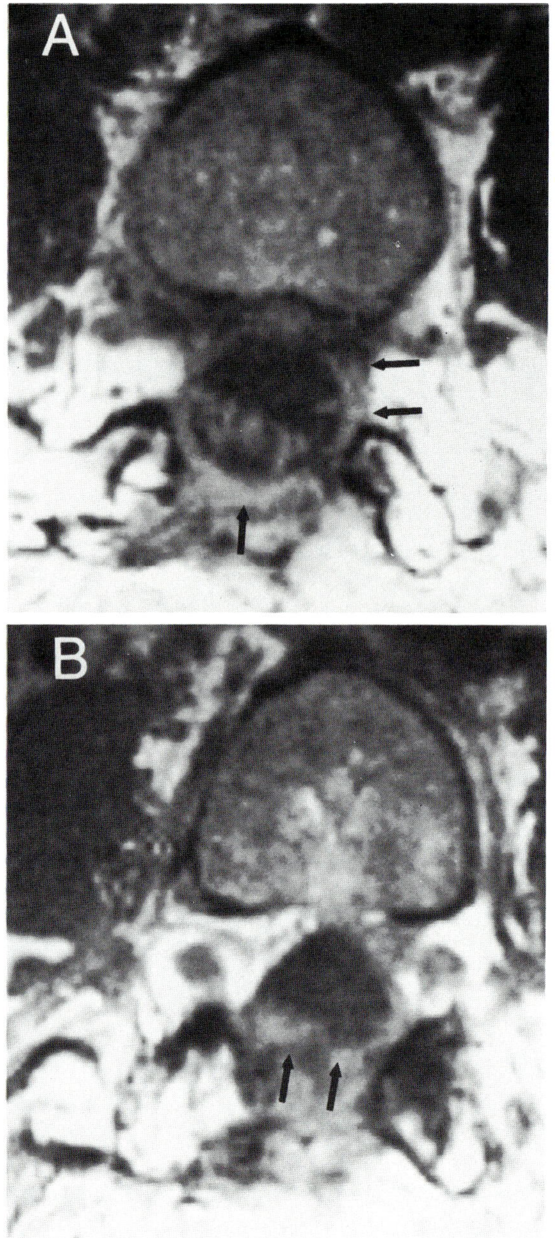

FIG 6–4.
Groups I and II arachnoiditis. Axial T_1-weighted MR at the L4 level (**A**) shows central clumping of the nerve roots. Peripherally, there is a rind of soft tissue comprised of thickened meninges and/or epidural fibrosis *(arrows)*. At the L5 level (**B**), the roots have become peripherally adhered to the meninges *(arrows)*. (From Ross J, Modic M, Masaryk T, et al: Postoperative lumbar spine. *Semin Roentgenol* 1988; 23:125–136. Used by permission.)

of iophendylate does decrease more rapidly than that of subcutaneous fat as images become progressively more T_2-weighted.

The literature concerning the appearance of arachnoiditis by MR is at the present time quite scarce and deals mainly with moderate to severe degrees of inflammation. Findings of subtle arachnoiditis have not yet been described. Nevertheless, for the diagnosis of moderate to severe arachnoiditis MR has excellent correlation with the CT myelographic and plain film myelographic findings.

DISK SPACE INFECTION

Prior to the advent of antibiotic therapy, spinal osteomyelitis was often an acute, virulent disease that caused death from septic complications. Patients who survived long enough to develop abscesses were generally treated by abscess drainage and immobilization. Since antibiotic therapy has become all pervasive, the character of the disease has changed to an insidious disorder of the geriatric population. Dilemmas may arise because clinical and laboratory findings can mimic a variety of neoplastic, traumatic, or inflammatory conditions. Reliance on conventional radiographs can allow extensive bony destruction to take place before therapy can be instituted.[13]

The sources for bacteremia that seed vertebral osteomyelitis are generally genitourinary (GU), dermal, and respiratory. The bacteria find their way to the vascularized disk in children where the destruction causes loss of disk space height. As the infection spreads to the adjacent end-plates, plain films will show the characteristic irregularity. Hematogeneous spread also occurs in adults, even though the disk has lost a great deal of its vascularity. The seeding is to the vascularized end-plates, with the disk and opposite end-plates infected secondarily. Spread to the spine via Batson's plexus from a GU source is no longer thought to be significant.

Infection may not be considered in the differential for back pain since it remains an uncommon disorder (less than 1% of all cases of osteomyelitis). Once infection is considered, accurate imaging is necessary to provide invasive tests for a microbiologic diagnosis or surgical drainage. Since abnormalities that appear on plain radiographs usually take days to weeks to become manifest, radionuclide studies have been the primary imaging modality for vertebral osteomyelitis.

Radionuclides most commonly used for detecting inflammatory changes of the spine are technetium 99m (^{99m}Tc) phosphate complexes, gallium citrate ^{67}Ga, and indium 111 labeled white blood cells. While scintigraphy with ^{99m}Tc and ^{67}Ga compounds is sensitive to infection, it is also quite nonspecific. Healing fractures, sterile inflammatory reactions, tumors, and loosened prosthetic devices can show increased uptake.[14–17] Studies of indium 111 labeled white blood cells (WBCs) have several advantages compared to the other radionuclides including higher target-to-background ratios, improved image quality (when compared to gallium), and intense uptake within abscesses. The main disadvantage of indium 111 is its accumulation within any inflammatory lesion, whether it is infectious or not.[18] The radionuclide study also takes time to perform—from hours to days. Computed tomography has played a minor role in cases with bony or soft tissue components and is not considered the mainstay for the diagnosis of disk space infection.[19,20] Literature comparing MR with the more conventional modalities in inflammatory processes continues to grow. It appears that in appropriate situations MR has a sensitivity for detecting vertebral osteomyelitis that exceeds that of plain films and CT and approaches or equals that of radionuclide studies.[21,22]

Pulse Sequences and Technical Considerations

For the evaluation of inflammatory changes in the spine, sagittal images are usually first obtained. Sagittal images are optimum for outlining a relationship of the involved area with the thecal sac and neural structures, and for determining the presence or absence of cord compromise. Also, the relationship and visibility of the disk space and end-plates (which is quite important for the proper diagnosis of disk space infection) is best appreciated in the sagittal plane. It is imperative to obtain both T_1-weighted and T_2-weighted images in at least the sagittal plane for optimum sensitivity to disease. The T_1-weighted spin-echo image allows detection of the increased water content or marrow fluid seen with inflammatory exudate or edema. Like most pathologic processes, disk space infections or vertebral osteomyelitis results in an increased signal intensity on T_2-weighted images secondary to an increased proton density or prolongation of the T_2 relaxation time. The diagnostic specificity of MR is provided by the signal intensity changes on T_1-weighted and T_2-weighted images, as well as by the anatomical pattern of disease involvement and the appropriate clinical situation.

Magnetic Resonance Findings: Pyogenic

Knowledge of the normal MR appearance of the intervertebral disk on T_2-weighted images is critical for the correct interpretation of disk space infections. On T_2-weighted images, the normal intervertebral disk usually shows an increased signal intensity within its central portion that is bisected by a thin horizontal line of decreased signal intensity. While the precise histologic correlation of this intranuclear cleft has not been conclusively proved, it appears to represent fibrous tissue secondary to fissuring (Fig 6–5). After the age of 30 years, this cleft is almost a constant feature of a normal intervertebral disk.[23]

Certain characteristic changes are seen by MR with disk space infections. T_1-weighted images will show confluently decreased signal intensity of the adjacent vertebral bodies and the involved intervertebral disk space when compared with the normal vertebral body marrow. A margin between the disk and adjacent vertebral bodies cannot be defined (Figs 6–5 and 6–6). Also, there is increased signal intensity at the vertebral bodies adjacent to the involved disk on T_2-weighted images. Finally, there is usually an abnormal configuration and increased signal intensity from the intervertebral disk itself. The abnormal configuration of the disk may take the form of streaky linear appearance or the absence of the intranuclear cleft on T_2-weighted images. These MR findings are much more typical of pyogenic, rather than tuberculous, spondylitis.[24] In a comparative study of patients with the clinical suspicion of vertebral osteomyelitis, MR had a sensitivity of 96%, specificity of 92%, and accuracy of 94%. Gallium 67 and technetium 99m bone scintigraphy had a sensitivity of 90%, specificity of 100%, and accuracy of 94% when combined. In this study, MR was as accurate and sensitive as radionuclide scanning for the detection of osteomyelitis.[21]

The decreased signal intensity seen on T_1-weighted images most likely results from increased water content of the exudative polymorphonuclear leukocyte response and local ischemia overwhelming and/or replacing the normal marrow signal. As the inflammatory process becomes more established, it will progress to involve the intervertebral disk and adjacent vertebral body and will result in the confluent decreased signal intensity that was noted in the majority of our cases.[25, 26]

The increased signal intensity on T_2-weighted images is a very nonspecific response, in and of itself, and is probably secondary to prolonged T_2 relaxation time of the inflammatory exudate or areas of ischemia.

The typical disk space infection represents no problem in diagnosis, provided that T_1-weighted and T_2-weighted images are obtained. However, atypical-appearing disk space infections do exist and complicate an unusually unequivocal diagnosis. One atypical form may be seen if DSI complicates a degenerated disk with an associated type II marrow change (i.e., increased signal from the end-plates on T_1-weighted images). In these cases, the T_1-weighted images may continue to show increased signal in the presence of DSI, in effect masking the usual characteristic confluent decreased intensity (Fig 6–7). The key in these cases is the abnormal disk signal intensity on the T_2-weighted images, something that does not occur in uncomplicated type II marrow change. Very early on in vertebral osteomyelitis, there may be decreased signal involving the end-plates without appreciable increased signal from the bodies or disk on T_2-weighted images.

Epidural infections can spontaneously occur as a result of extension of vertebral osteomyelitis. The most common organism is *Staphylococcus aureus.* Many other organisms may be the cause of the infection including *Streptococcus, Salmonella, Klebsiella,* and *Mycobacterium tuberculosis.* Any symptoms and signs of infection will depend on the extent of root and cord compression. These epidural abscesses are capable of producing rapid paraplegia or bowel and bladder symptomatology. Plain film findings are generally not helpful in diagnosing epidural abscesses unless one sees very typical changes of vertebral osteomyelitis. Myelography can show the extent of the epidural disease and reveal a partial or total block of the contrast column.

While at present no comparative studies exist between the more conventional imaging modalities in MR in the evaluation of epidural abscesses, MR certainly has the potential as a precise diagnostic tool and as a means for determination of the extent of the epidural disease.[27] Our limited experience with five cases showed that T_1- and T_2-weighted SE studies were excellent for the depiction of the site of epidural abscess and the degree of extension superiorly or inferiorly (Figs 6–8 through 6–10). These abscesses were uniformly seen as areas of high signal intensity in the anterior epidural space centered principally at the site of the disk space infection. High signal intensity material can be seen extending cephalad or caudad from the epicenter. The margin between the thecal sac and the abscess is usually quite well defined by a thin line of low signal intensity probably representing the leptomeninges. These T_2-weighted images also allow an accurate assessment of the degree of thecal sac compromise.

The differentiation of degenerative disease and tumor from vertebral osteomyelitis is easier by MR than on radionuclide studies or plain radiographs. Degenerated disks will show decreased signal intensity within their central portion on T_2-weighted images. This should be contrasted to the very high signal intensity seen with active inflammation. It may be difficult to differentiate metastatic disease, postoperative changes, or degenerative changes from osteomyelitis by scintigraphic means. These entities can usually be differentiated from osteomyelitis on MR by the lack of confluent decreased signal intensity of the vertebral body and disk on the T_1-weighted images. Likewise, metastatic disease can be distinguished from osteomyelitis by the lack of involvement of the disk space. This continues to be a reliable sign of benign disease in the overwhelming majority of cases, although rare instances of metastatic in-

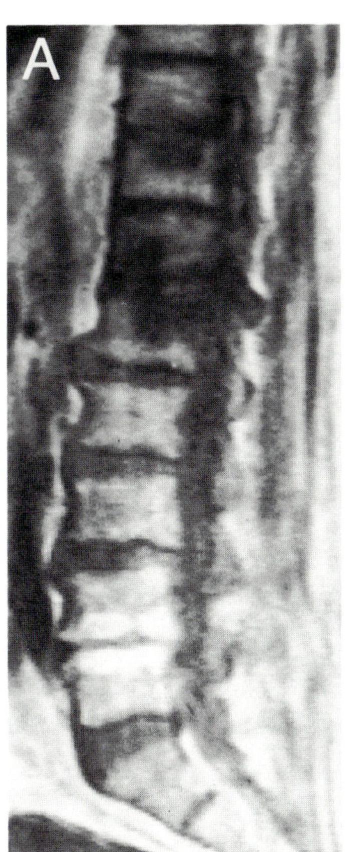

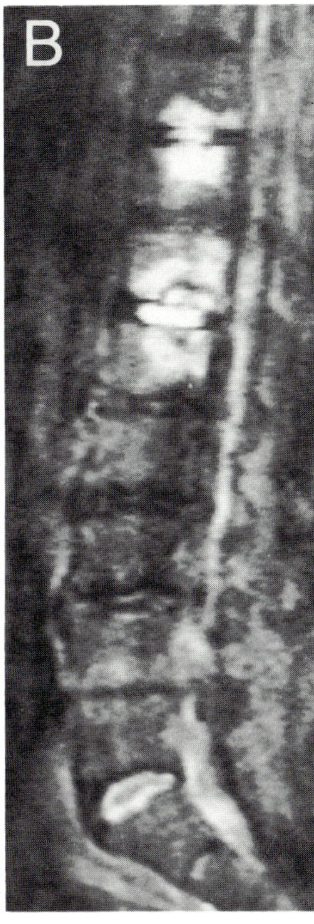

FIG 6–5.
Lumbar vertebral osteomyelitis. Sagittal T_1-weighted image (**A**) shows decreased signal intensity from the T10–11 and T12–L1 intervertebral disks and adjacent vertebral body end-plates involved with osteomyelitis. The disk margins are indistinct. The high signal intensity from the end-plates adjacent to the L4 disk denotes chronic degenerative change (type II marrow). The T_2-weighted image (**B**) shows characteristic findings of disk space infections at T10 and T12: (1) abnormal high signal intensity of the adjacent end-plates and (2) high signal intensity from the intervertebral disk without the intranuclear cleft. Compare T10 and T12 to the normal L5 disk with an intranuclear cleft. Disks L1 through L4 are degenerated as evidenced by the low signal on the T_2-weighted images.

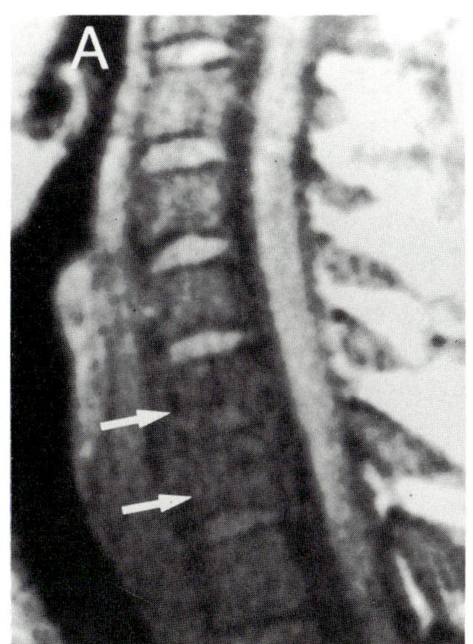

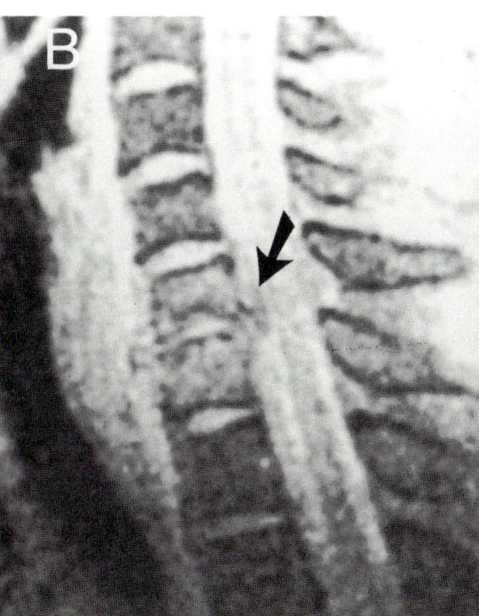

FIG 6–6.
Cervical disk space infection in a drug addict. Sagittal T_1-weighted SE image (**A**) shows decreased signal from the C6 and C7 vertebral bodies *(arrows)* and C6–7 disk space. The 10-degree fast low-angle shot (FLASH) image (**B**) shows abnormal high signal from the vertebral bodies with extension into the epidural space *(arrow).*

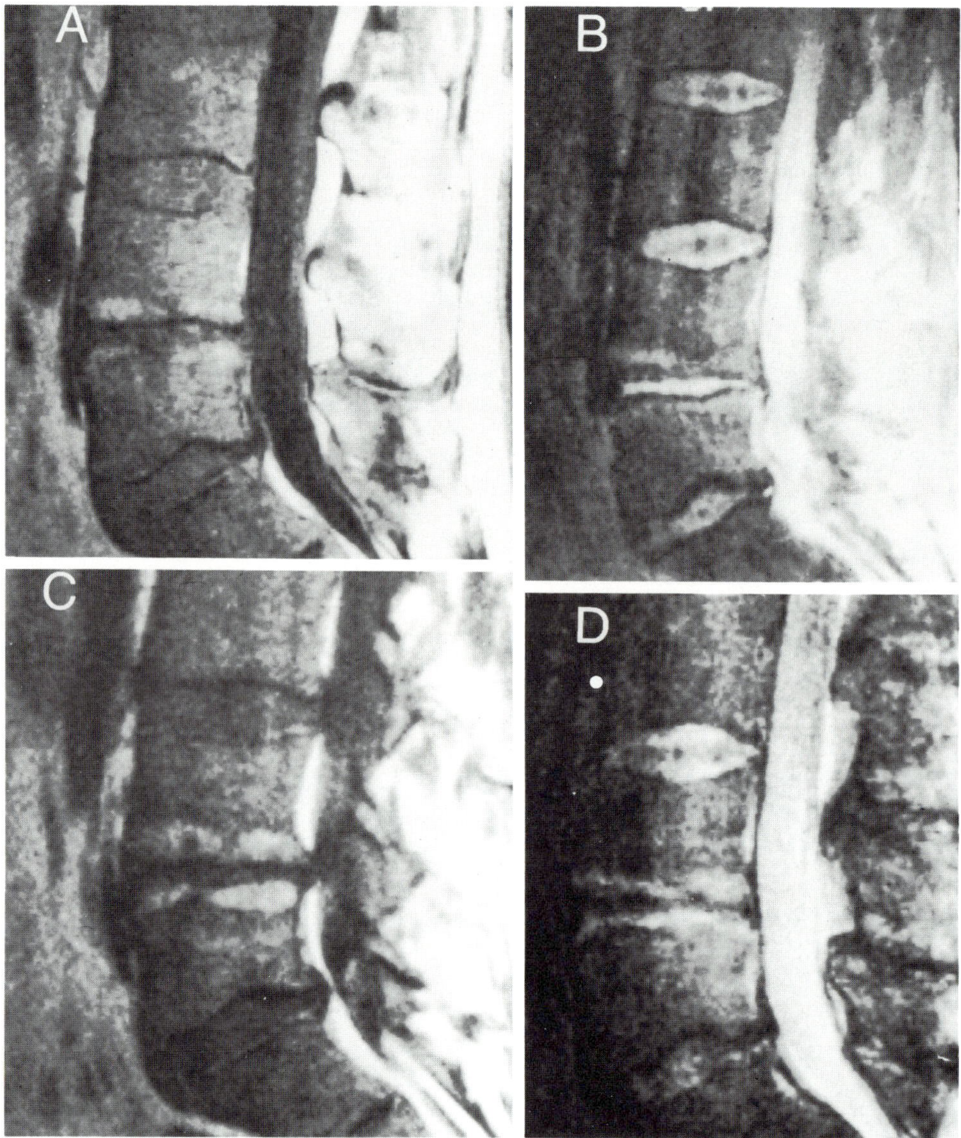

FIG 6–7.
Atypical disk space infection. Sagittal T_1-weighted images (**A**) shows increased signal from the L4–5 end-plates consistent with type II marrow change. Sagittal T_2-weighted image (**B**) shows abnormal increased signal from the L4–5 disk without an intranuclear cleft in the biopsy-proved disk space infection. There is very little increased signal from the adjacent end-plates. Posttreatment T_1-weighted image (**C**) shows more extensive type II marrow change. Sagittal T_2-weighted image after treatment (**D**) shows resolution of the increased signal from the disk space and more prominent marrow changes. The type II end-plate change likely masked the usual confluent low signal seen from marrow with pyogenic disk space infections.

volvement of the disk have been reported.[28, 29] In the initial stages of vertebral osteomyelitis, when the disk space is not yet involved, it may be difficult to exclude neoplastic disease or compression fracture from the differential diagnosis using only MR. Follow-up studies are usually necessary to further define the nature of the lesion.

Severe degenerative changes can produce changes similar to vertebral osteomyelitis on plain films and radionuclide studies. On MR, degenerative disk disease can occasionally show decreased signal intensity within the adjacent vertebral bodies on T_1-weighted images and increased signal intensity on T_2-weighted images. However, the disk space itself is always distinct from the adjacent vertebral body end-plate on T_1-weighted images. Also, the signal intensity of the disk is decreased on T_2-weighted images in degenerative disease, while inflammation will show high signal intensity.[30] Similar changes within the adjacent vertebral bodies can be

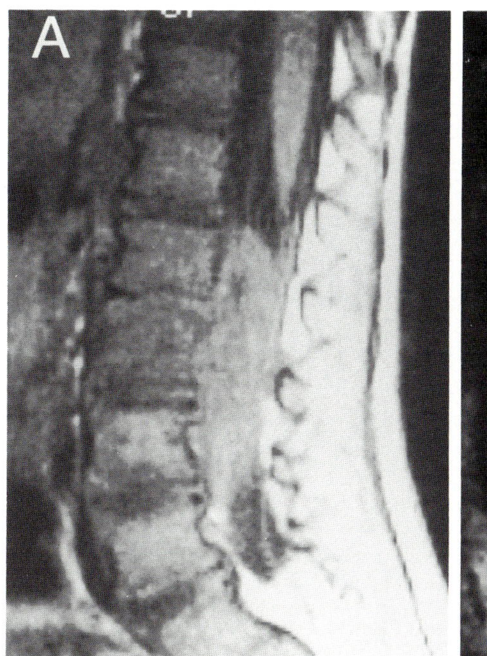

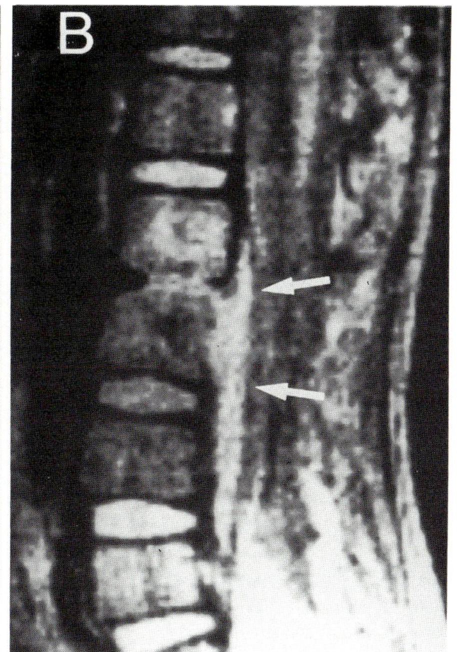

FIG 6–8.
Epidural abscess in a 10-year-old male. The T_1-weighted image (**A**) shows confluent decreased signal from the vertebral bodies and disk space. Epidural spread of infection is seen as intermediate signal mass compressing the anterior thecal sac. Spin-density image (**B**) shows high signal from the involved vertebral bodies and epidural abscess *(arrows).*

seen following surgical instrumentation or chymopapain injection into the intervertebral disk.[31] As with the changes seen with degenerative disk disease, the signal intensity of the disk usually remains decreased on both T_1- and T_2-weighted images, and the borders of the disk are maintained.

Radionuclide studies have several advantages over MR. These studies are not as sensitive to patient positioning, claustrophobia, or patient motion. Surface coil MR has a limited field of view, and involvement of the extravertebral osseous or soft tissue structures is better appreciated with the radionuclide studies. Also, images produced by ^{67}Ga scintigraphy may revert to normal following antibiotic therapy. This can be used as an indication of appropriate therapy and does not appear to be present with MR. The effects of antibiotics on MR signal intensity have not been described. While the MR findings are altered, they apparently are not obscured in the early stages of treatment as can occur with ^{67}Ga imaging. The findings of vertebral osteomyelitis with MR and ^{67}Ga appear approximately at the same time.

With treated osteomyelitis, any abnormal signal-intensity changes revert to normal in a time period ranging from 6 weeks to 1 year. Changes in signal intensity reflect the resolution of the inflammatory exudate or ischemia with fibrous scar tissue replacement and a small amount of new bone formation. Magnetic resonance imaging is sensitive to detection of inflammatory diseases in the spine, but because of the characteristic pattern of involvement, it can also be highly specific.

Tuberculous Spondylitis

Tuberculous spondylitis has been noted to demonstrate findings more typical of neoplasm than those described for pyogenic spondylitis.[32] These findings include (1) sparing of the intervertebral disk space with no abnormal increased signal on T_2-weighted images, (2) preferential involvement of the posterior elements and posterior portions of vertebral bodies, (3) involvement of more than two vertebral bodies, and (4) large paraspinal soft tissue masses (Fig 6–11).

Tuberculous spondylitis is described as beginning in the anterior/inferior portion of the vertebral body, with spread of infection beneath the longitudinal ligaments.[33] The intervertebral disk is commonly not involved. The lack of proteolytic enzymes in mycobacteria has been touted as the cause of intervertebral disk space preservation.[34]

With the predilection for multiple vertebral body involvement, and posterior element involvement, the distinction from metastatic disease may be impossible, except when correlated with history. In North America, spinal TB is most common in young adults (30 to 45

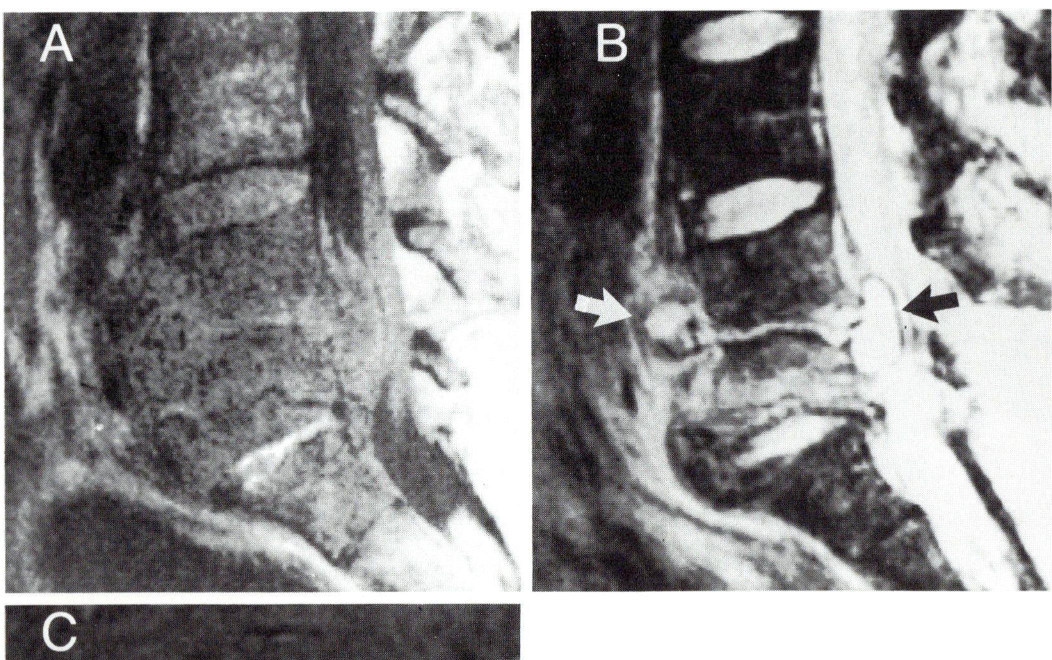

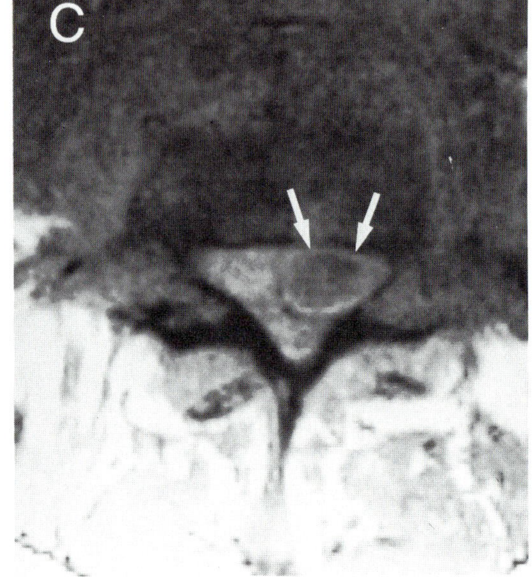

FIG 6–9.
Lumbar epidural abscess. T_1-weighted sagittal image (**A**) shows decreased signal from the L4 disk space. There is anterior and posterior extension of the infection with compression of the lumbar thecal sac. Sagittal T_2-weighted image (**B**) shows the anterior paravertebral *(white arrow)* and posterior epidural extensions *(black arrow)* as high signal intensity. Axial T_1-weighted image (**C**) also demonstrates the large epidural component *(arrows).*

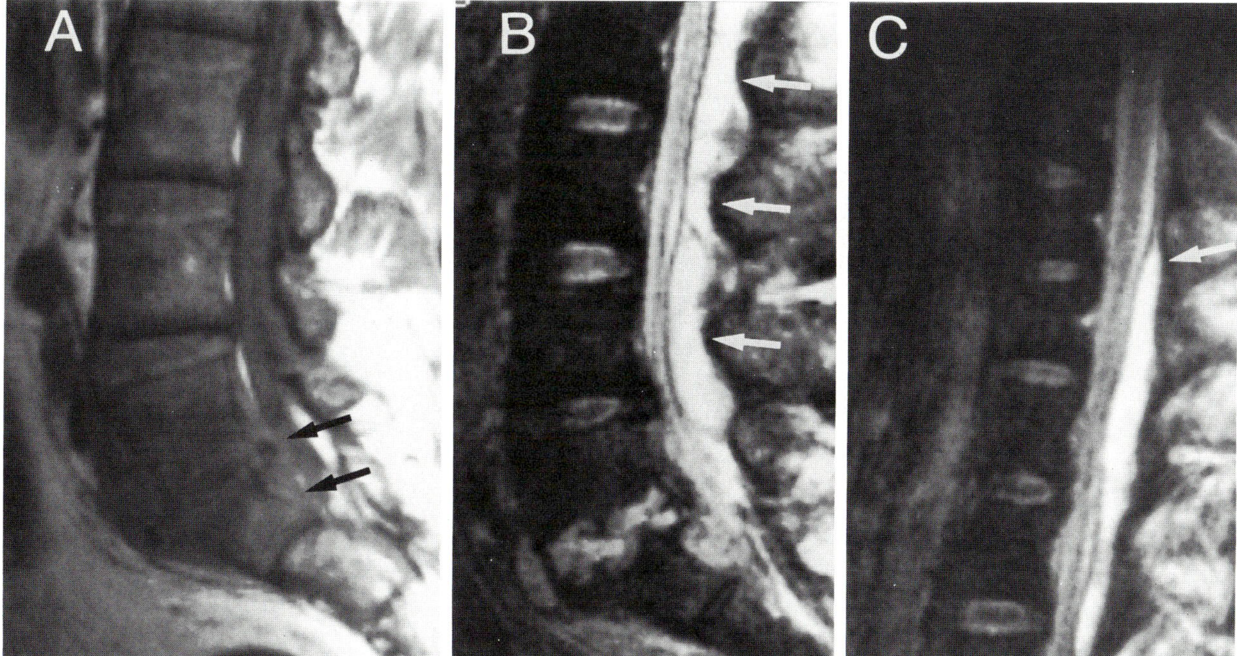

FIG 6–10.
Epidural abscess. Sagittal T_1-weighted image (**A**) shows confluent low signal intensity from the L5 and S1 vertebral bodies. There is an ill-defined anterior epidural mass *(black arrows)*. Sagittal T_2-weighted image (**B**) shows abnormal increased signal from the L5 disk as well as a large posterior epidural collection extending cephalad *(arrows)*. Sagittal T_2-weighted image of the upper lumbar spine (**C**) shows the high signal intensity fluid collection extending to the thoracolumbar junction (arrow).

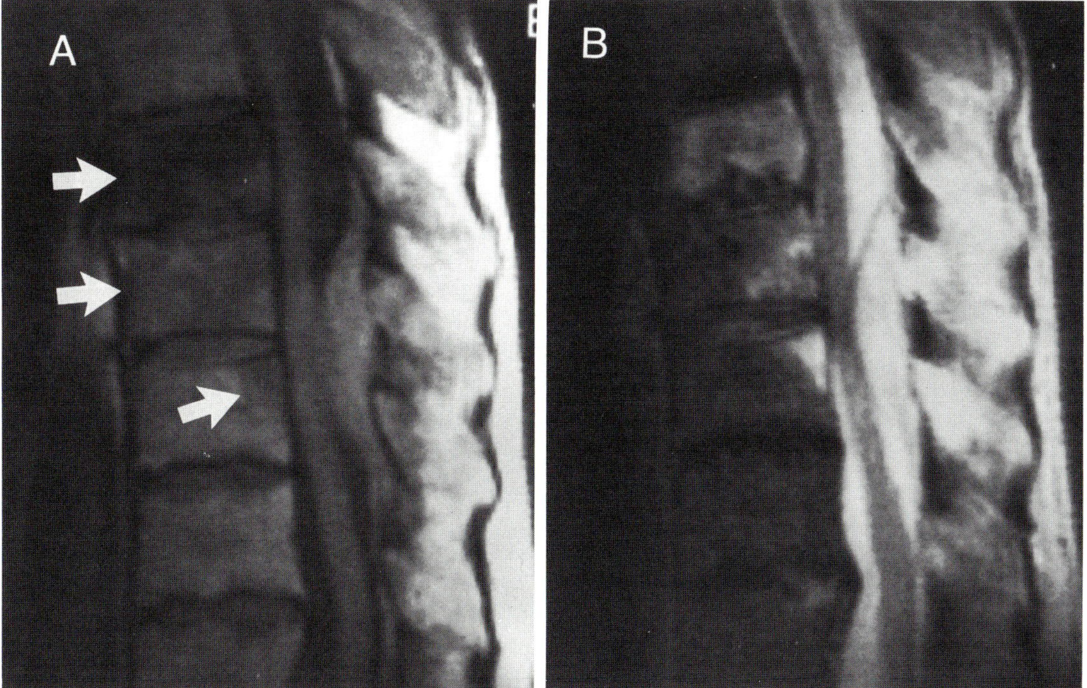

FIG 6–11.
Tuberculous spondylitis. Sagittal T_1-weighted image (**A**) shows areas of decreased signal intensity within the T7–9 vertebral bodies *(arrows)* with preservation of the intervertebral disks. A large posterior soft tissue mass displaces the cord anteriorly. Sagittal T_2-weighted image (**B**) shows abnormal increased signal from the involved vertebral bodies, without abnormal signal from the intervertebral disks. The posterior mass also shows high signal intensity. (From Smith AS, Weinstein MA, Mizushima A, et al: Tuberculous spondylitis: A contradiction to the MR characteristics of vertebral osteomyelitis. *AJNR,* in press. Used with permission.)

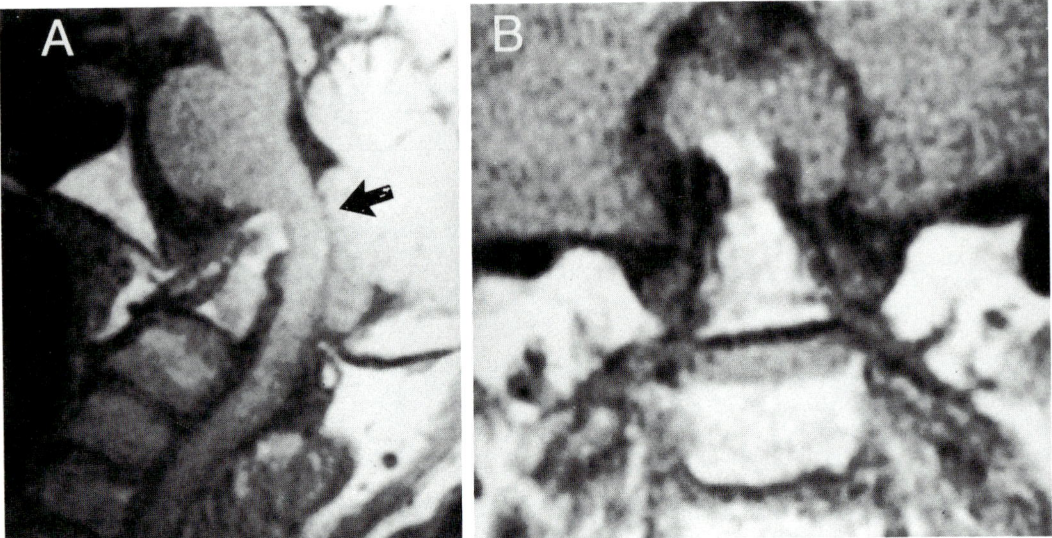

FIG 6–12.
Rheumatoid arthritis. **A,** there is severe upward translocation of a severely eroded dens, which compresses and kinks the pontomedullary junction *(arrow).* **B,** coronal T_1-weighted image shows the severely eroded dens outlined by pons superiorly.

years), and has an insidious onset (from months to years).[32,33] Also to be included in the differential diagnosis are other unusual infections such as actinomycosis, which can also spread in a subligamentous route, and hydatid disease, which can produce vertebral body destruction and a paraspinal mass. Type I vertebral body changes should also be considered, since both type I changes and spinal TB can show increased signal intensity from adjacent vertebral bodies, and a narrowed disk space without increased signal on T_2-weighted images.

RHEUMATOID ARTHRITIS

Rheumatoid arthritis is a disease that produces synovial inflammation and hyperemia with resultant destruction of the cartilage and subchondral bone by the pannus. Laxity of joint capsules and ligaments can result in a variety of deformities, subluxation, dislocation, fractures, and bony sclerosis. Sixty percent to 70% of rheumatoid patients develop symptoms related to the cervical spine disease during the course of their illness.

Five types of subluxations may occur at the atlantoaxial joint in rheumatoid arthritis:

1. Anterior atlantoaxial subluxation
2. Upward translocation of the dens
3. Lateral subluxation of the lateral masses of C1
4. Inferior subluxation of C1
5. Posterior atlantoaxial subluxation (associated with an eroded odontoid)

All of these subluxations appear to relate to seropositivity, duration of disease, steroid treatment, and the presence of rheumatoid nodules.[35,36]

While extensive upward translocation can be fatal, the intimate relationship of the dens and the CMJ is not necessarily more clinically important than anterior atlantoaxial subluxation.[37] Perhaps the abdundant pannus and erosion of the odontoid tip serve as a buffer against the cervicomedullary junction compression.

Bundschuh et al.[38] studied 15 patients with rheumatoid arthritis and compared MR images to plain films and tomography for defining subluxations and erosions (Figs 6–12 and 6–13). All patients with MR-derived cervicomedullary angles less than 135 degrees had brain stem compression, myelopathy, or C2 root pain. Surface coil T_1-weighted MR was as accurate as tomography in evaluating atlantodental interval (ADI), dens erosion, osteophytes, and the various C1–2 subluxations and subaxial subluxations. Magnetic resonance was not as efficient in evaluating basion-dental interval (BDI), apophyseal disease, and cystic changes of the C1–2 facets. In 70% of the cases, the dental opacity correlated well with the MR appearance, e.g., the sclerotic regions of the dens appeared dark and the osteopenic regions bright on T_1-weighted images. Pannus was most commonly found in a retrodental location as an increased amount of intermediate soft tissue material. Loss of a normal supraden-

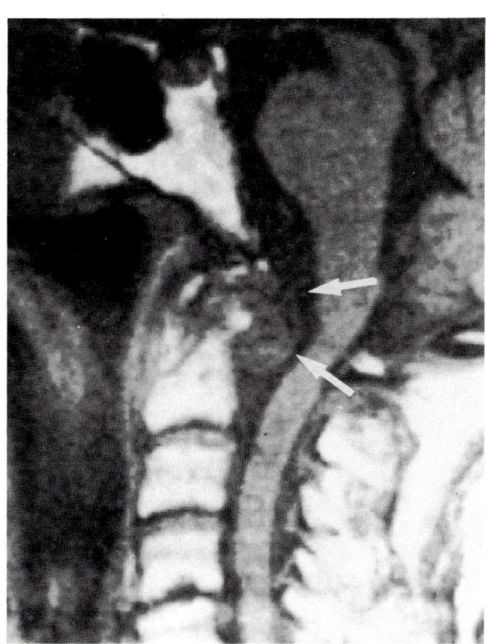

FIG 6–13.
Rheumatoid arthritis. A large mass of pannus *(arrows)* erodes the odontoid and extends posteriorly to encroach upon the cervicomedullary junction.

tal fat pad implies the presence of thickened ligaments or pannus. When brain stem symptoms are present, MR will consistently show marked craniovertebral junction (CVJ) abnormalities.[39]

REFERENCES

1. Burton CV, Kirkaldy-Willis WH, Yong-Hing K, et al: Causes of failure or surgery on the lumbar spine. *Clin Orthop* 1981; 157:191–199.
2. Smolik E, Nash F: Lumbar spinal arachnoiditis: A complication of the intervertebral disc operation. *Ann Surg* 1951; 133:490–495.
3. Jorgensen J, Hansen PH, Steenskrov V, et al: A clinical and radiological study of chronic lower spinal arachnoiditis. *Neuroradiology* 1975; 9:139–144.
4. Smith RW, Loesser JD: A myelographic variant in lumbar arachnoiditis. *J Neurosurg* 1972; 36:441–446.
5. Simmons JD, Newton TH: Arachnoiditis, in Newton TH, Potts DG (eds): *Computed Tomography of the Spine and Spinal Cord.* Calif, Clavadel Press, 1983, p 224.
6. Quencer RM, Tenner M, Rothman L: The postoperative myelogram. *Radiology* 1977; 123:667–679.
7. Reicher MA, Gold RH, Halboch VV, et al: MR imaging of the lumbar spine: Anatomic correlations and the effects of technical variations. *AJR* 1986; 147:891–898.
8. Ross JS, Masaryk TJ, Modic MT, et al: MR imaging of lumbar arachnoiditis. *AJNR* 1987; 8:885–892.
9. Mark AS, Andrews B, Sanches J, et al: MR imaging of Syringomyelia secondary to arachnoid adhesions, presented at the 73rd annual meeting of the Radiological Society of North America, Chicago, Nov 29–Dec 4, 1987.
10. Quiles M, Marchisello PJ, Tsairis P: Lumbar adhesive arachnoiditis, etiologic and pathologic aspects. *Spine* 1978; 3:45–50.
11. Braun IF, Malko JA, Davis PC, et al: The behavior of Pantopaque on MR: In vivo and in vitro analyses. *AJNR* 1986; 7:997–1001.
12. Marnourian AC, Briggs RW: Appearance of Pantopaque on MR Images. *Radiology* 1986; 158:457–460.
13. McHenry MC, Weinstein AJ: Lumbar vertebral osteomyelitis, in Hardy RW (ed): *Lumbar Disc Disease.* New York, Raven Press, 1982, pp 229–254.
14. Lisbona R, Rosenthal L: Observations on the sequential use of Tc-99m phosphate complex and Ga-67 imaging in osteomyelitis, cellulitis, and septic arthritis. *Radiology* 1977; 123:123–129.
15. Gelman MI, Coleman RE, Stevens PM, et al: Radiography radionuclide imaging and arthrography in the evaluation of total hip and knee replacement. *Radiology* 1978; 128:677–682.
16. Weiss PE, Mall JC, Hoffer PB, et al: Tc-99m methylene diphosphonate bone imaging in the evaluation of total hip prosthesis. *Radiology* 1979; 133:727–729.
17. Rosenthal L, Lisbona R, Hernandez M, et al: Tc-99m PP and Ga-67 imaging following insertion of orthopedic devices. *Radiology* 1979; 133:717–721.
18. McAfee JG, Samin A: In-111 labeled leukocytes: A review of problems in image interpretation. *Radiology* 1985; 155:221–229.
19. Golimbu C, Firooznia H, Rafii M: CT of osteomyelitis of the spine. *AJR* 1984; 142:159–163.
20. Jeffrey RB, Callen PW, Federle MP: Computed tomography of psoas abscesses. *J Comput Assist Tomogr* 1980; 4:639–641.
21. Modic MT, Feiglin DH, Piraino DW, et al: Vertebral osteomyelitis: Assessment using MR. *Radiology* 1985; 157–166.
22. Modic MT, Weinstein MA, Pavlicek W, et al: Nuclear magnetic resonance imaging of the spine. *Radiology* 1983; 148:757–762.
23. Aguila LA, Piraino DW, Modic MT: Magnetic resonance imaging of the intranuclear cleft. *Radiology* 1985; 155:155–158.
24. deRoos A, VanMeerten EL, Bloem JL, et al: MRI of tuberculosis spondylitis. *AJR* 1986; 146:79–82.
25. Fletcher BD, Scoles PV, Nelson AD: Osteomyelitis in children: Detection by magnetic resonance. *Radiology* 1984; 150:57–60.
26. Kahn DS, Pritzker KPH: The pathophysiology of bone infection. *Clin Orthop* 1973; 96:12–20.
27. Angtuaco EJC, McConnell JR, Chadduck WM, et al: MR Imaging of spinal epidural sepsis. *AJNR* 1987; 8:879–883.
28. Norman A, Kambolis CP: Tumors of the spine and their relationship to the intervertebral disc. *AJR* 1964; 92:1270–1274.
29. Resnick D, Niwayama G: Intervertebral disc abnormalities associated with vertebral metastases: Observations in pa-

tients and cadavers with prostatic cancer. *Invest Radiol* 1978; 13:182–190.

30. Modic MT, Steinberg PM, Ross JS, et al: Degenerative disk disease: Assessment of changes in vertebral body marrow with MR imaging. *Radiology* 1987; 166:193–199.
31. Masaryk TJ, Modic MT, Boumphrey F, et al: The effects of chemonucleolysis demonstrated by magnetic resonance imaging. *J Comp Assist Tomog* 1986; 10:917–923.
32. Smith AS, Weinstein MA, Mizushima A, et al: Tuberculous spondylitis: A contradiction to the MR characteristics of vertebral osteomyelitis. *AJNR*, in press.
33. Weaver P, Lifeso RM: The radiological diagnosis of tuberculosis of the adult spine. *Skeletal Radiol* 1984; 12:178–186.
34. Chapman M, Murray RO, Stoker DJ: Tuberculosis of the bones and joints. *Semin Roentgenol* 1979; 14:266–282.
35. Laasonen EM, Kankaanpaaa U, Pauku P: Computed tomographic myelography in atlanto-axial rheumatoid arthritis. *Neuroradiology* 1985; 27:119–122.
36. Winfield J, Cooke D, Brook AS, et al: A prospective study of the radiological changes in the cervical spine in early rheumatoid disease. *Ann Rheum Dis* 1981; 40:109–114.
37. Rana NA: Upward translocation of the dens in rheumatoid arthritis. *J Bone Joint Surg Br* 1973; 55B:471–477.
38. Bundschuh CV, Modic MT, Kearny F, et al: Rheumatoid arthritis of the cervical spine: Surface-coil MR imaging. *AJNR* 1988; 9:565–571.
39. Beltran J, Caudill JL, Herman LA, et al: Rheumatoid arthritis: MR imaging manifestations. *Radiology* 1987; 165:153–157.

7

Spine Tumors

Thomas J. Masaryk, M.D.

The crux of the diagnostic imaging evaluation of spine tumors lies with their physical location with respect to the neural axis. In conjunction with such information as age and past medical history, tumor location often enables the radiologist to predict a brief differential diagnosis and thus the mode of therapy and prognosis with a reasonable degree of confidence. Myelography has long been the diagnostic mainstay in the evaluation of spinal neoplasms by providing an indirect image of the spinal cord and nerve roots from the foramen magnum to the sacrum. Visualization of the negative shadow margins of the cord and its coverings as well as direct assessment of the integrity of the bony canal frequently enabled radiologists to predict the location of mass lesions as intramedullary, extramedullary intradural, and extramedullary extradural.[1] In addition, use of water-soluble intrathecal contrast material in conjunction with high-resolution computed tomography (CT) provided a second imaging plane to define the suspected location and thus increase the specificity of the radiographic workup.[2–4]

Magnetic resonance imaging (MRI) combines the best of both modalities with few (if any) of the disadvantages. Many early reports documenting the utility of MRI in the spine commented on its ability to image the spinal cord in multiple planes and thus accurately pinpoint neoplastic disease.[5–14] Additionally, MRI not only characterizes lesions based on morphology and location with respect to the cord, but also according to signal-intensity characteristics that reflect tissue T_1, T_2, and spin-density as well as paramagnetic or chemical-shift effects and motion. The subsequent implementation of surface coil technology, cardiac gating, gradient refocussing, and paramagnetic contrast agents has done much to improve the visualization of the spinal cord and surrounding tissues, as well as to increase sensitivity and specificity to disease.[15–28] The most recent innovations in pulse-sequence design such as saturation pulses and gradient echo volume imaging are likely to further refine the utility of MR imaging of spine neoplasms.[29,30]

EPIDEMIOLOGY

Tumors of the spinal cord and its coverings are fortunately rare; their frequency varies among different clinical series depending on histologic classification and whether masses related to congenital defects, vascular anomalies, and spinal extension of intracranial tumors and extraspinal metastases have been excluded. The annual incidence of primary spine neoplasms has been estimated at 2.5/100,000 population per year.[31] There is no significant sex difference for the development of spine neoplasia.[32]

In a review of numerous series, Nittner[33] suggested that approximately 1/5 of all central nervous system tumors occur in the spine.[33] The frequency at various levels of the spinal canal (cervical, thoracic, lumbar) is roughly proportional to the number (and length) of segments at that level.[34] Only 1% of primary spinal cord tumors involve multiple, separate levels—a finding that should suggest the possibility of neurofibromatosis.[35,36] In his 1976 review of 4,885 adult spinal cord tumors presented in the literature, Nittner[33] found neurilemomas (schwannomas) (23%), meningiomas (22%), glial (intramedullary) tumors (13.2%) and (extramedullary) ependymoma (2.5%), sarcoma (8.2%), and metastases (6.0%) most common. The remaining 25% of cases were dispersed among a wide variety of miscellaneous mass lesions. Pain is a significant presenting complaint among adults with spine tumors.[34]

Differences exist among series detailing spine neoplasms found in adults when compared to those dealing with children. As might be expected, lipomas, dermoids, and other embryonal tumors are more common earlier in life, increasing the percentage of lesions found in the lumbosacral region among pediatric patients.[37,38] In addition to developmental lesions, intramedullary (gliomas) and extradural (sarcomas) tumors occur more commonly in children, while intradural extramedullary masses (schwannomas, meningiomas) are uncommon.[39,40] Clinical presentation likewise differs from adults, with a preponderance of motor findings (gait disturbance, sphincter dysfunction) possibly related to the inability of very young patients to articulate their symptoms.[41]

INTRAMEDULLARY NEOPLASMS

Gliomas

The most common intramedullary neoplasms are the gliomas: ependymoma, astrocytoma (grades 1–4),

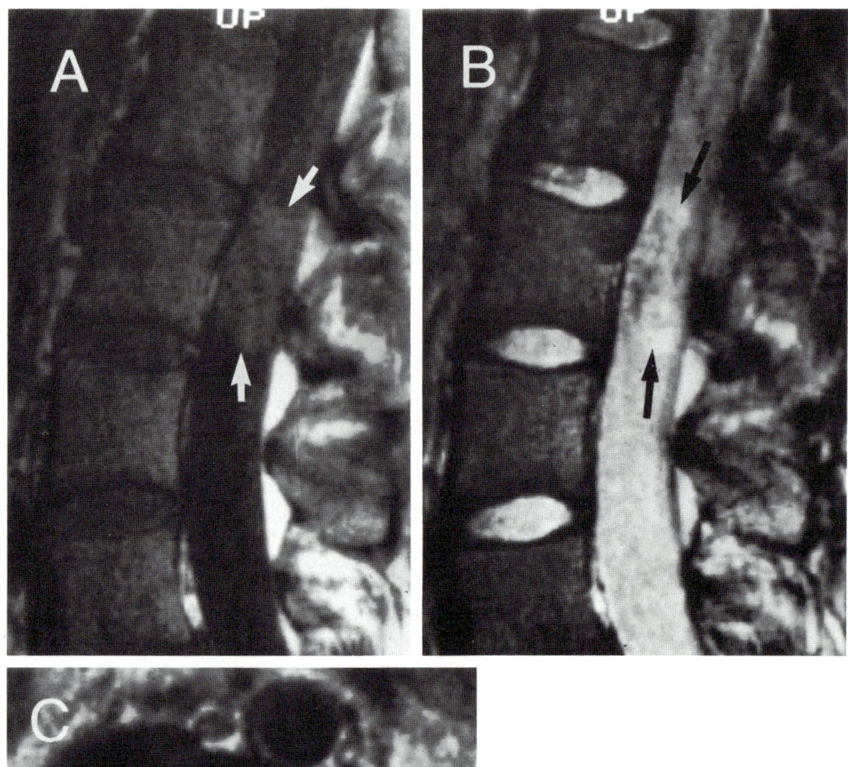

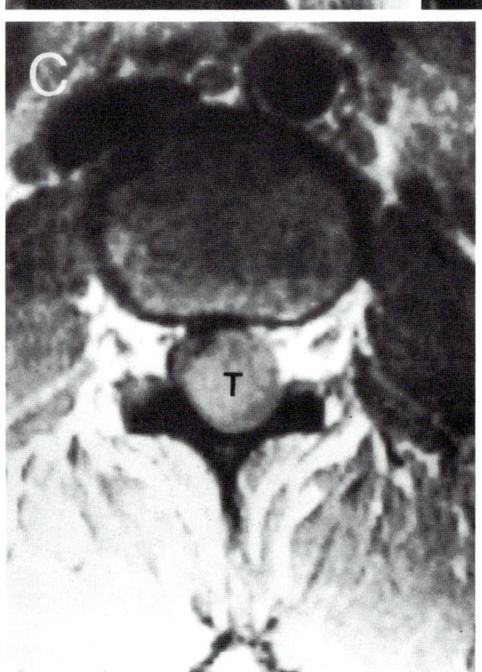

FIG 7–1.
A, 500-msec TR/17-msec TE midline sagittal image of the lumbar spine demonstrates a rounded, globular soft tissue mass present near the conus medullaris *(arrows)* of approximately the same signal intensity as the spinal cord. **B,** 2,000-msec TR/90-msec TE sagittal midline image of the lumbar spine again demonstrates a globular soft tissue mass *(arrows)*, now of increased signal intensity at the conus medullaris. **C,** axial T_1-weighted image confirms tumor mass (T) within the canal. Surgery confirmed the presence of an ependymoma of the conus medullaris.

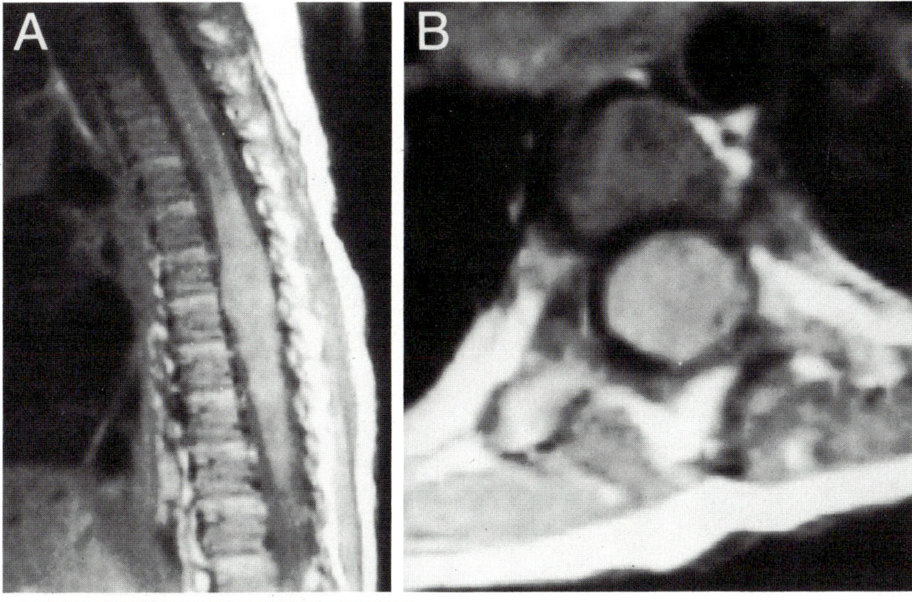

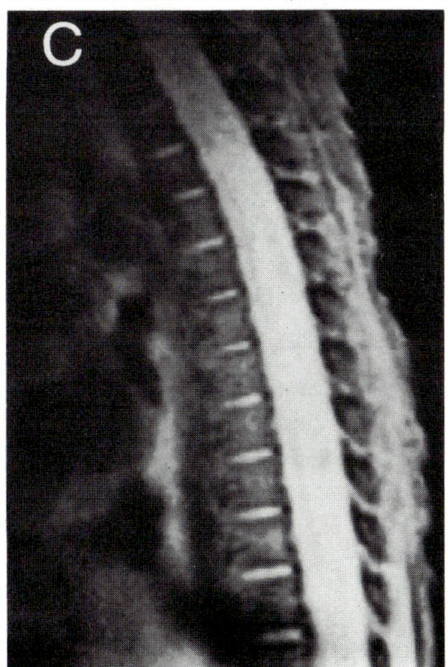

FIG 7–2.
A, 500-msec TR/17-msec TE midline sagittal slice of the thoracic spine in this child demonstrates marked fusiform enlargement of the thoracic spinal cord. **B,** 500-msec TR/17-msec TE axial image confirms the enlargement of the thoracic spinal cord. **C,** 2000-msec TR/90-msec TE midline sagittal T_2-weighted image (nonrefocussed) of the thoracic spinal cord demonstrates homogeneously increased signal intensity of the cord and the surrounding CSF that masks the previously noted thoracic spinal cord mass lesion. Surgery confirmed the presence of a thoracic astrocytoma.

oligodendroglioma, and medulloblastoma. Astrocytomas and ependymomas comprise the overwhelming majority of these lesions. Ependymomas are often cited as the most frequent in adults (65%), particularly at the conus medullaris and filum terminale.[34, 35, 42] Conversely, astrocytomas appear to dominate the pediatric population (59%), occasionally presenting as massive lesions involving the entire length of the spinal cord.[43, 44]

Ependymomas may involve any portion of the spinal cord, including the conus and filum terminale. Thus, they may appear as a fusiform enlargement of the spinal cord itself or as a lobulated extramedullary mass involving the filum terminale and cauda equina (Fig 7–1). Ependymomas are often amenable to surgical removable both within the cord and at the filum.[45] Prognosis following surgery and radiation therapy can be quite good.[45, 46]

Astrocytomas likewise appear as soft tissue masses within the substance of the spinal cord producing a focal enlargement; however, unlike ependymomas, there is rarely a surgically identifiable cleavage plane between the tumor and cord substance (Figs 7–2 and 7–3).[45] This fact, coupled with the relative resistance of this neoplasm to radiotherapy, accounts for the poor prognosis associated with these lesions.[45, 46]

Magnetic resonance imaging findings for all types of

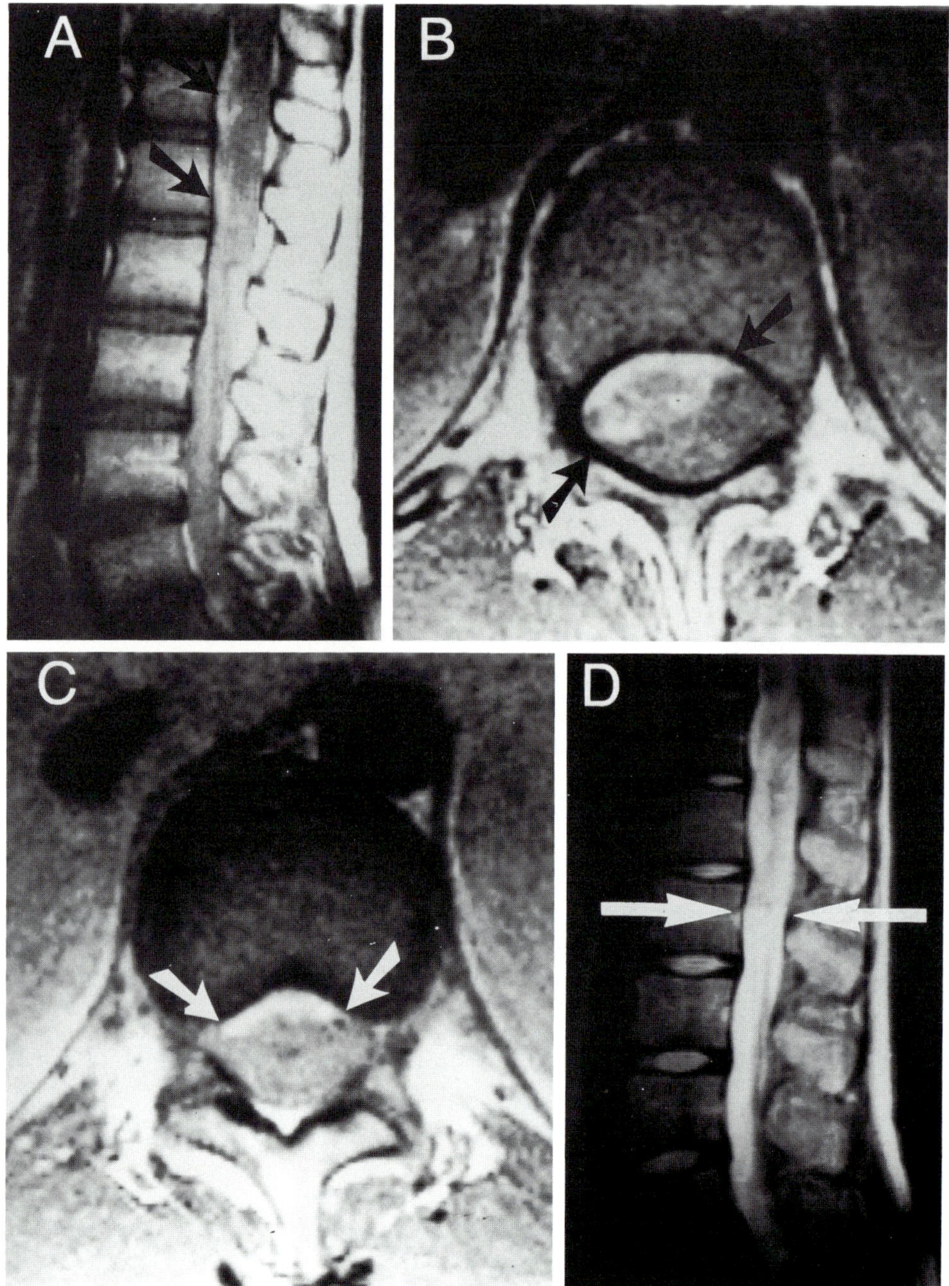

FIG 7–3.
A, 500-msec TR/17-msec TE midline sagittal image of the thoracolumbar junction demonstrates heterogeneous soft tissue signal in the region of the conus medullaris *(arrows)* but no obvious soft tissue mass. Also note, that the spinal cord itself is poorly visualized at this level. **B** and **C,** 500-msec TR/17-msec TE axial images through the thoracolumbar junction again demonstrate heterogeneous areas of signal intensity within the spinal canal *(arrows)* without a discernible spinal cord itself. Note the enlargement of the spinal canal in image **B. D,** 2,000-msec TR/90-msec TE midline sagittal image of the thoracolumbar junction demonstrates diffuse soft tissue enlargement of the conus medullaris. The CSF space below the level of the conus is completely blocked by the mass as evidenced by its high signal intensity and lack of CSF pulsation artifact in the phasing-encode direction *(arrows).*

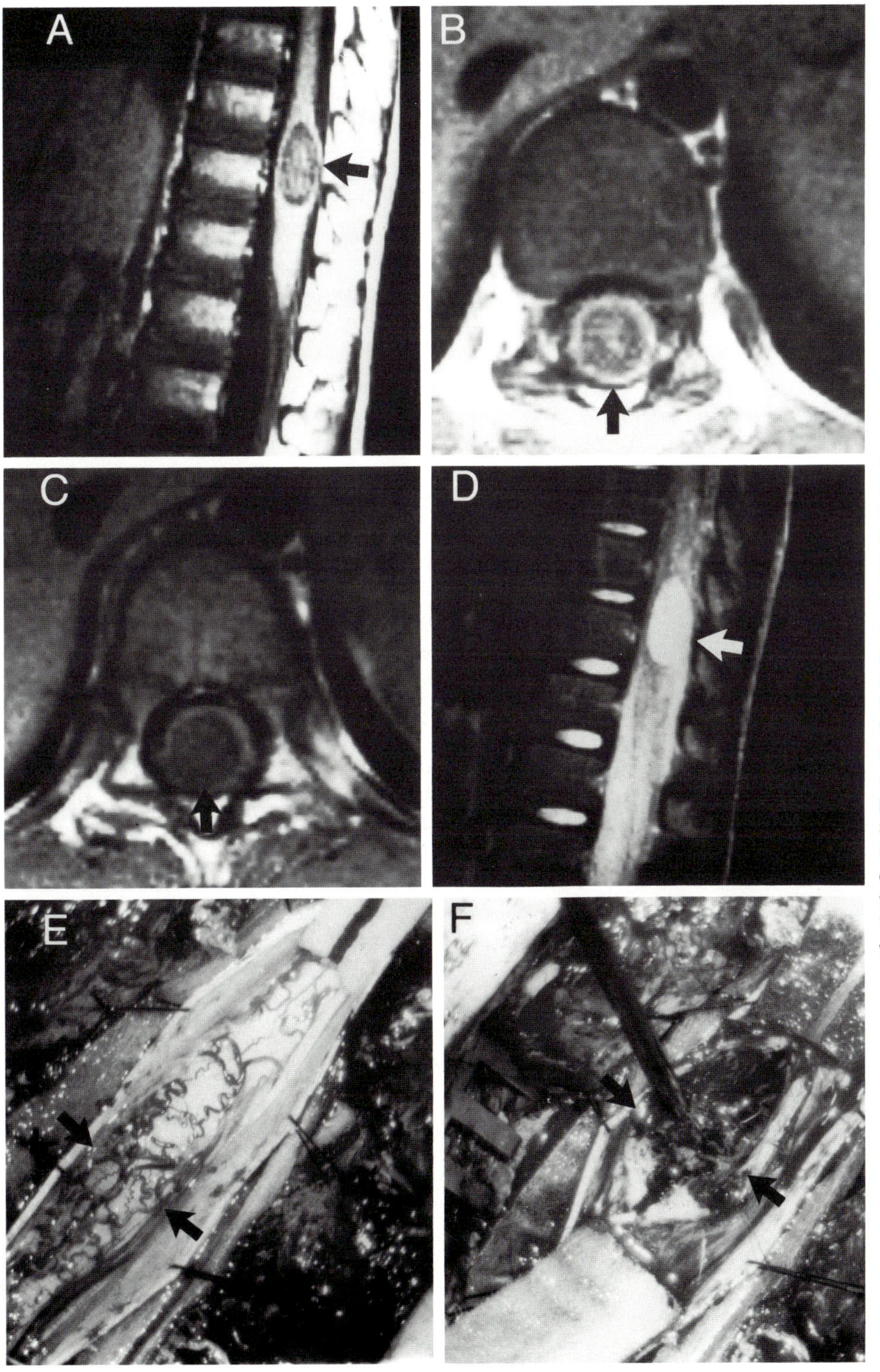

FIG 7–4.
A, 500-msec TR/17-msec TE midline sagittal image through the distal spinal cord demonstrates an intramedullary cystic mass lesion *(arrow)* in this young boy who presented only with paresthesia in one thigh. **B** and **C,** 500-msec TR/17-msec TE axial images through the level of the lesion again demonstrate its cystic nature *(arrows).* **D,** 2,000-msec TR/120-msec TE midline sagittal image through the level of the cystic mass of the conus again demonstrates high signal intensity emanating from the cyst *(arrow).* **E,** intraoperative photographs demonstrate diffuse swelling of the distal spinal cord with multiple enlarged vessels *(arrows)* overlying it. **F,** when the spinal cord was opened, a blood-filled "intratumoral cyst" *(arrows)* was found within this astrocytoma.

intramedullary gliomas are similar. T_1-weighted sagittal examination typically demonstrate fusiform enlargement of the spinal cord over one or several segments by a soft tissue mass of normal or slightly decreased signal intensity (see Figs 7–1 through 7–3). T_2-weighted sagittal and axial studies demonstrate focal areas of increased signal within the enlarged cord segment that represent neoplastic and edematous cord tissue (see Figs 7–1 through 7–3). The use of cardiac gating, even echo rephasing, or additional refocussing gradients during the acquisition of these T_2-weighted images will improve the visualization of these intramedullary signal derangements.

The MR appearance of intramedullary gliomas may vary from the above description with the presence of intramedullary cysts or cavitations. In the series of Sloof et al., 38% of astrocytomas and 46% of ependymomas demonstrated "syringomyelic" cavities at autopsy.[34] Cysts located rostral or caudal to the tumor are typically non-neoplastic with gliotic linings and filled with fluid similar to cerebrospinal fluid (CSF), while those within neoplastic masses are lined by abnormal glia and are xanthochromic or blood filled.[44] In an effort to avoid confusion between benign syringomyelia, Gay et al.[47] defined the rostral and caudal cavities as "tumor cysts" and those central areas of neoplastic cavitation as "intratumoral cysts"[47] (Fig 7–4). Reports of the accuracy of MR in demonstrating such cysts (long T_1, long T_2) vary depending on pulse sequence used and the presence of protein within the cysts that may alter relaxation times of the cyst fluid.[47–49] Also, in the case of large intratumoral cysts without an obvious soft tissue mass one may have difficulty distinguishing a neoplastic lesion from a benign syrinx cavity.[49] Morphologically, the presence of distinct margins with a sharp, smooth interface with cyst fluid that is isointense with CSF favors a diagnosis of benign syrinx.[49]

It must also be noted that motion effects on signal intensity within the syringomyelic or tumor cysts may help distinguish them from necrotic intratumoral cysts. It is postulated that derangements of intracranial and spinal venous and CSF pressure produce dissecting CSF shifts that result in and extend these cavities.[50,51] This motion within these non-neoplastic, glial-lined syringomyelic and tumor cysts can be recognized by the presence of CSF flow void signal loss on nonrefocussed, asymmetric echo, T_2-weighted scans.[52,53] Conversely, intratumoral cysts resulting from necrotic cavitation usually will not possess this fluid motion and thus have higher (than CSF) signal intensity on such T_2-weighted sequences.

Paramagnetic contrast has also been used with some success to accurately locate intramedullary mass lesions within the spinal cord on T_1-weighted images, separating tumor from surrounding edema or cystic cavitations.[26] Whether intravenous contrast enhancement will aid in the differentiation of benign, gliotic line cysts from areas of neoplastic cavitation remains to be seen.

Hemangioblastomas

Hemangioblastomas are uncommon. Frequent confusion with vascular malformations and other vascular tumors, as well as lack of uniformity in classification, make assessment of their incidence relative to other spine tumors difficult. In the review of Sloof of 1,322 primary tumors of the spinal canal, there were 300 intramedullary lesions, only four of which were hemangioblastomas.[34] These tumors have a predilection for the cervicothoracic and thoracolumbar regions, and while they can occur as isolated masses, they are often multiple and seen in association with posterior fossa hemangioblastomas as part of the von Hippel-Lindau syndrome.[54] This autosomal dominant congenital complex features hemangioblastomas of the posterior fossa and spinal neural axis; retinal angiomata; cysts or cyst adenoma of the pancreas, adrenals, kidneys and ovaries; and renal cell carcinoma.[54,55]

Hemangioblastomas are histologically similar to angioblastic meningiomas and apparently arise as small nodules from the pia.[55] They often present as intramedullary cysts containing a vascular nodule. Like the gliomas, these lesions may also produce syringomyelic tumor cysts or (characteristically) cord enlargement secondary to edema.[56,57] Magnetic resonance imaging is particularly suited to the evaluation of these lesions because of its superior ability to image not only the spinal cord, but also the posterior fossa structures. Additionally, because of their vascularity, they enhance vigorously with paramagnetic contrast material (Fig 7–5).

Embryonal Tumors

Lipomas, dermoids, and epidermoids may present as primary intramedullary mass lesions at any level of the spine[58–60] (Fig 7–6). However, they are most frequently recognized as intradural, intramedullary lesions at or near the conus medullaris in conjunction with dysraphic complexes. Regardless, they are congenital tumors arising from the implantation of embryonic rests during the closure of the neural tube between the sixth and eighth week of intrauterine life. Lipomas are characterized by their high signal intensity on T_1-weighted images that are less intense with more T_2 weighting.[7,61] Central nervous system (CNS) dermoids and epidermoids display a variety of noncharacteristic signal-inten-

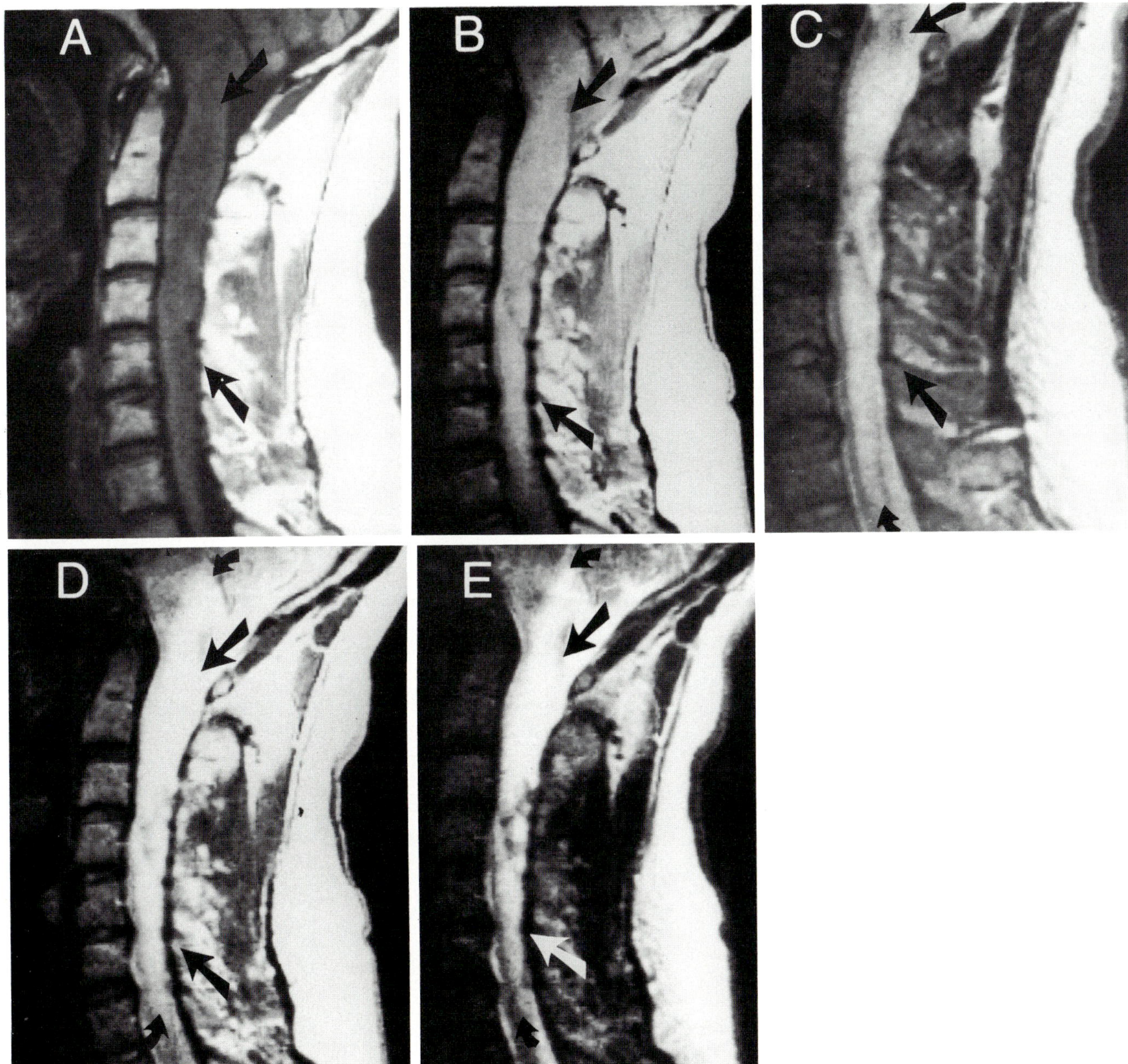

FIG 7–5.
A middle-aged college professor presented with signs and symptoms suggesting cervical myelopathy. Initial MR examination (**A–E**) suggested an intramedullary cervical tumor. **A,** 500-msec TR/17-msec TE midline sagittal image demonstrates diffuse enlargement of the upper cervical spinal cord *(arrows).* **B–E,** 2000-msec TR/30–60–90–120-msec TEs, respectively, demonstrate spinal cord enlargement *(slanted arrows)* with increased signal intensity within the mass lesion and high signal intensity edema extending above and below the mass *(small curved arrows). (Continued)*

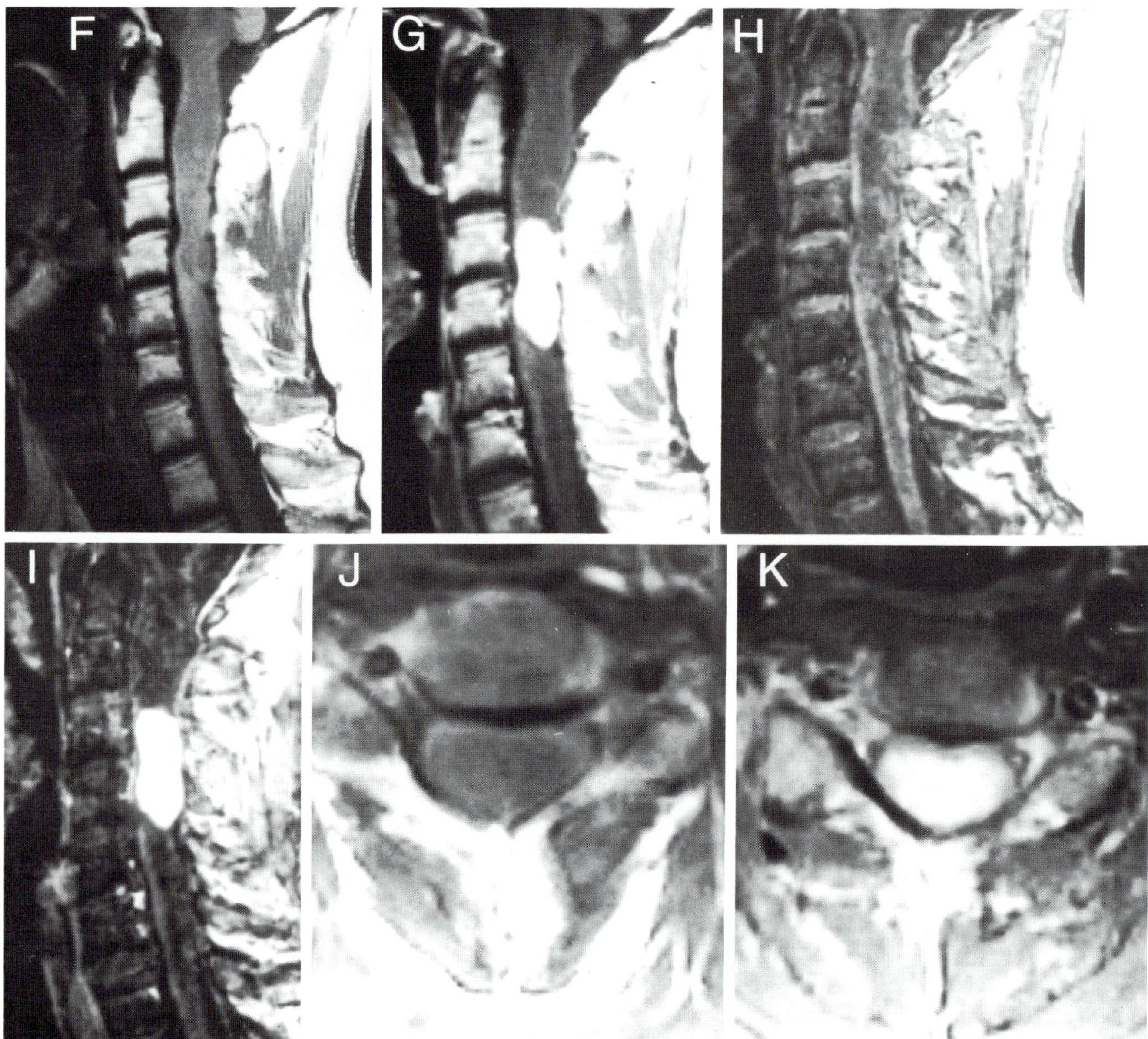

FIG 7–5 (cont.).

Follow-up examination over 1 year after the initial onset of symptoms (F–K) was performed with and without intravenous Gd-DTPA. **F,** midline sagittal 500-msec TR/17-msec TE image of the cervical spinal cord again demonstrates diffuse enlargement, suggesting extensive involvement of the upper cervical spinal cord. However, following the administration of Gd-DTPA (**G**), the actual tumor nidus is seen to be confined to a small, focal area of increased signal intensity representing enhancement at the C3–4 levels only. **H** and **I,** Gd-DTPA works equally well at demonstrating intramedullary lesions when gradient echo pulse sequences are used. These studies were performed using a fast low-angle shot (FLASH) 60-degree technique without (**H**) and with (**I**) Gd-DTPA. Axial 500-msec TR/17-msec TE scans without (**J**) and with (**K**) Gd-DTPA confirmed intramedullary location of the tumor nidus. Histologic studies were most consistent with a diagnosis of hemangioblastoma. Such diffuse cord enlargement with a focal nidus of tumor may commonly be seen with this tumor.

sity patterns on T_1- and T_2-weighted images between different lesions or within one tumor.[62,63] This may be related to the physical state (solid vs. liquid) and lipid content (cholesterol vs. fatty acid) of the cyst.

Metastases

Metastatic disease may also (rarely) present as an intramedullary mass lesion. Intracranial neoplasms such as medulloblastomas, ependymomas, and gliomas are known to spread via CSF seeding to the leptomeninges, which may lead to direct invasion of the spinal cord.[64–69] Primary tumors outside the CNS may spread to the cord hematogeneously.[70–73] Carcinoma of the lung and breast are most frequently identified, with melanoma, lymphoma, and adenocarcinoma also reported.[70–73] The thoracic spine is most frequently involved.[73] Also, while leptomeningeal disease may coexist with intramedullary foci, concomitant osseous metastatic implants are uncommon.[70–72] Like primary intramedullary tumors, metastatic lesions typically produce enlargement (best appreciated on T_1-weighted images) and signal-intensity alterations (low signal on T_1- and high signal on T_2-weighted images) of the cord[74] (Fig 7–7).

EXTRAMEDULLARY INTRADURAL MASS LESIONS

This category of primarily benign tumors comprises the largest single group of spinal mass lesions; meningiomas and nerve sheath tumors alone account for roughly half of all adult spine tumors.

Meningiomas

Meningiomas are unique in that there is a 4:1 female to male predominance, with most patients over 40 years of age.[33] Eighty percent of lesions can be found in the thoracic spine.[33] They are often located anterolaterally or posterolaterally in the canal as they are thought to arise in the region of the denticulate ligaments.[34,42] Meningiomas are also the most common tumor of the foramen magnum, where they are frequently located anteriorly or laterally.[33] Rarely, meningiomas are both intradural and extradural (6%) or purely extradural (7%).[33] Magnetic resonance evaluation of possible spinal meningiomas requires special attention to imaging technique. Because of the high frequency of meningiomas in the thoracic spine, care must be taken to reduce or eliminate ghosting artifact secondary to respiratory and cardiac motion that commonly plagues this region. Possible solutions include switching direction of the phase- and frequency-encode axes, cardiac and respiratory gating, refocussed or symmetric multiecho sequences, and saturation pulses. Additionally, one must be aware of the order of acquisition of images in the axial plane. Cerebrospinal fluid pulsations may produce entry-slice artifact on the initial superior-most image that may strongly resemble an intradural extramedullary soft tissue mass.

Like meningiomas of the cranial cavity, their appearance in the spinal canal can be variable. Sagittal and axial T_1-weighted images typically demonstrate a small soft tissue mass within the spinal canal that is isointense to the spinal cord and can be seen displacing it[26,27,75] (Figs 7–8 and 7–9). There may be widening of the adjacent neural foramen. T_2-weighted images most commonly depict the tumor as a low signal (isointense with spinal cord) intradural defect surrounded by high signal CSF (see Fig 7–8). However, personal experience has proved that this may not always be the case, as there have been instances in which signal from these lesions was relatively high on long repetition time (TR)/echo time (TE) images[25] (see Fig 7–9).

Nerve Sheath Tumors

Nerve sheath tumors appear under a variety of titles: schwannoma, neuroma, neurilemomas, perineurofibroblastoma, and neurofibroma. Classically, there are probably two types of tumors. Schwannomas are often solitary and composed solely of Schwann cells of peripheral sensory nerves, while neurofibromas are composed of both Schwann cells and fibroblasts and are almost universely seen in multiples with von Recklinghausen's neurofibromatosis.[42] These tumors are seen most commonly in adults between the ages of 20 and 50 years, with no predilection for either sex.[33] They may occur anywhere in the spine with the thoracic spine being most often implicated.[33] The majority of lesions are intradural extramedullary, 10% are intradural and extradural, while 11% are strictly extradural.[33]

Magnetic resonance imaging is particularly helpful in the diagnosis of these lesions by virtue of its ability to depict the extent of extradural disease. Like meningiomas, nerve sheath tumors appear as a soft tissue mass outlined by low signal CSF within the spinal canal on T_1-weighted images. Often, there is displacement of the spinal cord. More T_2-weighted images typically demonstrate these lesions as high signal masses outlined by lower signal spinal and paraspinal soft tissues[75–77] (Fig 7–10). These foci of high signal may possess a central area of lower signal intensity that may distinguish them from lateral meningoceles commonly found with neurofibromatosis.[76]

Alternatively, on intermediate scans (long TR/short

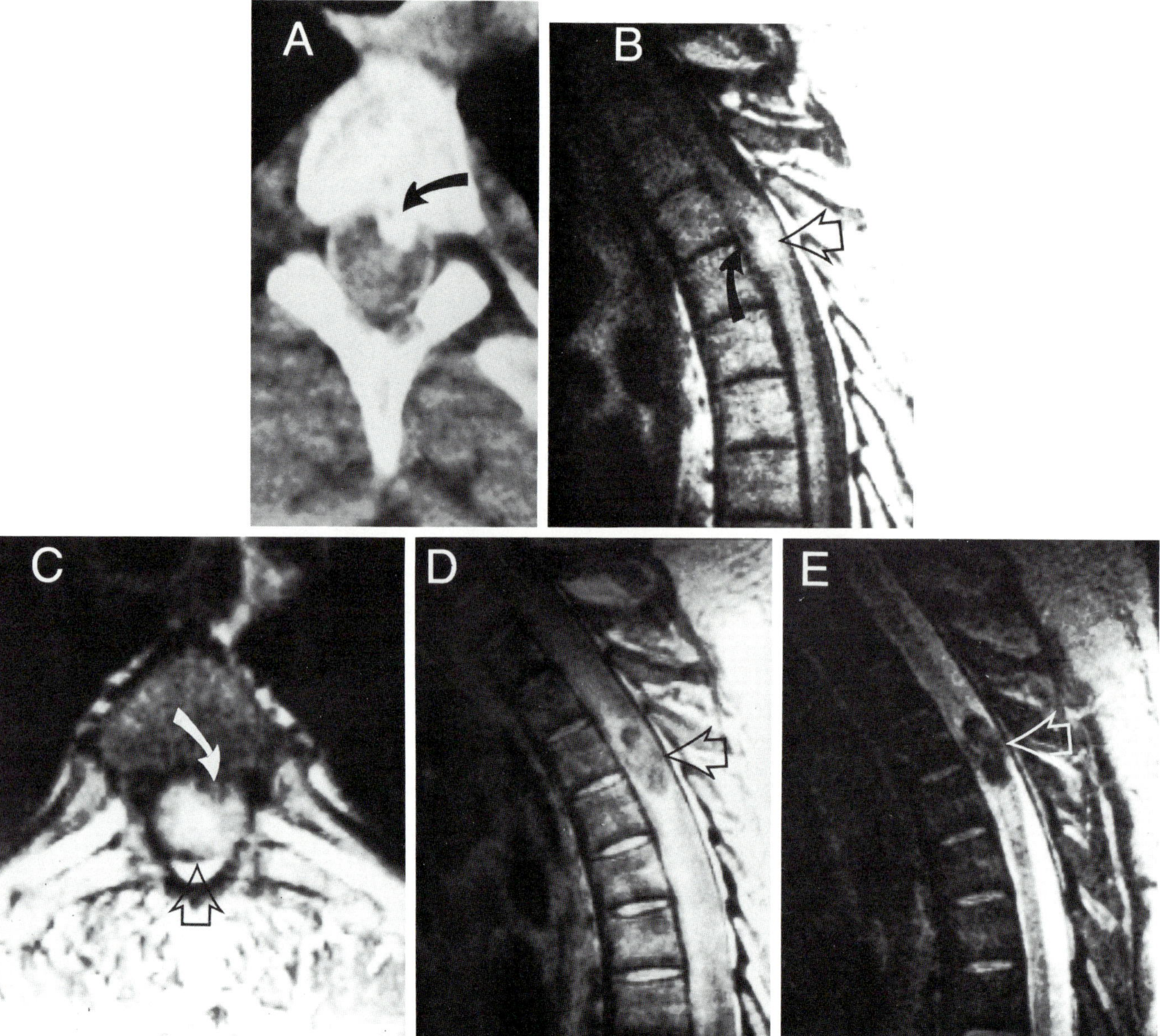

FIG 7–6.

A middle-aged man who presented with myelopathy at a thoracic sensory level was originally evaluated with myelography followed by high-resolution CT scan. **A,** an axial image from the CT scan at the level of the sensory deficit demonstrates enlargement of the thoracic spinal cord by a partially calcified mass *(arrow)* located anteriorly. **B,** subsequent MR study demonstrated focal intramedullary mass lesion on this 500-msec TR/17-msec TE sagittal scan. The mass is primarily of high signal intensity *(open arrow)* with a smaller, focal area of decreased signal intensity identified anteriorly, probably representing the calcification noted on the previous CT scan of the patient **C,** 500-msec TR/17-msec TE axial image through the level of the lesion again demonstrates an area of high signal intensity within the central portion of the thoracic spinal cord *(open arrow)* with a small, focal area of decreased signal intensity *(curved arrow)* in the region of the calcification. **D,** 2,000-msec TR/60-msec TE sagittal scan through the thoracic spine again demonstrates the intramedullary mass that now appears decreased in signal relative to the spinal cord *(open arrow).* **E,** 2,000-msec TR/120-msec TE midline sagittal image through the thoracic spinal cord demonstrates a focal, low signal enlargement of the spinal cord at the level of the mass lesion *(open arrow)* with a small amount of edema seen within the cord above and below the lesion. *(Continued)*

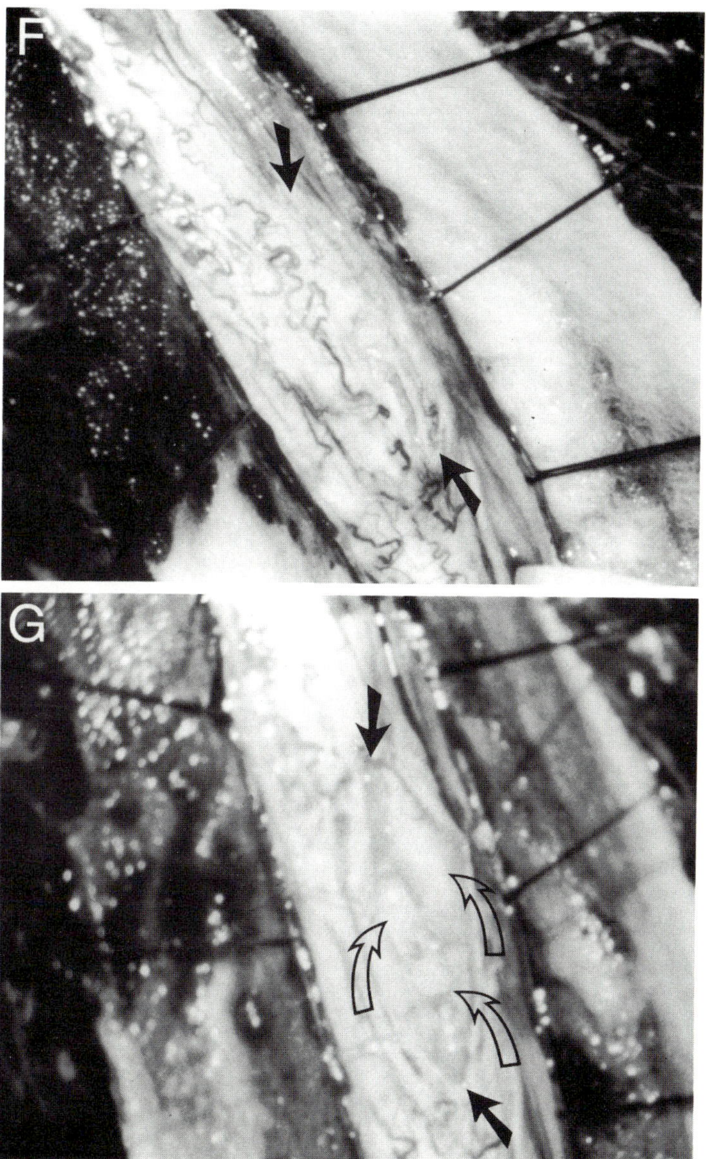

FIG 7-6 (cont.).
F and **G,** intraoperative photographs demonstrate focal enlargement of the thoracic spinal cord *(solid arrows)* that on myelotomy produced a white collection of material *(open arrows)* that histologically proved to be an intramedullary epidermoid.

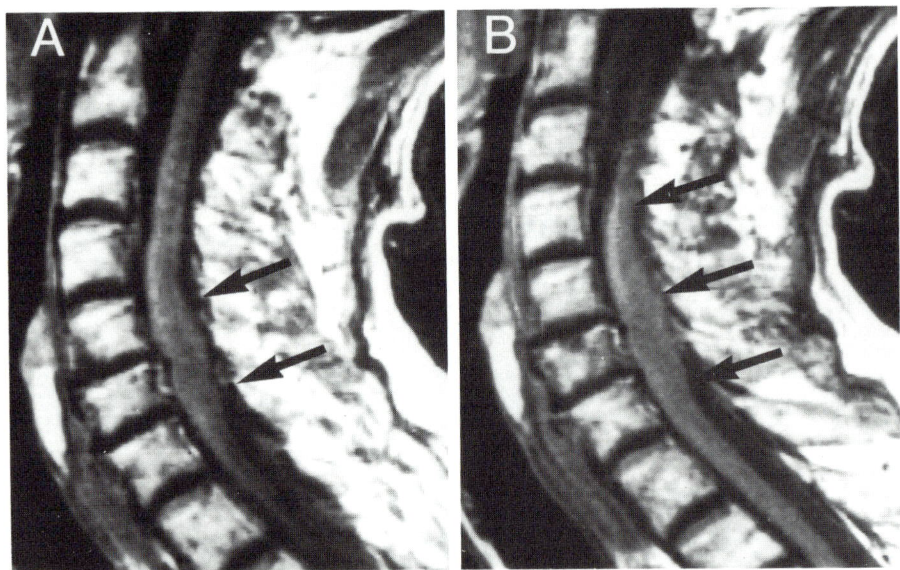

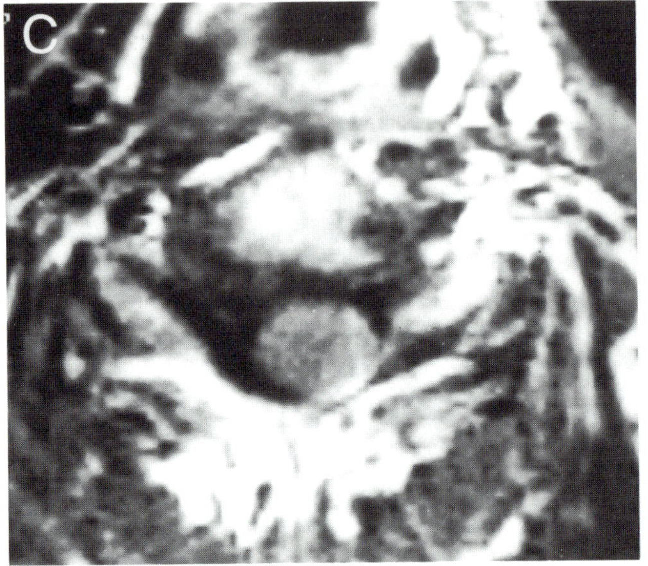

FIG 7–7.
A and **B,** 500-msec TR/17-msec TE sagittal images demonstrate focal enlargement of the cervical spinal cord in a patient with known metastatic carcinoma of the breast. **C,** 500-msec TR/17-msec TE axial image confirms the spinal cord enlargement representing an intramedullary metastatic focus.

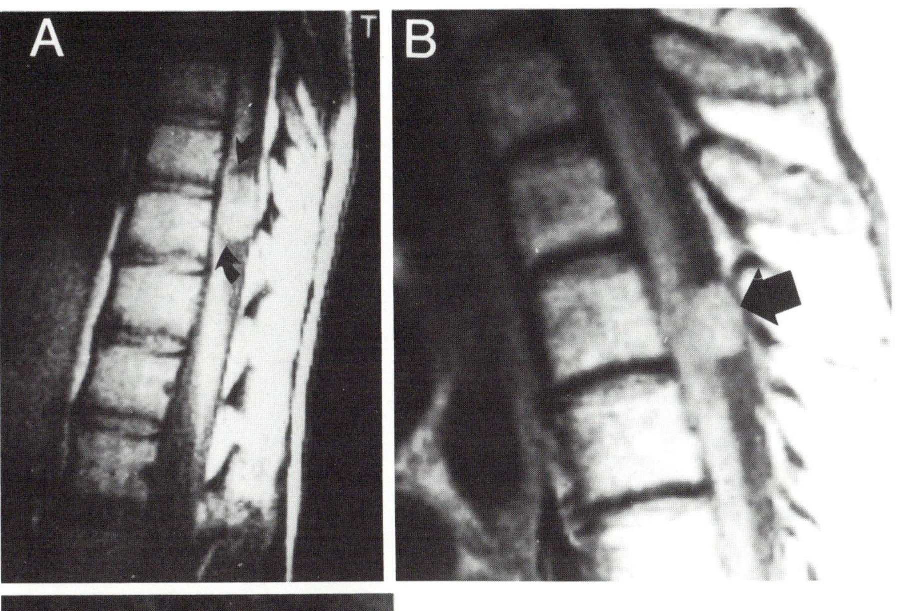

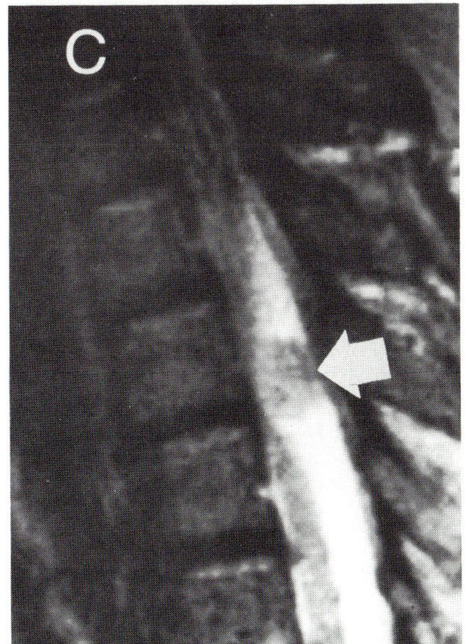

FIG 7–8.
500-msec TR/17-msec TE sagittal (**A**) and parasagittal (**B**) images through the thoracic spine demonstrate a soft tissue mass posterolateral to the thoracic spinal cord that is isointense in signal intensity with the spinal cord itself *(black arrows).* **C,** 2,000-msec TR/120-msec TE parasagittal scan through the region of the mass *(arrow)* again demonstrates it to be isointense with spinal cord (i.e., low signal intensity). The MR findings suggest a thoracic meningioma that was confirmed at the time of surgery.

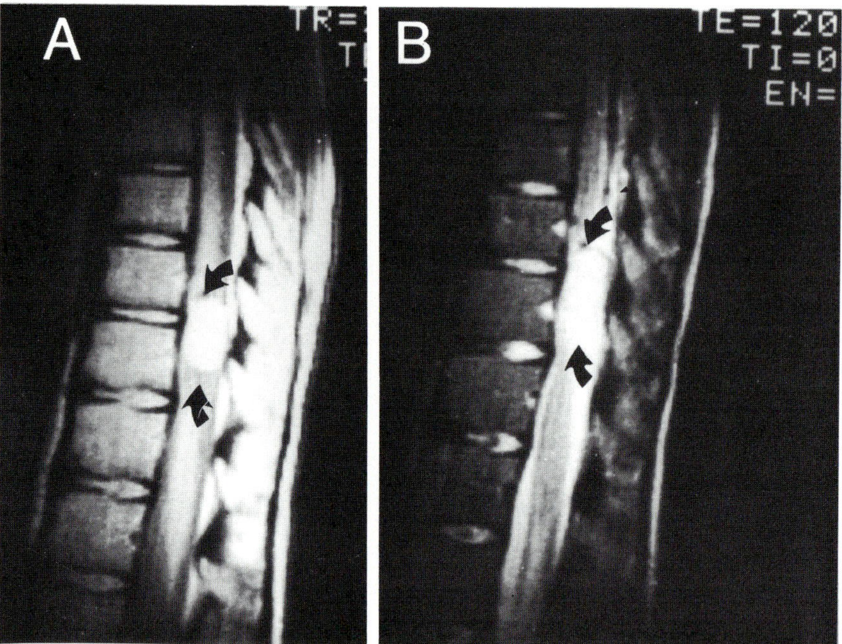

FIG 7–9.
A, 2,000-msec TR/30-msec TE parasagittal image of the thoracic spine demonstrates a soft tissue mass posterolateral to the spinal cord that is of approximately the same signal intensity as the cord itself *(arrows).* **B,** 2,000-msec TR/120-msec TE image through the region of the mass *(arrows)* demonstrates increase in signal of the mass relative to the spinal cord. On this image, the mass itself is obscured by the surrounding increased signal intensity of the spinal fluid. Surgery confirmed the presence of a meningioma.

TE), these masses will often have higher signal than CSF within the spinal canal, while meningoceles should remain isointense with CSF. Unfortunately, signal intensity characteristics in neurofibromas do not appear to be sensitive for the recognition of malignant degeneration.[77]

Two points concerning the MR imaging evaluation of both meningiomas and neuronomas are pertinent here. First, preliminary work indicates that intravenous paramagnetic contrast (gadolinium diethylenetriamine penta-acetic acid [DPTA]) significantly improves the conspicuity of these lesions on T_1-weighted images[25–27] (Figs 7–11 and 7–12). Secondly, cystic, syringomyelic cavities may occur locally in the spinal cord secondary to these lesions—a complication MR is ideally suited to detect.[78] Much like the tumoral cysts found with intramedullary lesions, CSF pulsations in regions of microcystic degeneration produced by the tumor may lead to enlarged cord cavities.[79]

Embryonal Tumors

The developmental tumors (epidermoids, dermoids, lipomas, and teratomas) have been previously discussed but are reintroduced to reinforce their association with lower spine dysraphic states or lumbar puncture and thus their frequent intradural extramedullary location.[58, 62, 80] Such tumors may be suggested by congenital cutaneous stigmata (subcutaneous lipoma, hairy patch, sacral dimple, or sinus tract and unusual pigmentation); however, these need not necessarily be present.[80, 81]

Lipomas possess the most characteristic MR appearance: high signal intensity, globular mass on T_1-weighted images (less intense on T_2) frequently in conjunction with a tethered cord or some form of lipomyelomeningocele[61] (Fig 7–13). It is noteworthy that fat may be present within the distal conus medullaris and filum terminale in normal subjects (5%). Thus it is likely that this represents a developmental spectrum, the significance of which lies with the level of the conus (normally L1-2 in adults) and the clinical history.

Epidermoids, dermoids, and teratomas have a variable appearance on MRI reflecting the variety of tissues comprising a single mass.[62, 63, 82] Epidermoids arise from heterotopic ectoderm, dermoids arise from embryonic rests of ectoderm and mesoderm, while teratomas are formed from all three germ layers. Liquid fat, solid keratin or cholesterol, fibrous tissue, muscle, or bone may be present within a single lesion.[82]

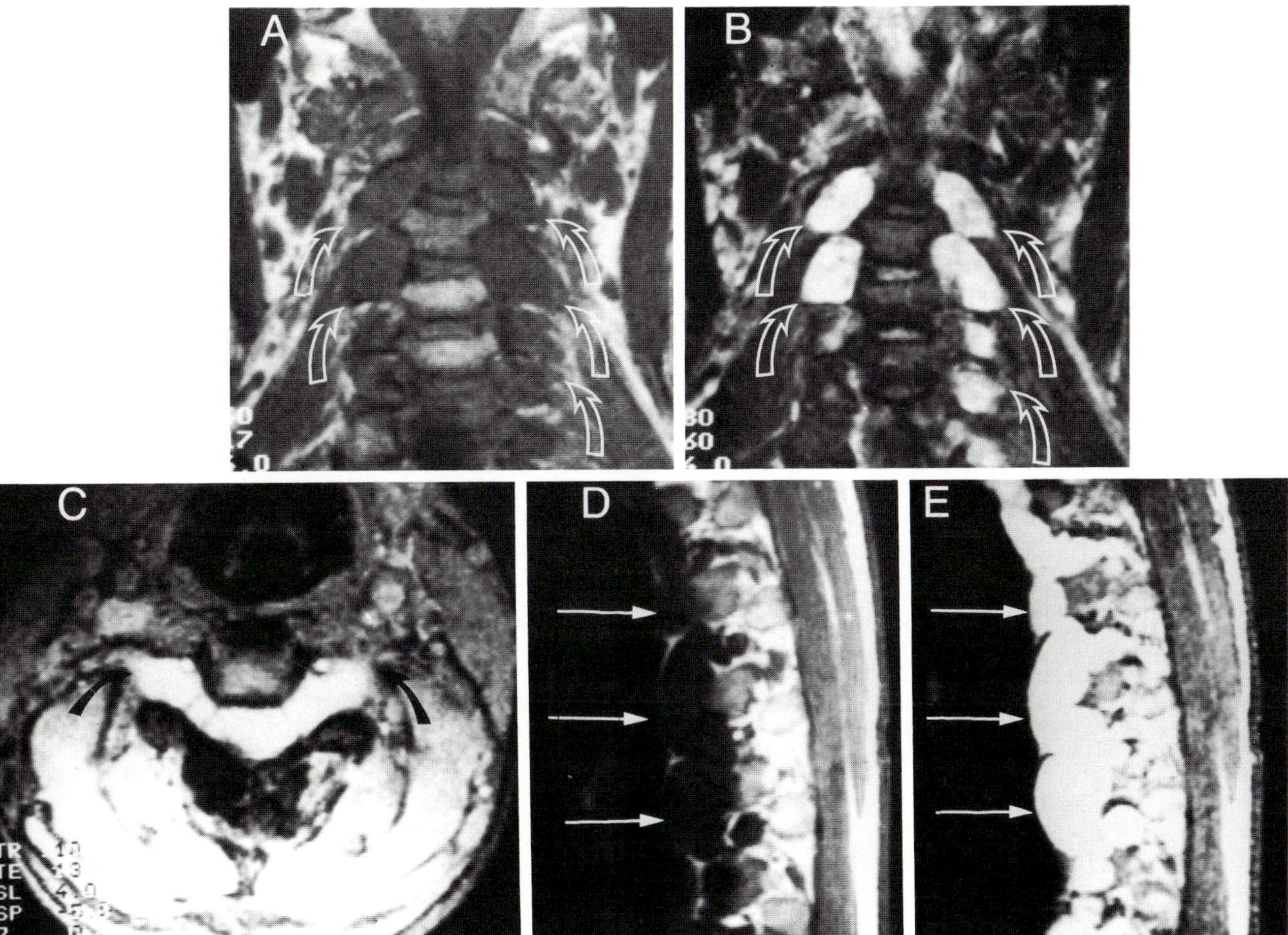

FIG 7–10.
A young patient with a known history of von Recklinghausen's neurofibromatosis. **A,** 500-msec TR/17-msec TE coronal image through the cervical spine demonstrates multiple, soft tissue masses emanating from the spinal canal consistent with numerous fibromas that are both intradural and extradural in location *(arrows).* **B,** 1,800-msec TR/60-msec TE image through the region of **A** demonstrates increased signal intensity within the mass lesions. Some of these have ill-defined areas of decreased signal intensity within them, again characteristic of neurofibromas *(arrows).* **C,** 100-msec TR/13-msec TE FLASH 10-degree scan demonstrates widening of the cervical neural foramen by the high signal intensity neurofibromas *(arrows).* **D,** 500-msec TR/17-msec TE parasagittal image through the thoracic spine demonstrates multiple, septated cavities just lateral to the spinal canal *(arrows).* **E,** 1,800-msec TR/60-msec TE scan in the same plane as **D** now demonstrates the cyst as having homogeneously increased signal intensity consistent with thoracic meningoceles. *(Continued)*

Metastases

Like the spinal cord, the spinal subarachnoid space may lend itself to secondary invasion by malignancy, primarily CSF seeding from cranial ependymomas, glioblastomas, and medulloblastomas. In adults, carcinoma of the lung and breast as well as lymphoma may also present in this fashion.[70–73] T_1-weighted images often demonstrate nodular masses of soft tissue signal intensity in the distal thecal sac or diffuse thickening of the cauda equina. Intravenously administered paramagnetic contrast greatly increases the conspicuity of such lesions[28] (Fig 7–14). T_2-weighted images are less helpful not only because of their lower signal-to-noise, but also low contrast-resolution between tumors (long T_2) and CSF (long T_2).

EXTRADURAL TUMORS

Extradural tumors are comprised of primary or metastatic, benign and malignant neoplasms involving vertebrae, adjacent soft tissue, nerve roots, and dura. These lesions account for approximately 30% of all spine neoplasms.[33] The primary benign soft tissue tumors are

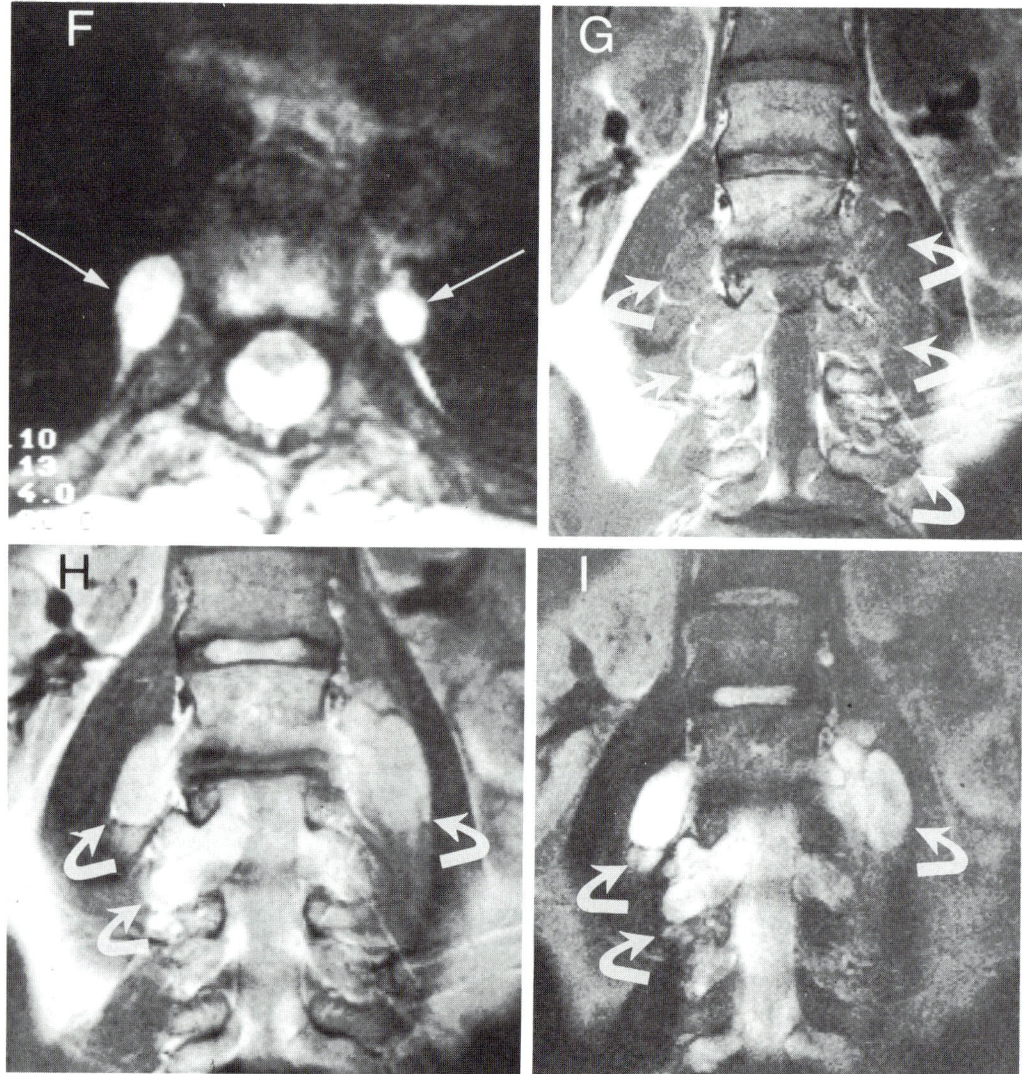

FIG 7–10 (cont.).
F, 100-msec TR/13-msec TE FISP 10-degree axial study again demonstrates the lateral meningoceles. **G,** 500-msec TR/17-msec TE coronal image through the lumbar spine again demonstrates multiple, intradural, and extradural "dumbbell" neurofibromas that have signal intensity of soft tissue *(arrows).* **H,** 2,000-msec TR/30-msec TE coronal scan through the lumbar spine again demonstrates the dumbbell neurofibromas that now are of increasing signal intensity *(arrows).* **I,** 2,000-msec TR/120-msec TE coronal scans through the lumbar spine now demonstrate high signal intensity neurofibromas, some of which have lower signal intensity within *(arrows).*

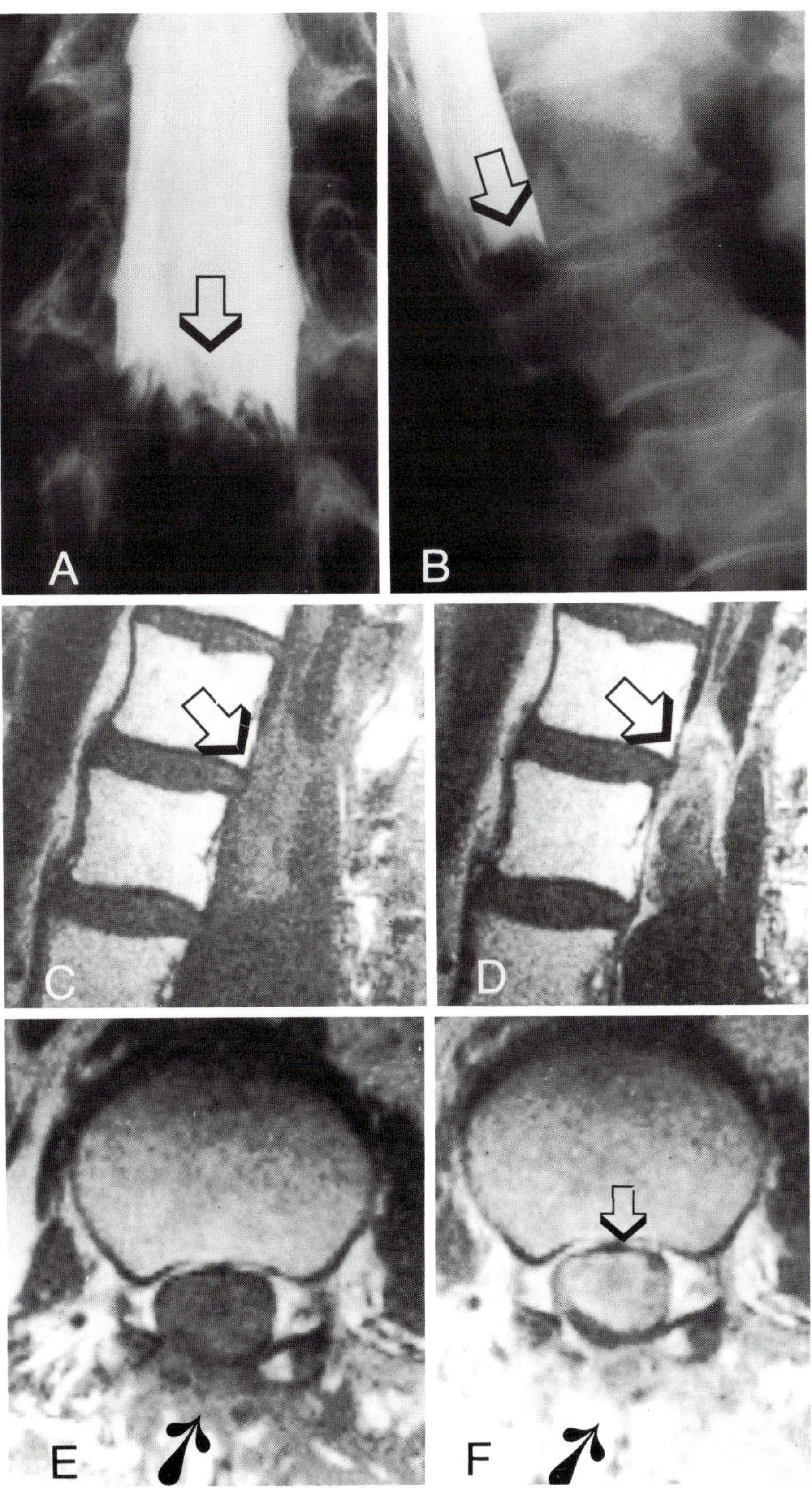

FIG 7–11.
An elderly man who has previously been operated on for an intradural lumbar neuroma, now presents with recurrent symptoms. Initial evaluation by water-soluble contrast myelography (**A** and **B**), showed complete block *(arrow)* to the caudad flow of contrast material below the upper lumbar spinal canal. **C,** 500-msec TR/17-msec TE sagittal image through this region demonstrates an ill-defined area *(arrow)* of increased signal intensity within the subarachnoid space. **D,** 500-msec TR/17-msec TE midline sagittal scan through the region of question following the administration of intravenous Gd-DTPA demonstrates diffuse enhancement of a soft tissue mass within the spinal canal of the upper lumbar spine. **E,** 500-msec TR/17-msec TE axial scan through the level of the previous laminectomy defect demonstrates low signal intensity epidural fibrosis *(arrow)* posteriorly as well as some heterogeneity of the signal intensity within the spinal canal itself. **F,** 500-msecTR/17-msec TE axial scan following the intravenous administration of Gd-DTPA demonstrates enhancement of the epidural fibrosis *(closed arrow)* as well as the intradural soft tissue mass *(open arrow).*

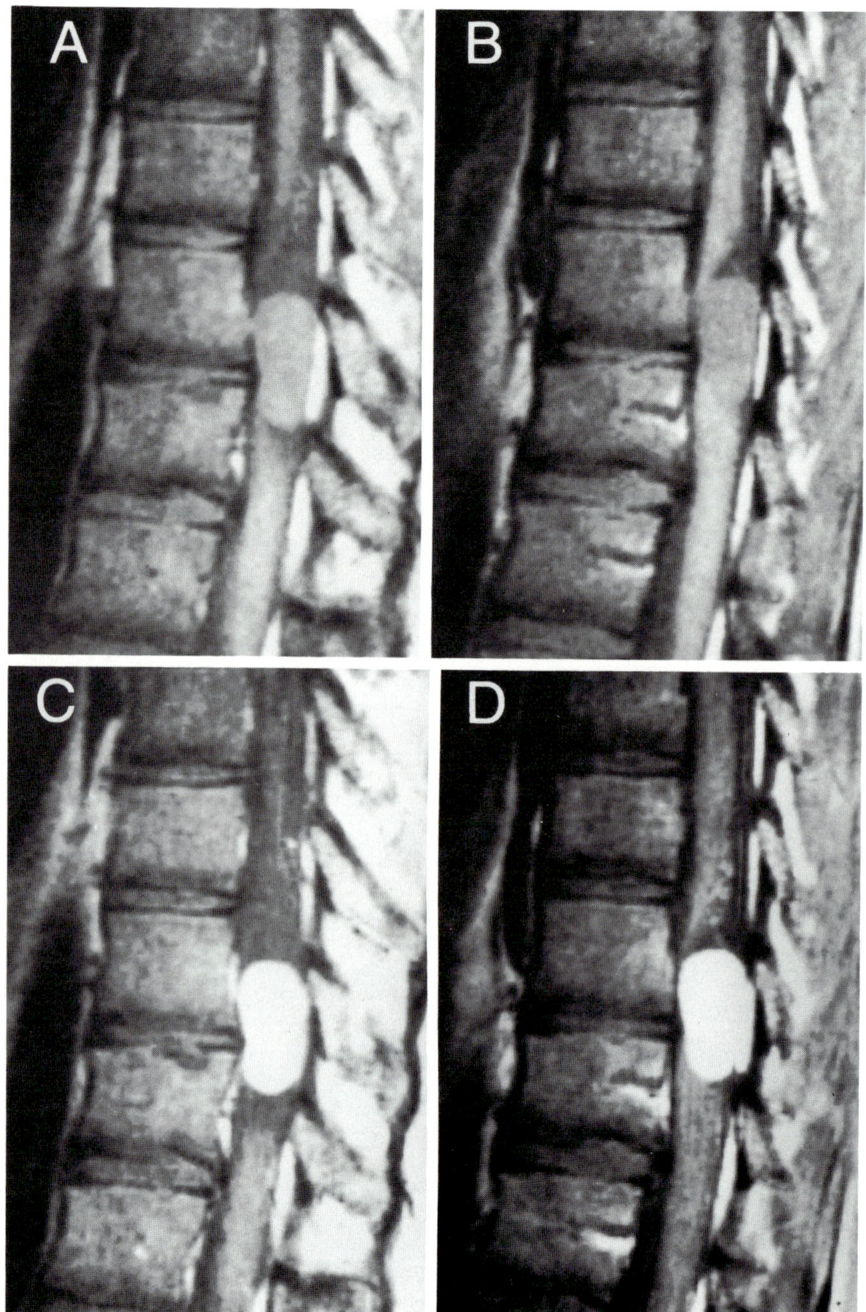

FIG 7–12.
A and **B,** 500-msec TR/17-msec TE sagittal image in a patient with an intradural extramedullary schwannoma demonstrates a soft mass adjacent to and isointense with the thoracic spinal cord. **C** and **D,** following administration of intravenous Gd-DTPA, there is marked increase in signal in this 500-msec TR/17-msec TE image secondary to uptake of contrast.

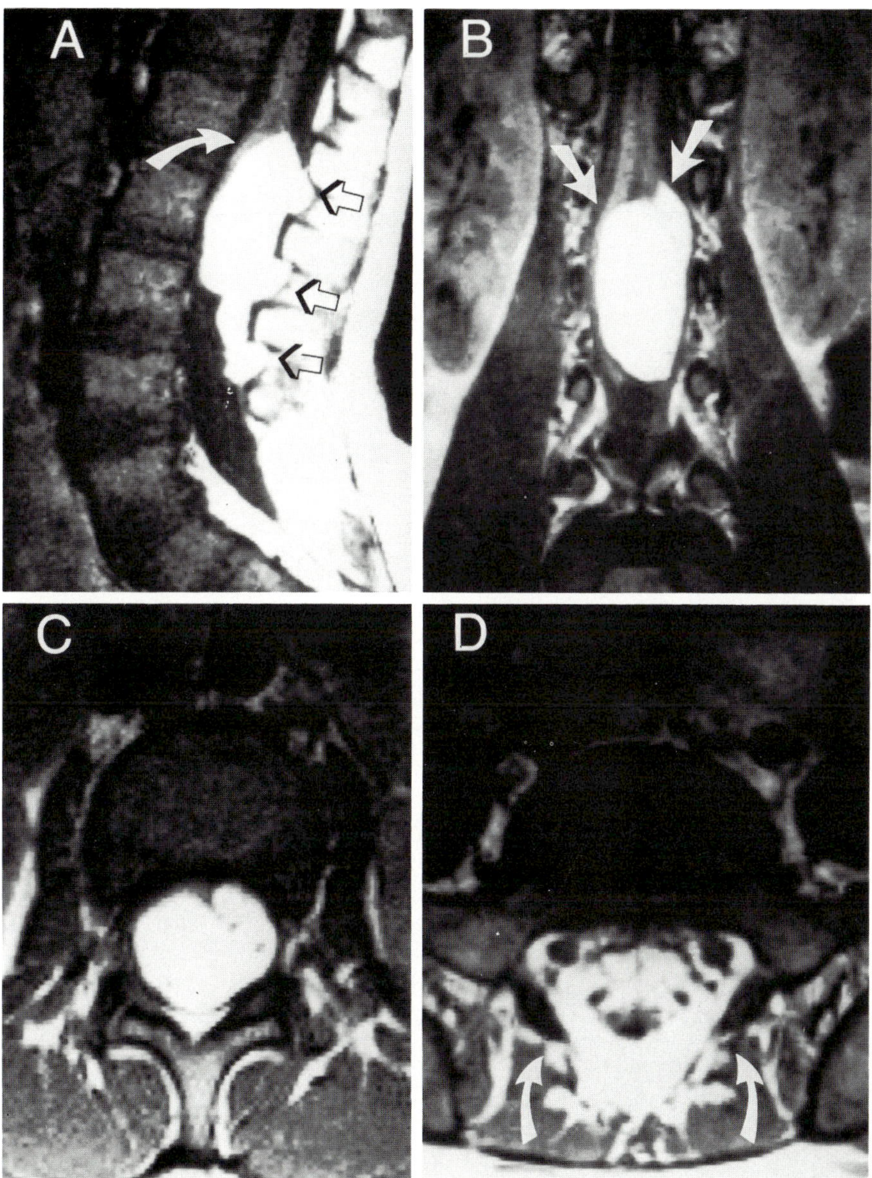

FIG 7–13.

A, 500-msec TR/17-msec TE midline sagittal image through the lower lumbar spine demonstrates a lipomeningocele *(open arrows)* that extends into the thecal sac and is attached to a tethered conus medullaris *(curved arrow).* **B,** 500-msec TR/17-msec TE coronal image through this region again demonstrates the intradural location of this high signal intensity lipoma *(arrows).* **C,** axial 500-msec TR/17-msec TE image through the region of the lipoma demonstrates the spinal canal completely occupied by the high signal intensity fat lesion. **D,** 500-msec TR/17-msec TE axial image through the level of S1 demonstrates spina bifida *(arrows)* emphasizing the frequent association of these lesions with dysraphic states.

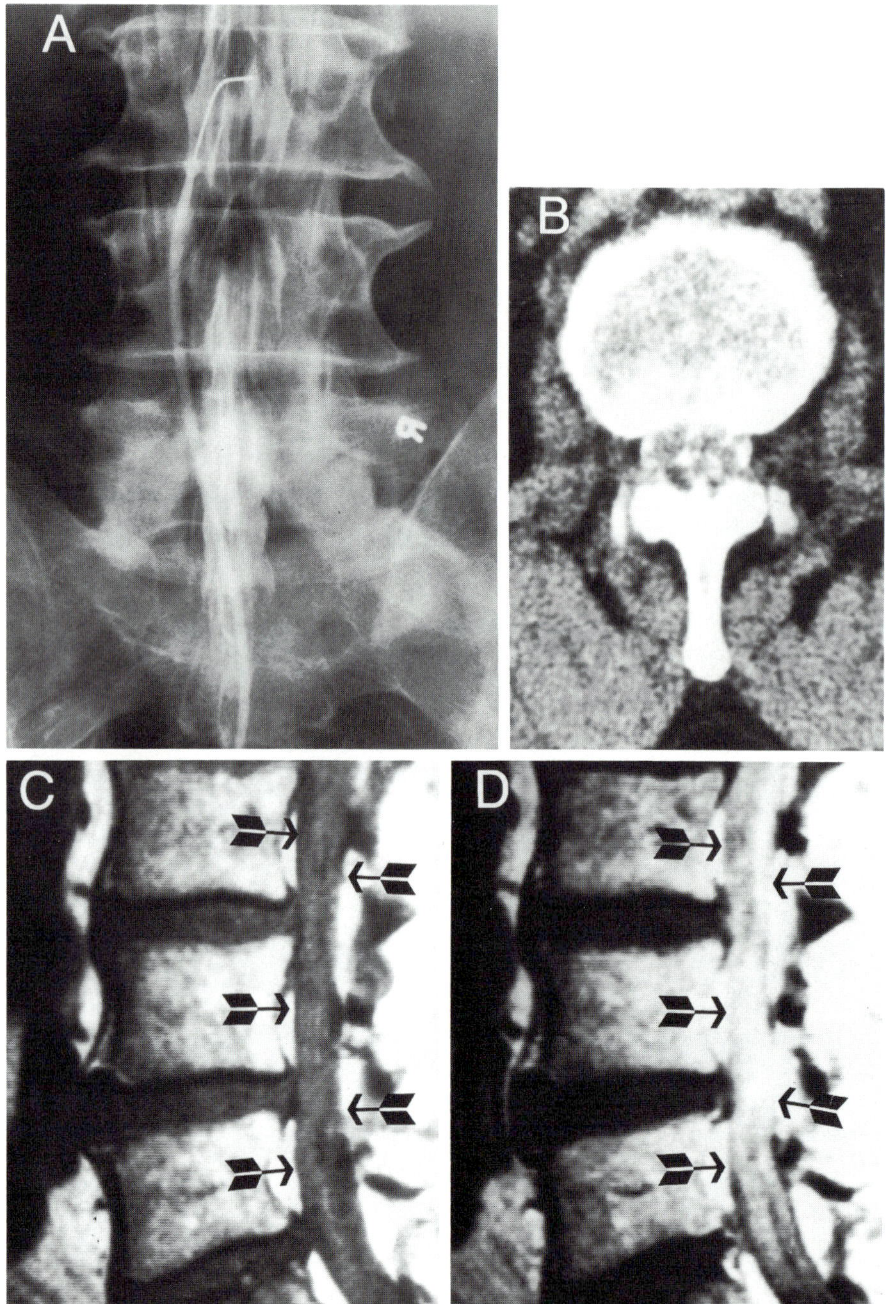

FIG 7–14.
This elderly, retiree experienced acute onset of sciatica following a round of golf. **A,** initial evaluation included a water-soluble contrast myelogram that demonstrated diffuse thickening of the nerve roots of the cauda equina. **B,** follow-up high-resolution CT scan again demonstrates thickened nerve roots of the cauda equina within the distal thecal sac. **C,** 400-msec TR/15-msec TE midline sagittal image of the lumbar spine demonstrates some slight heterogeneity of the signal intensity within the thecal sac *(arrows).* **D,** 400-msec TR/15-msec TE midline sagittal image through the lumbar spine following the intravenous administration of Gd-DTPA demonstrates diffuse, intense enhancement of the intrathecal nerve roots. *(Continued)*

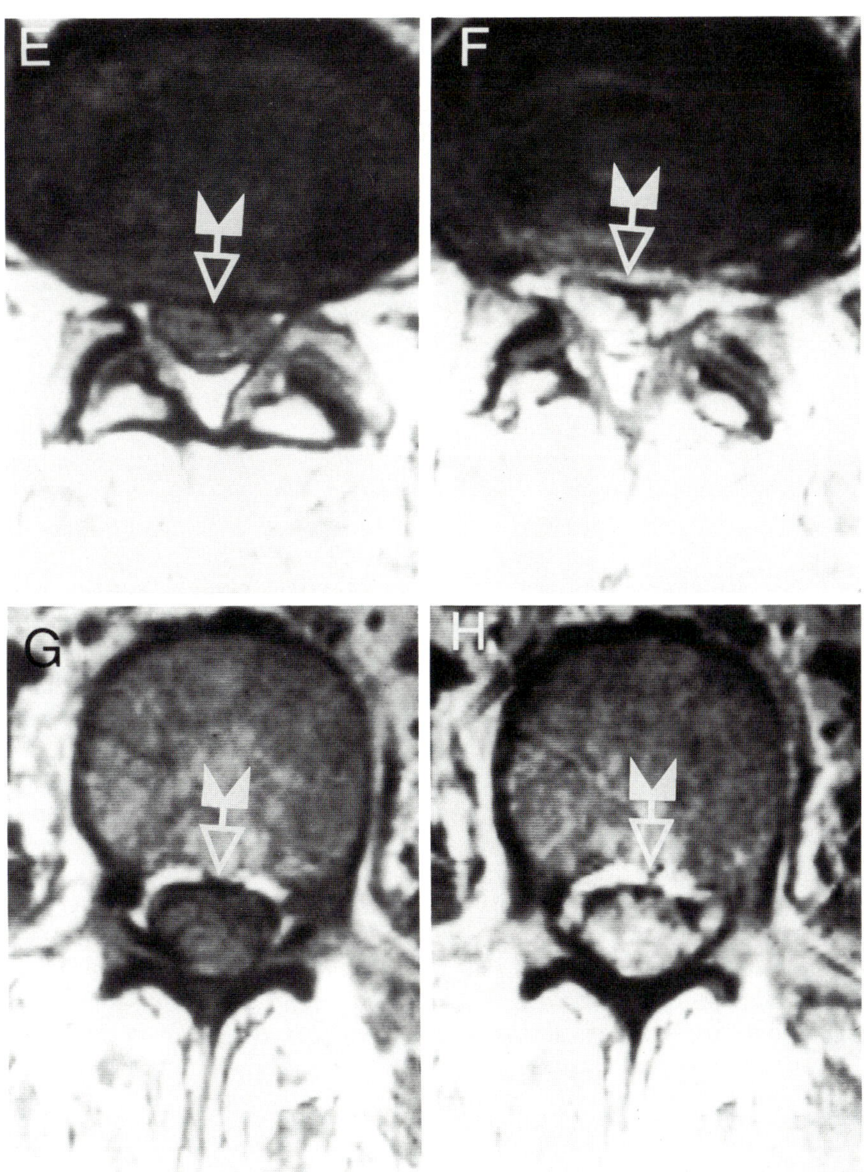

FIG 7–14 (cont.).
E, 600-msec TR/15-msec TE axial image through the midline lumbar spine is essentially normal. *Arrow* indicates nerve roots within the thecal sac. **F,** 600-msec TR/15-msec TE axial image through the level of **E** again demonstrates diffuse, intense enhancement of the nerve roots of the cauda equina *(arrow).* **G** and **H,** additional axial T_1-weighted images again demonstrate diffuse enhancement of the intradural contents following the intravenous administration of Gd-DTPA. Histologic examination of the spinal fluid obtained at the time of myelography was positive for histiocytic lymphoma.

comprised of the small minority of extradural meningiomas, neurinomas, and developmental tumors that have already been addressed. Thus, this section will specifically focus on a few benign tumors arising from the vertebrae and a range of malignant neoplasms.

Unlike plain film radiographs, myelography, and computed tomography (which primarily focus on the bony architecture of the spinal canal and its adjacent soft tissues), MR images the vertebral marrow space and its nearby soft tissues. To some extent, this puts MR at a disadvantage when primary vertebral tumors that are best known to radiologists on the basis of location, integrity of cortical bone, pattern of cancellous bone involvement, as well as presence and type of calcified matrix are evaluated. The terms osteolytic and osteoblastic have no meaning with MRI. Nonetheless, certain primary lesions involving the vertebrae have been noted to have unique appearances with MR.

Hemangiomas

Vertebral hemangiomas are slow-growing benign lesions that have been demonstrated in 11% of spines at autopsy but are only rarely symptomatic.[83–85] Histopathologically, they appear as collections of thin-walled blood vessels or sinuses lined by endothelium that are interspersed among bony trabeculae and abundant adipose tissue.[86] They most commonly occur in the thoracic spine and have a distinctive appearance on magnetic resonance scans.[87] On T_1-weighted images, the intraosseous portions appear as mottled increased signal intensity secondary to the adipose tissue interspersed among thickened bony trabeculae.[88] An extraosseous matrix often displays lower (soft-tissue) signal on T_1-weighted images.[88] On T_2-weighted images, both intraosseous and extraosseous tumor demonstrates increased signal intensity, possibly related to more cellular components of the tumor[88] (Fig 7–15). Flow-related effects are not thought to significantly contribute to the MR appearance of these lesions. Focal fat deposition within the spine may mimic vertebral hemangiomas on T_1-weighted images but fail to have the same increased signal intensity on T_2-weighted studies.[89]

Aneurysmal Bone Cyst

Like vertebral hemangiomas, aneurysmal bone cysts have a characteristic MR appearance. Commonly, they manifest as expansile, benign mass lesions with multiple blood-filled cysts contained by thin calcified or noncalcified periosteal membranes.[90] MRI typically demonstrates numerous well-defined cystic cavities that are surrounded by a rim of low signal intensity and may demonstrate multiple fluid-fluid levels.[91–94] These cavities may show a wide range of signal intensities on both T_1- and T_2-weighted images depending on the various blood products present, their paramagnetic properties, and the field strength of magnet utilized[93, 94] (Fig 7–16). Only 20% of aneurysmal bone cysts involve the spine.[95] These lesions are considered benign but may compromise the vertebral canal resulting in neurologic dysfunction.[96]

Chordomas

Chordomas are uncommon, aggressive extradural lesions of the bony spine arising from remnants of the primitive notochord and representing approximately 3% to 5% of primary bone tumors.[97] Although notochord remnants are found distributed equally along the neural axis, chordomas are found predominantly in the sacrococcygeal area (50%), with 30% to 40% arising from the basisphenoid region and the remainder from the vertebral bodies (Fig 7–17).[98] Ectopic notochord tissue may be present intradurally (2% of all autopsies) as small nodules (known as ecchondrosis physaliphora) that have only rarely been reported to degenerate into purely intradural chordomas.[99]

Such lesions typically present in adults as destructive or expansile lesions involving two or more vertebrae with a sclerotic rim.[100] The intravertebral disk is commonly affected, and there is often a paraspinal soft tissue mass that may possess a calcified matrix.[100]

Sze et al.[101] have reviewed the MR findings in 20 cases of histologically verified chordoma. They found such lesions isointense (75%) or hypointense (25%) on T_1-weighted images. On T_2-weighted studies all chordomas demonstrated increased signal intensity, and the majority (70%) possessed low signal septa. While MR is superior to CT scanning in delineating the extent of chordomas and the relationship to adjacent vasculature or neural structures, it was inferior to CT in its ability to detect bone destruction and/or calcification. The authors also pointed out that MR may be able to distinguish chondroid chordomas from typical chordomas based on the shorter T_1 and T_2 relaxation times of chondroid chordomas.[101] This is of some clinical significance in as much as chondroid chordomas have a significantly better prognosis than do typical chordomas.

Extradural Malignancy

While magnetic resonance imaging is sensitive in the detection of most other primary or secondary extradural spine neoplasms, their appearance with MR is generally nonspecific. Typically, such lesions are recognized by their involvement with one or more vertebrae and

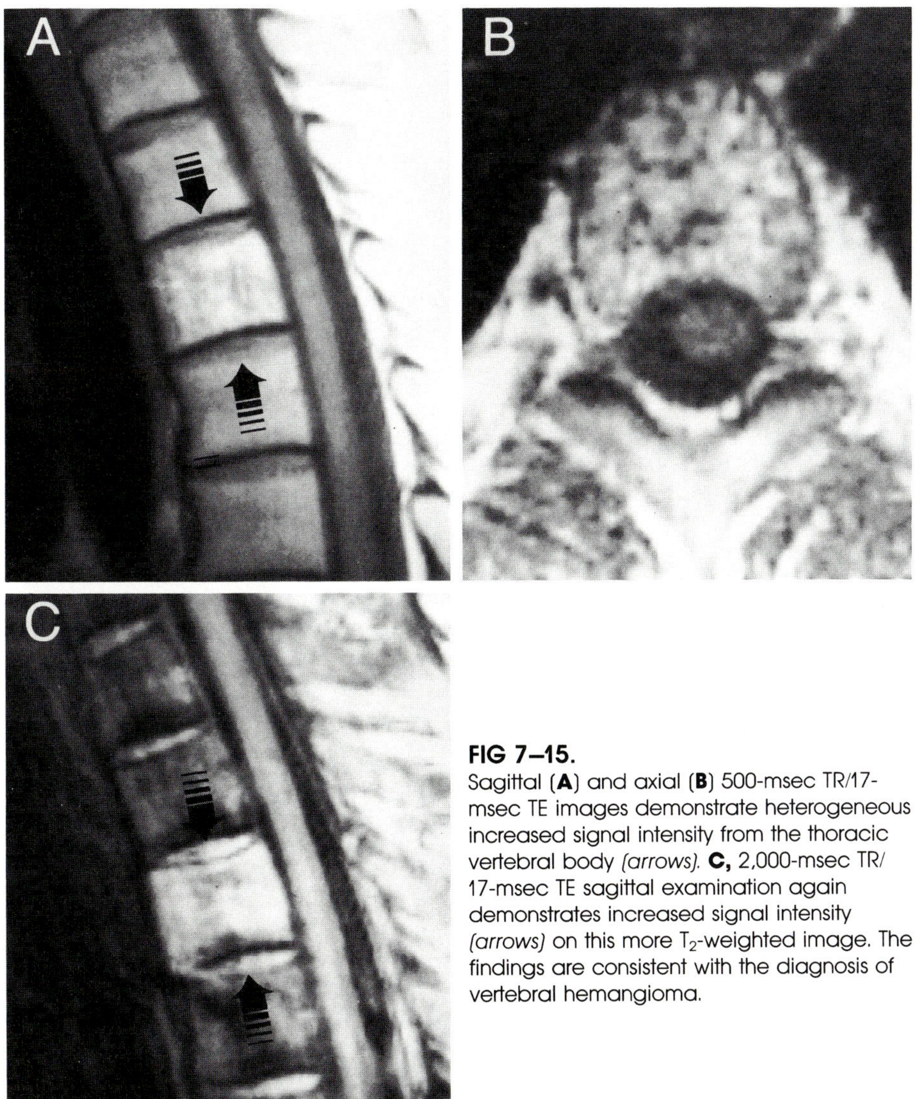

FIG 7–15.
Sagittal (**A**) and axial (**B**) 500-msec TR/17-msec TE images demonstrate heterogeneous increased signal intensity from the thoracic vertebral body *(arrows)*. **C,** 2,000-msec TR/17-msec TE sagittal examination again demonstrates increased signal intensity *(arrows)* on this more T_2-weighted image. The findings are consistent with the diagnosis of vertebral hemangioma.

the adjacent soft tissues. Most neoplasms possess a long T_1 relative to the fat normally present within the bone marrow and are thus recognized as focal areas of decreased signal intensity on T_1-weighted images within the bony spine. On T_2-weighted study, these lesions demonstrate variable degrees of increased signal and consequently may be less conspicuous relative to adjacent normal marrow than on the T_1-weighted study (Figs 7–18 through 7–21). In adults, the vast majority of such lesions are represented by metastatic foci that frequently involve the bony canal (e.g., lung, breast, prostate). Malignant lymphoma, (Hodgkin's disease and reticulum cell sarcoma) may also manifest in this fashion, particularly in its later stages. However, in the majority of cases, vertebral bone involvement is minimal in comparison to the epidural and paravertebral disease.[102]

Among secondary intraspinal malignancies in children, neuroblastoma is most common. Seventy percent of patients are under 4 years of age, and there is a male predominance.[103, 104] While commonly appearing as an extension from a paraspinal mass in the sympathetic chain or adrenal medulla, neuroblastoma may arise primarily from the intramedullary posterior root ganglion primordia.[105] Thus it is often difficult, if not impossible, to discern if the mass arose from the spinal canal or secondarily invaded it. With MR, the tumor appears as a soft tissue mass expanding the spinal canal and adjacent neural foramen on T_1-weighted images. Unlike x-ray CT, calcification may not be discernible. The tumor will demonstrate increased signal intensity on T_2-weighted

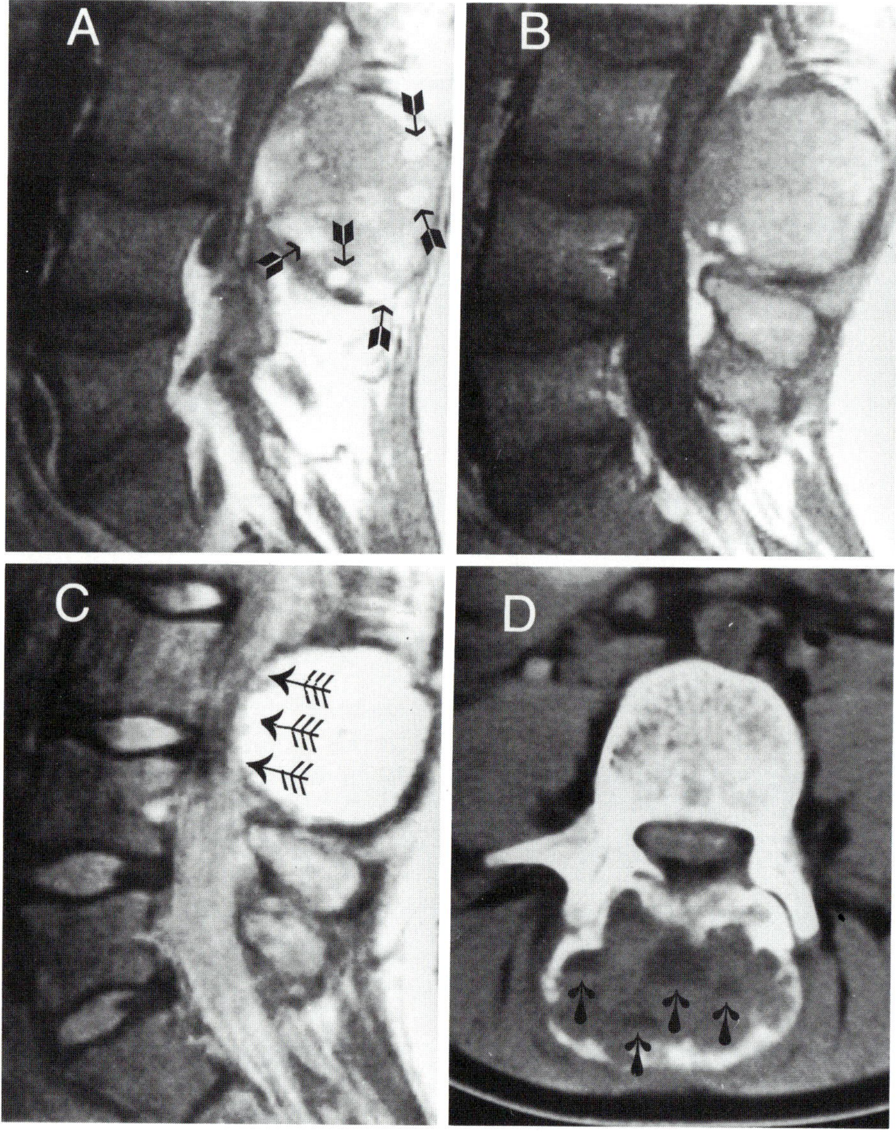

FIG 7–16.

A, 500-msec TR/17-msec TE parasagittal image to the lower lumbar spine demonstrates diffuse enlargement of the posterior elements of the L3 vertebral body. Heterogeneous, focal cystic areas of high signal intensity are noted within this expansile lesion *(arrows)*. **B,** 500-msec TR/17-msec TE midline sagittal image of the lumbar spine again demonstrates an enlarged, expansile mass within the spinous process of L3 that is compressing the thecal sac. **C** 2,000-msec TR/90-msec TE demonstrates the expansile lesion to have increased signal intensity with more T_2-weighting. Again, notice the compression of the thecal sac *(arrows)*. **D,** axial CT scan through the region of the lesion demonstrates an expansile, cystic mass within the posterior elements of L3. *Arrows* indicate the presence of fluid-fluid levels within multiple cysts of the mass lesion. Surgery confirmed the presence of an aneurysmal bone cyst.

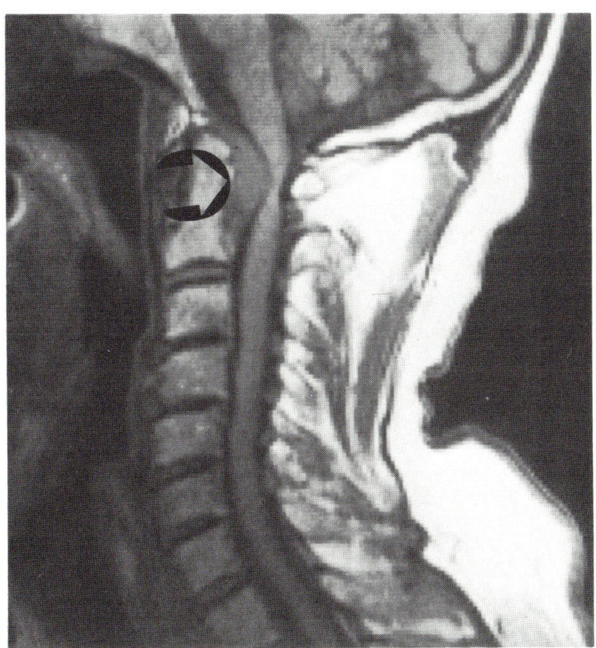

FIG 7–17.
500-msec TR/17-msec TE midline sagittal image through the cervical spine demonstrates a soft tissue mass arising from the body of C2 that is compressing the cervicomedullary junction *(arrow)*. Diagnostic considerations would include meningioma vs. chordoma. Surgery confirmed the presence of a C2 chordoma. (Courtesy of A. Smith, M.D.)

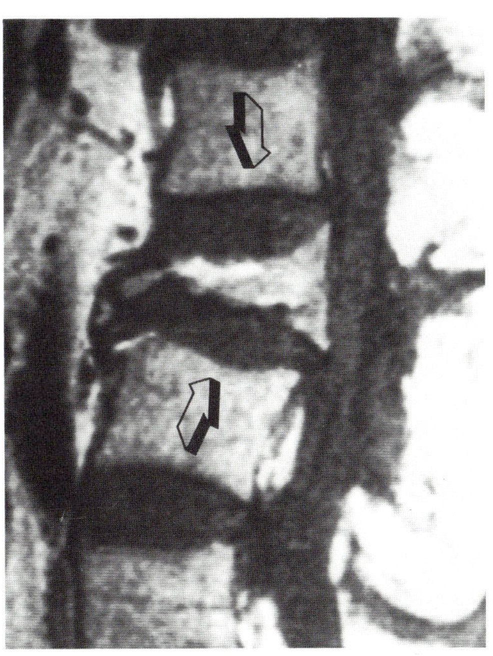

FIG 7–19.
500-msec TR/17-msec TE midline sagittal image through the lumbar spine demonstrates a wedge compression fracture of one of the upper lumbar vertebral bodies. Notice that on this T_1-weighted image the compression fracture has relative high signal intensity. Such findings are most consistent with a compression fracture secondary to senile osteoporosis rather than a pathologic fracture secondary to metastatic disease that more typically has low signal intensity on T_1-weighted images.

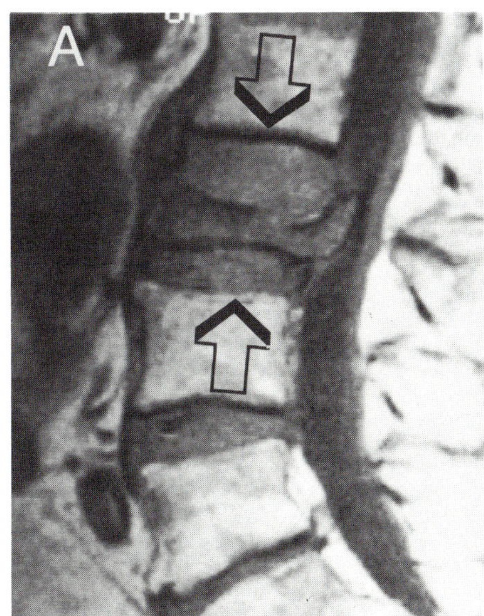

FIG 7–18.
A, 500-msec TR/17-msec TE midline sagittal image through the lumbar spine demonstrates compression of L3 *(open arrows)* that is of low signal intensity on this T_1-weighted image. The findings are most consistent with a pathologic fracture. **B,** 2,000-msec TR/120-msec TE sagittal image again demonstrates a pathologic compression fracture that has a somewhat higher signal intensity on this more T_2-weighted image.

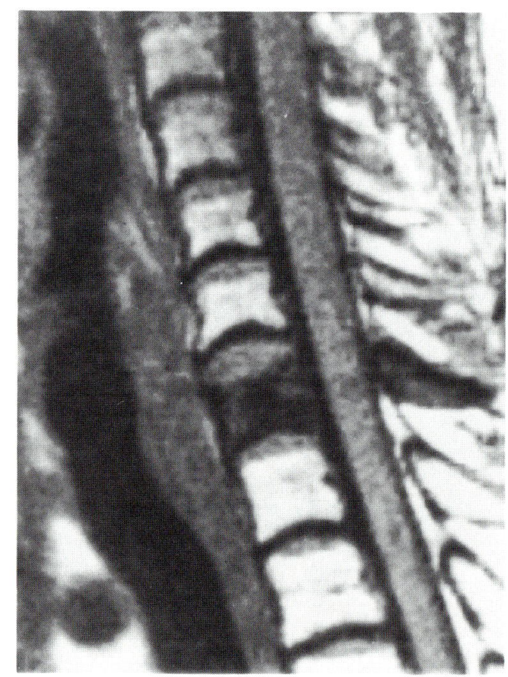

FIG 7–20.
Midline sagittal 500-msec TR/17-msec TE sagittal image through the cervical spine demonstrates diffuse replacement of marrow of C6 metastatic neoplasm. Consequently, the vertebral body and spinous process are diffusely low in signal intensity on this T_1-weighted image.

studies. Despite its malignant nature, long-term survival with neuroblastoma has occurred presumably due to spontaneous regression or maturation to a benign, nonprogressive state.[106]

The role of paramagnetic contrast in the evaluation of malignant extradural disease is less clearly defined than the indications for its use with intradural mass lesions. The preliminary experience of Sze et al.[107] suggests that intravenous Gd-DPTA may actually mask osseous spine implants by making them isointense with normal vertebral marrow. However, contrast may increase the specificity of MR for extradural masses (e.g., distinguishing metastases from disk fragment) and aid in directing needle biopsy.[107]

CHEMICAL-SHIFT IMAGING

As noted above, MR is often sensitive to the presence of extradural tumor by its ability to detect signal changes in the vertebral marrow space. In magnetic resonance imaging, T_1 and T_2 are different for each subpopulation of protons (i.e., water protons, methylene protons, lactate protons, etc.). Relaxation times determined for tissues containing both methylene (fat) and water protons are composite values resulting from both components.[108] T_1 relaxation times for vertebral marrow

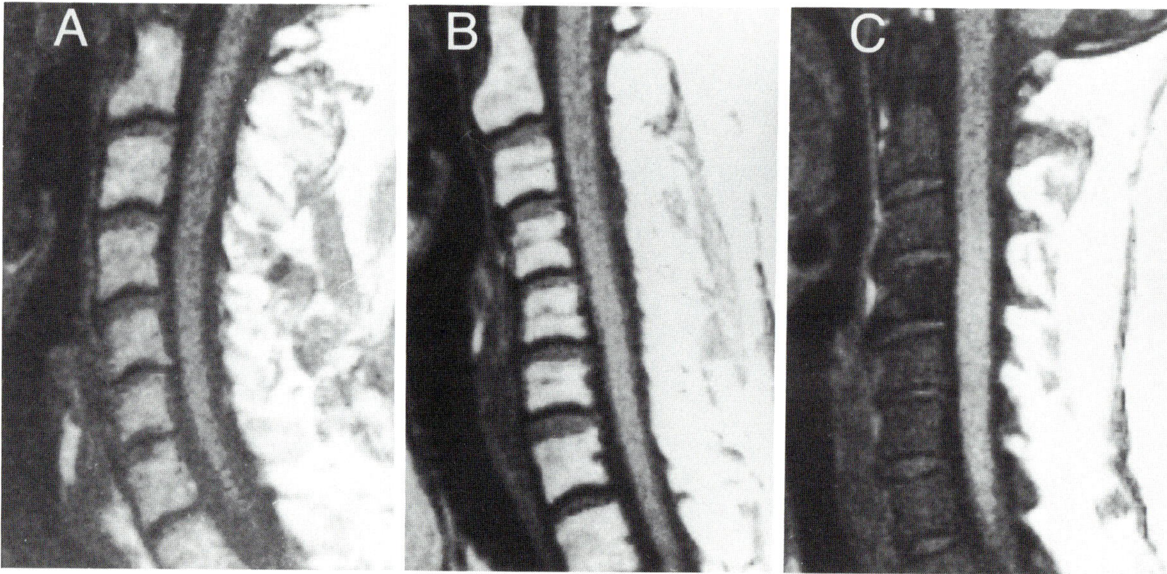

FIG 7–21.
Serial sagittal 500-msec TR/17-msec TE T_1-weighted images in three different patients to demonstrate the variability of marrow signal in normal subjects and various disease states. **A,** normal signal intensity from the cervical body marrow space in this patient with cervical disk disease. **B,** increased signal intensity within the cervical vertebral bodies indicative of previous radiation therapy. Radiation therapy results in replacement of normal hematopoietic elements by vertebral body fat. **C,** diffuse decrease in signal intensity of the vertebral body marrow space in this patient with leukemia suggests neoplastic invasion.

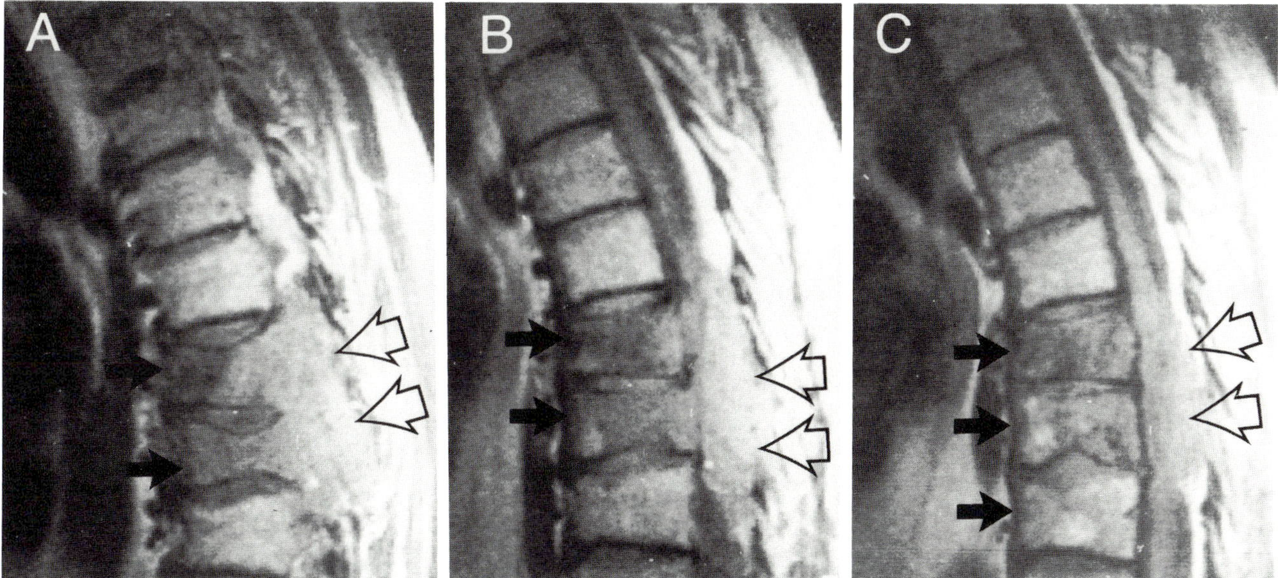

FIG 7–22.
500-msec TR/17-msec TE sagittal images through the midthoracic spine in a patient with known metastatic disease. Multiple areas of low signal intensity and with compression fractures are noted within the vertebral bodies *(closed arrows)* consistent with metastatic invasion. Additionally, a soft tissue mass can be seen surrounding the spinal canal and directly invading the thoracic spinal cord *(open arrows)*.

normally decrease with age, while T_2 relaxation times increase with age due to replacement of hematopoietic elements by fat.[108] This phenomenon is more prominent in women and is exaggerated in patients who have had radiation therapy.[109, 110] In contrast, neoplastic invasion of a vertebra significantly prolongs T_1 and T_2 due to the replacement of marrow fat by increasing amounts of tissue water protons.[111–114] With conventional spin-echo proton imaging, such derangements are most often manifest on T_1-weighted images.[111–114] In addition to the difference in relaxation times, tissue water and methylene (fat) protons actually resonate at slightly different frequencies within the same applied magnetic field secondary to different local fields induced by nearby nuclei and electrons. While conventional imaging uses the total signal generated by the spectrum of resonance frequencies, numerous methods exist that selectively image certain hydrogen spectral peaks.[115] These techniques are collectively known as chemical-shift imaging.[115] Chemical-shift imaging has been applied to the study of axial bone marrow in normal subjects and patients with neoplastic disease.[116] To date, such methods appear to be most helpful for the detection of diffuse, sometimes insidious changes in bone marrow signal over time. For example, McKinstry et al.[117] have serially studied patients with chronic granulocytic leukemia and aplastic anemia with chemical-shift imaging and were able to effectively demonstrate marrow response to therapy using their technique.

SPINAL CORD COMPRESSION AND BLOCK

While primary or metastatic, tumors of the spine are evaluated in terms of their biologic activity, they are also (and possibly more urgently) evaluated with respect to the degree of mechanical compression they produce on the spinal cord. Classically, the clinical manifestations of spinal cord compression have been divided into three stages.[33, 118] The first stage (neuralgic stage) is characterized by root pain and segmental sensory and motor loss. The second stage (transitional stage or incomplete transsection syndrome) is heralded by the onset of Brown-Séquard syndrome as a result of incomplete transsection. The final stage is that of complete transsection in which the complete deficit often begins in the distal extremities and ascends as the lesion progresses. Unfortunately, it may be clinically difficult to determine what stage of compression a patient is experiencing at the time of presentation, and it is certainly impossible to predict the rate of progression from stage to stage (and thus eminent risk of permanent neurologic deficit). Historically, such clinical questions have been answered by myelography (occasionally aided by CT) where the com-

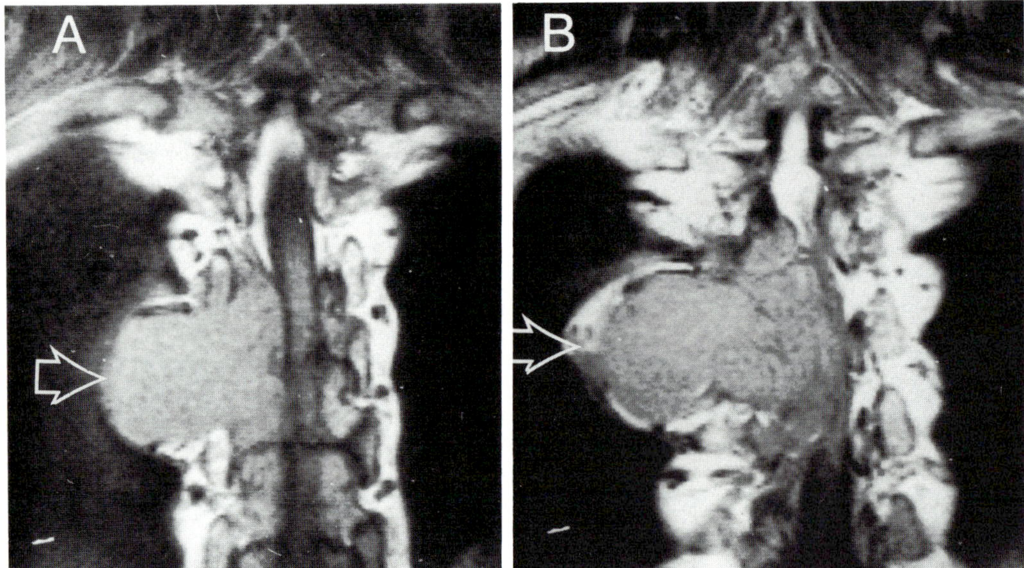

FIG 7–23.
500-msec TR/17-msec TE coronal images in a thoracic spine demonstrate direct invasion of the spinal canal by a carcinoma of the lung *(open arrow)*.

plete obstruction to flow of contrast material in the subarachnoid space is considered an indication for emergent therapy.[1] Unfortunately, CSF pressure shifts induced by lumbar puncture in the presence of complete subarachnoid block may lead to rapid neurologic deterioration in a significant percentage of these patients.[119] Other potential pitfalls include (1) puncture site hematoma, (2) inability to examine the entire spine in the presence of multiple compression sites, and (3) inability to demonstrate paravertebral disease.[120–122] In a retrospective review of 58 patients with suspected epidural metastases, Smoker, et al.[123] found MR to be diagnostic in 60 of 64 examinations performed. Additionally, MR was as diagnostic as myelography in 22 cases on which both studies were performed. Magnetic resonance was felt to provide additional information in 13 of 22 patients.[123] Because MR is also noninvasive, it was considered the examination of choice for the evaluation of spinal metastases and possible cord compression. The MR examination may be tailored specifically toward the question of cord compression by obtaining a localizing sagittal T_1 body coil image through the midline, followed by rapid, serial sagittal and axial studies over the length of the spinal cord (Figs 7–22 and 7–23). If tumor is found but the clinical question of a "complete block" lingers, it may be possible to perform a magnetic resonance version of Queckenstedt's test. More specifically, a nongated, nonrefocussed long TR/long TE sagittal image through a suspected compressive lesion will not demonstrate ghosting artifact secondary to CSF pulsation in the presence of complete block. This will be more apparent when the phase-encode direction is oriented perpendicular to the spine.

REFERENCES

1. Shapiro R: Tumors, in Shapiro R (ed): *Myelography*. Chicago, Year Book Medical Publishers, 1984, pp 345–421.
2. Aubin ML, Jardin C, Bar D, et al: Computerized tomography in 32 cases of intraspinal tumor. *J Neuroradiol* 1979; 6:81–92.
3. Hammerschlag SB, Wolpert SM, Carter BL: Computed tomography of the spinal canal. *Radiology* 1976; 121:361–367.
4. Nakagaaia H, Auang YP, Malis LI, et al: Computed tomography of intraspinal and paraspinal neoplasm. *J Comput Assist Tomogr* 1977; 1:377–390.
5. Modic MT, Weinstein MA, Pavlicek W, et al: Nuclear magnetic resonance imaging of the spine. *Radiology* 1983; 148:757–762.
6. Modic MT, Weinstein MA, Pavlicek W, et al: Magnetic resonance imaging of the cervical spine: Technical and clinical observations. *AJR* 1983; 141:1129–1136.
7. Han JS, Kaufman B, El Yousef SJ, et al: NMR Imaging of the spine. *AJR* 1983; 141:1137–1145.
8. Norman D, Mills CM, Brant-Zawadski M, et al: Magnetic resonance imaging of the spinal cord and canal: Potentials and limitations. *AJR* 1983; 141:1147–1152.
9. Modic MT, Hardy RW, Weinstein MA, et al: Nuclear magnetic resonance of the spine: Clinical potential and limitation. *Neurosurgery* 1984; 15:582–592.

10. Bradley WG, Waluch V, Yadley RA, et al: Comparison of CT and MR in 400 patients with suspected disease of the brain and cervical spinal cord. *Radiology* 1984; 152:695–702.
11. Hyman RA, Edwards JH, Vacinca SJ, et al: 0.6 T MR imaging of the cervical spine: Multislice and multiecho techniques. *AJNR* 1985; 6:229–236.
12. Kucharczyk W, Brant-Zawadzki M, et al: Central nervous system tumors in children: Detection by magnetic resonance imaging. *Radiology* 1985; 155:131–136.
13. Di Chiro G, Doppman JL, Dwyer AJ, et al: Tumors and arteriovenous malformations of the spinal cord: Assessment using MR. *Radiology* 1985; 156:689–697.
14. Haughton VM, Rimm AA, Sobocinski KA, et al: A blinded clinical comparison of MR imaging and CT in neuroradiology. *Radiology* 1986; 160:751–755.
15. Axel L: Surface coil magnetic resonance imaging. *J Comput Assist Tomogr* 1984; 8:381–384.
16. Fisher MR, Barker B, Amparo EG, et al: MR imaging using specialized coils. *Radiology* 1985; 157:443–447.
17. Kulkarni MV, Patton JA, Price RR: Technical considerations for the use of surface coils in MRI. *AJR* 1986; 147:373–378.
18. Enzmann DR, Rubin JB, Wright A: Use of cerebrospinal fluid gating to improve T_2 weighted images: I. The spinal cord. *Radiology* 1987; 162:763–767.
19. Enzman DR, Rubin JB, Wright A: Cervical spine MR imaging: Generating high signal CSF in sagittal and axial images. *Radiology* 1987; 163:233–238.
20. Rubin JB, Enzman DR: Optimizing conventional MR imaging of the spine. *Radiology* 1987; 163:777–783.
21. Rubin JB, Enzman DR, Wright A: CSF-gated MR imaging of the spine: Theory and clinical implementation. *Radiology* 1987; 163:784–792.
22. Rubin JB, Enzman DR: Harmonic modulation of proton MR precessional phase by pulsatile motion: Origin and spinal CSF flow phenomena. *AJR* 1987; 148:983–994.
23. Haacke EM, Lenz GW: Improving MR image quality in the presence of motion by using rephasing gradients. *AJR* 1987; 148:1251–1258.
24. Brasch RC: Contrast enhancement in NMR imaging, in Newton TH, Potts DG (eds): *Advanced Imaging Techniques: Modern Neuroradiology*. San Anselmo, Clavadel Press, 1983, vol 2, pp 63–79.
25. Bydder GM, Kingsley DPE, Brown J, et al: MR imaging of meningiomas including studies with and without gadolinium-DTPA. *J Comput Assist Tomogr* 1985; 9:690–697.
26. Bydder GM, Brown J, Niendorf HP, et al: Enhancement of cervical intraspinal tumors in MR imaging with intravenous gadolinium-DTPA. *J Comput Assist Tomogr* 1985; 9:847–85.
27. Schroth G, Thron A, Guhl L, et al: Magnetic resonance imaging of spinal meningiomas and neurinomas: Improvement of imaging by paramagnetic contrast enhancement. *J Neurosurg* 1987; 66:695–700.
28. Sze G, Abramson A, Krol G, et al: Gadolinium-DTPA in the evaluation of intradural extra-medullary spinal disease. *AJNR* 1988; 9:153–163.
29. Edelman RR, Atkinson DJ, Silver Loaiza FL, et al: FRODO pulse sequences: A new means of eliminating motion, flow and wraparound artifacts. *Radiology* 1988; 166:231–236.
30. Tyrrell RL, Deimling M: Fast 3D imaging—clinical application. *J NMR Med* 1987; 6:240–252.
31. Kurland LT: The frequency of intraspinal neoplasms in the resident population of Rochester, Minnesota. *J Neurosurg* 1958; 15:627–641.
32. Perry AK, Elveback LR, Okazaki H, et al: Neoplasms of the central nervous system: Epidemiologic considerations. *Neurology* 1972; 22:40–48.
33. Nittner K: *Spinal meningiomas, neurinomas and neurofibromas and hourglass tumors,* in Vinken PJ, Bruyn GW (eds): *Handbook of Clinical Neurology*. New York, Elsevier North-Holland Inc, 1976, vol 20, pp 177–322.
34. Sloof JL, Kernohan JW, MacCarty CS: *Primary Intramedullary Tumors of the Spinal Cord and Filum Terminale.* Philadelphia, WB Saunders Co, 1964.
35. Kernohan JW, Sayre GP: Tumors of the central nervous system, in National Research Council, *Atlas of Tumor Pathology*. Washington DC, Armed Forces Institute of Pathology, 1952.
36. Lombardi G, Passerini A: Spinal cord tumors. *Radiology* 1961; 76:381–392.
37. Mosbery WH: Spinal tumors diagnosed during the first year of life. *J Neurosurg* 1951; 8:220.
38. Okazaki H: *Fundamentals in Neuropathology*. New York, Igaku-Shoin, 1983.
39. Alter M: Statistical aspects of spinal cord tumors, in Vinken PJ, Bruyn GW (eds): *Handbook of Clinical Neurology*. New York, Elsevier North-Holland Inc, 1975, vol 19, pp 1–22.
40. DiLorenzo N, Giuffre R, Fortuna A: Primary spinal neoplasms in childhood: Analysis of 1,234 published cases (including 56 personal cases) by pathology, sex, age, and site: Differences from the situation in adults. *Neurochirurgia (Stuttg)* 1982; 25:153–164.
41. DeSousa AL, Kalsbeck JE, Mealey J, et al: Intraspinal tumors in children. *J Neurosurg* 1979; 51:437–445.
42. Russell DS, Rubinstein LJ: Pathology of tumors of the nervous system. London, EA Pall, 1977; pp 190–191; 204–219.
43. Epstein F, Epstein N: Intramedullary tumors of the spinal cord, in Shillito J Jr, Matson DD (eds): *Pediatric Neurosurgery of the Developing Nervous System*. New York, Grune & Stratton, 1982, pp 529–539.
44. Epstein F, Epstein N: Surgical treatment of spinal cord astrocytomas of childhood. *J Neurosurg* 1982; 57:685–689.
45. Guidetti B, Mercuri S, Vagnozzi R: Long term results of surgical treatment of 129 intramedullary spinal gliomas. *J Neurosurg* 1981; 54:323–330.
46. Kopelson G, Linggood RM, Kleinman GM, et al: Management of intramedullary spinal cord tumors. *Radiology* 1980; 135:473–479.
47. Gay AMC, Pinto RS, Raghavendra BN, et al: Intramedul-

lary spinal cord tumors: MR imaging with emphasis on associated cysts. *Radiology* 1986; 161:381–386.
48. Rubin JM, Hisen A, DiPictro MA: Ambiguities in MR imaging of tumoral cysts in the spinal cord. *J Comput Assist Tomogr* 10:395–398.
49. Williams AL, Haughton VM, Pojunas KW, et al: Differentiation of intramedullary neoplasms and cysts by MR. *AJR* 1987; 149:159–164.
50. Williams B: On the pathogenesis of syringomyelia: A review. *J R Soc Med* 1980; 73:798–806.
51. Ball MJ, Dayan AD: Pathogenesis of syringomyelia. *Lancet* 1972; 2:799–801.
52. Sherman JL, Barkovich AJ, Citrin CM: The MR appearance of syringomyelia: New observations. *AJR* 1987; 148:381–391.
53. Enzman DR, O'Donohue J, Rubin JB, et al: CSF pulsations within non-neoplastic spinal cord cysts. *AJR* 1987; 149:149–157.
54. Sato Y, Waziri M, Smith W, et al: Hippel-Landau Disease: MR imaging. *Radiology* 1988; 166:241–246.
55. Wyburn Mason R: The vascular abnormalities and tumors of the spinal cord and its membranes. London, Kimpton, 1943.
56. Poser CM: The relationship between syringomyelia and neoplasm, in American lecture series No. 262: *American Lectures in Neurology*. Springfield, Ill, Charles C Thomas Publishers, 1956.
57. Solomon RA, Stein BM: Unusual spinal cord enlargement related to intramedullary hemangioblastoma. *J Neurosurg* 1988; 68:550–553.
58. Thomas JE, Miller RH: Lipomatous tumors of the spinal canal. *Mayo Clin Proc* 1973; 48:393–400.
59. Alves AM, Norrell H: Intramedullary epidermoid tumors of the spinal cord. *Int Surg* 1970; 54:239–243.
60. Bailey IC: Dermoid tumors of the spinal cord. *J Neurosurg* 1970; 33:676–681.
61. Barnes PD, Lester PD, Yamanashi WS, et al: Magnetic resonance imaging in infants and children with spinal dysraphism. *AJNR* 1986; 7:465–472.
62. Phillips J, Chiu L: Magnetic resonance imaging of intraspinal epidermoid cyst. *J Comput Assist Tomogr* 1987; 11:181–183.
63. Davidson HD, Ouchi T, Steiner RE: NMR imaging of congenital intracranial germ layer neoplasms. *Neuroradiology* 1985; 27:301–303.
64. Wood EH, Taveras JM, Pool JL: Myelographic demonstration of spinal cord metastases from primary brain tumors. *AJR* 1953; 69:221–230.
65. Sagerman RH, Bayshaw MA, Hanbery J: Considerations in treatment of ependymoma. *Radiology* 1965; 84:401–408.
66. Smith DR, Hardman JM, Earle KM: Metastasizing neuroectodermal tumors of the central nervous system. *J Neurosurg* 1969; 31:50–58.
67. Puljic S, Batnitzky S, Yang WC, et al: Metastases to the medullar of the spinal cord: Myelographic features. *Radiology* 1975; 117:89–91.
68. Erlich SS, Davis RL: Spinal subarachnoid metastasis from primary intracranial glioblastoma multiforme. *Cancer* 1978; 42:2854–2864.
69. Deutsch M, Reigel DH: The value of myelography in the management of childhood medulloblastoma. *Cancer* 1980; 45:2194–2197.
70. Benson DF: Intramedullary spinal cord metastasis. *Neurology* 1960; 10:281–287.
71. Jellinger K, Kothbauer P, Sunder-Plassmann E, et al: Intramedullary spinal cord metastases. *J Neurol* 1979; 202:31–41.
72. Costigan DA, Winkleman MD: Intramedullary spinal cord metastasis: A clinico-pathological study of 13 cases. *J Neurosurg* 1985; 62:227–233.
73. Grem JL, Burgess J, Trump DL: Clinical features and natural history of intramedullary spinal cord metastases. *Cancer* 1985; 56:2305–2314.
74. Donovan Post JM, Quencer RM, Green BA, et al: Intramedullary spinal cord metastases, mainly of non-neurogenic origin. *AJR* 1987; 148:1015–1022.
75. Scotti G, Scialfa G, Colombo N, et al: MR imaging of intradural extramedullary tumors of the cervical spine. *J Comput Assist Tomogr* 1985; 9:1037–1041.
76. Burk DL, Brunberg JA, Kanal E, et al: Spinal and paraspinal neurofibromatosis: Distinction from benign tumors using imaging techniques. *AJR* 1987; 149:1059–1064.
77. Levine E, Huntrakoon M, Wetzel LH: Malignant nerve sheath neoplasms in neurofibromatosis: Distinction from benign tumors using imaging techniques. *AJR* 1987; 149:1059–1064.
78. Custillo M, Quencer RM, Green BA, et al: Syringomyelia as a consequence of compressive extra-medullary lesions: Postoperative clinical and radiological manifestations. *AJNR* 1987; 8:973–978.
79. Quencer RM, EL Gammal T, Cohen G: Syringomyelia associated with intradural extramedullary masses of the spinal canal. *AJNR* 1986; 7:143–148.
80. Choremis C, Economos D, Papadatos C, et al: Intraspinal epidermoid tumors (cholesteatomas) in patients treated for tuberculous meningitis. *Lancet* 1956; 2:437–439.
81. Sachs E, Horrax G: A cervical and lumbar pilonidal sinus communicating with intraspinal dermoids: Report of 2 cases and review of the literature. *J Neurosurg* 1949; 6:97–112.
82. Monajati A, Spitzer RM, LaRue Wiley J, et al: MR imaging of a spinal teratoma. *J Comput Assist Tomogr* 1986; 10:307–310.
83. Feuerman T, Divan PS, Young RF: Vertebrectomy for treatment of vertebral hemangioma without preoperative embolization. *J Neurosurg* 1986; 65:404–406.
84. Mohan V, Gupta SK, Tuli SM, et al: Symptomatic vertebral hemangiomas. *Clin Radiol* 1980; 31:575–579.
85. Paige ML, Hemmati M: Spinal cord compression by vertebral hemangioma. *Pediatr Radiol* 1977; 6:43–45.
86. Murray RO, Jacobson HG: *Radiology of Skeletal Disorders,* ed 2. New York, Churchill Livingstone, 1977, p 578.

87. Wilmer D: *Radiology of Bone Tumors and Allied Disorders*. Philadelphia, WB Saunders Co, 1982; p 664.
88. Ross JS, Masaryk TJ, Modic MT, et al: Vertebral hemangiomas: MR imaging. *Radiology* 1987; 165:165–169.
89. Hajck PC, Baker LL, Goober JE, et al: Local fat deposition in axial bone marrow: MR characteristics. *Radiology* 1987; 162:245–249.
90. Hudson TM: Fluid levels in aneurysmal bone cysts: A CT feature. *AJR* 1984; 142:1001–1004.
91. Zimmer WD, Berquist TH, McLeod RA, et al: Bone tumors: Magnetic resonance imaging versus computed tomography. *Radiology* 1985; 155:709–718.
92. Zimmer WD, Berquist TH, Sim FH, et al: Magnetic resonance imaging at aneurysmal bone cysts. *Mayo Clin Proc* 1984; 59:633–636.
93. Hudson TM, Hamlin DJ, Fitzsimmons JR: Magnetic resonance imaging of fluid levels in an aneurysmal bone cyst and in anticoagulated human blood. *Skeletal Radiol* 1985; 13:267–270.
94. Beltran J, Simon DC, Levy M, et al: Aneurysmal bone cysts: MR imaging at 1.5 T. *Radiology* 1986; 158:689–690.
95. Hay MC, Paterson D, Taylor TKF: Aneurysmal bone cysts of the spine. *J Bone Joint Surg [Br]* 1978; 60:406–411.
96. Nosrat OA, Abbassioun K, Saleh H, et al: Aneurysmal bone cyst of the spine. *J Neurosurg,* 1985; 63:685–690.
97. Dahlin DC: *Bone tumors: General Aspects and Data on 6,221 Cases*. Springfield Ill, Charles C Thomas, 1978, pp 329–43.
98. Higinbothan NL, Phillips RF, Farr HW, et al: Chordoma: Thirty-five-year study at Memorial hospital. *Cancer* 1967; 20:1841–1850.
99. Mapstone TB, Kaufman B, Ratcheson RA: Intradural chordoma without bone involvement: Nuclear magnetic resonance (NMR) appearance. *J Neurosurg* 1983; 59:535–537.
100. Firooznia H, Pinto RS, Lin JP, et al: Chordoma: Radiologic evaluation of 20 cases. *AJR* 1976; 127:797–805.
101. Sze G, Vichanco LS, Brant-Zawadzki MN, et al: Chordomas: MR imaging. *Radiology* 1988; 166:187–191.
102. Friedman M, Kim TH, Panahon A: Spinal cord compression in malignant lymphoma. *Cancer* 1976; 37:1485–1491.
103. Boulian M: Neuroblastoma. *Pediatr Clin North Am* 1959; 6:449–472.
104. Gross RE, Farber S, Martin LW: Neuroblastoma sympatheticum: A study and report of 217 cases. *Pediatrics* 1959; 23:1179–1191.
105. Balakrishan V, Rice MG, Simpson DA: Spinal neuroblastomas: Diagnosis, treatment and prognosis. *J Neurosurg* 1974; 40:631–638.
106. Koop CE, Hernandez JR: Neuroblastoma experience with 100 cases in children. *Surgery* 1964; 56:726–733.
107. Sze G, Krol G, Zimmerman RD, et al: Malignant Extradural Spinal Tumors: MR Imaging with Gd-DTPA. *Radiology* 1988; 167:217–223.
108. Rosen BR, Carter EA, Pykett IL, et al: Proton chemical shift imaging: An evaluation of its clinical potential using an in vivo fatty liver model. *Radiology* 1985; 154:469–472.
109. Deom GC, Fisher MR, Hricak H, et al: Bone marrow imaging: Magnetic resonance studies related to age and sex. *Radiology* 1985; 155:429–432.
110. Ramsey RG, Zacharias CE: MR imaging of the spine after radiation therapy: Easily recognizable effects. *AJR* 1985; 144:1131–1135.
111. Daffner RH, Lupetin AR, Dash N, et al: MRI in the detection of malignant infiltration of bone marrow. *AJR* 1986; 146:353–358.
112. Olson DO, Shields AF, Scheurich CJ, et al: Magnetic resonance imaging of the bone marrow in patients with leukemia, aplastic anemia and lymphoma. *Invest Radiology* 1986; 21:540–546.
113. Moore SG, Gooding CA, Brasch RC, et al: Bone marrow in children with acute lymphocystic leukemia: MR relaxation times. *Radiology* 1986; 160:237–240.
114. Sugimura K, Yamusaki K, Kitagaki H, et al: Bone marrow diseases of the spine: Differentiation with T1 and T2 relaxation times in MR imaging. *Radiology* 1987; 165:541–544.
115. Brateman L: Chemical shift imaging: A review. *AJR* 1986; 146:971–980.
116. Wismer GL, Rosen BR, Buxton R, et al: Chemical shift imaging of bone marrow: Preliminary experience. *AJR* 1985; 145:1031–1037.
117. McKinstry CS, Steiner RE, Young AJ, et al: Bone marrow in leukemia and aplastic anemia: MR imaging before, during and after treatment. *Radiology* 1987; 162:701–707.
118. Oppenheim H: *Lehrbuch der Nervenkrankheiten Fur Arzte und Studierende,* ed 6. Berlin, S Karger, 1923, vol 1.
119. Hollis PM, Malis LI, Zappulla RA: Neurologic deterioration after lumbar puncture below complete spinal subarachnoid block. *J Neurosurg* 1986; 64:253–256.
120. Mapstone TB, Rekate HL, Shurin SB: Quadriplegia secondary to hematoma after lateral C1-2 puncture in a leukemic child. *Neurosurgery* 1983; 12:230–231.
121. Rengachary SS, Murphy D: Subarachnoid hematoma following lumbar puncture causing compression of the cauda equina: Case report. *J Neurosurg* 1974; 41:252–254.
122. Rogers LA: Acute subdural hematoma and death following lateral cervical spinal puncture: Case report. *J Neurosurg* 1983; 58:284–286.
123. Smoker WRK, Godersky JC, Knutzon RK, et al: The role of MR imaging in evaluating metastatic spinal disease. *AJNR* 1987; 8:901–908.

8

Spine Trauma

Thomas J. Masaryk, M.D.

The primary concern in the diagnostic evaluation of spine trauma is the recognition of actual or potential permanent spinal cord injury. While the estimated annual incidence of spinal cord injury in the United States is only 40 to 50 cases per million, the resultant loss and hardships placed on the patients, their families, and society cannot be overemphasized.[1–4] Medical care of these patients is directed at preventing the progression of cord injury, either by relieving compression or stabilizing the patient's condition to facilitate healing. This chapter reviews fundamental pathologic and diagnostic concepts of spine trauma with respect to present and future roles of magnetic resonance imaging (MRI) in the management of these injuries.

Spine trauma can typically be classified as (1) lesions or defects resulting from sharp or penetrating injury, and (2) blunt trauma. The pathologist might further characterize traumatic lesions as "primary," "secondary," "late sequelae," and "late complications." Primary lesions are those resulting from direct mechanical force on tissue. Secondary or reactive alterations are most commonly post-traumatic vascular disruptions. Late sequelae are the natural results of healing (e.g., scar, myelomalacia), while late complications would include such entities as infection or syringomyelia.

PENETRATING (OPEN) TRAUMA

The incidence of open or penetrating spine trauma ranges from over 75% of spine casualties in wartime, to 12% of civilian spine injuries.[1, 5, 6] The majority of civilian missile injuries are produced by bullets from handguns. Injuries by other types of missiles, such as fragments of metal, rocks, or debris from explosions are relatively rare. Classification schemes for such injuries are based on type (direct vs. indirect) of damage to the spinal cord and location of the missile after impact.[7, 8] Direct lesions result from passage of the missile across the spinal canal. Under such circumstances, cord transsection is not uncommon and has been reported even in the absence of significant osseous disruption.[7] More commonly, however, the cord escapes direct damage but is compressed or contused by bony fragments or blast effects (Fig 8–1). As one might expect, civilian missile injuries are less extensive than wounds inflicted during military combat.[5, 6, 9]

By contrast, puncture or stab wounds involving the spine are typically well-defined cuts, most commonly located in the thoracic spine (74%).[10] This type of clearly delimited lesion attracts considerable clinical interest owing to the close correlation between lesion and symptoms.[11] The degree of damage to the cord varies according to the level of injury, character of the weapon, and force of delivery. As the vertebral laminae protect the spinal cord dorsally, stab wounds typically enter lateral to the midline and produce asymmetric dorsolateral lesions (Fig 8–2).

Pathologically, penetrating wounds produce slits or tears of the meninges that are frequently hemorrhagic. The ends of the torn dura will tend to approximate, while the margins of the cord wound separate (see Fig 8–2). Histologically, there are three zones constituting the spinal cord wound: (1) a debris zone with total liquefaction necrosis and hemorrhage; (2) a petechial zone with indirect but irreversible damage, as evidenced by vacuolization and decreased stainability; and (3) a zone of reversible, peritraumatic intracellular edema composed of swollen astroglia.[12, 13] The central area of primary debris rapidly undergoes dissolution and clearing of blood pigments, while the petechial zone accumulates red blood cells over the first 24 hours. Astroglial edema is maximal between 2 and 12 hours.

After the immediate post-traumatic necrosis (36 to

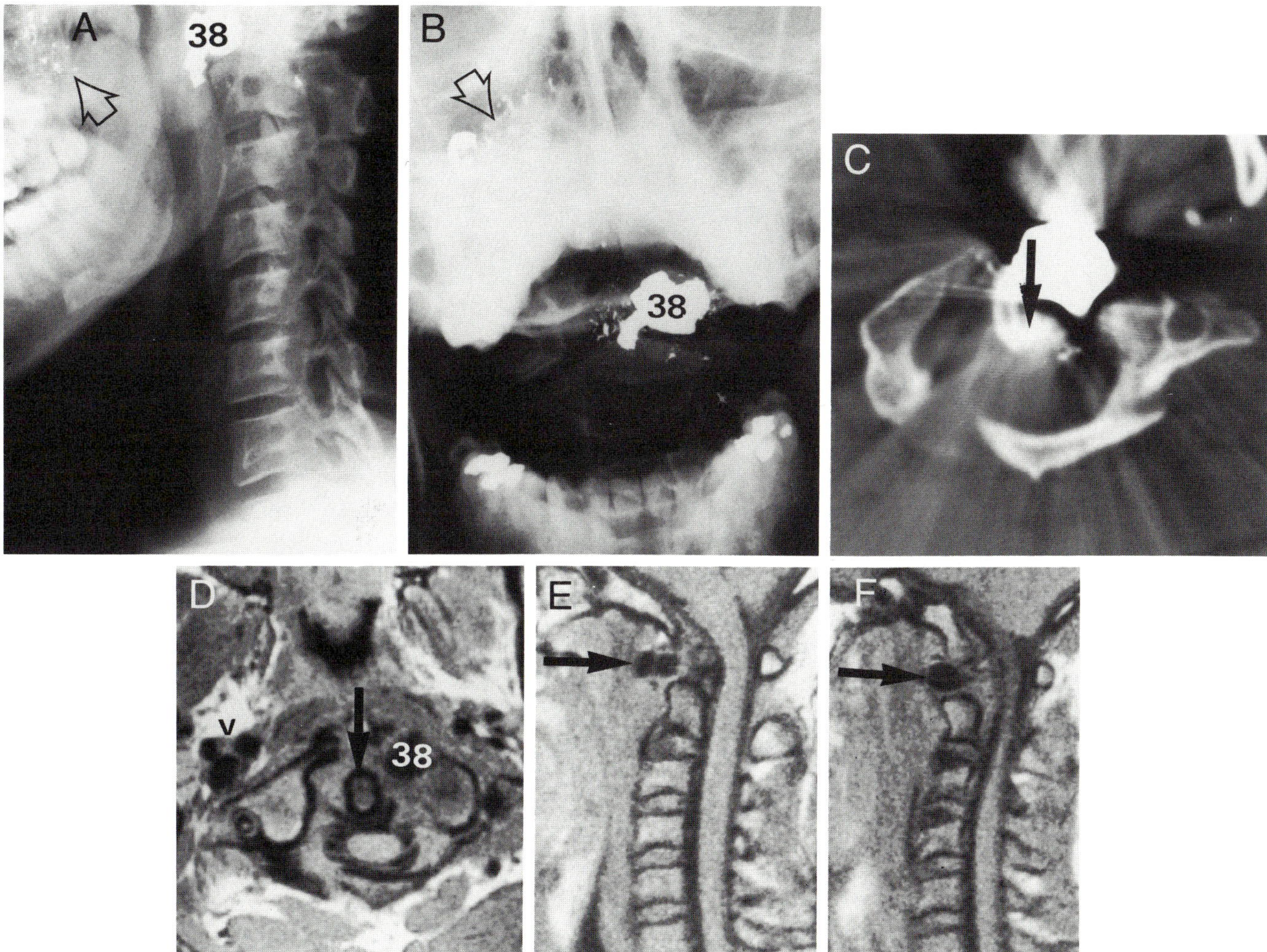

FIG 8–1.
A, lateral radiograph of the cervical spine in a victim of an armed robbery, in which the weapon was fired point-blank into the nose. Lead fragments remain within the nasal cavity *(open arrow)* while the majority of the .38-caliber slug can be seen against the dens. **B,** open-mouth view, again demonstrating debris within the right nasal cavity and maxillary antrum *(open arrow)* as well as the bulk of the bullet *(38)* just left of midline. **C,** axial CT scan performed on the level of the dens demonstrates fracture of the atlas with posterior displacement of the odontoid *(arrow).* **D,** similar axial MR scan performed using 500-msec TR/17-msec TE spin-echo technique likewise demonstrates fracture of the atlas with the signal void immediately anterior to the displaced dens *(arrow)* representing the bullet fragment *(38).* Notice that it is difficult to distinguish the neurovascular bundle *(v)* from additional bullet fragments. **E,** sagittal 500-msec TR/17-msec TE midline image demonstrates displaced, fractured dens abutting the cervicomedullary junction with the bullet fragment *(arrow)* seen immediately anterior. Notice the significant amount of soft tissue swelling present within the oropharynx. **F,** parasagittal 500-msec TR/17-msec TE image of the cervical spine just left of midline again demonstrates the bulk of the bullet fragment *(arrow)* completely replacing the anterior arch of C1.

48 hours), there is reabsorption and organization by phagocytes and microglia, with astroglial and mesenchymal proliferation at the wound margins. Subsequently, damaged spinal cord is replaced by gliofibrous scar at 3 to 4 weeks. Grossly, incompletely transsected cord segments are thin and hard secondary to the union of meninges to cord and spinal canal by collagenous scar. The meninges may demonstrate local hemosiderin deposition in this region and may also become thickened to the point of mimicking an extradural mass that extends over several segments.[14, 15] Similar cicatrization may occur in the arachnoid, producing CSF cavities and "adhesive arachnoiditis." Following complete cord transsection there may be dehiscence of the disrupted ends, with thickening of the meninges adherent to the dura and stump.

Secondary lesions and late sequelae include intramedullary cysts secondary to remote liquefaction necro-

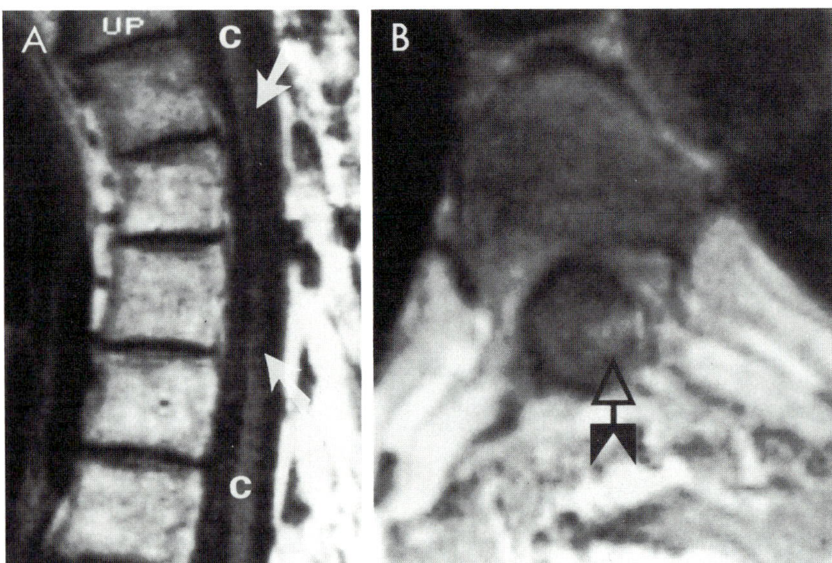

FIG 8–2.
A, midline sagittal 500-msec TR/17-msec TE image of the thoracic spine in a patient with Brown-Sequard syndrome following a stab wound to the spine. The cord is identified *(c)* above and below an area of extreme of thinning of the spinal cord at the site of the lesion *(arrows).* **B,** axial 500-msec TR/17-msec TE image of the same patient demonstrates remaining half of the cord unaffected by the stab wound on the left *(arrow).*

sis or dissecting CSF pressure shifts, as well as secondary degeneration of ascending and descending fiber tracts at areas of transsection (see Fig 8–2).

Late complications generally are inflammatory lesions such as extradural or subdural empyema, leptomeningitis, and cord infection. However, such sequelae are rare even in the presence of bullets, knife fragments, or splinters, which are often surrounded by dense collagenous connective tissue with fibrous reactive change.[5, 6, 16]

Concerning management of such injuries, surgical intervention rarely changes neurologic outcome in cases of direct, penetrating trauma. In the absence of a communication between the wound, foreign bodies, and skin, the chance of infection is rare with appropriate antibiotic therapy.[5, 6, 9] Thus, without spine instability or blunt cord compression, immediate interventional therapy is usually limited to debridement.[9] If a more extensive surgical procedure is required, preoperative imaging beyond plain radiographs and tomography may be necessary. Should MRI be considered, it is necessary for the consulting radiologist to be aware of the presence and composition of metallic foreign bodies. For example, bullets may be homogeneous (e.g., lead, zinc, magnesium, plastic), "coated" (e.g., lead covered by a thin layer of copper or brass) and "jacketed" (core of lead or steel surrounded by a thicker layer of copper or steel)[17] (Fig 8–3). Patients with such metallic foreign bodies may be at risk for ferromagnetic interactions with the imager, including (1) local tissue heating secondary to radiofrequency (RF) deposition, (2) motion of the foreign fragment related to the static or gradient magnetic fields, and (3) eddy current effects secondary to the applied gradient fields that may locally degrade the image (military ammunition is more commonly ferromagnetic) (see Fig 8–3). Reports already exist for complications resulting from ferromagnetic-induced motion of a foreign body within the CNS.[18] Our personal experience with a small number of civilian gunshot wounds has indicated that MRI may safely produce valuable information concerning the location of bullet fragments with respect to the spinal cord, without significant artifact (unlike x-ray CT). However, it may be difficult to distinguish the signal void of lead bullets from nearby vessels or densely calcified structures (see Fig 8–1).

CLOSED TRAUMA

Mechanism of Injury

Closed spine trauma is the result of both blunt forces transmitted to the spine and penetrating injuries that do not pierce the canal. Due to the static condition of the spine and neural axis, the lower cervical region and thoracolumbar junction are the most frequent sites of traumatic damage, although the frequency distribution at the level of the traumatic lesion varies in different series.[19–21] While there is no ideal classification of closed spinal cord injuries in terms of pathogenesis, the anatomic deformities (with or without neurological deficit) are most often described in terms of the forces that produced the trauma relative to the salient anatomic features of the vertebral level involved. Thus, there are general patterns of spine trauma that recur and merit separate descriptions. Most commonly an attempt is made to classify an injury as (1) flexion, (2) extension, (3) vertical compression (axial loading), or (4) rota-

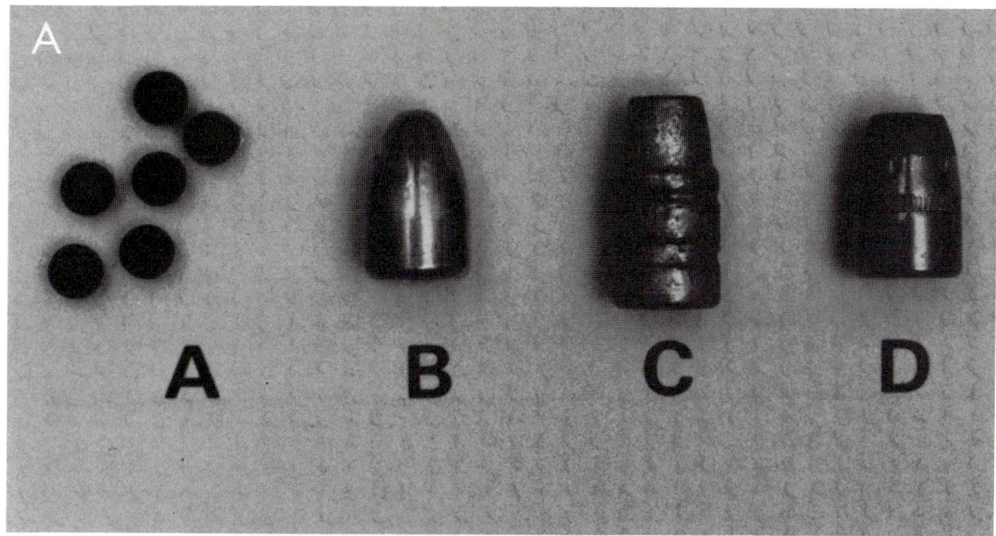

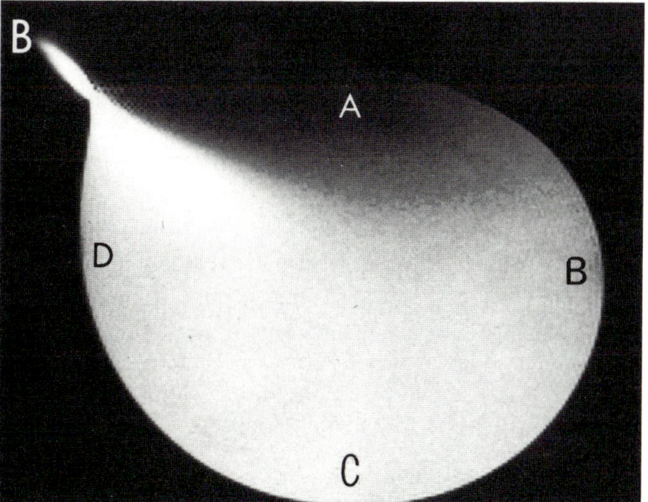

FIG 8–3.
A, examples of various civilian ammunition includes steel BBs *(A)*, 9-mm round with full copper jacket *(B)*, .38-caliber lead slug *(C)*, and hollow point, semi–copper jacketed .357 round *(D)*. **B,** phantom study performed with ammunition demonstrated in **A** placed symmetrically about the phantom. Note that the most significant distortion of the image occurs at the site of the steel BBs *(A)*. Only minimal local field distortion can be seen at the site of the full copper jacket 9-mm round *(B)*, while the .357 and .38-caliber ammunition *(C)* leaves the image relatively unaffected. (Ballistics courtesy of Gregory Group.)

tion.[22–24] Frequently, the mechanism of insult is actually a combination of the above.[25]

Craniovertebral Junction

Physiologic motion of the craniovertebral junction (i.e., occiput, atlas, axis) includes flexion, extension, rotation, axial loading, and lateral bending.[26–28] The integrity of the atlanto-occipital articulation is maintained by the tectorial membrane, posterior atlanto-occipital membrane and the alar and apical ligaments. The atlantoaxial joint is reinforced by the apical, alar, and (the especially durable) transverse ligaments.[29] Added support is lent by the anterior and posterior longitudinal ligaments.

The most common mechanism of injury at the craniovertebral junction is flexion. Extreme flexion and rotation injuries are not uncommon in newborn infants; acute hemorrhage or hemorrhagic cord necrosis may occur even in the absence of fracture (Figs 8–4 and 8–5).[30] However, flexion fracture-dislocation of the atlanto-occipital articulation is rarely seen in adults, primarily because these patients seldom survive.[31] Upper cervical spine flexion trauma most commonly manifests in fracture or (less frequently) dislocation of the dens. Odontoid fractures are classified as type I (avulsion), type II

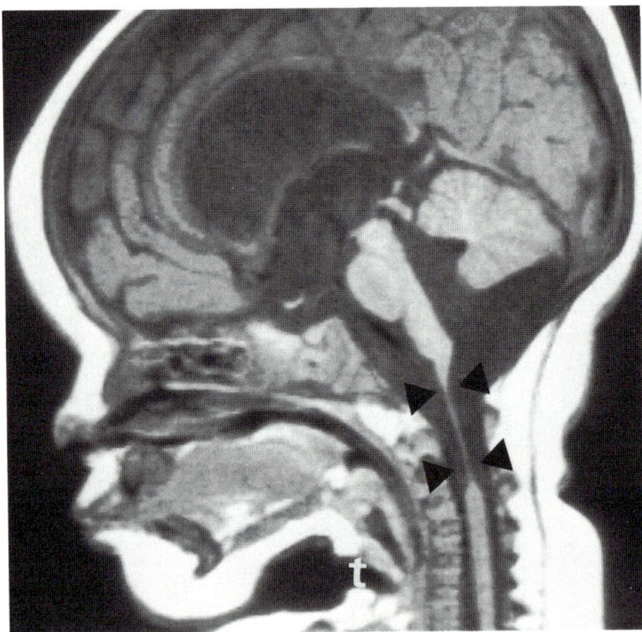

FIG 8–4.
Sagittal 50-msec TR/17-msec TE in an infant following flexion injury during delivery. Note the marked thinning of the upper cervical spinal cord *(arrowheads)*. Tracheostomy tube (t) is identified inferiorly.

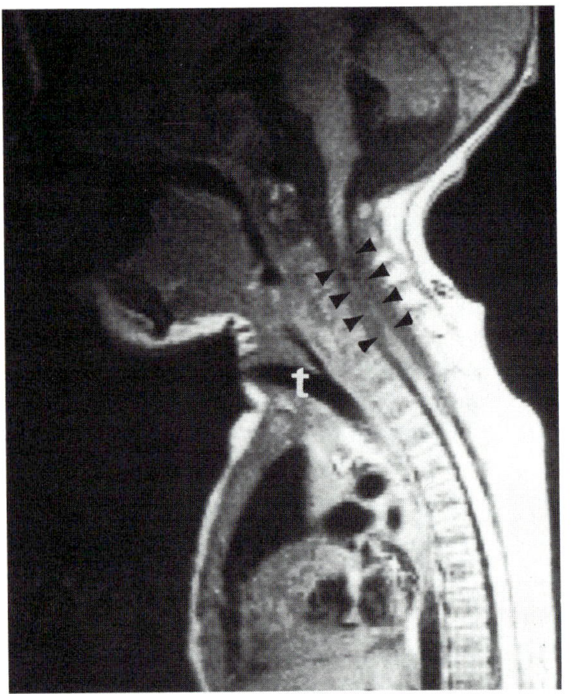

FIG 8–5.
Another example of flexion birth injury demonstrated on a 500-msec TR/17-msec TE midline sagittal image. There appears to be complete transsection of the cervical spinal cord *(arrowheads)*. Again, tracheostomy tube is seen in place *(t)*.

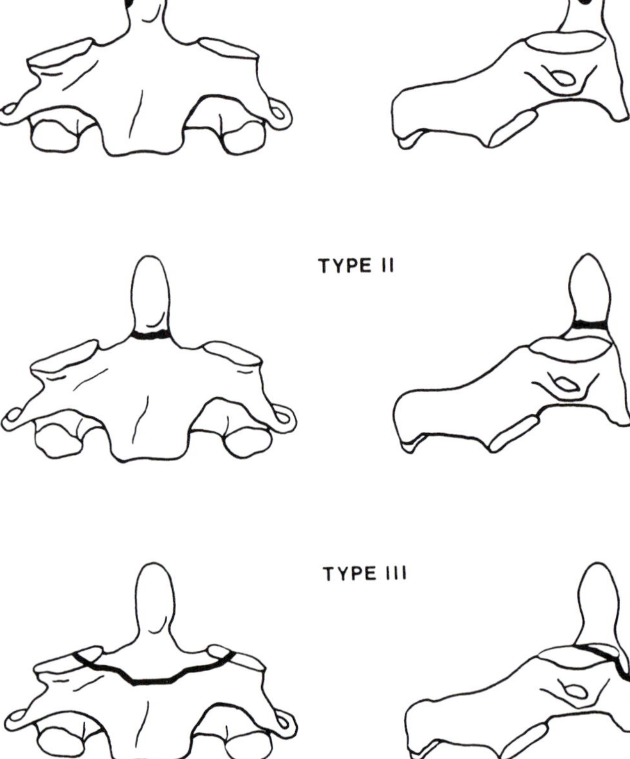

FIG 8–6.
Three types of odontoid fractures.

(involving the body), and type III (basilar) (Fig 8–6).[32] It is worth noting that type II fracture demonstrates the highest incidence of non-union and delayed instability (Fig 8–7).

Extension injuries have also been reported to fracture the odontoid, but this is unusual. More commonly, extension produced through sudden deceleration results in fracture of the posterior ring of the atlas or bilateral fracture of the pedicles of the axis.[33] Anterior avulsion fractures of the axis with severe extension injury may also be seen.

Direct axial loading with forces transmitted through the lateral masses of the atlas typically produce bilateral fractures that spread the lateral masses.[34]

Rotational injury to the craniovertebral junction is uncommon, as are neurological deficits with upper cervical injuries.[34,35]

Lower Cervical Spine

In the lower cervical spine, stabilizing soft tissue and bone may be divided into anterior and posterior columns. The anterior group is composed of vertebral bodies, intervertebral disks, and anterior and posterior

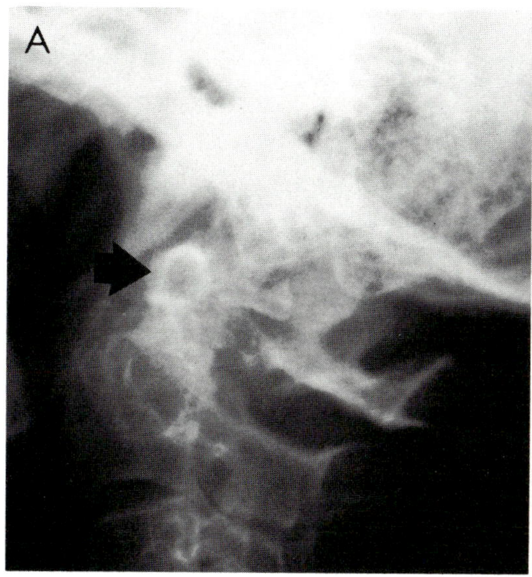

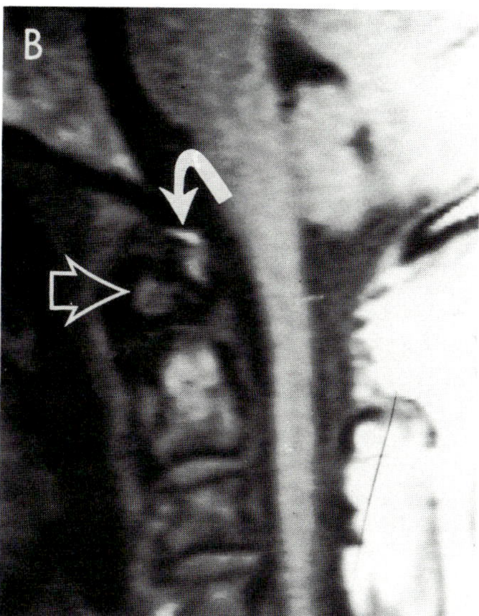

FIG 8–7.
A, lateral plain film radiographs of patient with remote odontoid fracture. The dens is not well visualized, while the body of C2 can be seen directly beneath the anterior arch of C1 *(arrow)*. **B,** sagittal 500-msec TR/17-msec TE demonstrates non-union of a remote type II odontoid fracture with partial reabsorption of the dens *(curved arrow)* and subluxation of the body of C2 beneath the anterior arch of the atlas *(open arrow)*.

longitudinal ligaments. The posterior apparatus is formed from the spinous processes and interspinous ligaments, laminae and ligamentum flavum, facet joints and vertebral body pedicles. Instability of this complex results from the disruption of these columns and is defined as the loss of the relationship between vertebrae such that there is damage or subsequent irritation of the spinal cord or nerve roots, or, in addition, the development of incapacitating deformity or pain due to structural changes.[36] More objective criteria include the displacement of two adjacent vertebrae greater than 3.5 mm and angulation greater than 11 degrees.[36]

Flexion injuries of the lower cervical spine may result in disk protrusion, vertebral body wedge compression fracture, tears of the posterior ligaments, subluxation of the articular processes, fracture-dislocation, or severe central cord necrosis or hemorrhage (Fig 8–8).

Subluxation resulting from flexion produces tears of the articular joint capsules, posterior ligaments, and posterior annulus. In the past, these were infrequently recognized by radiologists, but are significant for their relatively high incidence of delayed instability (Figs 8–9 and 8–10).[37] More dramatic forward displacement may result in bilateral interfacet dislocation (bilateral "locked" or "perched" facets). The dislocated facets pass upward and forward over the inferior facets of the joint and come to lie in the intervertebral foramina. Bilateral facet dislocation is associated with a high incidence of cord damage resulting from a compression between the

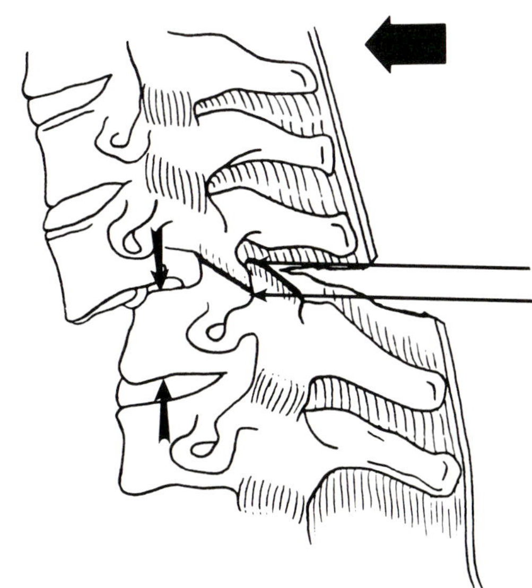

FIG 8–8.
Diagramatic representation of flexion injury of the cervical spine. Such injuries typically result from force applied in the posterior to anterior direction in the upper cervical spine *(thick black arrow)*. As the spine is driven forward, such force may be transmitted vertically to produce compression of a more inferior vertebral body *(vertical arrows)*. With extreme forward motion of the upper spine, there may be disruption of the interspinous ligament, and/ or the joint capsule of the articular facets *(long horizontal arrows)*.

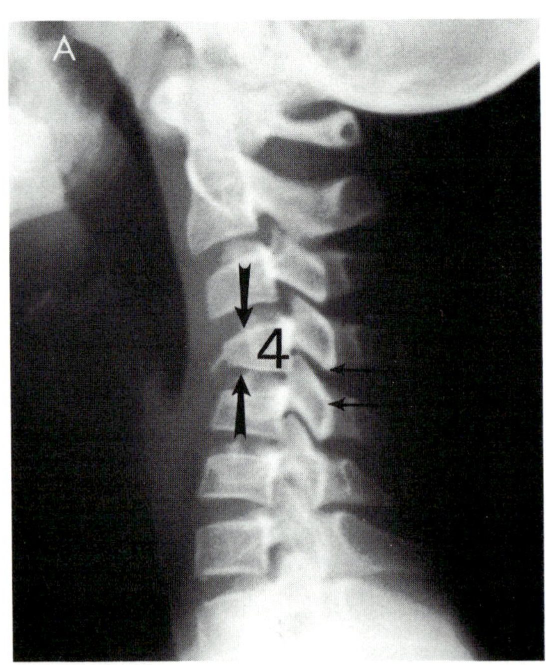

FIG 8–9.
A, lateral radiograph of the cervical spine in a patient with flexion injury at C4–5. Notice the wedge compression of the C4 vertebral bodies *(vertical arrows)* and mild distraction of the C4 and C5 facets *(horizontal arrows).* Flexion films failed to demonstrate any significant instability. **B,** sagittal 500-msec TR/17-msec TE image likewise demonstrates wedge compression of C4 *(vertical arrows).* **C,** parasagittal 500-msec TR/17-msec TE image again demonstrates slight distraction of the facet joints at this level *(arrows).* **D** and **E,** similar findings are observed on these 10-degree FISP sagittal and parasagittal scans. There is no evidence of posterior ligamentous disruption on the MR examination.

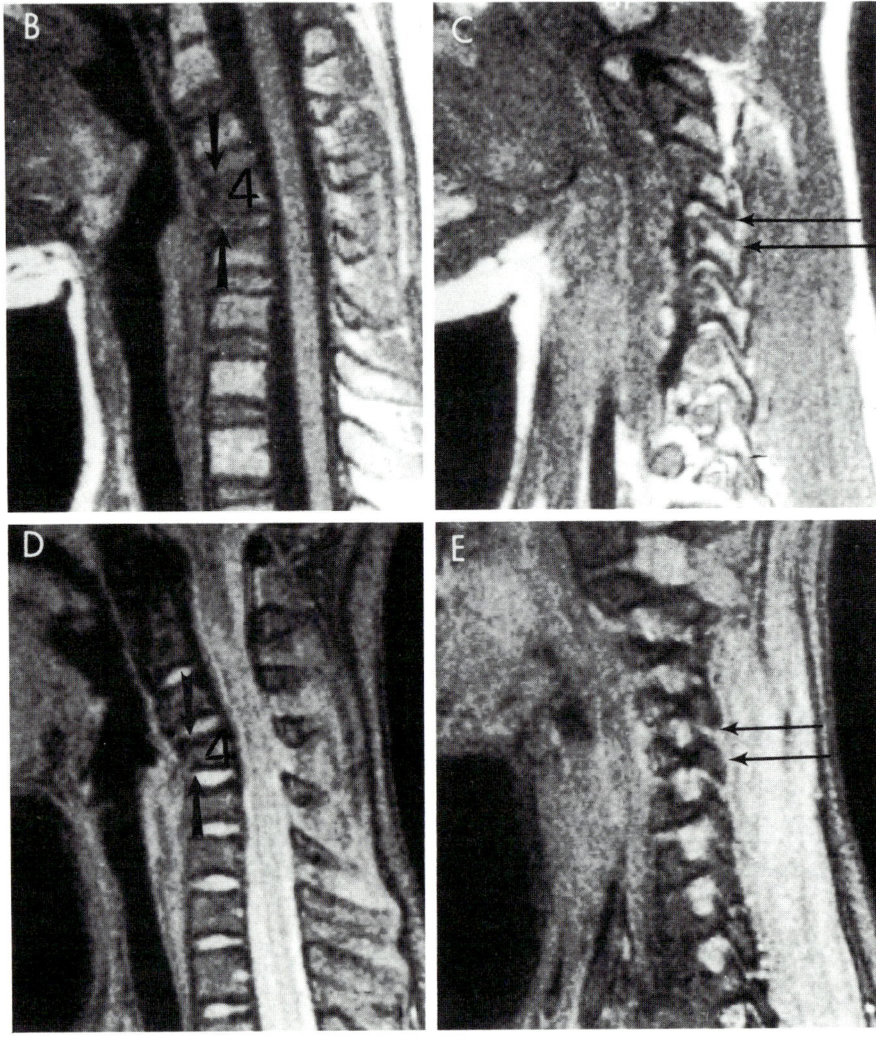

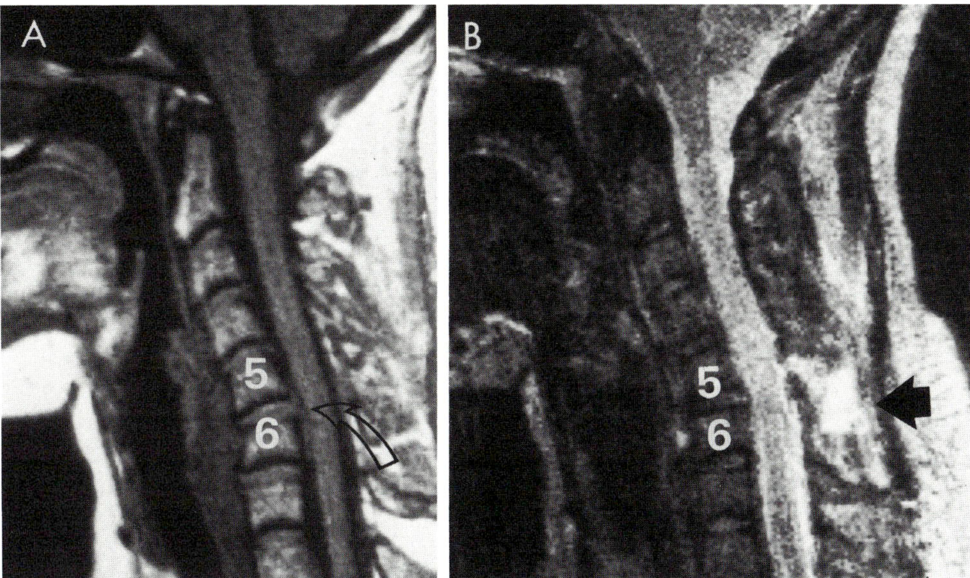

FIG 8–10.
A, sagittal 500-msec TR/17-msec TE image in a patient with a flexion injury and anterior cord syndrome. Given point of flexion was at C5–6. Notice the traumatic disk herniation at this level *(open arrow).* A less prominent disk herniation is also noted at C4–5. **B,** midline sagittal 2,000-msec TR/120-msec TE scan does not demonstrate the traumatic disk herniation as well as the T_1-weighted study. However, this T_2-weighted examination points out a previously unsuspected disruption of the intraspinous ligaments, which can be seen as a wedge-shaped area of increased signal intensity behind C5–6 *(arrow).*

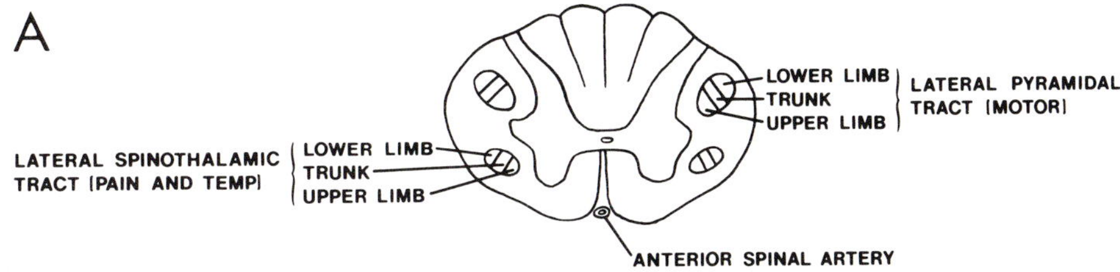

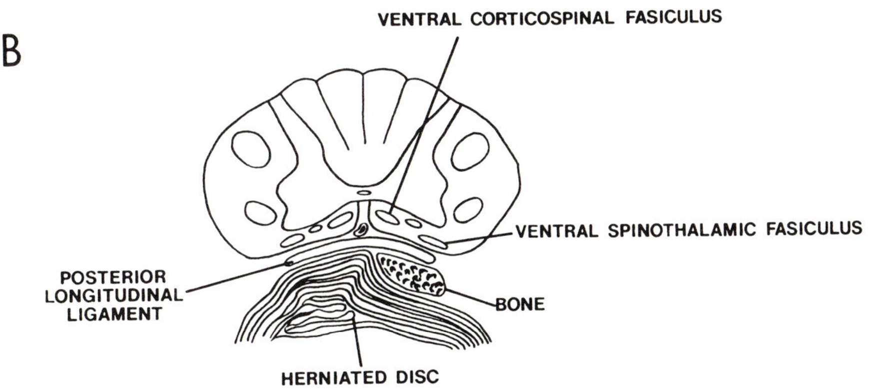

FIG 8–11.
A, schematic representation of a cross section of the cervical spinal cord demonstrating the relative positions of the ascending and descending fiber tracts. **B,** schematic representation of the affected portions of the cord in the so-called anterior cord syndrome.

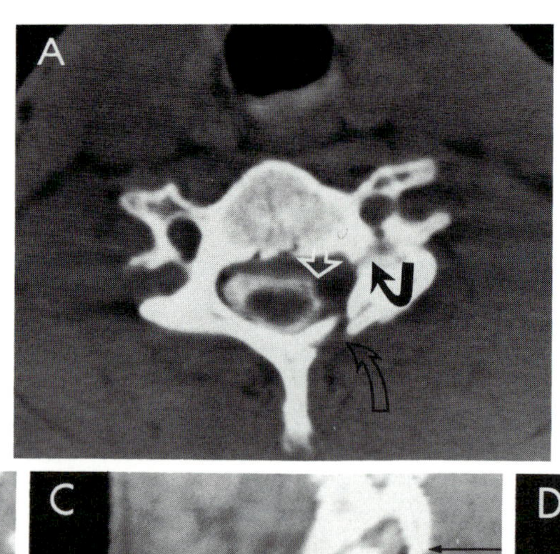

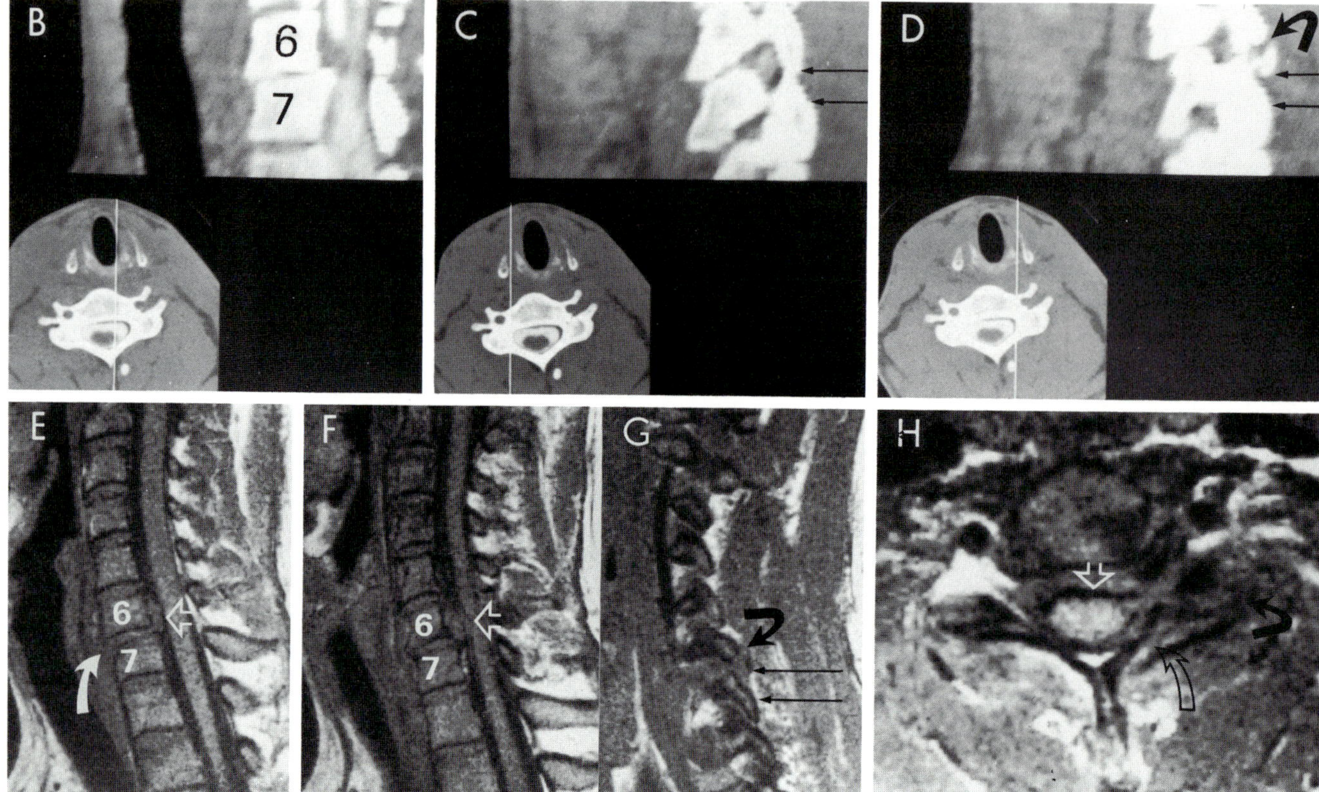

FIG 8–12.

Flexion-rotation injury. **A,** axial CT scan through the level of the C6 pedicle in a patient with a flexion-rotation injury. As the patient's head and upper cervical spine were flexed over C6, additional right-to-left rotation forces were applied, causing the spine to pivot (and thus crush) the left C6 pedicle and facet while producing subluxation on the contralateral side. This scan demonstrates fractures of the left pedicle and lamine *(curved arrow)* as well as a traumatic disk herniation *(open arrow)* in the lateral recess on the left. **B,** sagittal reconstruction of the post-myelogram CT demonstrates C6–7 subluxation as well as a soft tissue mass anterior to the thecal sac. **C,** right parasagittal reconstruction of this examination demonstrate subluxation of the right C6–7 facets. *(arrows).* **D,** left parasagittal reconstructions demonstrate the fractured C6 facet *(curved arrow)* and distraction of the joint itself *(straight arrow),* indicating instability. **E,** midline sagittal 500-msec TR/17-msec TE image demonstrates a traumatic disk herniation at C6–7 with an anterior extradural mass immediately behind the body of C6 *(open arrow).* Notice that there has been disruption of the anterior longitudinal ligament at C6–7 *(curved arrow).* F left parasagittal 500-msec TR/17-msec TE image again demonstrates the traumatic disk herniation at C6–7 *(open arrow).* **G,** parasagittal 500-msec TR/17-msec TE image at C6–7 on the left demonstrate some distraction of the facet joints *(horizontal arrows)* as well as fracture of the C6 facet *(curved arrow)* secondary to the pivoting action of the flexion-rotation force. **H,** axial 500-msec TR/17-msec TE image through the C6 vertebral body again demonstrates a fractured lamina *(open curved arrow),* disrupted facet joint (curved arrow), and traumatic disk herniation *(open straight arrow).*

posterior part of the inferior vertebral body and the dislocated/fractured posterior arch of the upper vertebrae.[38, 39]

A flexion teardrop fracture-dislocation is the most severe injury of the lower cervical spine.[40] It consists of vertebral body fracture with forward subluxation or dislocation of the posterior elements and ligamentous disruption. It is often associated with the anterior cord syndrome, which is defined as complete motor paralysis with loss of pain and temperature sensation, but with sparing of the sense of position, vibration, and motion in the posterior column[41] (Fig 8–11).

In conjunction with rotational forces, flexion may produce unilateral facet dislocation. The rotational force is directed about one facet, which acts as a pivot point, while flexion causes the contralateral facet to dislocate (Fig 8–12). This condition is characterized by mechanical stability, even though the posterior ligament complex is disrupted.[42]

Severe extension trauma to the cervical spine forces the spinous and articular processes of the midcervical vertebrae together. The posterior column becomes a fulcrum separating the vertebral body and subjacent intervertebral disk (Fig 8–13), and resulting in dislocation or ventral fracture dislocation with concomitant compression or fracture of the articular processes and disruption (and displacement) of the disk. With sufficient force, the separation may proceed and rupture the anterior and posterior longitudinal ligaments. The buckling of the posterior longitudinal ligament may decrease the anteroposterior dimensions of the spinal canal, producing complete or partial cord transsection[43] (Fig 8–14). This squeezing mechanism frequently produces the most extensive hemorrhage and necrosis within the central part of the cord[44] (Fig 8–15).

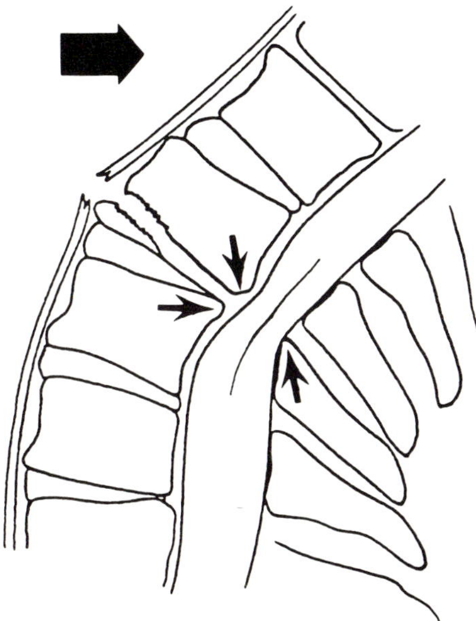

FIG 8–13.
Schematic representation of a cervical extension injury. With the force of the injury directed from anterior to posteior *(thick horizontal arrow)* there can be disruption of the antherior longitudinal ligament and disk, with pinching of the spinal cord as the superior vertebral body is driven toward the posterior elements at the lower level.

Thoracic Spine

Compressive (axial loading) forces secondary to vertical impact (e.g., diving accidents) are absorbed by the vertebral bodies, resulting in vertical or burst fractures. Ligaments are typically intact. As mentioned previously, spine injuries are more commonly seen in the upper cervical or thoracic spine, but between T2 and T10, flexion and axial loading are the most common mechanisms of injury. In general, however, because of the stability provided by the rib cage, costovertebral ligaments, and intervertebral disks, the thoracic spine is resistant to all but the most violent trauma.[45] Also, even in the presence of fracture or fracture-dislocation the upper thoracic spine remains quite stable by virtue of these supporting structures. The sagittally placed facet joints in the thoracic spine limit the potential for rotational forces to produce trauma. Nevertheless, it is worth mentioning that the actual thoracic vertebral canal is quite small, with only marginal allowance for traumatic disk herniations or fracture fragments prior to cord compression.

Lumbar Spine

Unlike the upper thoracic spine, which is braced by adjacent ribs, the thoracolumbar junction acts as a fulcrum for spine motion and is thus susceptible to unstable traumatic injury. While the thick, sagittally oriented facets may minimize rotational components to injury; flexion, or flexion-dislocation, and axial loading injury are common (Figs 8–16 and 8–17). These forces frequently combine to produce flexion-compression injury or the so-called "burst fractures," which are significant for (1) motion instability and (2) a predisposition for displacing fracture fragments and causing cord compromise, respectively[24, 26] (Figs 8–18 and 8–19).

An analogous lumbar spine injury associated with rapid-deceleration motor vehicle accidents is the so-called "seat-belt" or "Chance" fracture. Hyperflexion occurs with the fulcrum occurring at the level of the seat belt, while the upper lumbar spine experiences tensile loading. The result is a horizontal fracture through both the anterior and posterior elements.[47, 48]

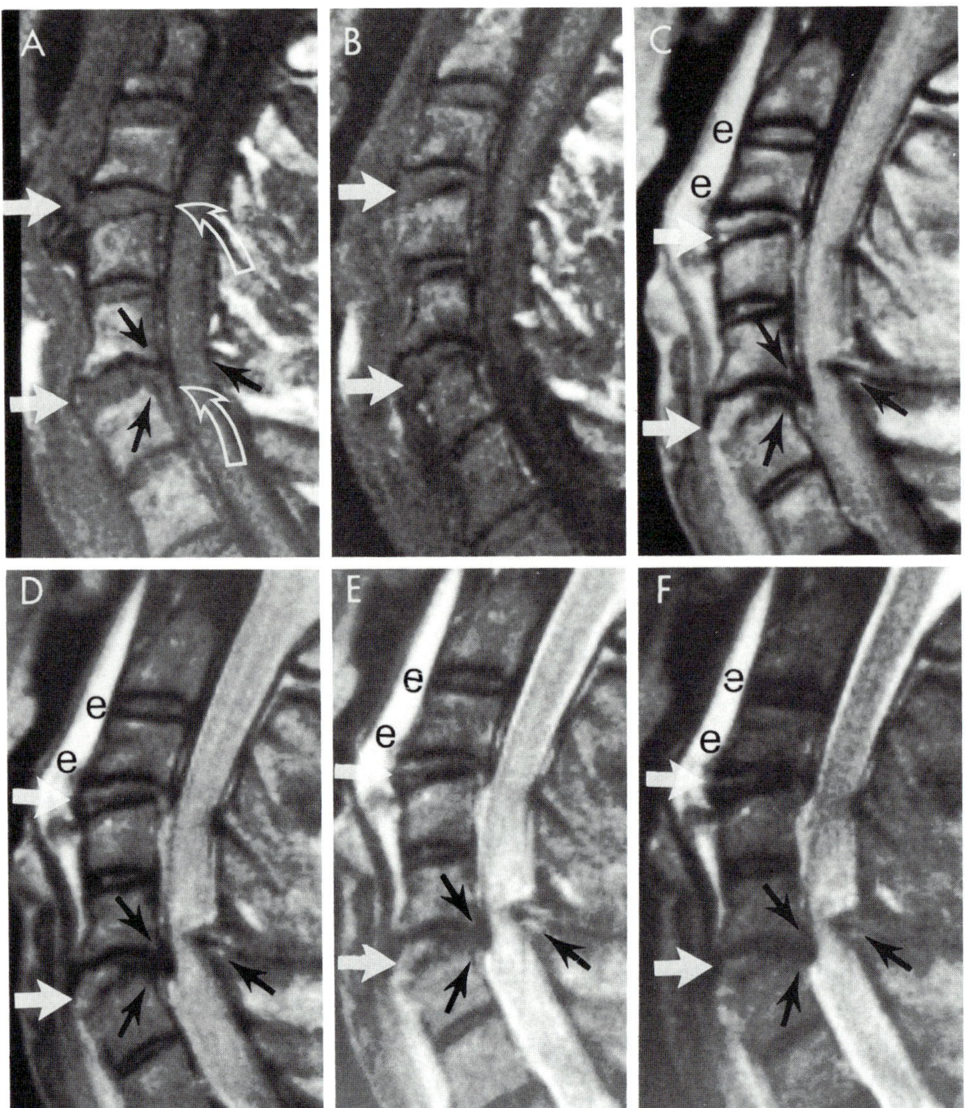

FIG 8–14.

A, 500—sec TR/17-msec TE sagittal image in a patient who sustained a cervical extension injury. Notice the disruption of the anterior longitudinal ligament at multiple levels *(solid white arrows)* as well as the traumatic disk herniations *(open arrow).* Pinching action takes place at the C5–6 level *(black arrows).* **B,** parasagittal 500-msec TR/17-msec image again demonstrates the anterior longitudinal ligament disruption *(arrows).* Notice the prevertebral soft tissue swelling as well. **C,** midline sagittal 2,000-msec TR/30-msec TE 7-mm image again demonstrates the ligamentous disruption *(white arrows),* prevertebral edema *(e)* and pinching action at C5–6 *(black arrows).* Notice that the compromise of the canal appears more serious on this 7-mm sagittal image, most likely related to partial volume effect from the lamina laterally. **D,** 2,000-msec TR/60-msec TE midline sagittal image demonstrates similar findings again with prevertebral edema *(e),* ligamentous disruption *(white arrows)* as well as some vague increase in signal intensity of the spinal cord at the site of compression *(black arrows).* **E** and **F,** 2,000-msec TR/90- and 120-msec TE images, respectively. Similar findings as previously noted, although the increased signal intensity within the spinal cord secondary to edema is more obvious on these more T_2-weighted scans. The absence of any significant focal areas of decreased signal intensity within these regions indicate a relative absence of intramedullary hemorrhage (contusion) and a more favorable prognosis. Despite initially severe neurologic deficit, this patient went on to recover significant function.

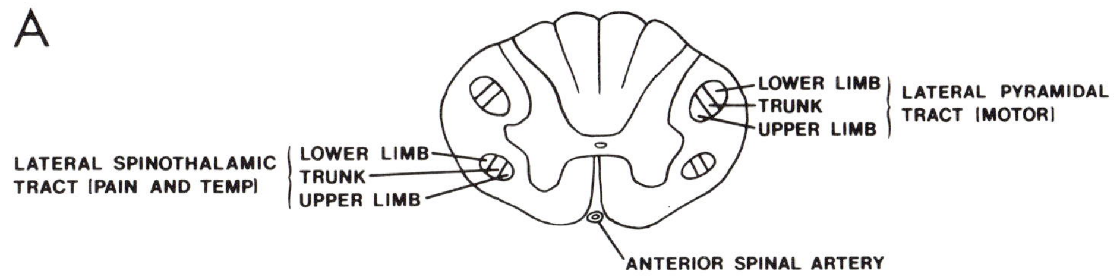

B

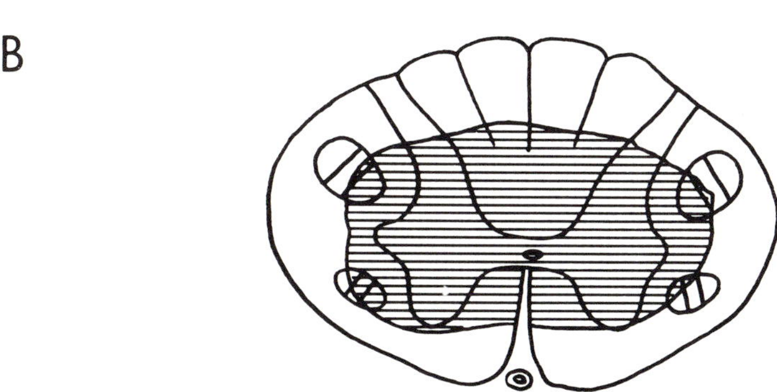

CENTRAL CORD SYNDROME

FIG 8–15.
A, schematic representation of the relative positions of the ascending and descending fiber tracts of the cervical spinal cord. **B,** schematic representation of those tracts involved in central cord syndrome, frequently the result of severe cervical extension injury. This may be aggravated by pre-existing cervical spondylosis, or posterior osteophytes.

SPINAL CORD INJURY

Concussion, Contusion, Compression

There is a wide range of reaction of the spinal cord, roots, coverings, and vasculature to closed injuries. Primary spinal cord lesions can be related to the site, intensity, and distribution of impact, biochemical and electrophysiological derangements, and hemodynamic changes.[49, 50]

Concussion of the spinal cord implies a purely functional derangement, attributed to a variety of conditions and etiologies. This loosely defined condition is a reversible disorder of the spinal cord that has been attributed to temporary changes in function of interneuronal transmitters or, possibly, transient deficiencies in the spinal cord microcirculation.[8, 51–53]

Spinal contusion includes all injuries (in the absence of continuing compression) that exceed the reversible, functional disturbance known as concussion.[13] Grossly, such contusion injuries range in severity from mild intramedullary (petechial) hemorrhage with edema, to extensive pulverization and rhexic bleeding, to complete transsection. Of note is the role played by the cord microvasculature in the pathophysiology of such lesions.[54–57] The early stages feature intramedullary hemorrhage involving the central gray matter, which extends centrifugally with the severity of trauma.[54, 55] Edema, in conjunction with hemorrhagic necrosis and liquefaction necrosis is also present within the central gray matter.[54, 55] Although edema, necrosis, and hemorrhage are often localized to the region of direct trauma, the bleeding may extend in a tapering fashion, cephalocaudad over several segments, to produce the condition known as hematomyelia. Alterations in cord microcirculation with bleeding and hemorrhagic necrosis maximize at 24 to 48 hours, while post-traumatic edema peaks at 3 to 6 days.

After 1 to 2 weeks, the edema has subsided and the blood pigments are absorbed while the damaged segment undergoes demyelination. Eventually there is cystic dissolution of the central necrotic area.[58] The margins of the injured region are characterized by reactive gliosis and vascular proliferation. As with open wounds, there may be dense fibrous scarring of the leptomeninges at the site of fracture-dislocation that may adhere to the damaged cord.

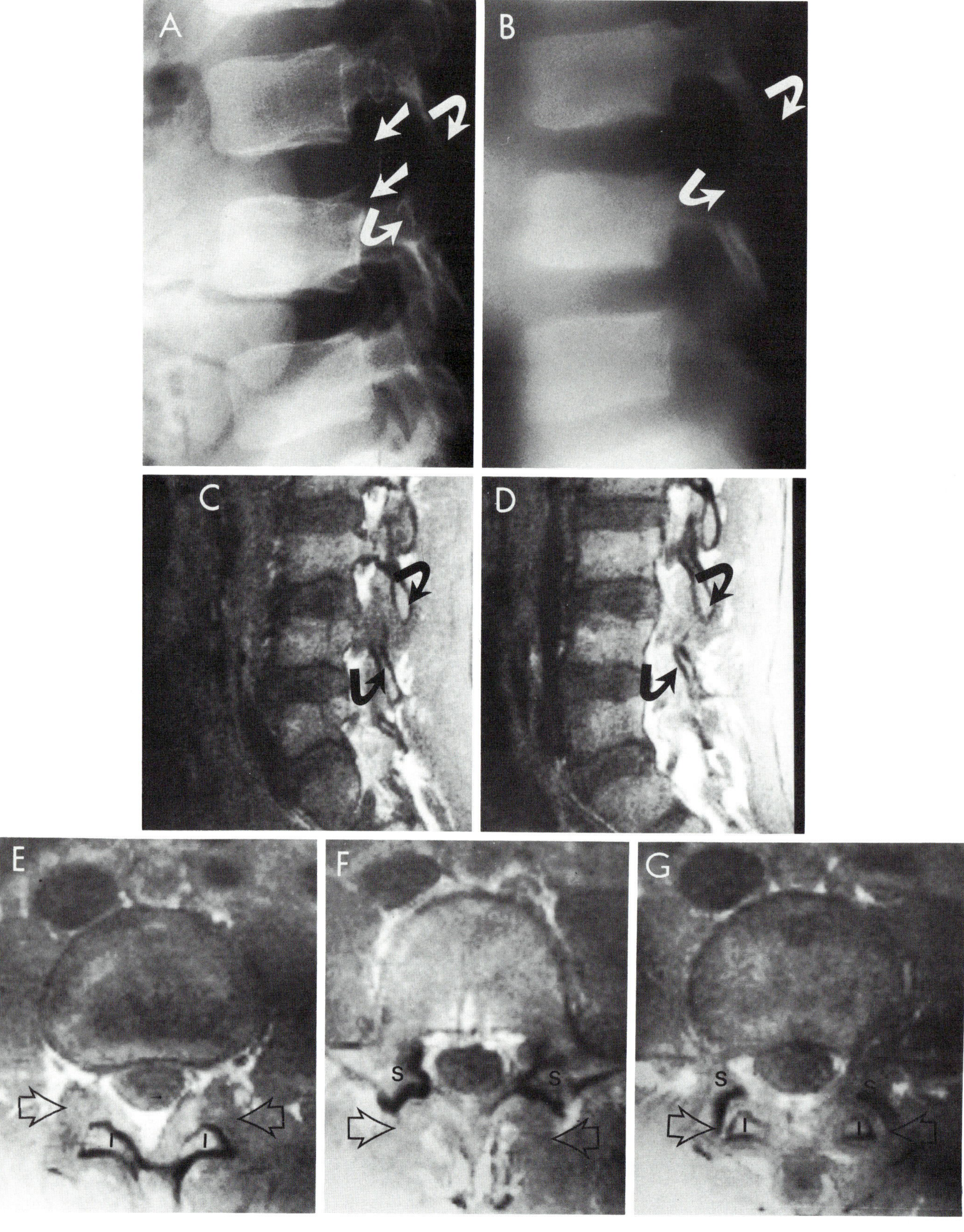
A
B
C
D
E
F
G
S
S
S
S
I
I
I
I

Sequelae or complications of cord contusion (particularly in the cervical spine) may result in post-traumatic myelopathy.[58, 59] Potential etiologies in the delayed development of myelopathy include (1) narrowing of the spinal canal (e.g., in cervical spondylosis) with cord compression, (2) secondary arachnoid adhesions, (3) cystic degeneration leading to syringomyelia, and (4) late-onset vascular compromise.

The term "cord compression" is self-explanatory. It may result from fracture-dislocation, dislocation, traumatic herniated disks, or pre-existing exostoses and spondylitic bars (see Fig 8–13). While compression in the thoracic and lumbar spine most frequently results from direct, persistent mechanical impingement, it may be a transitory "pinching" event in the cervical spine. A sudden or permanent loss of up to 50% of the anteroposterior dimension of the spinal canal is necessary for such cord compressions.[60] This condition may be aggravated by extensive intramedullary hemorrhage as described previously with cord contusion. The pathologic changes in the cord caused by pressure may be transient or permanent, including necrosis with or without hemorrhage. If the cord is compressed for a short period, the pathologic findings will be the same as those of a simple contusion, while longer, more intense compression will result in more severe damage. Several experimental models have given information concerning the separate and sometimes additive effects of compression and contusion.[61, 62] The cause of reversible neurologic deficit produced by cord compression has been attributed to direct mechanical distortion of the tissue, as well as impairment of the spinal cord circulation.[63–65]

FIG 8–16.
A, lateral radiograph of the lumbar spine in a patient with a flexion-dislocation injury. Notice the separation of the intervertebral disk posteriorly *(straight arrows)* as well as the distraction of the facet joints posteriorly *(curved arrows)*. These injuries result from the same forces and produce analogous defects to those observed in the cervical spine. **B,** parasagittal tomograms of the lumber spine again demonstrates marked distraction of the facet joints at this level *(curved arrows)*. **C** and **D,** parasagittal 500-msec TR/17-msec TE image of the lumbar spine demonstrates widely separated facet joints at the L3–4 level bilaterally *(curved arrows)*. **E,** axial 500-msec TR/17-msec TE image through the L3–4 intervertebral disk demonstrates the inferior facets *(I)* of L3 posteriorly, but no superior facets *(s)* of L4 articulating with it anteriorly, only soft tissue and hemorrhage *(open arrows)*. **F,** axial 500-msec TR/17-msec TE image through the upper L4 vertebral body demonstrates the inferior facets of L3 *(I)* barely articulating with the superior facets of L4 *(s)*. Notice the joint just barely maintained *(open arrows)*. **G,** axial 500-msec TR/17-msec TE image through the L4 vertebral body demonstrates the superior facets of L4 *(s)*, which no longer articulate with the distracted inferior facets of L3 *(I)*. This gives the appearance of the so-called "naked facets" *(open arrows)*.

TRAUMA MANAGEMENT

The management of spinal cord injury begins at the scene of the accident. When spine injury is suspected, instability is assumed and immediate immobilization of the spine is mandatory. Optimal oxygen and blood flow to the spinal cord should be provided. Strict attention should be paid to maintaining a good airway and oxygenation, as well as providing the support necessary to maintain blood pressure within normal limits. Nasogastric and urinary catheters are often inserted to minimize distension. A neurologic examination must be performed to assess motor and sensory function of the cord, as well as reflex changes and autonomic function. Unfortunately, it is difficult to assess the extent of spinal cord pathologic impairment from examination of initial neurologic deficit. Various clinical classification schemes of spinal cord injury have been developed as a means with which to document efficacy of treatment.[66, 67] However, such classifications have little predictive value in assessing initial deficits with respect to recovery of neurologic function.

The Role of MRI

As mentioned at the beginning of this chapter, medical care of patients sustaining spine injury is directed at stabilization and relief of cord compression. Confirmation of unstable fracture or fracture dislocation is obtained with plain film radiography. Should the preliminary studies prove negative, flexion/extension views may reveal otherwise nascent ligamentous disruption. Positive findings (with or without neurologic deficit) usually warrant further evaluation, with computed tomography (CT) directed to the region of interest.

A number of studies have documented the ability of CT to demonstrate fractures and suggest soft tissue injury to better advantage than plain film radiographs.[68–75] Preliminary studies comparing CT and MRI in the evaluation of spine stability suggest that while CT is superior for the demonstration of fractures (particularly of the posterior elements) MR is capable of direct demonstration of ligamentous tears (see Figs 8–11, 8–16, and 8–18).[76, 77] For example, flexion-compression fractures are well-demonstrated on sagittal T_1- and T_2-weighted images with intermediate and decreased signal respectively.[76] Disruption of the interspinous ligaments may also be visualized (see Figs 8–10 and 8–17). Axial images display concentric rings of heterogeneous signals, which represent the expanded, fractured body. The outermost ring represents the anterior longitudinal ligament and associated fragments; the middle ring represents avulsed dark end-plate cortex; and the innermost ring repre-

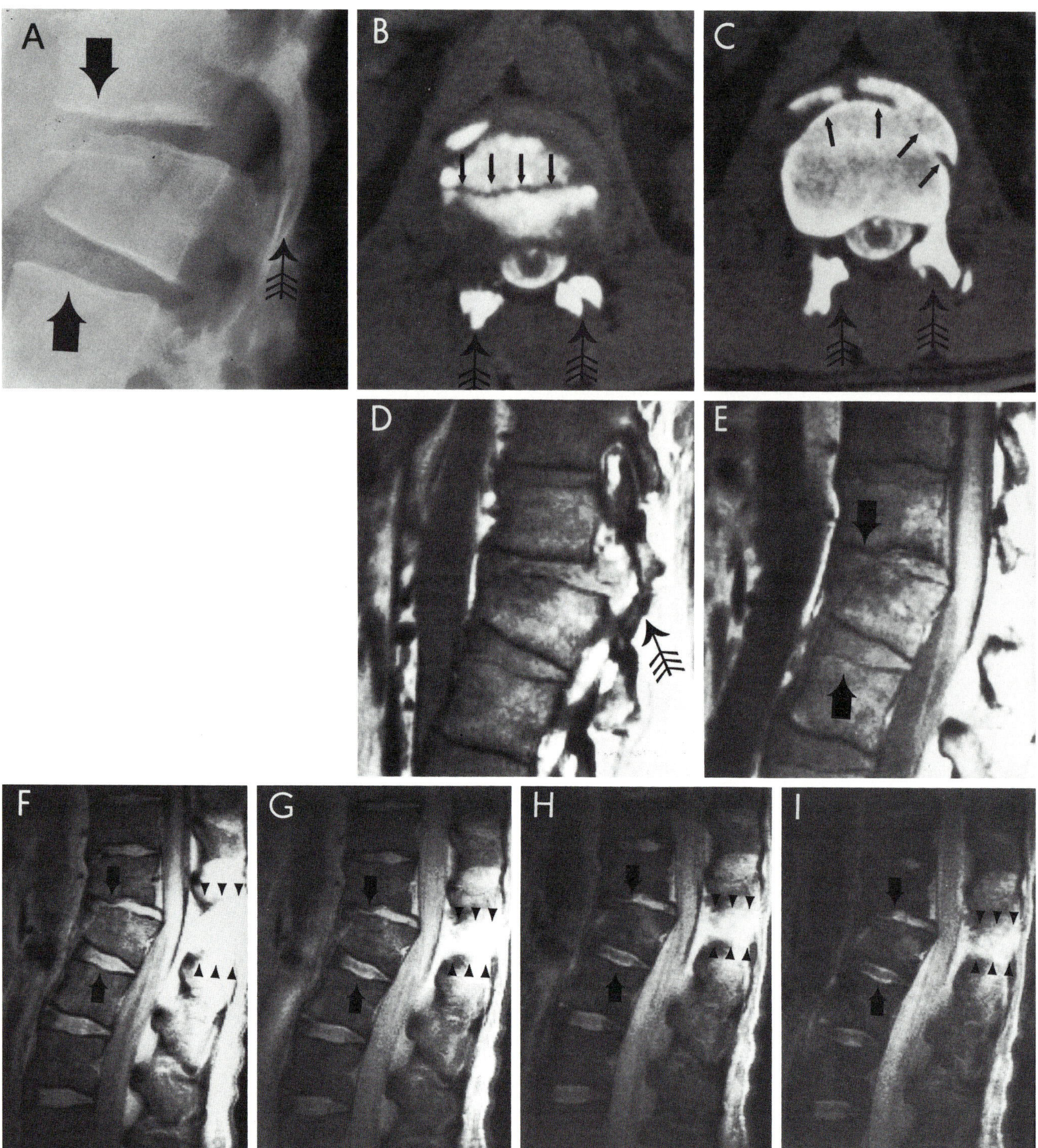

FIG 8–17.

A, lateral radiograph from a flexion-dislocation injury at the thoracolumbar junction. There is mild compression of the L1 vertical body *(solid arrows)* as well as distraction of the facets posteriorly *(tailed arrow).* **B,** axial CT scan following a myelogram at the level of the T12-L1 disk demonstrates horizontal fracture of the end-plate *(arrows)* and minimal articulation of the facets as well as facet malalignment *(tailed arrows).* **C,** more inferior axial scan demonstrates the naked facets of L1 *(tailed arrows)* as well as adjacent end-plate fractures anteriorly *(arrows).* **D,** parasagittal 500-msec TR/17-msec TE image demonstrates malalignment and dislocation of the facet joints *(tailed arrow).* **E,** midline sagittal 500-msec TR/17-msec TE image demonstrates dislocation and compression at T12-L1 *(arrows).* **F–I,** 2,000-msec TR/30- 60- 90- 120-msec TE images, respectively, demonstrate vertical compression and dislocation of T12-L1 *(arrows).* More important in these T_2-weighted studies, however, is the ability to detect the disruption of the interspinous ligament posteriorly *(arrowheads)* with increasing T_2 weighting.

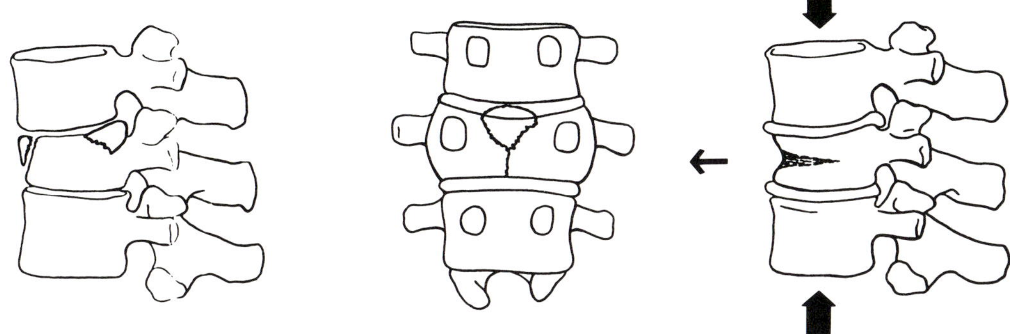

FIG 8–18.
Schematic representation of axial loading injury. With the application of vertical or axial force, the nucleus pulposus above is driven through the end-plate and into the vertebral body below, resulting in the so-called burst fracture. Typically, this produces fragmentation of the superior end-plate, often compromising the vertebral canal.

sents the cortex of the superior end-plate (see Fig 8–19).[76] Fractured bodies demonstrate diffuse increased signal intensity on T_2-weighted images but may be isointense (acutely) or increased in signal (subacute) depending on their age and the presence of traumatic hemorrhage.[76] Actual fracture lines are best demonstrated on high signal-to-noise T_1 or spin-density images as either increased or decreased signal relative to adjacent cortex or cancellous (marrow-filled) bone (see Figs 8–12 and 8–19). Fractures and fracture dislocations of the posterior elements can also be visualized on sagittal MR studies. However, characterization of the fractures with axial studies may be inferior to that possible with CT.[76] Rupture of the anterior and posterior longitudinal ligaments, ligamentum flavum, and interspinous and supraspinous ligaments can frequently be recognized as high-signal discontinuities of these low-signal structures on sagittal T_2-weighted images (see Fig 8–10, 8–14, and 8–17).[76–78]

With respect to actual spinal cord deficit, the importance of recognizing and distinguishing traumatic cord compression from contusion with MRI has been documented in numerous case series, which describe improvement or resolution of both acute and chronic neurologic deficits with surgical decompression of compressive lesions.[79, 80] However, it should be mentioned that similar clinical series have failed to demonstrate significant change in clinical outcome between operative and nonoperative cases.[81, 85] Such discrepancies in treatment philosophy are not trivial inasmuch as early surgery has been associated with increased risk of neurologic deterioration. Conversely, some experimental evidence indicates that degree of permanent neurologic deficit may be a direct function of the duration of cord compression.[86–89] Possible explanations for these controversies and the variability in outcome with surgical treatment include the following: (1) inaccurate criteria used to define significant cord compression as well as satisfactory decompression; (2) the type of operative procedure performed (anterior vs. posterior, stabilizing vs. decompressing); (3) inaccurate initial assessment of neurologic deficit secondary to concomitant head injury; and (4) inability of preoperative imaging studies to accurately characterize type of cord trauma (i.e., concussion vs. contusion).

In the past, the presence of acute, incomplete traumatic neurologic deficit (with or without fracture-dislocation) justified the administration of intrathecal contrast material to evaluate cord integrity and rule out potentially reversible cord compression. Computed tomographic myelography is preferred over plain film myelography because of its ability to outline the anterior spinal cord, determine the etiology of block, and visualize the vertebral canal below points of obstruction.[90]

Preliminary reports of MRI in the evaluation of acute spinal cord trauma list similar virtues (discriminating compression from contusion) with the added advantage of being noninvasive.[76–78] MRI signal intensities on T_1- and T_2-weighted images have also proved reliable in discriminating spinal cord edema and hemorrhage.[90, 91] Kulkarni et al.[92] have described three patterns of intramedullary signal changes observable with MRI in patients with acute trauma. Traumatic lesions acutely demonstrating foci of hypointensity on T_1- and T_2-weighted images are consistent with cord contusion with intramedullary hemorrhage (composed of deoxyhemoglobin) and a poor prognosis. Subsequently, degradation of deoxyhemoglobin to intracellular methemoglobin produces high signal on T_1-weighted images (beginning at the periphery) and low signal on T_2-weighted images. Eventual red blood cell lysis and the release of extracellular methemoglobin produces high signal on both T_1- and T_2-weighted images (Fig 8–20).

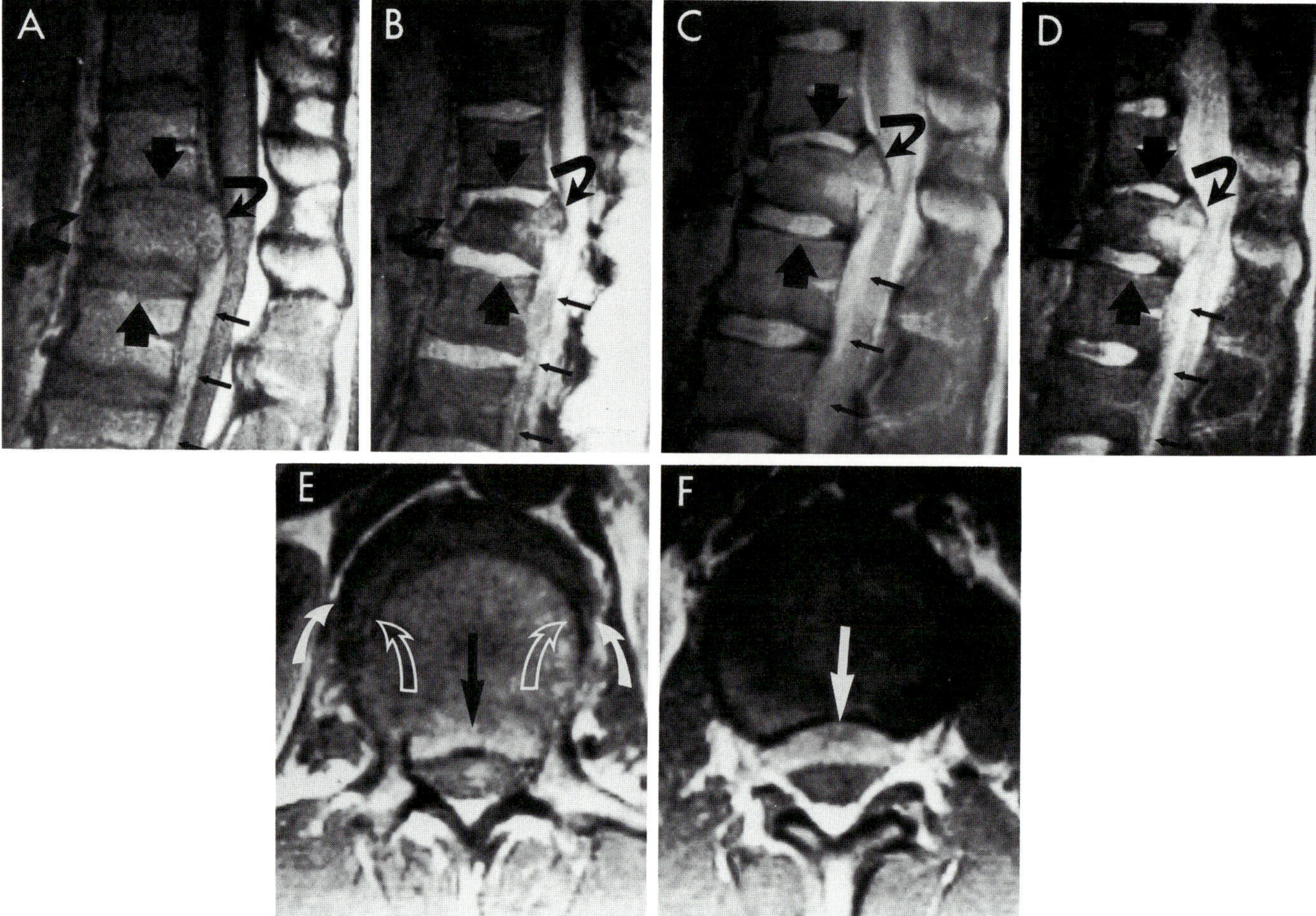

FIG 8–19.

A, 500-msec TR/17-msec TE sagittal image at the lower thoracolumbar junction following axial loading *(vertical arrows).* Notice the displaced fracture fragments *(curved arrows)* as well as the soft tissue immediately anterior to the canal, probably an epidural hematoma *(thin straight arrows).* **B,** FLASH 60 degree midline sagittal image following axial loading *(vertical arrows)* again demonstrates displaced fracture fragments *(curved arrows)* as well as an anterior epidural mass *(small, straight arrows).* Notice the low signal intensity of the hemorrhage on this gradient echo scan, probably related to magnetic susceptibility effect. **C** and **D,** 2,000-msec TR/30- and 120-msec TE images, respectively. Note with more T_2 weighting the increase in signal intensity from the fractured vertebral body when compared to the relatively low signal at this site on the T_1-weighted image. This is characteristic of acute fractures. Again, note displaced fragment *(curved arrow)* and epidural hematoma. **E,** axial 500-msec TR/17-msec TE image through the region of the fragment demonstrates the central, retropulsed fragment *(black arrow),* the outer dark ring represents the anterior longitudinal ligament *(curved white arrow)* while the inner ring represents the cortex of the superior end-plate *(open arrows).* **F,** axial 500-msec TR/17-msec TE image through a lower intervertebral disk continues to demonstrate what was believed to be an epidural hematoma *(solid arrow).*

FIG 8–20.

A and **B,** sagittal 500-msec TR/17-msec TE spin-echo and 20 degree FISP gradient-echo scans, respectively, demonstrate focal areas of low signal intensity within the conus medullaris of a young woman following spinal cord trauma. The findings are consistent with subacute intramedullary hemorrhage. In particular, the loss of signal from this region on the gradient-echo study is highly suggestive of magnetic susceptibility effect secondary to hemorrhage. **C** and **D,** 2,000-msec TR/60- and 120-msec TE images, respectively, in the same patient following spinal cord trauma. The focal area of decreased signal intensity represents intramedullary hemorrhage while the peripheral area of increased signal intensity within the conus medullaris suggests edema. MR scans obtained 1 week after the initial study. **E,** 500-msec TR/17-msec TE sagittal image through the level of the conus medullaris demonstrates a focal area of increased signal intensity consistent with intracellular methemoglobin. **F,** axial 500-msec TR/17-msec TE through the same region again demonstrates a focal hematoma composed of intracellular methemoglobin. **G,** 2,000-msec TR/120-msec TE demonstrates focal area of low signal within the cord at the site of the hematoma, again consistent with the signal-intensity characteristics of intracellular methemoglobin on this T_2-weighted scan. **H,** follow-up 2,000-msec TR/20-msec TE axial image several weeks after the initial injury demonstrates a focal area of increased signal intensity within the cord, consistent with extracellular methemoglobin.

→

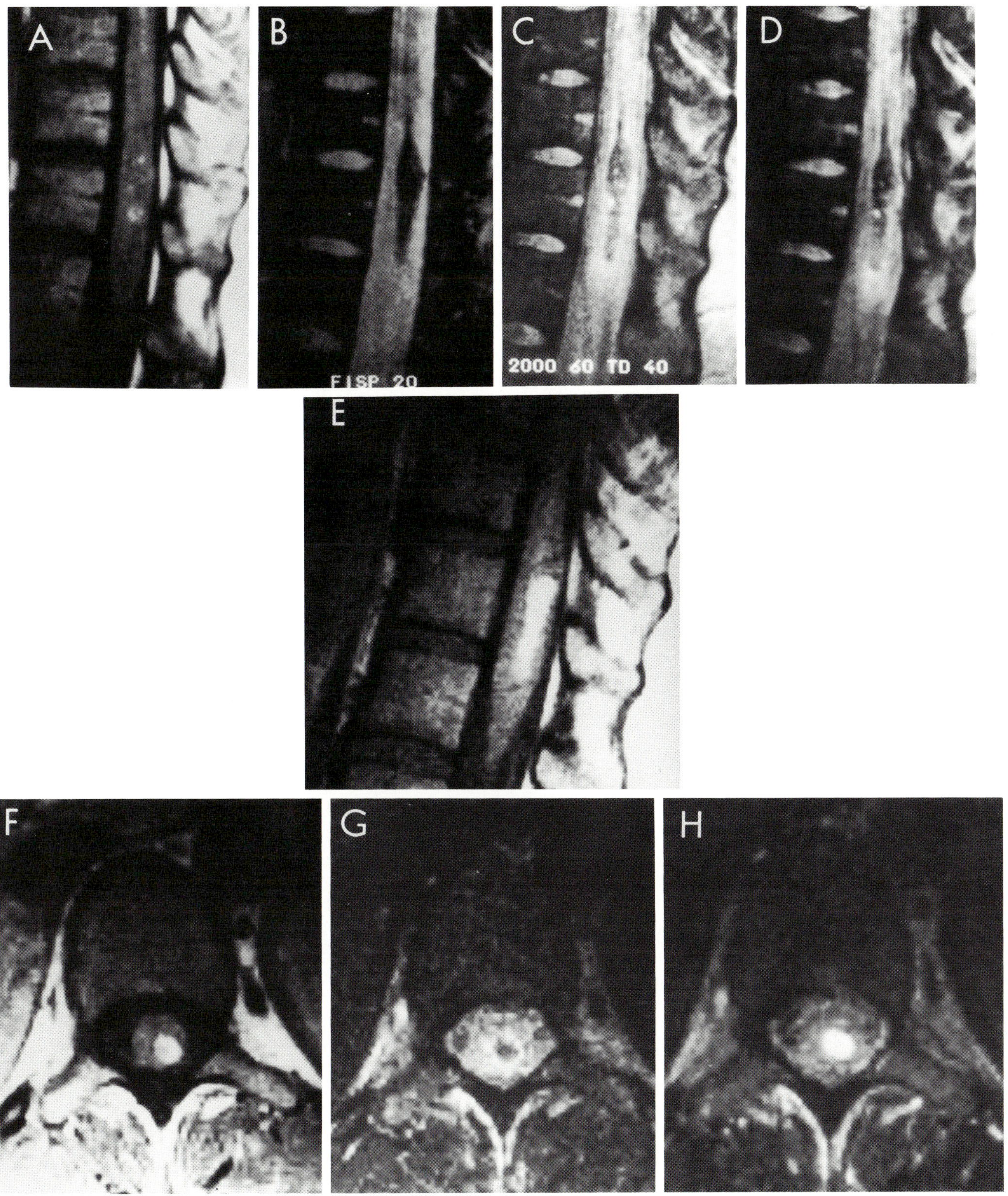
A
B
C
D
FISP 20
2000 60 TD 40
E
F
G
H

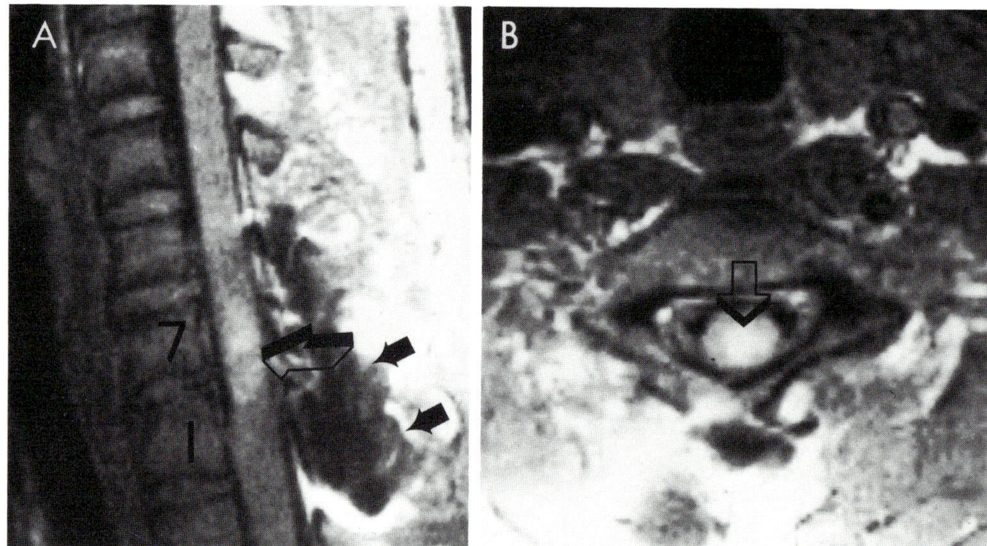

FIG 8–21.
Sagittal (**A**) and axial (**B**) 500-msec TR/17-msec TE images in a patient who sustained flexion dislocation injury at C7-T1 several weeks earlier. Patient has undergone posterior wire fusion for stabilization *(closed arrows)*. Residual petechial hemorrhage within the spinal cord *(open arrows)* is represented as ill-defined areas of increased signal intensity on these T_1-weighted images.

The second pattern of acute spinal cord injury is recognized as low or normal signal on T_1-weighted images and a spindle-shaped region of high signal on T_2-weighted images.[91,92] Such lesions are consistent with the edema of cord concussion and carry a more favorable prognosis. The third pattern represents a mixture of the first two, the low-signal center surrounded by peripheral ring of high signal on T_2-weighted images. Patients with type III lesions may be capable of neurologic improvement with appropriate treatment (Fig 8–21).

While accurate, efficient, noninvasive imaging of ligamentous disruption, traumatic disk herniation with cord compression, cord concussion, and cord contusion is desirable, the potential for ferromagnetic interactions

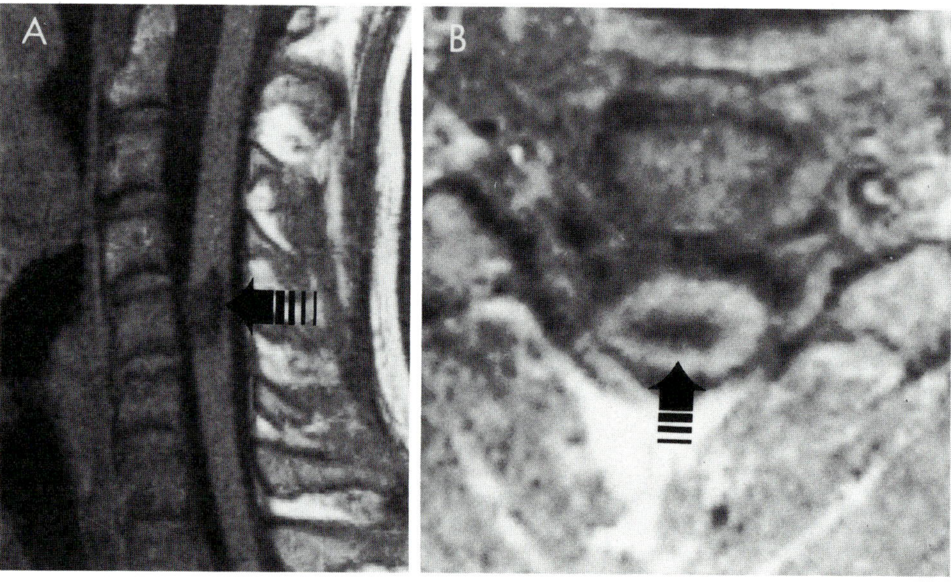

FIG 8–22.
Sagittal (**A**) and axial (**B**) 500-msec TR/17-msec TE images in a patient with previous cervical spine trauma. There was no evidence of bony disruption or fracture at the time of the original injury, which rendered the patient quadriparetic. Neurologic deficit persisted. Subsequent MR examination demonstrated this focal cystic region within the spinal cord *(arrow)*.

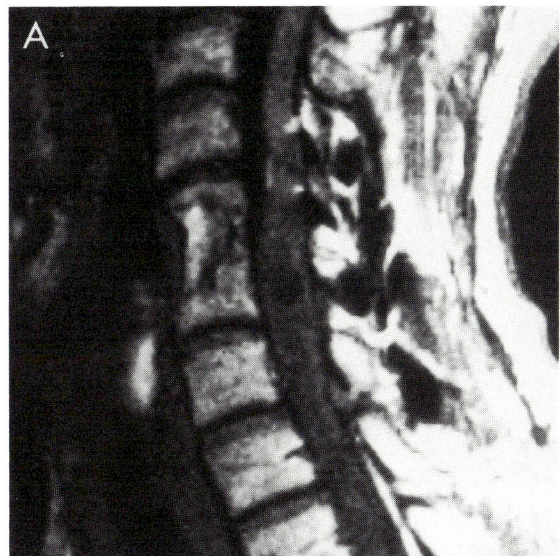

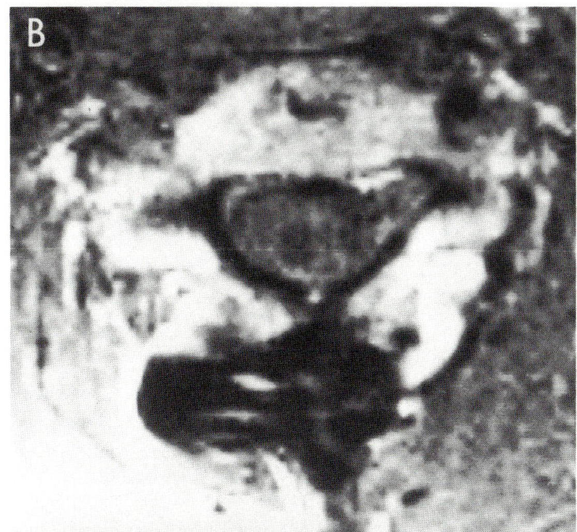

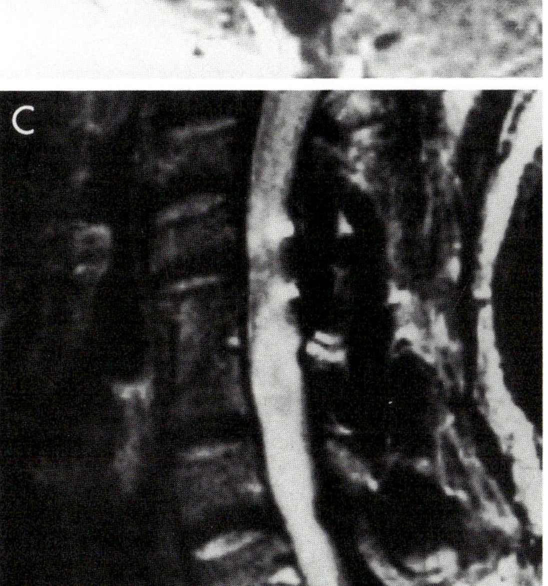

FIG 8–23.
A, sagittal 500-msec TR/17-msec TE image in a patient who had a remote cervical spinal cord injury. Patient has undergone both anterior interbody fusion and posterior fusion (wiring) procedure. Notice the cystic area within the spinal cord immediately posterior to the interbody fusion. **B,** axial 500-msec TR/17-msec TE image through this region again demonstrates what appears to be a cystic region within the spinal cord. In the presence of worsening clinical symptoms in the patient, there was clinical suspicion of post-traumatic syringomyelia. **C,** however, on this 2,000-msec TR/30-msec image it can be seen that the area of traumatic cord damage has increased signal intensity, consistent with a diagnosis of myelomalacia rather than syringomyelia.

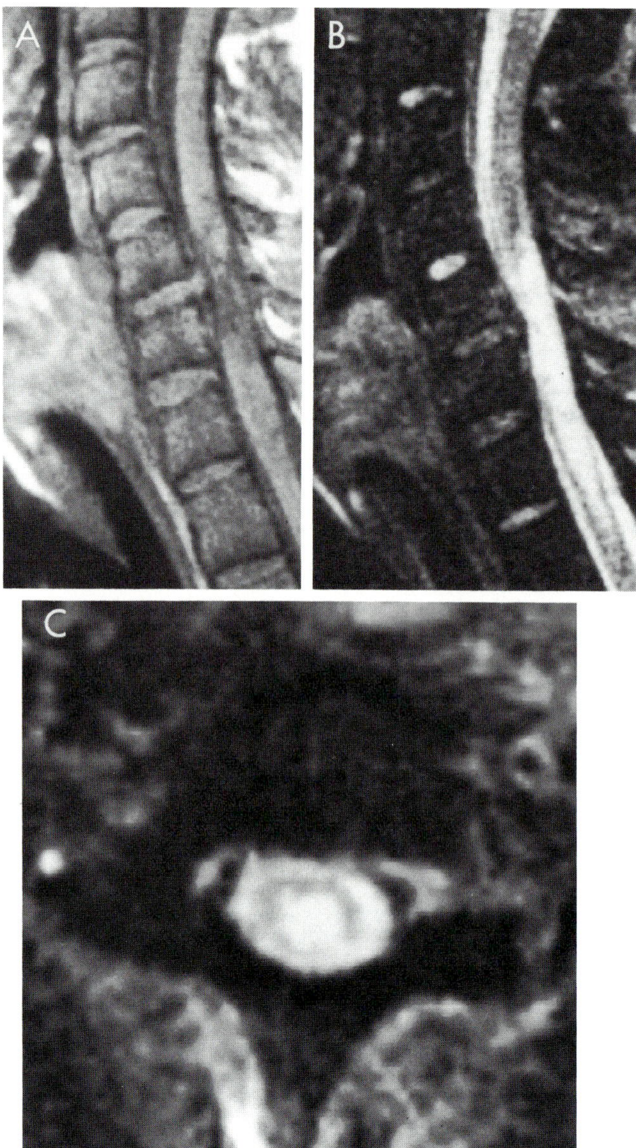

FIG 8–24.
A, 500-msec TR/17-msec TE image in a patient who has sustained flexion-dislocation injury remotely at C5–6. Note the persistent cord compression by the traumatic disk. Also, there are ill-defined areas of low signal intensity within the spinal cord in this region. Sagittal (**B**) and axial (**C**) 2,000-msec TR/120-msec TE images through the region of chronic cord damage demonstrate increased signal intensity, also consistent with myelomalacia.

between imager and spine stabilization devices, electronic monitoring equipment, and respiratory support devices have muted the enthusiasm for the use of MR in the evaluation of acute spinal cord trauma. Fortunately, steady progress has been made in overcoming these obstacles.

Spine traction or stabilization devices cannot be strongly ferromagnetic because they may be displaced in the imaging bore or may distort the image.[93] These risks can be reduced by appropriate selection of materials for such devices (such as titanium, tantalum, or high-nickel stainless steel alloys).[93] At least two manufacturers have made an effort to accommodate MR imagers in the design of their halo stabilization devices (Ace Medical Company, Los Angeles, and Bremmer Orthopedics, Jacksonville, Fla). Additionally, McArdle et al.[94] have described an inexpensive and effective traction system for MR imagers to be used in conjunction with such halo devices. We prefer the Trippi-Wells traction device with such vests, since it allows for closer application of spine surface coils.

It is important to remember that patients with acute spinal cord trauma may be subject to hemodynamic instability and/or ventilatory compromise. Safe and effective imaging of such patients within the confines of high–field strength, whole-body imagers requires use of reliable monitoring equipment for heart rate, blood pressure, and respiratory rate. As with traction devices, such equipment must not be ferromagnetic. It is desirable to place monitoring instruments as remotely from the magnet as possible, either through the use of telemetric or fiberoptic transmission.[95, 96] Appropriate selection of monitoring equipment operated at frequencies outside the imager's field strength–dependent RF spectrum will minimize any distortion of signal.[97] Arterial blood pressure must frequently be monitored outside the scanner by lengthening the rubber tubing connected to the blood pressure cuff, as it may be difficult to carry out auscultation in the presence of the actively scanning imager.[95, 98] Decisions concerning the necessity and/or type of ventilatory support are best left to the anesthetist; however, pneumatically driven volume- and pressure-cycled fluidic ventilators that are MRI-compatible are available commercially.[99, 100] Similarly, there are numerous reports in the literature describing several ventilatory circuits and anesthesia techniques for use with MRI.[101–103] One important note: laryngoscopes are nonmagnetic but can only be employed at an imager when batteries with paper or plastic casings are used.[98]

LATE COMPLICATIONS OF SPINAL CORD TRAUMA

For a patient who has incurred spinal cord injury with permanent neurologic deficit, the acquisition of new, debilitating symptoms can be catastrophic. This clinical entity has been termed post-traumatic progressive myelopathy, and may be secondary to syringomyelia (i.e., post-traumatic cystic myelopathy) or noncystic post-traumatic lesions such as myelomalacia.[104] This distinction is significant inasmuch as the cystic form of myelopathy may be remediable by surgical shunting.[104–108]

In 1966, Barrett et al. drew attention to a progressive post-traumatic spinal cord syndrome that, on the basis of clinical presentation and surgical findings, closely resembled syringomyelia.[109] Numerous clinical series provide an estimated incidence of 2% or less in all post-traumatic spinal cord injury patients.[110–113] Patients typically present with spinothalamic symptoms (i.e., pain and/or sensory loss), which occur months or years following the injury. This cystic degeneration does not appear to be related to the site or severity (incomplete/complete) of the original cord lesion (Fig 8–22).[104–113] Cysts may occur either above or below the level of the original spinal cord lesion.[106]

The exact mechanism of post-traumatic cyst formation and extension is not known. McLean et al.[114] have suggested that at the time of traumatic contusion a necrotic blood-filled space develops within the spinal cord that in the course of normal healing results in a glial-lined cavity.[114] Alternatively, post-traumatic arachnoid adhesion at the site of injury may tether the cord such that it is subject to unusual stresses by common CSF pressure changes associated with the Valsalva maneuver, coughing, sneezing, or motion above or below the site of injury.[108, 113, 114]

Until recently, delayed high-resolution CT scanning with water-soluble contrast material was the examination of choice for preoperative detection of post-traumatic spinal cord cystic myelopathy.[107, 108, 116] It could determine the presence of post-traumatic cysts in enlarged or atrophic spinal cords, locate them dorsally or ventrally above or below the lesion, and determine if they were single or multiple.[107, 108, 116] Unfortunately, delayed-contrast CT suffers from its invasiveness and nonspecificity (i.e., inability to distinguish some spinal cord cysts from myelomalacia).[104, 107, 108]

More recently, MRI using T_1- and T_2-weighted images has been shown to be the examination of choice for the preoperative evaluation of post-traumatic myelopathy.[104, 117] It is noninvasive and capable of distinguishing myelomalacia from post-traumatic cysts. On T_1-weighted images both myelomalacia and post-traumatic syringes are low in signal intensity with respect to the surrounding cord parenchyma. On spin-density (intermediate) weighted images, post-traumatic syringes continue to have a low signal with respect to the cord (paralleling CSF), while myelomalacia is isointense or higher in signal when compared to normal cord parenchyma (Fig 8–23). On T_2-weighted images, both post-traumatic cysts and myelomalacia may have hyperintense signal with respect to normal cord parenchyma, but the syrinx should follow CSF signal[104, 117] (Fig 8–24). Occasionally, sagittal and axial imaging may fail to confirm this "characteristic" progression of signal-intensity changes because of CSF pulsation–induced signal loss seen in some large cysts on T_2-weighted images.[118] Such cyst fluid motion may also be recognized on axial gradient echo scans by the flow-related enhancement it produces.[118] Absence of these motion-induced signal changes following surgical shunting may have prognostic significance, i.e., indicating successful decompression.

REFERENCES

1. Krause JF, Franti CE, Riggins RS, et al: Incidence of traumatic spinal cord lesions. *J Chron Dis* 1975; 28:471–492.
2. Bracken MB, Freeman DH, Hellenbrand K: Incidence of acute traumatic hospitalized spinal cord injury in the United States, 1970–1977. *Am J Epidemiol* 1981; 113:615–622.
3. Anderson DW, Mclauren RL (eds): The national head and spinal cord injury survey. *J Neurosurg* 1980; 53(suppl):S1–S43.
4. Young JS, Burno PE, Bowen AM, et al: *Spinal Cord Injury Statistics Systems.* Phoenix, Good Samaritan Medical Center, 1982.
5. Wannamaker GJ: Spinal cord injuries: A review of early treatment in consecutive cases during the Korean conflict. *J Neurosurg* 1954; 11:517–524.
6. Jacobson SA, Bors E: Spinal cord injury in Vietnamese combat. *Paraplegia* 1970; 7:263–281.
7. Klaw R: Beitrag zur pathologischen Anatomie der Verletzungen des Ruckenmarkes mit besonderer Brucksichtig ungder Ruckenmark skontusion. Ein Vergleisch zwischen Ruckenmarks—und Hirnverletzungen. *Arch Psychiatr Nervenkr* 1948; 180:206–270.
8. Guttmann L: *Spinal Cord Injuries: Comprehensive Management and Research.* Oxford-London, Blackwell Scientific Publications, 1973.
9. Yashon D, Jane JA, White RJ: Prognosis and management of spinal cord and cauda equina bullet injuries in 65 civilians. *J Neurosurg* 1970; 32:163–170.
10. Lipschitz R: Stab wounds of the spinal cord, in Vinken PJ, Bruyn GW (eds): *Handbook of Clinical Neurology,* vol 25. Amsterdam, Elsevier-North Holland, 1976, pp 197–207.
11. Brown-Sequard CE: Lectures on the physiology and pathology of the nervous system and on the treatment of organic nervous affections. *Lancet* 1868; 2:593, 659, 755, 821.
12. Wolman L: The neuropathology of traumatic paraplegia. A critical historical review. *Paraplegia* 1954; 2:233–251.
13. Jellinger K: Neuropathology of cord injuries, in Vinken PJ, Bruyn GW (eds): *Handbook of Clinical Neurology,* vol 25. Amsterdam, Elsevier-North Holland, 1976, pp 43–121.
14. Elsburg CA (quoted by Wolman L, 1964): *Ann Surg* 1919; 69:239.
15. Marburg O: Zur Pathologie der Kreigsshadigurgen des Ruckenmarks. *Arb Neurol Inst Univ Wien* 1919; 1:498–556.
16. Wolf SM: Delayed traumatic myelopathy following transfixation of the spinal cord by a knife blade. *J Neurosurg* 1973; 38:221–225.
17. Finck PA: Ballistic and forensic pathologic aspects of missile wounds. Conversion between Anglo-American and metric-system units. *Milit Med* 1965; 130:545–569.
18. Kelly WM, Payle PG, Pearson JA, et al: Ferromagnetism of intraocular foreign body causing untilateral blindness after MR study. *AJNR* 1986; 7:243–245.
19. Adams AE: Uber Grundlagen und Klinische Beurteilung der Stumpfen Traumen des Ruckenmarkes. *Nervenartz* 1969; 40:579–585.
20. Wilcox NE, Staufner EF, Nickel VL: A statistical analysis of 423 consecutive patients admitted to the spinal cord injury center Rancho Los Amigos Hospital. *Paraplegia* 1970; 8:27–35.
21. Hardy AG, Rossier AB: Tetia and paraplegie, in Nigst H (ed): *Spezielle Frakturen-and Luxationslehre,* vol I/z. Stuttgart, Tieme, 1972, pp 64–140.
22. Beatson TR: Fractures and dislocations of the cervical spine. *J Bone Joint Surg* [*Br*] 1963; 45:21–25.
23. Felding JW, Hawkins RJ: *Roentgenographic Diagnosis of the Injured Neck,* instructional course lectures, American Academy of Orthopedic Surgeons, vol 25. St Louis, CV Mosby, 1976, chap 7, p 149.
24. Holdsworth F: Fractures, dislocations and fracture-dislocations of the spine. *J Bone Joint Surg* [*Am*] 1970; 52:1534–1551.
25. Roaf R: International classification of spine injuries. *Paraplegia* 1972; 10:78–84.
26. Felding JW: Cineroentgenography of the normal cervical spine. *J Bone Joint Surg* [*Am*] 1957; 39:1280–1288.
27. Holm: Normal motions of the upper portion of the cervical spine. *J Bone Joint Surg* [*Am*] 1964; 46:1777–1779.
28. Holh M, Baker HR: The atlanto-axial joint. Roentgenographic and anatomic study of normal and abnormal motion. *J Bone Joint Surg* [*Am*] 1964; 46:1739–1752.
29. Bohlman HH, Ducker TB, Lucas JT. Spine and spinal cord injuries, in Rothman RH, Simeone FA (eds): *The Spine,* vol 2. Philadelphia, WB Saunders, 1982, pp 661–756.
30. Jellinger K, Schwingshackel A: Birth injury of the spinal cord. *Neuropaediatr* 1973; 4:111–123.
31. Bohlman HH: Acute fractures and dislocations of the cervical spine: An analysis of 300 hospitalized patients and a review of the literature. *J Bone Joint Surg* [*Am*] 1979; 61:1119–1142.
32. Anderson LD, D'Alonzo RT: Fractures of the odontoid process of the axis. *J Bone Joint Surg* [*Am*] 1974; 56:1663–1691.
33. Schneider RC, Livingston KE, Cav AJ, et al: "Hangman's fracture" of the cervical spine. *J Neurosurg* 1965; 22:141–154.
34. Jefferson G: Fractures of the atlas vertebrae. Report of four cases and a review of those previously recorded. *Br J Surg* 1920; 7:407–422.
35. Eismont FJ, Clifford S, Goldberg M, et al: Cervical sagittal spinal canal size in spine injury. *Spine* 1984; 9:663–666.
36. White AA, Panjabi MM: *Clinical Biomechanics of the Spine.* New York, JB Lippincott Co, 1978.
37. Cheshire DJ: The stability of the cervical spine following

treatment of fractures and fracture-dislocations. *Paraplegia* 1969; 7:193–203.
38. Barnes R: Paraplegia in cervical spine injuries. *J Bone Joint Surg* [*Br*] 1948; 30:234–244.
39. Penning L: *Functional Pathology of the Cervical Spine*. Amsterdam, Excerpta Medica, 1968.
40. Schneider RC, Kahn EA: Chronic neurological sequelae of acute trauma to the spine and spinal cord: I. The significance of the acute flexion or "tear-drop" fracture-dislocation of the cervical spine. *J Bone Joint Surg* [*Am*] 1956; 38:958–997.
41. Schneider RC: Chronic neurological sequelae of acute trauma to the spine and spinal cord: V. The syndrome of acute central cervical spinal cord injury followed by chronic anterior cervical cord injury (or compression) syndrome. *J Bone Joint Surg* [*Am*] 1960; 42:253–260.
42. Braakman R, Vinken PJ: Unilateral facet interlocking in the lower cervical spine. *J Bone Joint Surg* [*Br*] 1967; 49:249–257.
43. Braakman R, Penning L: *Injuries to the Cervical Spine*. Amsterdam, Excerpta Medica, 1971.
44. Gosch H, Gooding HE, Schneider RC: An experimental study of cervical spine and cord injuries. *J Trauma* 1972; 12:510–576.
45. Bohlman HH, Freehafer A, Dejak J: The results of treatment of acute injuries of the upper thoracic spine with paralysis. *J Bone Joint Surg* [*Am*] 1985; 67:360–369.
46. Atlas SW, Regenbogen V, Rogers LF, et al: The radiographic characterization of burst fractures of the spine. *AJR* 1986; 147:575–582.
47. Chance GQ: Note on a type of flexion fracture of the spine. *Br J Radiol* 1948; 21:452–453.
48. Smith WS, Kaufer H: Patterns and mechanisms of lumbar injuries associated with lap seat belts. *J Bone Joint Surg* [*Am*] 1969; 51:239–254.
49. Saul TB, Ducker TB: Treatment of spinal cord injury, in Cowley RA, Trump B (eds): *Cellular Injury in Shock, Anoxia and Ischemia: Pathophysiology, Prevention and Treatment*. Baltimore, Williams & Wilkins, 1981.
50. De La Torre JA: Spinal cord injury: Review of basic and applied research. *Spine* 1981; 6:315–335.
51. Dohrmann GJ, Wagner FC, Buey PC: The microvasculature in transitory traumatic paraplegia. An election microscopic study in the monkey. *J Neurosurg* 1971; 35:263–271.
52. Dohrmann GJ, Wick KM, Buey PC: Blood flow patterns in the intrinsic vessels of the spinal cord following contusion. *Trans Am Neurol Assoc* 1972; 97:189–192.
53. Dohrmann GJ, Wick KM, Buey PC: Spinal cord blood flow patterns in experimental traumatic paraplegia. *J Neurosurg* 1973; 38:52–58.
54. Ducker TB, Assenmacher D: Microvascular response to experimental spinal cord trauma. *Surg Forum* 1969; 20:428–430.
55. Ducker TB, Kindt GW, Kempe LG: Pathological findings in acute experimental spinal cord trauma. *J Neurosurg* 1971; 35:700–708.
56. Assenmacher DR, Ducker TB: Experimental traumatic paraplegia. The vascular and pathological changes seen in reversible and irreversible spinal cord lesions. *J Bone Joint Surg* [*Am*] 1971; 53:671–680.
57. Wolman L: The disturbances of circulation in traumatic paraplegia in acute and late stages. A pathological study. *Paraplegia* 1965; 2:231–236.
58. Dohrmann GJ, Wagner FC, Buey PC: Transitory traumatic paraplegia: Electron microscopy of early alteration in myelinated nerve fibers. *J Neurosurg* 1972; 367:407–415.
59. Jellinger K: Traumatic vascular disease of the spinal cord, in Vinkin PJ, Bruyn GW (eds): *Handbook of Clinical Neurology: II. Vascular Disease of the Nervous System,* vol 12. Amsterdam, Elsevier North-Holland Inc, 1972, pp 556–630.
60. Scarff, JE: Injuries of the vertebral column and spinal cord, in Brock S (ed): *Injuries of the Brain and Spinal Cord and Their Coverings,* ed 4. London, Cassell, 1960, pp 530–589.
61. Tarlov IM: *Acute Spinal Cord Compression*. Springfield, Ill, Charles C Thomas, 1957.
62. Bohlmann HH, Bahniuk E, Raskulineez G, et al: Mechanical factors affecting recovery from incomplete spinal cord injury: A preliminary report. *Johns Hopkins Med J* 1979; 145:115–125.
63. Tarlov IM: Acute spinal cord compression paralysis. *J Neurosurg* 1972; 36:10–20.
64. Doppman JL, Girton M: Angiographic study of the effect of laminectomy in the presence of acute anterior epidural masses. *J Neurosurg* 1976; 45:195–202.
65. Hukuda S, Wilson CB: Experimental cervical myelopathy. *J Neurosurg* 1972; 37:631–652.
66. Frankel HL, Hancock DO, Hyslop G, et al: The value of posteral reduction in the initial management of closed injuries of the spine with paraplegia and tetraplegia. *Paraplegia* 1969; 7:179–192.
67. Lucas JT, Ducker TB. Motor classification of spinal cord injuries with mobility morbidity and recovery indices. *Am Surg,* 1979, pp 151–158.
68. Brant-Zawadski M, Miller EM, Federle MP: CT in the evaluation of spine trauma. *AJR* 1981; 136:369–375.
69. Donovan Post MJ, Green BA, Quencer RM, et al: The value of computed tomography in spinal trauma. *Spine* 1982; 7:417–431.
70. Keene JS, Goletz TH, Lilleas F, et al: Diagnosis of vertebral fractures: A comparison of conventional radiography convention tomography and computed axial tomography. *J Bone Joint Surg* [*Am*] 1982; 64:586–595.
71. McAfee PC, Yuan HA, Frederickson BE, et al: The value of computed tomography in thoracolumbar fractures. *J Bone Joint Surg* [*Am*] 1983; 65:461–473.
72. Kilcoyne RF, Mack LA, King HA, et al: Thoracolumbar spine injuries associated with vertical plunges: Reappraisals with computed tomography. 1983; 146:137–140.
73. Handel SF, Lee Y: Computed tomography of spinal fractures. *Radiol Clin North Am* 1981; 19:69–89.
74. Cooper PR, Cohen W: Evaluation of cervical spinal cord

injuries with metrizamide myelography-CT scanning. *J Neurosurg* 1984; 61:281–289.
75. Faerber EN, Wolpert SM, Scott RM, et al: Computed tomography of spinal fractures. *J Comput Assist Tomogr* 1979; 3:657–661.
76. McArdle CB, Crafford MJ, Mirfakhraee M, et al: Surface coil MR of spinal trauma: Preliminary experience. *AJNR* 1986; 7:885–893.
77. Tarr RW, Drolshagen LF, Kerner TC, et al: MR imaging of recent spinal trauma. *J Comput Assist Tomogr* 1987; 11:412–417.
78. Mirvis SE, Geisler FH, Jelinek JJ, et al: Acute cervical spine trauma: Evaluation with 1.5T MR imaging. *Radiology* 1988; 166:807–816.
79. Larson SJ, Hobst RA, Hemmy DC, et al: Lateral extracavitary approach to traumatic lesions of the thoracic and lumbar spine. *J Neurosurg* 45:628.
80. Brodkey JS, Miller CF, Harmody RM. The syndrome of acute cervical spinal cord injury revisited. *Surg Neurol* 1980; 14:251–257.
81. Maynard FM, Reynolds GG, Fountain S, et al: Neurologic prognosis after traumatic quadriplegia. *J Neurosurg* 1979; 50:611–616.
82. Heiden JS, Weiss MH, Rosenberg AW, et al: Management of cervical spinal cord trauma in Southern California. *J Neurosurg* 1975; 43:732–736.
83. Dickson JH, Harrington PR, Erwin WD: Results of reduction and stabilization of severely fractured thoracic and lumbar spine. *J Bone Joint Surg [Am]* 1978; 60:799–805.
84. Wagner FC, Chehrazi B: Early decompression and neurological outcome in acute cervical spinal cord injuries. *J Neurosurg* 1982; 56:699–705.
85. Harris P, Karmi MZ, McClemont E, et al: The prognosis of patients sustaining severe cervical spine injury. *Paraplegia* 1980; 18:324–330.
86. Marshall LF, Knowlton S, Gartin SR, et al: Deterioration following spinal cord injury: A multicenter study. *J Neurosurg* 1987; 66:400–404.
87. Dolan EJ, Tator CH, Endrenyi L: The value of decompression for acute experimental spinal cord compression injury. *J Neurosurg* 1980; 53:749–755.
88. Tarlov IM, Klinger H: Spinal cord compression studies: II. Time limits for recovery after acute compression in dogs. *Arch Neurol Psychiatr* 1954; 71:271–290.
89. Tarlov IM: Spinal cord compression studies: III. Time limits for recovery after gradual compression in dogs. *Arch Neurol Psychiatr* 1954; 71:588–597.
90. Brant-Zawadzki M, Post MJD: Trauma, in Newton TH, Potts DG (eds): *Computed Tomography of the Spine and Spinal Cord: Modern Neuroradiology,* vol 1. San Anselmo, Calif, Clavadel Press, 1983, pp 149–186.
91. Hackney DB, Asato R, Joseph PM, et al: Hemorrhage and edema in acute spinal cord compression: Demonstration by MR imaging. *Radiology* 1986; 161:387–390.
92. Kulkarni M, McArdle CB, Kopanicky D, et al: Acute spinal cord injury: MR imaging at 1.5T. *Radiology* 1987; 164:837–843.
93. New PFJ, Rosen BR, Brady TJ, et al: Potential hazards and artifacts of ferromagnetic and nonferromagnetic surgical and dental materials and devices in nuclear magnetic resonance imaging. *Radiology* 1983; 147:139–148.
94. McArdle CB, Wright JW, Prevost WJ, et al: MR imaging of the acutely injured patient with cervical traction. *Radiology* 1986; 159:273–274.
95. Roth JL, Nugent M, Gray JE, et al: Patient monitoring during magnetic resonance imaging. *Anesthesiology* 1985; 62:80–83.
96. Higgins CB, Lanzer P, Stark D, et al: Imaging by nuclear magnetic resonance in patients with chronic ischemic heart diseases. *Circulation* 1984; 69:523–531.
97. McArdle CB, Nicholas DA, Richardson CJ, et al: Monitoring of the neonate undergoing MR imaging: Technical considerations. *Radiology* 1986; 159:223–226.
98. Geiger RS, Cascorbi HF: Anesthesia in an NMR scanner. *Anesth Analg* 1984; 63:622–623.
99. Dunn V, Coffman CE, McGowan JE, et al: Mechanical ventilation during magnetic resonance imaging. *Magnetic Resonance Imaging* 1985; 3:169–172.
100. Mirvis SE, Borg V, Belzberg H: MR imaging of ventilator-dependent patients: Preliminary experience. *AJR* 1987; 149:845–846.
101. Nixon C, Hirsch NP, Ormerod IEC, et al: Nuclear magnetic resonance: Its implications for the anesthetist. *Anaesthesia* 1986; 41:131–137.
102. Smith DS, Askey P, Youing ML, et al: Anesthetic management of acutely ill patients during magnetic resonance imaging. *Anesthesiology* 1986; 65:710–711.
103. Boutros A, Pavlicek W: Anesthesia for magnetic resonance imaging. *Anesth Analg* 1987; 66:367.
104. Gebarski SS, Maynard FW, Gabrielsen TO, et al: Posttraumatic progressive myelopathy. *Radiology* 1985; 157:379–385.
105. Edgar RE: Surgical management of spinal cord cysts. *Paraplegia* 1976; 14:21–27.
106. Tator CH, Meguro K, Rowed DW. Favorable results with syringosubarachnoid shunts for treatment of syringomyelia. *J Neurosurg* 1982; 56:517–523.
107. Quencer RM, Green BA, Eisemont FJ. Posttraumatic spinal cord cysts: Clinical features and characterization with metrizamide computed tomography. *Radiology* 1983; 146:415–423.
108. Quencer RM, Morse BMM, Green BA, et al: Intraoperative spinal sonography: An adjunct to metrizamide CT in assessment and surgical decompression of spinal cord cysts. *AJNR* 1984; 5:71–79; *AJR* 1984; 142:593–601.
109. Barrett HJM, Botterell EH, Jousse AT, et al: Progressive myelopathy as a sequel to traumatic paraplegia. *Brain* 1966; 89:159–173.
110. Williams B, Terry AF, Jones F, et al: Syringomyelia as a sequel to traumatic paraplegia. *Paraplegia* 1981; 19:67–80.
111. Griffiths ER, McCormic CC: Posttraumatic syringomyelia (cystic myelopathy). *Paraplegia* 1981; 19:96–97.

112. Watson N. Ascending cystic degeneration of the cord after spinal cord injury. *Paraplegia* 1981; 19:9–95.
113. Vernon JD, Chir B, Silver JR, et al: Post-traumatic syringomyelia. *Paraplegia* 1982; 20:339–364.
114. McLean DR, Miller JPR, Allen PBR, et al: Posttraumatic syringomyelia. *J Neurosurg* 1973; 39:485–492.
115. duBoulay G, Shah SH, Currie JC, et al: The mechanism of hydromyelia in Chiari type I malformations. *Br J Radiol* 1974; 47:579–587.
116. Seibert CE, Dreisbach JN, Swanson WB, et al: Progressive posttraumatic cystic myelopathy: Neuroradiologic evaluation. *AJR* 1981; 136:1161–1165.
117. Quencer RM, Sheldon JJ, Donovan Post MJ, et al: MRI chronically injured cervical spinal cord. *AJNR* 1986; 7:457–464, *AJR* 1986; 147:125–132.
118. Enzmann DR, O'Donohoe J, Rubin JB, et al: CSF Pulsations within non-neoplastic spinal cord cysts. *AJNR* 1987; 8:517–525; *AJR* 149:149–157.

9

The Pediatric Spine: Normal Anatomy and Spinal Dysraphism

Bonnie D. Flannigan-Sprague, M.D.

Michael T. Modic, M.D.

Traumatic, neoplastic, inflammatory, and degenerative processes—while not as common as in the adult population—are encountered in the pediatric age group and usually entail similar differential and pulse-sequence considerations. In addition, while the pediatric spine is essentially a miniature version of its adult counterpart, it is somewhat unique in its normal anatomy and disease processes, which are developmental in nature. To appreciate the normal anatomy and developmental disorders, the main subject of this chapter, an understanding of the basic embryonic developmental sequence is necessary.

NORMAL ANATOMY AND DEVELOPMENT

The internal architecture of the spinal cord develops from the ectoderm of the embryonic disk, which forms the neural plate (Fig 9–1). The neural plate deepens into a groove and fuses posteriorly, a process called neurulation. This process begins in the cervical area and proceeds cranially and caudally to form the neural tube, which contains the ventricles and central canal of the spinal cord. This process is usually completed by the fourth week of gestation. The most cephalic end of the neural tube, the anterior neuropore, closes first at the lamina terminalis. The caudal end, the posterior neuropore, closes next (probably in the sacral region) and heralds the end of the stage of neurulation. The process of canalization then occurs, which results in elongation of the neural tube caudal to the posterior neuropore; this in turn produces an ependyma-lined tubular structure, which unites with the neural tube above. The final phase, retrogressive differentiation, results in a decrease in the size of the cell mass and central lumen of the caudal neural tube via cell necrosis. This process produces the filum terminale and distal conus as well as a focal dilatation of the central canal, the ventriculus terminalis, at the tip of the conus medullaris. Concomitant with the process of neurulation, the closing neural tube separates from the overlying ectoderm, a process designated as disjunction. The overlying ectoderm fuses in the midline posterior to the neural tube. Perineural mesenchyme then surrounds the neural tube and is induced to form the meninges, bone, and muscles. Normally, the closure of the neural tube, concomitant with disjunction, results in isolation of the mesenchyme from the newly formed central canal of the cord. This process is extremely critical, and abnormalities during this stage are thought to result in a number of important developmental lesions.[1–3]

During these early stages of development, there is no specific boundary between the brain and spinal cord, with the latter being defined as beginning at the level of the first pair of cranial nerves. The spinal cord, from its beginnings as a thick-walled tube, enlarges at or about 4 months at the levels of nerve root plexes for the upper and lower limbs, resulting in a cervical and lumbosacral enlargement. While the development of the bony spine closely follows that of the spinal cord, after the third month the vertebral column grows faster. Thus, in normal circumstances the spinal cord appears to recede up the vertebral canal with its terminal portion at the level of L3 at birth, gradually receding to its adult position behind the body of L1 by age 2 to 3 months. The central canal of the cord, particularly in the region of the ven-

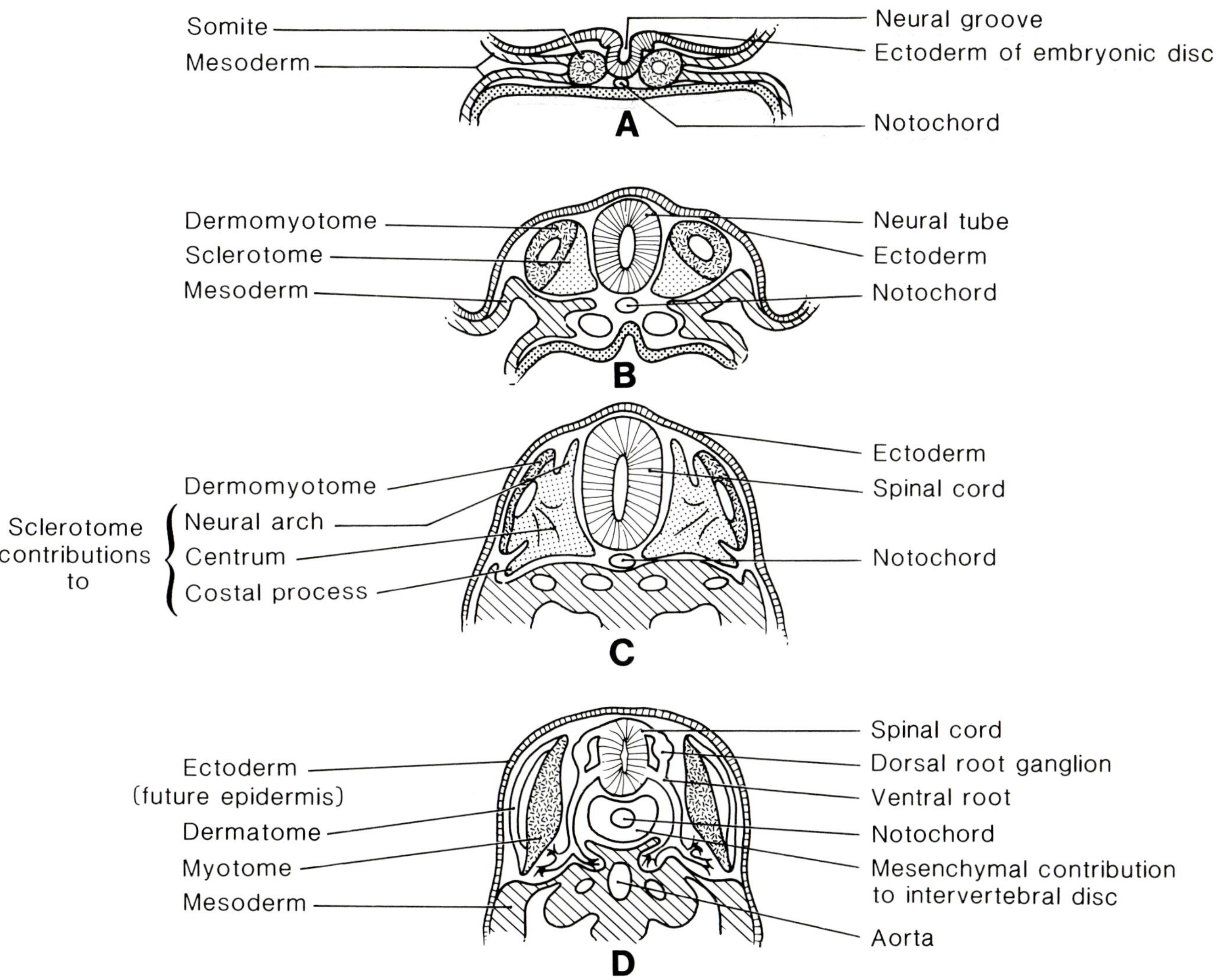

FIG 9–1.
Diagrams illustrating formation of the neural tube and spinal cord and differentiation of somites into sclerotomes and dematomyotomes. **A–D,** transverse sections at about 18, 22, 27, and 30 days, respectively.

triculus terminalis, is more prominent in the child than in the adult and frequently can be identified on normal studies; this may be of use in identifying the level of the conus in cases of tethering (Fig 9–2). The tip of the neural tube retains its terminal connection, being stretched and differentiated into a slender fibrous strand, the filum terminale. In the infant, the cord is positioned in the center of the canal, but its relative position changes as a normal thoracic kyphosis develops.[2,3]

THE BONY SPINE

The development of the bony spine is best understood in terms of nodocord and sclerotome morphology (Fig 9–3). The notocord begins within a mass of ectoderm called Hensen's node and develops into a slender chain of cells between the neural tube and developing gut. At about 3 weeks, the notocord separates from the primitive gut and neural tube. It appears to act as a framework for the developing spine and induces and controls the appropriate formation of vertebral bodies.[2,3] Once this process is under way, the notocordal cells begin to disappear, except at certain sites. They form the nucleus pulposus and notocordal rests may persist in any portion of a track along the basisphenoid, basiocciput, odontoid, and vertebral bodies caudally to the conus; this is why chordomas can arise along this line later in life.[2,4]

The mesenchyme lateral to the closing neural tube

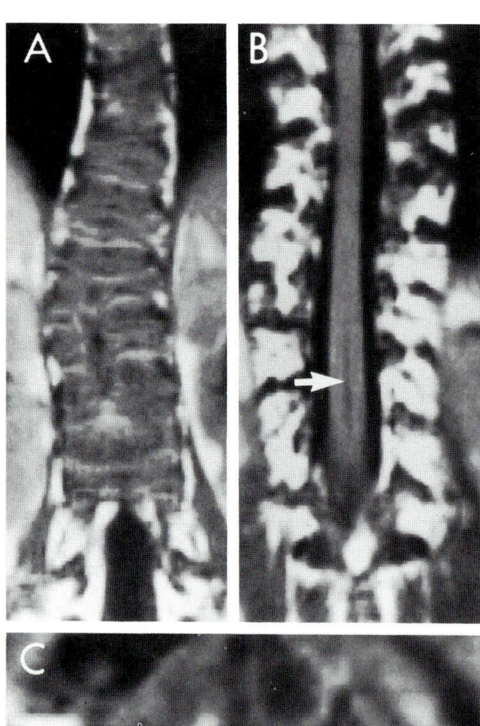

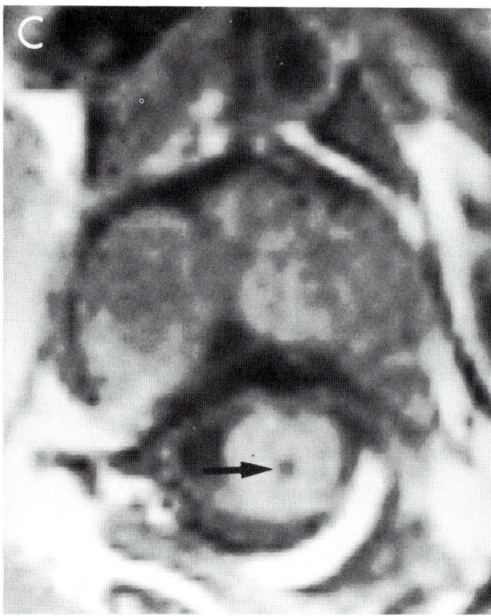

FIG 9–2.
Hemivertebrae and scoliosis in a 2-year-old child. **A** and **B,** coronal (500/20) spin echo images through the thoracolumbar spine. Note the thin slit-like structure representing dilation of the terminal central canal (ventriculus terminalis) *(arrow).* **C,** axial image through the region of the ventriculus terminalis *(arrow).* Note the mildly asymmetric clefted hemivertebrae.

organizes into paraxial mesoderm, which is the forerunner of the somites. The somites then differentiate into a ventral medial and a dorsal lateral compartment. The former, ventral medial, gives rise to the sclerotomes, which consist of cephalic and caudal masses of cells that develop into the vertebral bodies and ribs; the latter, the dorsal lateral dermomyotome, will give rise to the paraspinal musculature. As the spinal cord develops, this process occurs first in the cervical region and from there proceeds cephalad and caudad. The caudal and cranial sclerotomes, while initially separated by intersegmental vessels, divide in half transversely along the sclerotomic fissures. Adjacent halves of contiguous sclerotomes then unite to form one vertebra and the intersegmental vessels become incorporated within the center of the vertebral bodies.[2,3,5] (see Fig 9–3). This zone, composed of a cartilaginous plate, is identified on plain films as a lucent band (Hahn's notch) and on magnetic resonance imaging (MRI) as a horizontal band of intermediate or low signal intensity dividing the vertebral body into cranial and caudal portions (Fig 9–4). These can be identified in infants younger than 2 months.

The normal pediatric spine reveals distinct differences when compared with the adult spine. In young infants, the spine has a straight or slightly C-shaped configuration due to the fact that there is less cervical and lumbar lordosis at this stage of life. This lends itself to direct coronal as well as sagittal imaging for optimal display of the entire spinal cord.

Once an infant begins to hold its head up, a cervical lordosis develops; a lumbar lordosis develops subsequently, when the infant begins to bear weight. Before weight bearing, the intervertebral disks are thicker and have a more spherical shape. The adjacent vertebral bodies have a biconcave contour, which accomodates the spherical disk (see Fig 9–4). The general vertebral body size is small in comparison with the spinal canal in a newborn. This is quite obvious on sagittal T_1-weighted images of the lumbar spine, on which the epidural fat behind L5 and S1 can appear very prominent and the thecal sac looks very capacious in relationship to the bodies of L5 and S1. As the vertebral bodies grow, this discrepancy becomes less apparent. In infants, the overall signal intensity of the vertebral bodies on T_1-weighted images is noted to be less than in older children or adults. This reflects the abundance of red (hematopoietic) mararow as compared with yellow (fat) marrow at this stage of life. With increasing age, the vertebral marrow increases in signal intensity on T_1-weighted images until it obtains an intensity similar to that of the adult spine.

TECHNICAL CONSIDERATIONS IN PEDIATRIC MRI

The biggest challenge in pediatric MRI is to obtain high-quality, motionless images. This is achieved with the use of sedation when required, and by choosing

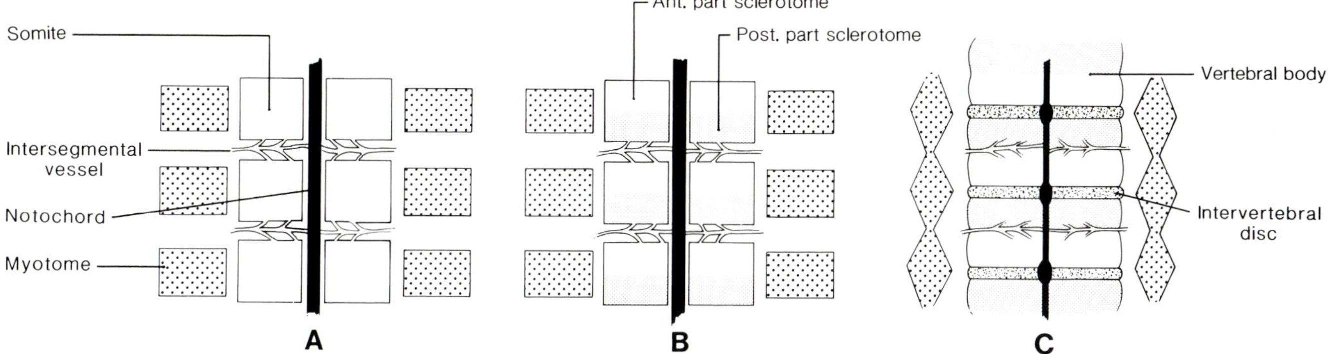

FIG 9–3.
Diagrammatic representation of the development of the vertebral body and intervertebral disk. The vertebral bodies are formed by fusion of adjacent portions of sclerotomes. The intervertebral disk develops both from these sclerotomes and from the incorporation of remnants of the notocord. The intersegmental vessels are incorporated into the areas of fusion and become the basivertebral vessels.

scan parameters that will allow adequate images to be obtained with a relatively short imaging time.

The importance of adequate sedation cannot be overemphasized. Regimens that have been commonly employed include chloral hydrate, 50 to 100 mg given orally, a mixture of meperidine, 2 mg/kg, Phenergan, 1 mg/kg, and chlorpromazine, 1 mg/kg IM (DPT), rectal thiopental, 20 to 30 mg/kg, or pentobarbital, 2 to 6 mg/kg IM. In the newborn, feeding just prior to the examination will also help.

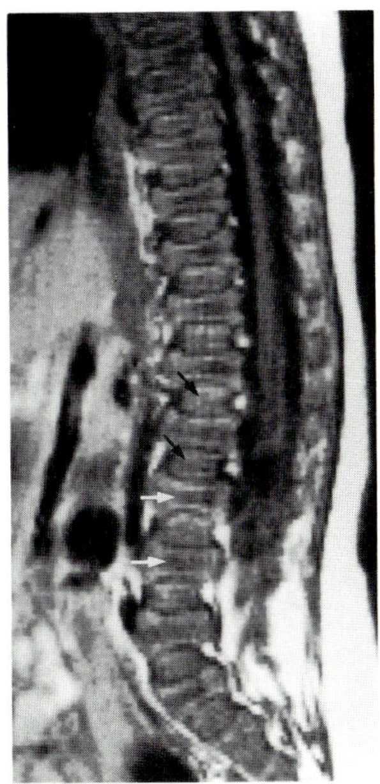

FIG 9–4.
Hahn's notch. Note the area of decreased signal intensity in the central portion of the vertebral bodies which represents the cartilaginous plates at the sites of fusion of the sclerotomes *(white arrows)*. The intervertebral disks are thick and spherical in shape *(black arrows)* (2-month-old normal male infant).

The use of sedation necessitates monitoring of respiratory function. At a minimum, this would consist of direct visual monitoring of the patient by an accompanying parent or nurse in the scanning suite. Affixing an object such as a paper cup to the child's chest can be a useful indicator of respiratory motion. Other devices that produce a more reliable means of monitoring the patient include respiratory, ECG, and pulse-oximeter monitoring for more critical evaluation of thoracic excursion, cardiac electrical activity, and oxygen saturation.

Coil selection will be mandated by the patient's size and by the type of examination desired. An effort should always be made to match the smallest coil possible with the field of view needed. In the very young the entire infant can usually be placed in the head or extremity coil or if a surface coil is mandated, an orbit or small planar coil can be employed. As the patient size increases, more routine adult-sized surface coils can be utilized.

The child should be placed in the supine position in the center of the chosen coil and strapped or padded securely in place. A short localizing scan (300/15) T_1-weighted spin-echo images with relatively thick slices (10 mm) is recommended to verify positioning and for minor adjustments if necessary before longer scan sequences begin. T_1-weighted images (short TR/short TE) are generally the most useful for screening purposes. Repetition times are chosen to obtain the optimal number of slices to cover the area of interest. The number of excitations will be dictated by the slice thickness in order to maintain an adequate signal-to-noise ratio. In general however, thin 2- to 4-mm slices, either contiguous or with a minimal gap (40% or less), will be required. In addition to routine sagittal and axial images, coronal images may play an important role in the screening evaluations for scoliosis and spinal dysraphism. In the very young, the lack of a cervical and lumbar lordosis can often result in depiction of the entire neural axis on a single slice in the coronal plane. Gradient-echo sequences, gating, refocussing, saturation pulses, and other technique modifications (discussed elsewhere) are also useful in optimizing the examination. Despite the smaller size found in the pediatric population, the examination is often as long if not longer than in the adult, as it is crucial to evaluate the entire spinal column from the foramen magnum to the sacrum if the examination is being carried out for the evaluation of congenital abnormalities.

SPINAL DYSRAPHISM

Spinal dysraphism is defined as incomplete or absent fusion of parts that normally unite, and designates the group of congenital disorders of the spine that involve, in part, imperfect fusion of midline mesenchymal, bony, and neural structures.[1] Magnetic resonance is an ideal tool for screening of these disorders as its noninvasive nature and multidimensional imaging capability allows depiction of the entire spinal axis with excellent discrimination of the extradural, intradural, and intramedullary compartments. Because of the complexity of developmental disorders, it is critically important to tailor each examination to the clinical question, which may necessitate additional imaging techniques such as plain films, CT, or ultrasound for definitive resolution of specific considerations.

SPINA BIFIDA

This term refers to incomplete fusion of the neural arch, which usually occurs in the midline involving the spinous process. Uncommonly, asymmetrical defects have been noted in the presence of a well-developed spinous process. The term *spina bifida occulta,* although commonly taken to indicate a minimal defect in fusion of the spinous process or lamina, actually implies a focal defect in the vertebral canal, often with associated neural defect but without obvious protrusion of the spinal contents. If a mass is present with spina bifida occulta, it is usually local and secondary to a lipoma.[1]

The term *spina bifida aperta* on the other hand, implies a herniation of all or part of the spinal contents through a posterior spina bifida to form an obvious protrusion, such as meningocele, myelocele, or meningomyelocele. These may be associated with other forms of dysraphism, such as syringomyelia, hydromyelia, and diastematomyelia, in other portions of the spinal axis.

The development of spina bifida may result from adhesion of ectodermal and neural ectodermal tissue during disjunction, which could prohibit mesenchyme from extending between the neural ectoderm and cutaneous ectoderm, producing a focal spina bifida.[1]

MENINGOCELES

Meningoceles represent a midline skin-covered protrusion of dura and arachnoid through a spinal defect without neural tissue; these are much less common than myelomeningoceles or lipomyelomeningoceles. Males and females are equally affected and they can occur anywhere in the central nervous system from the nasal cavity to the sacral coccygeal region. The lumbar region is the most common location. Although by definition meningoceles should contain no neural elements, occasionally a herniation of a loop of nerve may occur, which may even become adherent to the wall of the sac. Lesions that are posterior are usually easily diagnosed clinically and require imaging merely for confirmation and better definition of the extent of the lesion. Lateral meningoceles and anterior sacromeningoceles (Fig 9–5), can be a more difficult diagnostic and differential problem, but can usually be distinguished from other paraspinal or pelvic masses by identifying the communication to the thecal sac via a neck, which may be either narrow or wide. T_1-weighted images in the sagittal or covonal plane provide the best definition of this communication, but the signal intensity of the CSF within the meningocele may appear brighter than that within the lumbosacral canal because of dampened CSF pulsations.

MYELOCELE AND MYELOMENINGOCELE

A myelocele represents a midline herniation of neural tissue that lies exposed at the skin surface and is flush with it. The surrounding skin is deficient. A myelomeningocele is a myelocele that protrudes above the skin surface secondary to enlargement of the subarachnoid space and represents the most common significant form of spinal dysraphism. The exposed plaque-like neural structure that opens dorsally is referred to as the placode. The placode may be looked upon as a cord that has a sagittal split and is open from the back, with the posterior surface representing the inside of the open cord adherent to the skin or dura. The anterior side of the placode is the entire outer surface of the cord. Thus, nerve roots that would typically arise from the ventral surface of the cord now exit off the central portion of the placode. The dorsal roots exit off the lateral edges

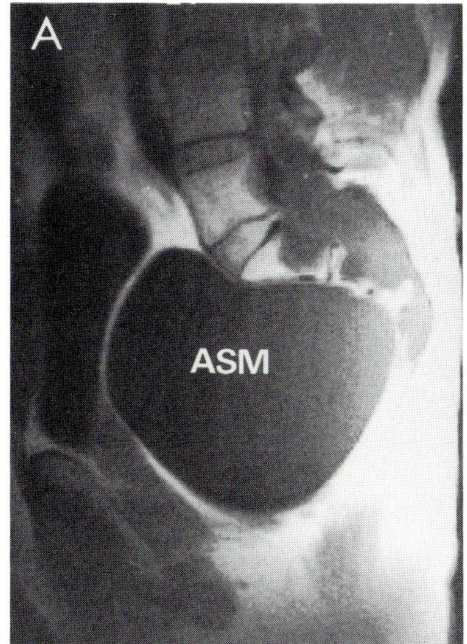

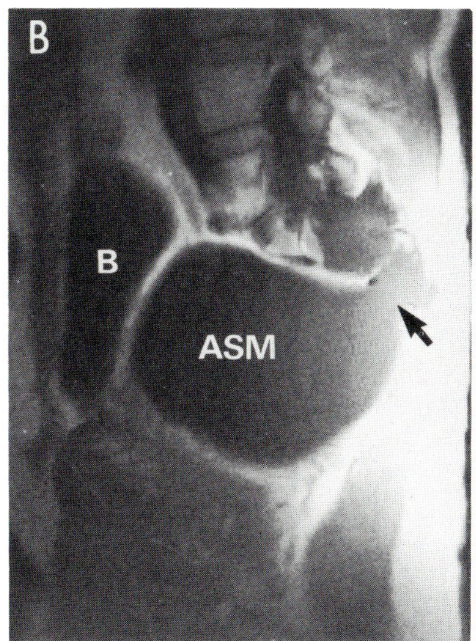

FIG 9–5.
Anterior sacral meningocele. **A** and **B,** sagittal (500/20) T_1-weighted spin-echo images through the lower lumbar and sacral regions. There is a low CSF signal intensity cystic mass anterior to the sacrum that communicates *(arrow)* with the sacral CSF space. (ASM = anterior sacral meningocele. B = bladder).

of the placode. Posterior bony defects usually extend over long segments, sometimes involving the entire lumbar canal.[1, 6–8]

Currently, the etiologic theory held in highest favor is one that suggests that the myelomeningocele represents a disturbance in the closure of the neural tube leaving it in its embryonal plaque-like state. The hydrocephalus and Chiari type II deformities invariably seen in this abnormality do not appear to develop at the same time, but later in fetal life.[1, 9, 10]

Initially, imaging modalities are usually contraindicated in the neonate with myelomeningocele as immediate surgical closure is the primary consideration to prevent infection. Following surgical closure, a baseline MR may be indicated because of the variable association of Chiari type II malformations, the frequent development of hydrocephalus and/or hydromyelia and the common association of other developmental anomalies (Fig 9–6).

Symptoms can be progressive, as the placode is usually tethered to the dura, and may become manifest as other associated congenital abnormalities become symptomatic. The cord is often split either above or—uncommonly—at the placode. The placode, if tethered to the dura, blends with it and is difficult to define. If the myelomeningocele occurs at a region higher than the lumbar region, there may be reconstitution of the cord inferiorly into a seemingly normal conus.[1, 11, 12]

On sagittal and axial T_1-weighted MR, the level of the neural placode or conus medullaris can generally be identified. It is, however, difficult to define the exact nature and/or existence of tethering if the placode is flat and not clearly distinct from the adjacent thecal sac in its dorsal position. Postoperatively, it is not uncommon to identify the conus medullaris and/or neural placode below the L2 level.[12] The diagnosis of tethering requires identification of an adherent scar at the repair site or of a thickened filum terminale and/or associated mass. Again, imaging of the entire spine is necessary because of the high incidence of associated abnormalities such as diastematomyelia or hydromyelia. Sagittal T_1-weighted imaging of the craniovertebral junction will demonstrate the constant association of Chiari type II malformations (see Fig 9–6). Hydromyelia often occurs near the level of the placode and may extend cephalad for variable distances.[12] Magnetic resonance imaging is particularly well suited to the evaluation of the latter complication, although the appearance of hydromyelia on MRI may be variable. When the central cavity is well delineated, with signal intensity similar to that of adjacent CSF, the diagnosis is rarely in doubt. However, a hydromyelia cavity may present as an enlarged cord with a signal intensity similar to that of the adjacent neural tissue. The reasons for this are thought to be related either to the proteinacious content of the CSF fluid or, what is more likely, to reduced CSF pulsations, which produce less spin dephasing and as a result, a higher signal intensity. Unrefocussed or intentionally dephased sequences may prove more useful in evaluating the pulsatile CSF within a hydromyelia cavity than the more commonly employed refocussing or motion compensated techniques. Care should be taken in this evaluation, as solid tumors

FIG 9–6.
Postoperative myelomeningocele in a 1-month-old boy. **A,** sagittal (500/20) T_1-weighted spin-echo images, which demonstrate deformity of the lower thoracic and upper lumbar spine at the site of the surgical repair *(large arrow)*. Hydromyelia is noted within the lower thoracic cord *(small arrow)*. **B–E,** axial (500/17) T_1-weighted spin-echo images passing cranially to caudally to just above the region of the placode. There is hydromyelia of a single cord *(arrows)* (**B**) passing asymmetrically into the left hemicord (**C**) above the level of a bony spur producing diastematomyelia (**D**). There is no evidence of hydromyelia at this level. Below the level of the spur *(E)*, the hemicords reunite, again with evidence of hydromyelia. **F,** sagittal (500/20) T_1-weighted image through the cervical medullary junction demonstrating a Chiari type II malformation *(arrows)*.

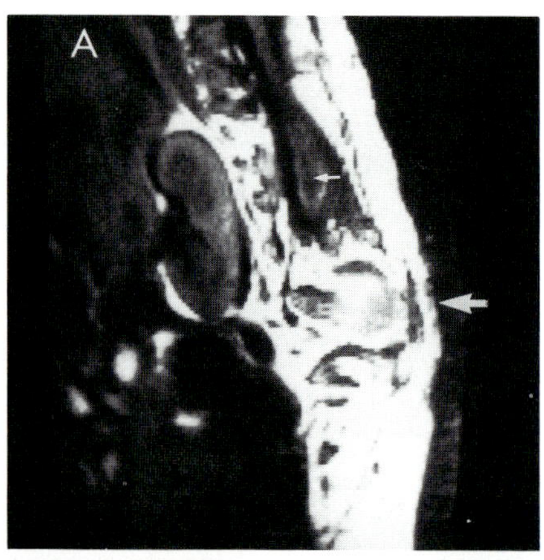

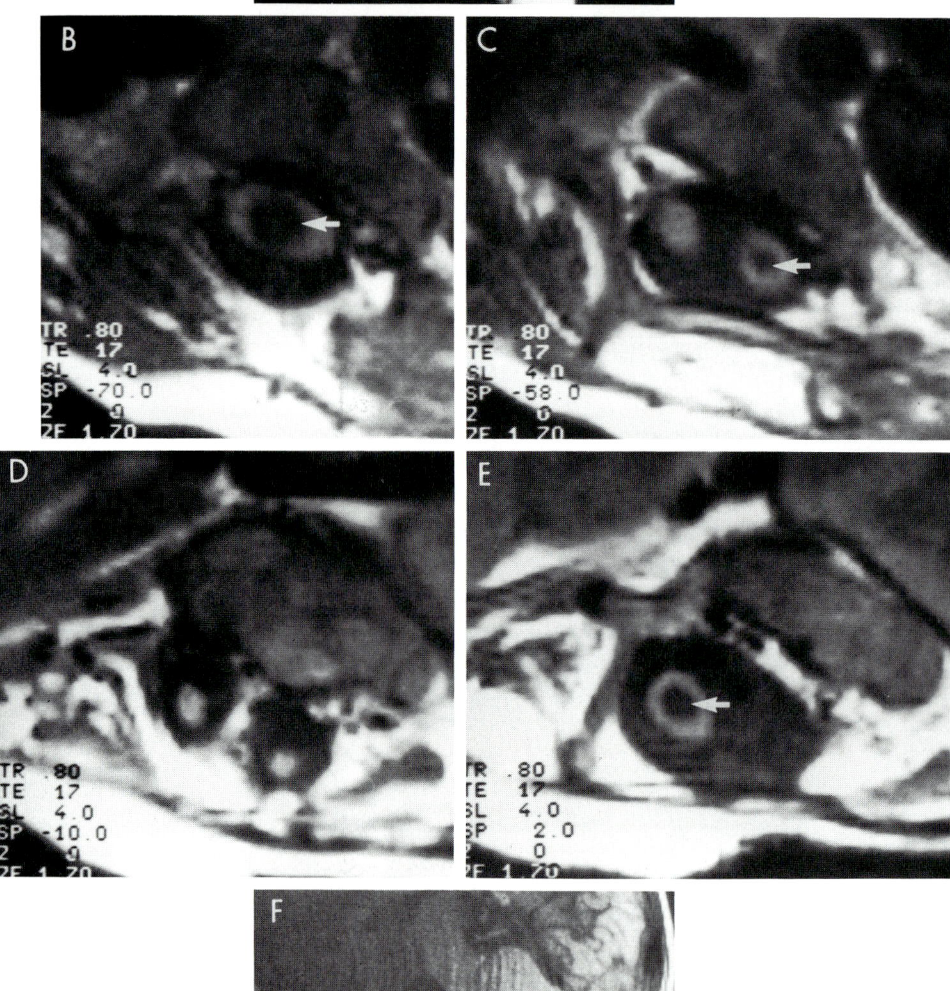

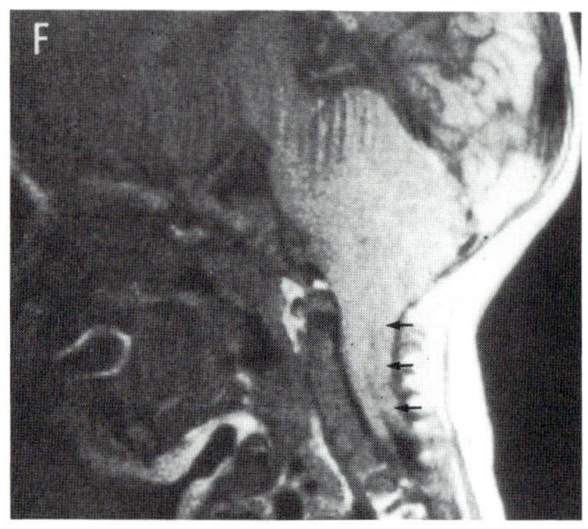

may occasionally produce signal intensity similar to that of an intramedullary cyst. If there is any question and surgery is contemplated, intraoperative ultrasound would provide the diagnostic distinction.

LIPOMYELOSCHISIS

This term refers to dorsal dysraphism with lipoma, of which intradural lipoma and lipomyelomeningocele are two forms (Figs 9–7 and 9–8). This abnormality has been well defined by Naidich et al.[13] who describe it as "consisting of skin-covered, focal spina bifida; focal partial clefting of the dorsal half to the spinal cord; continuity of the dorsal cleft with the central canal of the cord above (and occasionally below) the cleft; deficiencies of the dura underlying the spina bifida; deep extension of the subcutaneous lipoma through the spina bifida and the dural deficiency to insert directly into the cleft on the dorsal half of the cord; variable cephalic extension of the lipoma into the contiguous central canal of the cord; and variable ballooning of the subarachnoid space to form an associated meningocele."[13]

The etiology is thought to be related to premature disjunction, which would allow the neural ectoderm to separate before closure of the neural tube and allow access of mesenchyme to the interior of the neural tube; this appears to induce production of lipomatous tissue. This mechanism would explain the occurrence of lipomas throughout the CNS as well as lipomyeloschisis.[1]

Cutaneous stigmata include a soft tissue mass in the midline (which usually extends asymmetrically toward one side), hypertrichosis, dermal sinus, dimple, or hemangioma.[14]

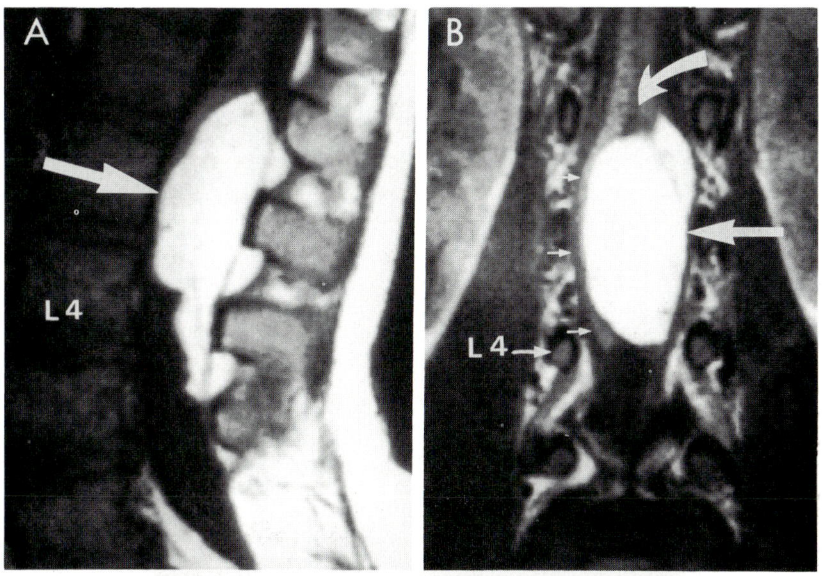

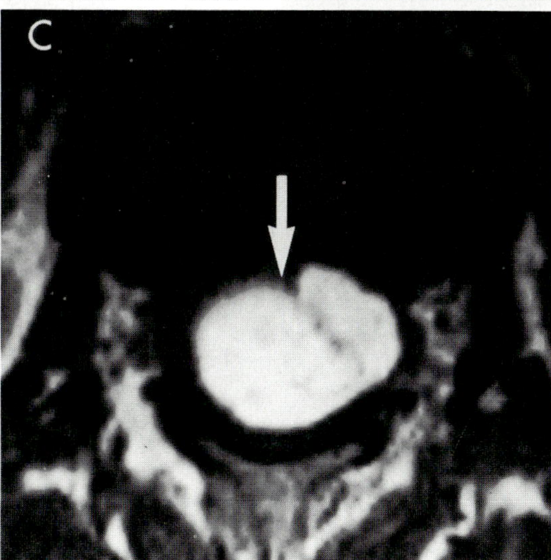

FIG 9–7.
Intradural lipoma. **A–C,** sagittal, coronal, and axial (500/20) T_1-weighted spin-echo images through the lumbar spine. There is an intradural and intramedullary lipoma (**B**) *(large arrow)* producing partial clefting *(curved arrow)* and tethering of the distal cord *(small arrows),* which, while filling almost the entire spinal canal, lies primarily posterior *(arrow)* to the neural elements.

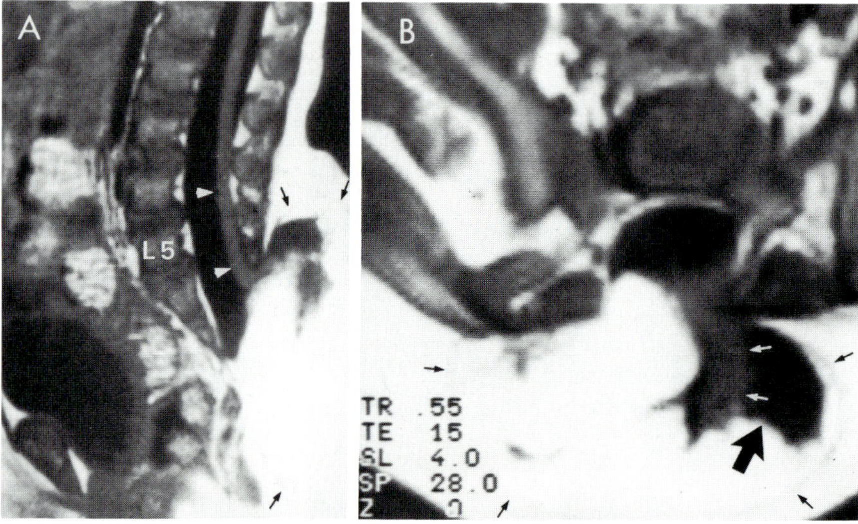

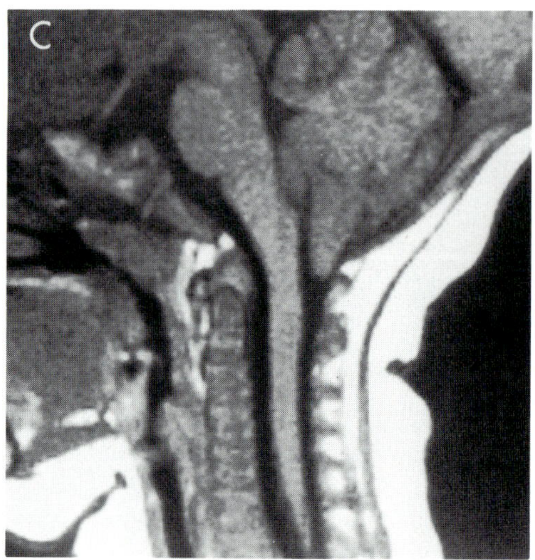

FIG 9–8.
Lipomyelomeningocele. Sagittal (**A**) and axial (**B**) (500/20) T_1-weighted spin-echo images through the region of a lipomyelomeningocele. Note the tethering of the spinal cord at the L5-S1 level *(small white arrows),* kinking, and posterior herniation of the neural elements into a lipomyelomingocele (*large black arrow*), filled primarily with fat (*black arrows* outline extent of sac). **C,** sagittal (500/20) T_1-weighted spin echo images through the cranial vertebral junction demonstrating an associated Chiari malformation.

Deep to the subcutaneous soft tissue mass there is usually a relatively focal spina bifida, most commonly in the lumbosacral spine. The transition from normal to abnormal vertebrae may be abrupt or gradual. A fibrovascular band connects the lamina of the most cephalic normal vertebra with the widely bifid lamina. When the spinal canal below the spina bifida is normal, there is often a caudal fibrovascular band as well. The meningocele and spinal cord herniation occur posteriorly in the subcutaneous tissue beneath the fibrovascular band and appear to tether the meningocele sac and neural tissue. The site of the band, as well as the superior kink in the meningocele sac and point of herniation, can usually be predicted on plain radiographs by identifying the level of the most cephalic widely bifid lamina.[13]

These abnormalities are often accompanied by fewer neurological symptoms than myelomeningoceles, and because there is usually reasonable preservation of neurological function the patient is usually fully evaluated before any surgery. Surgery itself is aimed at the release of the tethered spinal cord. The importance in defining the anatomy is that proper presurgical radiological assessment is critical for guiding surgical repair.[13] High-resolution CT and plain films may be more accurate in documenting the presence and site of the spina bifida and the size and asymmetry of the widely bifid lamina. Magnetic resonance imaging, on the other hand, provides a noninvasive means of evaluating the lipomyeloschisis, the site and size of the lipoma, the degree of extension of the lipoma within the extra-arachnoid space and in the central canal of the cord, the position of the herniated placode, and the course and length of dorsal and ventral nerve roots.

DORSAL DERMAL SINUS

The dorsal dermal sinus is a midline epithelium-lined sinus tract extending variable distances from the skin inward. It frequently connects the body surface

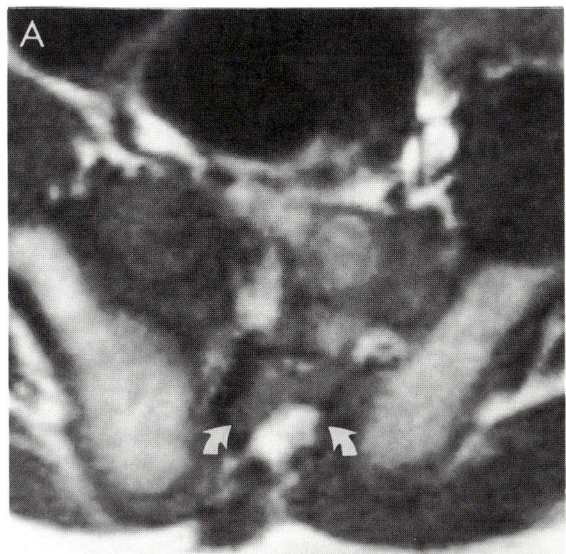

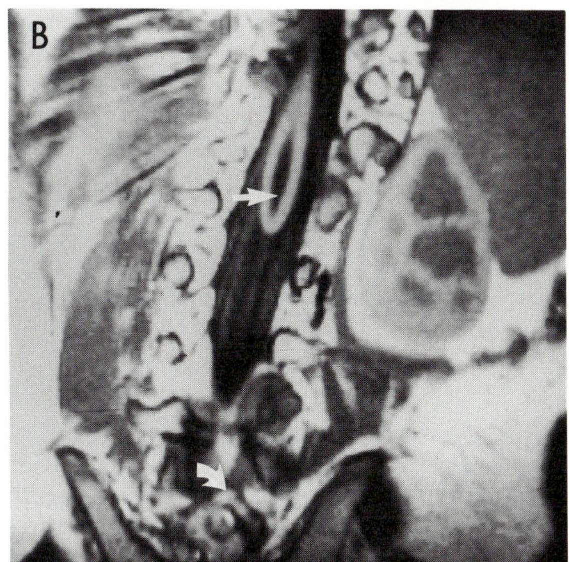

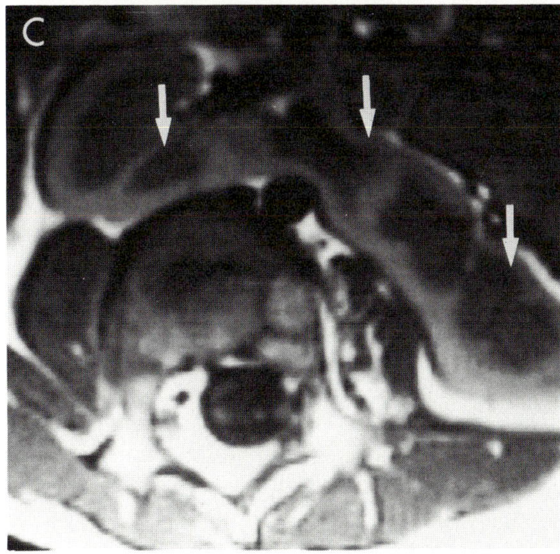

FIG 9–9.
Sacral agenesis. **A,** coronal (500/20) T_1-weighted spin-echo images through the lumbosacral region. Note the dilatation of the distal central canal *(straight arrow),* scoliosis, and absence of the sacrum *(curved arrow).* **B,** axial (500/20) T_1-weighted spin-echo image through the region of the ilia demonstrating absence of the sacrum *(curved arrows).* **C,** axial (500/20) T_1-weighted spin-echo image through the upper lumbar region demonstrating mild deformity of the vertebral body and associated horseshoe kidney *(arrows).*

with the CNS or its coverings. It presents as a midline dimple or pinpoint osteum and is usually associated with local stigmata such as hyperpigmentation, hairy nevus, or capillary angioma. The overwhelming majority are lumbosacral. The inner aspect of the sinus may be associated with the development of congenital inclusion masses such as dermoid or epidermoid cysts in 30% to 50% of cases. Not all cysts, however, are connected to sinus tracts. The sinus tracts may be associated with tethering, as may the mass.[1, 15] Magnetic resonance imaging is capable of identifying the sinus tract, but experience to date is too small to compare the accuracy of MRI with that of other modalities. Nevertheless, it is highly accurate in identifying tethering and/or the presence of an epidermoid or dermoid mass, and is therefore the most reasonable first test in patients who present with a cutaneous sinus or stigmata suggestive of this abnormality.

CAUDAL REGRESSION

This term defines a spectrum of anomalies, which includes maldevelopment and/or absence of the caudalmost spine. It may be associated with anal atresia, malformed external genatalia, renal dysplasia or aplasia, and pulmonary hypoplasia. This is a rare anomaly and the degree of spinal agenesis is variable. When limited to the coccygeal segment, agenesis is usually an incidental finding without symptoms. The most common type consists of partial bilateral symmetrical sacral agenesis, often with stable articulation between the ilia[1] (Fig 9–9).

DIASTEMATOMYELIA AND DIPLOMYELIA

This form of dysraphism is characterized by sagittal clefting of one portion (rarely two or more) of the spinal cord, conus medullaris, and/or filum terminale. This results in two frequently asymmetrical hemicords, each of which contains a central canal and a single dorsal and ventral horn giving rise to ipsilateral nerve roots. This cleft frequently contains a fibrous or osteocartilagenous spur. Overlying bony and/or soft tissue anomalies are invariably present[1, 16, 17] (Figs 9–10 and 9–11).

Diplomyelia is a more or less perfect duplication of the spinal cord, with each hemicord containing the central canal and two dorsal and two ventral horns and their corresponding nerve roots. In both, the conus medullaris is usually low and the cleft is most often encountered in the lower thoracic or upper lumbar region. With higher clefting, the hemicords frequently reunite into a more or less normal cord below. In 50% of cases, the hemicords lie side by side within a single subarachnoid space and a single arachnoid and dural tube.[17] There is usually no fibrous septum extending through this cleft, but there may be fibrolipomatous tissue at its dorsal aspect. In the other 50%, each hemicord is surrounded by an individual arachnoid and dural sheath.

Diastematomyelia is usually associated with tethering of the conus, often with lipoma (Figs 9–7 and 9–12). It may also be associated with other types of spinal dysraphism. When associated with lipomyelomeningocele or myelomeningocele it is usually cranial to the placode (see Figs 9–6 and 9–11). Clinically, the symptomatology is often similar to that of a tethered cord. Hydromyelia may be associated with one or both of the hemicords. Orthopedic deformities such as clubfoot, cutaneous manifestation such as hairy patches, and segmental anomalies such as butterfly vertebrae or hemivertebrae with scoliosis and kyphosis are the most common clinical findings. Magnetic resonance imaging can noninvasively identify the position and division of the cord as well as the site and length of the abnormality and assess any additional changes, such as hydromyelia.[12, 18, 19] Plain radiographs and CT scans are better at showing the bony abnormalities as well as the nature of the cartilaginous, osteocartilaginous, or fibrous spur.

THE TIGHT FILUM TERMINALE/TETHERED CORD

This abnormality refers to a variety of neurologic and orthopedic deformities associated with a thick filum terminale and low position of the conus medullaris. Clinical symptoms are thought to be secondary to stretching of the spinal cord, as they are aggravated by exercise and increase during periods of rapid growth. The normal filum terminale measures 2 mm or less in diameter. Dysraphism is usually less severe and the degree of tethering is variable. The filum may appear normal in size or thick. Sometimes it is difficult, when there is marked tethering, to distinguish between a stretched conus and the filum terminale. Lipomas are frequently associated distally and are located posteriorly (see Fig 9–12).

SCOLIOSIS

Scoliosis in the pediatric age group, while usually idiopathic, may be an indicator of an underlying spinal abnormality. Magnetic resonance imaging serves as a reasonable noninvasive imaging tool to evaluate this latter possibility. The presence or absence of cord abnor-

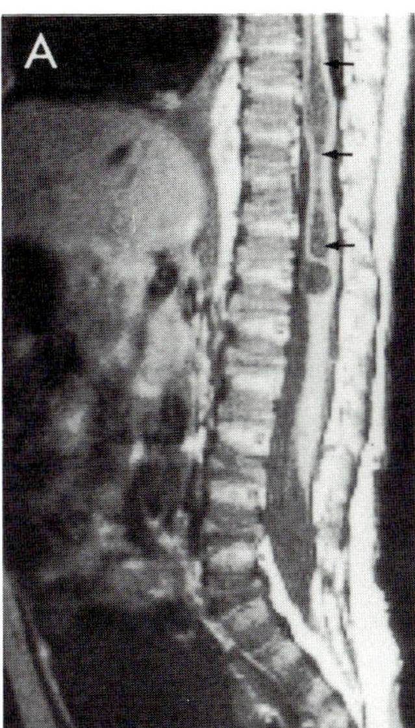

FIG 9–10.
Tethered cord, hydromyelia, and diastematomyelia. **A,** sagittal (500/20) T_1-weighted spin-echo image demonstrating tethering of the spinal cord at the L4 level. There is evidence of hydromyelia, but not of diastematomyelia on the sagittal image *(arrows).* **B** and **C,** contiguous coronal (500/17) sagittal T_1-weighted images through the thoracolumbar region. The central cystic dilatation is well appreciated as are asymmetrical hemicords below the level of the hydromyelia *(arrows).* Axial (500/20) images through the level of the hydromyelia superiorly (**D,** *arrow*) and diastematomyelia inferiorly (**E,** *arrow*). (Note the asymmetrical hemicords in **E** above the level of tethering.)

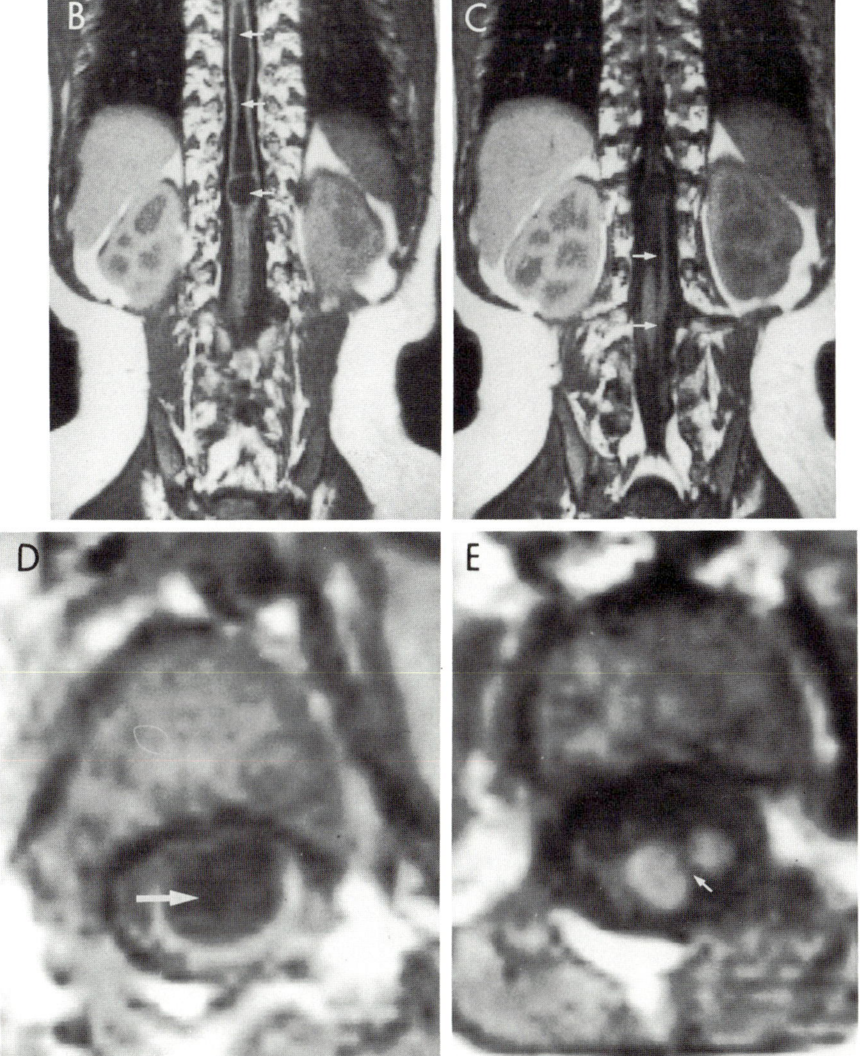

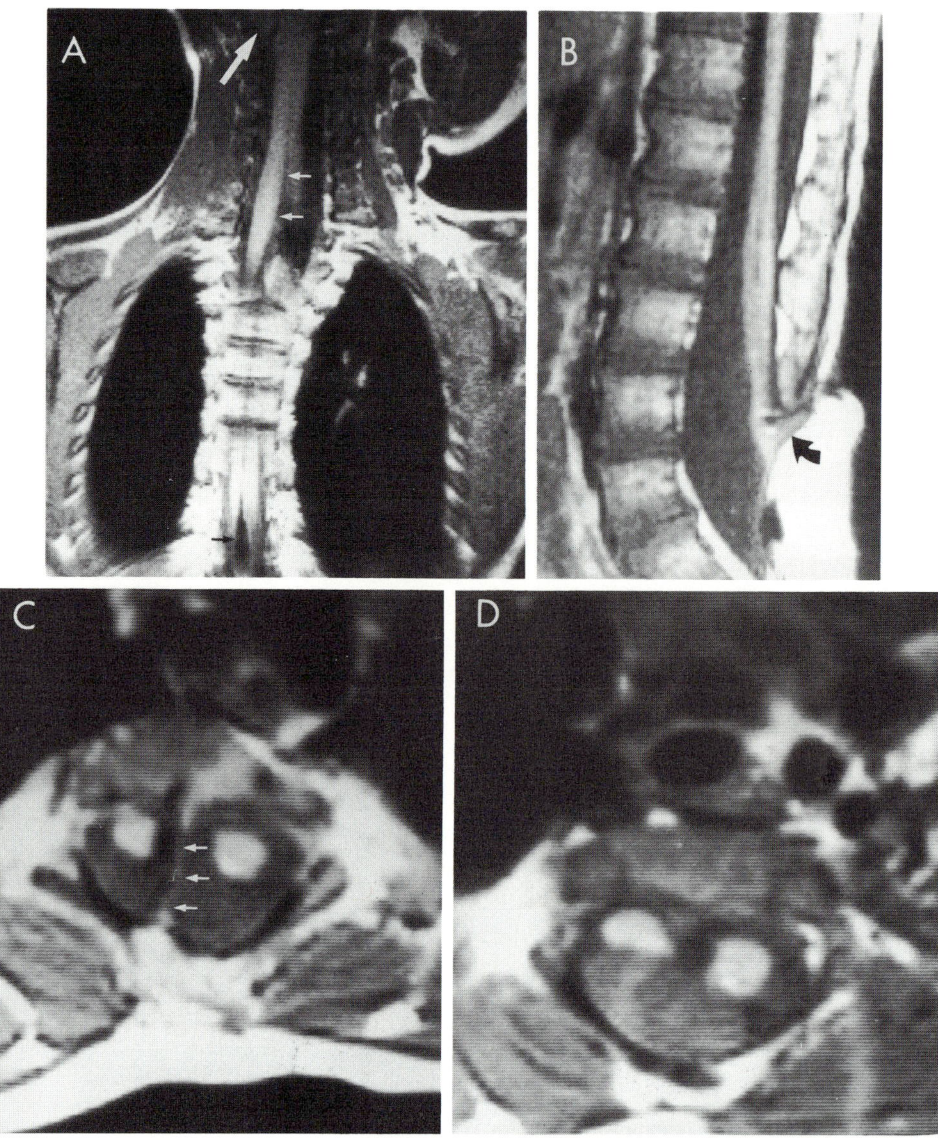

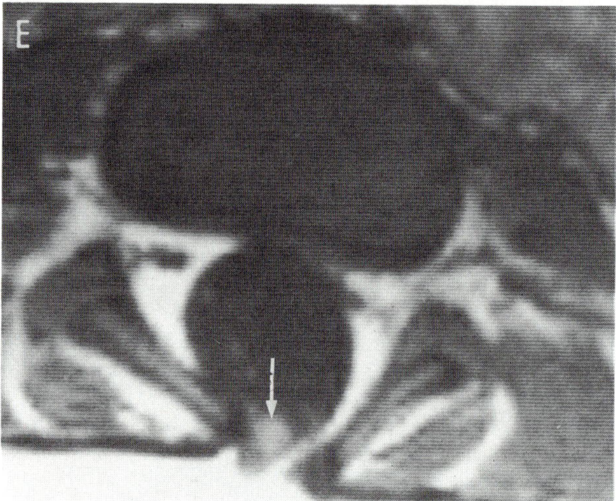

FIG 9–11.
Postoperative lipomyelomeningocele and diastematomyelia. **A,** coronal (500/20) T_1-weighted spin-echo image to the cervical and thoracic spine. A Chiari malformation is noted *(large white arrow).* The cord splits in the upper thoracic region and continues down into the lumbar region *(small arrows).* **B,** sagittal (500/17) T_1-weighted spin-echo image through the lumbar region. The distal cord is noted to be adherent posteriorly at the site of surgical repair of the lipomyelomeningocele at the inferior aspect of L4 *(arrow).* **C,** axial (500/17) T_1-weighted spin-echo image at the level of the fibrous septum in the upper thoracic region (*arrows*). Representative axial images through the midthoracic (**D**) and site of the tethered cord distally (**E**). Note the slight asymmetry of the hemicords in **D** and the posterior location of the tethered distal cord at the level of the spina bifida in **E** (*arrow*).

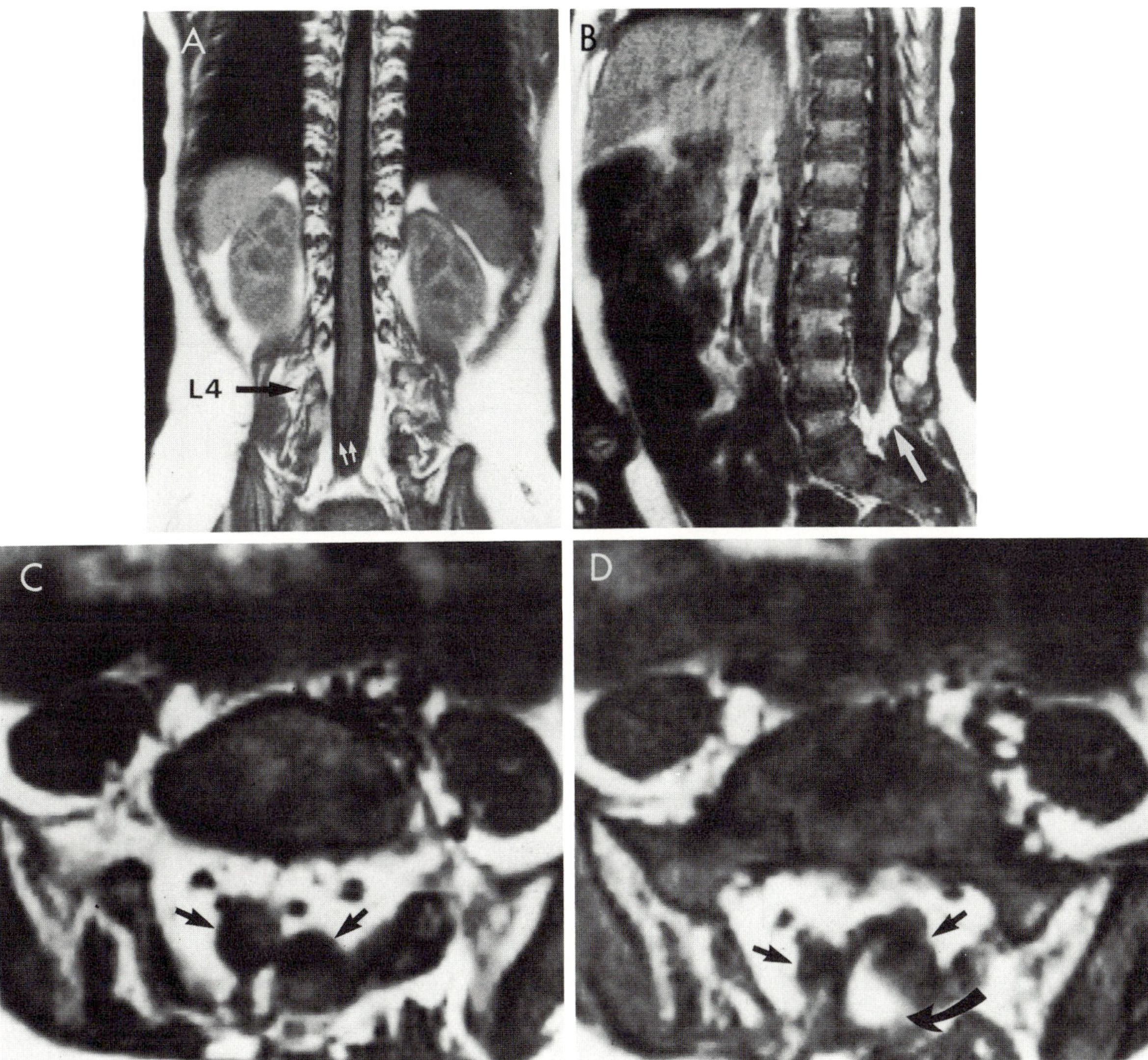

FIG 9–12.

Tethered cord, diplomyelia, and lipoma. **A,** coronal (500/20) T_1-weighted spin-echo image through the thoracolumbar spine. The conus medullaris is tethered at the L4–5 level. **B,** sagittal (500/20) T_1-weighted spin-echo image, which demonstrates a lipoma posteriorly at the L5-S1 level, the site of tethering. The distal cord is slightly out of plane on this image. **C** and **D,** axial (500/20) T_1-weighted spin-echo image at the L5-S1 level. Note the lipoma posteriorly *(curved arrow)* and distal splitting of the cord at this level *(small arrows).*

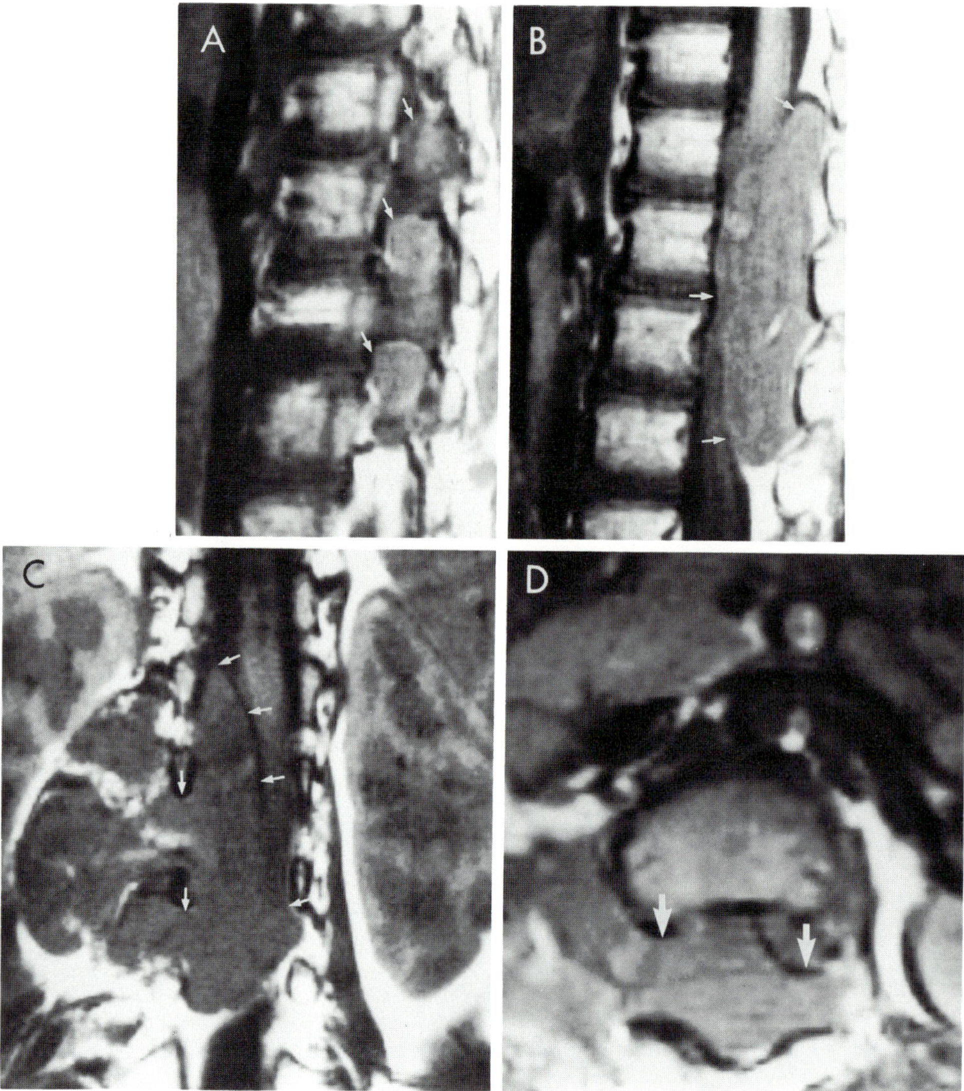

FIG 9–13.

Ganglioneuroblastoma. **A–C,** parasagittal, sagittal, and coronal (500/20) T_1-weighted spin echo images through the thoracolumbar spine. Soft tissue mass is noted expanding the neural foramen on the parasagittal images and occupying the posterior lateral aspect and the neural canal on the midline sagittal images *(arrows).* **D,** axial (500/20) T_1-weighted spin-echo image, which demonstrates this soft tissue mass within the neural canal extending through the neural foramen into the paravertebral soft tissue *(arrows).* At surgery this lesion was found to be entirely extradural.

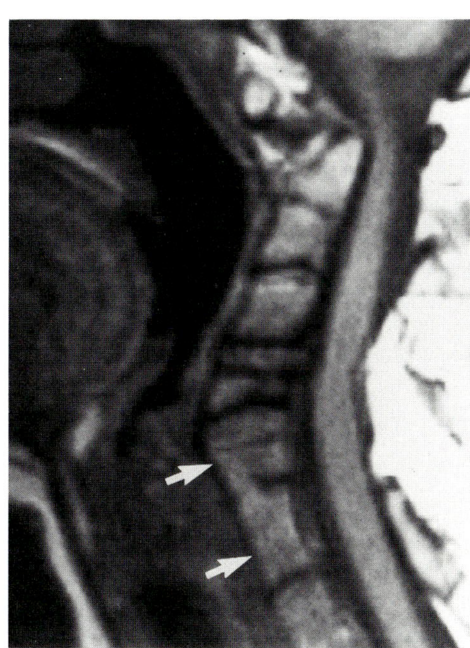

FIG 9–14.
Klippel-Feil syndrome. Sagittal (500/20) T_1-weighted spin-echo image through the cervical spine. Note the fused "block" vertebrae (*arrows*) as well as malformed C4. There is evidence of C1 and C2 malalignment.

malities, paravertebral masses (Fig 9–13), and vertebral body abnormalities, such as segmentation failure, can be identified. This last group would include blocked vertebrae, the Klippel-Feil syndrome (short neck, limitation in neck movement, and low posterior hairline) (Fig 9–14), and hemivertebrae (see Fig 9–2), all of which can lead to scoliosis (see Figs 9–2 and 9–14). Severe scoliosis requires multiple planes of imaging and sequences to evaluate the entire cord and spinal canal and to unravel the complex anatomy.

While clinical studies with MR are still accumulating, it is already apparent that T_1-weighted spin-echo MR examinations are extremely useful in defining both normal and abnormal pediatric spinal anatomy.[12, 20–22] The oft-quoted radiologic maxim regarding orthogonal views is again extremely applicable. In addition, the frequent cross-association of the various types of developmental abnormalities and their occurrence at different locations within the spine requires that the entire spinal axis, from the foramen magnum to sacrum, be studied in any patient suspected of having a congenital abnormality.

REFERENCES

1. Naidich TP, McLone DG, Harwood-Nash DC: Spinal dysraphism, in Newton TH, Potts DG (eds): *Modern Neuroradiology: Computed Tomography of the Spine and Spinal Cord,* vol 1. San Anselmo, Calif, Clavidel Press, 1983.
2. Sarwar M, Kier EL, Virapongse C: Development of the spine and spinal cord, in Newton TH, Potts DG (eds): *Modern Neuroradiology: Computed Tomography of the Spine and Spinal Cord,* vol 1. San Anselmo, Calif, Clavidel Press, 1983.
3. Arey LB: *Developmental Anatomy: A Textbook and Laboratory Manual of Embryology,* ed 7. Philadelphia, WB Saunders, 1965.
4. Peacock A: Observation of the prenatal development of the intervertebral disk in man. *J Anat* 1951; 85: 260–274.
5. Parke WW: Development of the spine, in Rothman RH, Simmone FA (ed): *The Spine.* Philadelphia, WB Saunders Co, 1975.
6. Fitz CR: Congenital anomalies of the spine and spinal cord, in Latchaw R (ed): *Computed Tomography of the Head, Neck, and Spine.* Chicago, Year Book Medical Publishers, 1985.
7. Humphreys RP: Spinal dysraphism, in Wilkins RH, Rengachary SS (eds): *Neurosurgery,* vol 3. New York, McGraw Hill Book Co, 1985.
8. Page LK: Occult spinal dysraphism and related disorders, in Wilkins RH, Rengachary SS (eds): *Neurosurgery,* vol 3. New York, McGraw Hill Book Co, 1985.
9. Osaka K, Matsumoto S, Tinimura T: Myeloschisis in early human embryos. *Childs Brain* 1978; 4:347–359.
10. Osaka K, Tinimura T, Hirayama A, et al: Myelomeningocele before birth. *J Neurosurg* 1978; 49:711–724.
11. Mori K: Spinal dysraphism (spina bifida), in Mori K, Harwood Nash DC (eds): *Anomalies of the Central Nervous System: Neuroradiology and Neurosurgery.* New York, Thieme-Stratton, 1985, pp 111–125.
12. Davis PC, Hoffman JC, Ball TI, et al: Spinal abnormalities in pediatric patients: MR imaging findings compared with clinical, myelographic and surgical findings. *Radiology* 1988; 166:679–685.
13. Naidich TP, McLone DG, Mutluer S: A new understanding of dorsal dysraphism with lipoma (lipomyeloschisis): Radiologic evaluation and surgical correction. *AJR* 1983; 140:1065–1078.
14. Zimmerman RA, Bilaniuk LT: Applications in magnetic resonance imaging and diseases of the pediatric central nervous system. *MRI Pediatr* 1986; 4:11–24.
15. Wright RL: Congenital dermal sinus. *Prog Neurol Surg* 1971; 4:175–191.
16. James CCM, Lassman LP: Diastematomyelia: A critical survey of 24 cases submitted to laminectomy. *Arch Dis Child* 1964; 39:125–130.
17. Naidich TP, Harwood-Nash DC: Diastematomyelia: Hemicords and meningeal sheaths: Single and double arachnoid and dural tubes. *Am J Neuroradiol* 1983; 4:633.
18. Han JS, Benson JE, Kaufman B, et al: Demonstration of diastematomyelia and associated abnormalities with MR imaging. *AJNR* 1985; 6:215–219.

19. Schlesinger AE, Naidich TP, Quencer RM: Concurrent hydromyelia and diastematomyelia. *AJNR* 1986; 7:473–477.
20. Lee BC, Lipper E, Nas R, et al: MRI of the central nervous system in neonates and young children. *AJNR* 1986; 7:605–616.
21. Walker HS, Dietrich RB, Flanagan BD, et al: Magnetic resonance imaging of the pediatric spine. *Radiographics* 1987; 7:1129–1152.
22. Barnes PD, Lester PD, Yamanashi WS, et al: Magnetic resonance imaging in infants and children with spinal dysraphism. *AJNR* 1986; 7:465–472.

10

Miscellaneous Topics

Thomas J. Masaryk, M.D.

INTRAMEDULLARY CYSTIC CAVITIES

Despite the minor variability in nomenclature as well as considerable debate surrounding the pathophysiology of intramedullary cystic cavities, magnetic resonance imaging (MRI) has significantly facilitated the diagnosis, treatment, and understanding of these lesions.[1–11] The distinction between hydromyelia and syringomyelia was first articulated by Simon in 1875.[12] Hydromyelia is the term reserved to specifically designate cystic dilatation of the ependymal lined central canal of the spinal cord by cerebrospinal fluid (CSF). The term syringomyelia refers to the state characterized by the presence of glial lined (central or eccentric), longitudinally oriented CSF cavities within the spinal cord. In as much as it is frequently difficult to distinguish between these two conditions, there has been a recent trend to combine the two terms ("syringohydromyelia") or refer to them generically as "syrinx cavities." Such lesions may be idiopathic or occur in association with congenital malformations (e.g., Chiari malformation), trauma, arachnoiditis, or intradural intramedullary and intradural extramedullary neoplasms. As might be expected from their varied etiology, these cavities are sporadic but are most frequently seen in young adults. While these cavities commonly involve the cervical and/or thoracic spinal cord, the precise clinical picture depends on the cross-sectional and vertical extent of cord destruction. Common presenting signs and symptoms include brachial amyotrophy with dissociative anesthesia in a "cape" or "vest" distribution. Paradoxically, pain is a frequent symptom in syringomyelia. Deep tendon reflexes are commonly diminished or absent; Horner's syndrome may be present.

Pathogenesis

Multiple theories have been offered to explain the pathophysiology that produces cystic cavitations of the spinal cord. Gardner[13, 14] initially attempted to explain the mechanism behind syrinx cavities from his work in treating patients with Chiari malformation. He maintained that in such patients normal CSF egress from the fourth ventricle is prevented by congenital obstruction of the foramina of Magendie and Luschka. As a result, he postulated that systolic CSF pressure pulsations generated by the choroid plexus were transmitted to the central canal of the cord via the obex of the fourth ventricle. Thus, the syrinx consists of a dilated central canal and/or diverticula of the central canal that extend by dissecting along the spinal cord fiber tracts. However attractive, this theory fails to explain those cavities in patients where the foramina of the fourth ventricle are patent, those without hindbrain malformations, and those instances in which the syrinx and fourth ventricle do not communicate.[15–17]

Williams[18, 19] modified Gardner's theory by considering intracranial and spinal venous and CSF pressure shifts. He maintained that coughing, sneezing, Valsalva maneuver, etc. increased intraspinal venous distension thus raising intraspinal CSF pressures. In the presence of partial spinal block (e.g., at the foramen magnum in Chiari malformation) a ball-valve phenomenon exists. When CSF pressure is increased below the lesion, fluid is forced temporarily above the point of obstruction. However, when venous pressure returns to normal, CSF pressure remains elevated above the site of block, which then forces fluid into the central canal below the block until the pressures equalize. Such cavities involving the central canal were termed communicating syringomyelia (rather than hydromyelia), while those not connecting to the central canal were termed noncommunicating syringomyelia. Pulsations of the epidural venous plexus induced by changes in intra-abdominal pressure were thought to produce shifts ("slosh") that extend these cavities.[20]

These theories have been questioned on other grounds by Ball and Dayan.[15] They calculated the pulse pressure wave transmitted to the cord substance under the circumstances described above to be such that it would be unlikely to produce cord cavitation. Instead, they maintained that CSF under pressure secondary to subarachnoid obstruction tracts into the spinal cord by way of the Virchow-Robin spaces. Subsequently small collections of CSF coalesce to form larger syrinx cavities that may or may not connect to the central canal. Quencher et al.[21] have invoked an analogous theory to explain the development of syrinx cavities in patients with previous intradural extramedullary neoplasms. He maintains that long-standing compression secondary to such mass lesions results in permanent enlargement or microcystic change of the perivascular space that predisposes to the development of syrinx cavities.

A similar mechanism for the development of syrinx cavities was subsequently proposed by Aboulker[22] and Aubin et al.[23] who claim that increased spinal CSF pressure forces CSF into the cord parenchyma along the posterior nerve rootlets.

Despite the lack of a comprehensive theory on the pathogenesis of spinal cord cystic cavities, a unifying theme among all the hypotheses put forth to date is the presence of dissecting, moving cerebrospinal fluid shifts. This is important to appreciate because such CSF motion may have significant impact on the MRI appearance of the syrinx cavity.[9,10]

Magnetic Resonance Evaluation

That MR is the safest, most efficient, and sensitive diagnostic imaging examination for the detection of intramedullary cystic cavities is no longer questioned. The majority of the literature on this subject describes examinations performed on patients with sagittal and/or axial short TR/short TE (T_1-weighted) spin-echo and sagittal long TR/long TE (T_2-weighted) spin-echo pulse sequences. Particular attention must be paid to the orientation of the phase and read gradients of such scans, as well as to the number of y-steps to avoid truncation error (Gibbs phenomenon), which may mimic syrinx cavities on sagittal images.[24,25] The typical appearance of a simple syrinx is that of a well-defined linear area of low signal within the spinal cord on T_1-weighted images that parallels the signal intensity of CSF with progressively more T_2-weighting. As radiologists have become increasingly sophisticated with respect to determining the effect of CSF motion on MR images of the spine, low signal (flow-void) has been recognized as a frequent finding within syrinx cavities on T_2-weighted images.[9,10] It is appealing to correlate the fluid shifts observed on MR (recognized as signal loss in the syrinx cavities on T_2-weighted images) with the theories proposed by Gardner, Williams and others.[9,10] Whether resolution of these motion-induced signal changes with surgical shunting of the syrinx cavities equates with a favorable clinical outcome will be decided with future, long-term studies.

Other variations from the simple MR description of syrinx cavities provided above arise with chronic cavities that may demonstrate multiple loculi secondary to gliosis, or variable signal intensities secondary to proteins present in solution. Such circumstances may lead to problems with interpretation of the MR study, particularly with respect to underlying etiology of the syrinx. More specifically, difficulty may arise in two instances: (1) the exclusion of an underlying cavitary neoplasm from an otherwise idiopathic, complicated syrinx and (2) differentiation of post-traumatic myelomalacia from syringomyelia.

With respect to the first diagnostic dilemma, Williams et al. found that while the appearance of a simple syrinx with distinct margins and signal intensity paralleling CSF correlated favorably with a non-neoplastic etiology, there were few additional clues on the MR examination to distinguish atypical idiopathic, post-traumatic, or congenital cavities (Figs 10–1 and 10–2). While areas of high signal-intensity tissue within adjacent cord parenchyma on T_2-weighted images may appear as an ominous finding, this can easily be explained on the basis of reactive gliosis and does not indicate the presence of an underlying tumor.[9,10] Whether the use of intravenous paramagnetic contrast material will facilitate the distinction between neoplastic and non-neoplastic cord cavities remains to be seen.

While the distinction between post-traumatic myelomalacia and syringomyelia is somewhat less problematic, it may occasionally be confusing. Both entities demonstrate long T_1 and T_2 relaxation times; that is, low signal intensity on short TR/short TE images and high signal intensity on long TR/long TE studies. If the signal intensity within the area of question parallels CSF on both T_1- and T_2-weighted scans, the lesion is probably a syrinx cavity.[11] Myelomalacia on the other hand, while demonstrating low signal on T_1-weighted images, is isointense or hyperintense to spinal cord on long TR/short TE images and less intense than CSF on long TR/

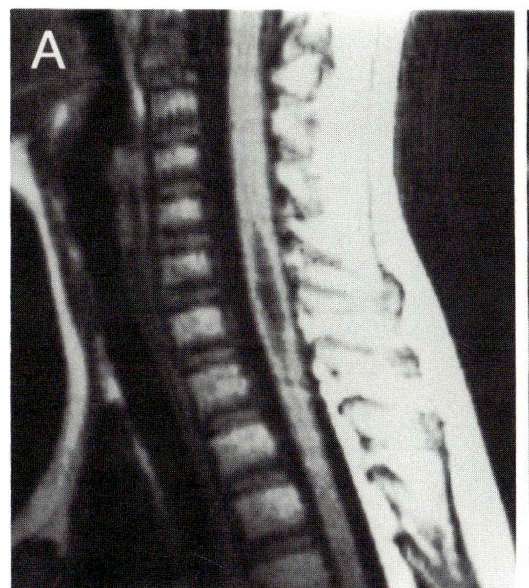

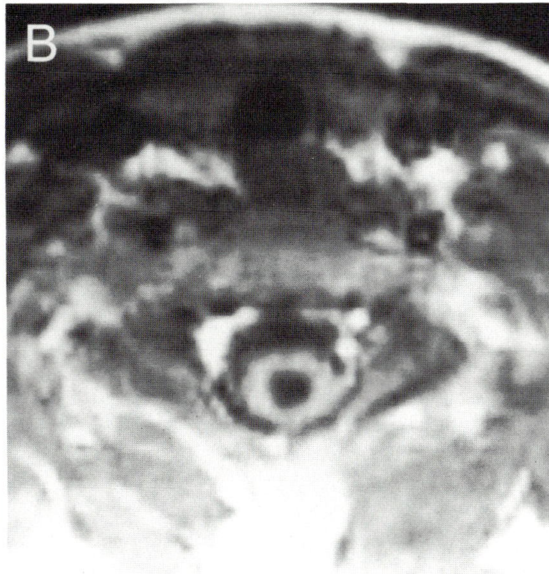

FIG 10–1.
A, 500-msec TR/17-msec TE midline sagittal image of the cervical spine in a patient with a simple syrinx cavity. The contents of the cavity are essentially isointense with CSF, and the cavity has smooth, well-marginated borders. **B,** 500-msec TR/17-msec TE axial image through the level of the syrinx.

long TE images. However, if motion-induced signal changes were present within a syrinx cavity, similar findings to those of myelomalacia might also be anticipated on long TR/long TE scans. The distinction between myelomalacia and syringomyelia may still be possible, however, through the use of axial gradient echo scans that should demonstrate flow-related enhancement in a syrinx cavity but not in an area of solid spinal cord tissue.[10]

EXTRAMEDULLARY CYSTIC CAVITIES (OF THE MENINGES)

Unlike the intramedullary cysts, which are generally accepted under the unifying, generic heading of "syrinx," extramedullary cysts of the meninges have long been mired in a loosely defined, confusing array of eponyms and synonyms. Mercifully, Nabors et al.[28] have recently introduced a lucid, concise, and unambiguous classification system for these lesions that not only lends perspective and insight to the previous literature but also encompasses knowledge gained through modern spine imaging modalities.[28] Spinal meningeal cysts are congenital diverticula of the dural sac, nerve root sheaths, or arachnoid that according to this classification can be categorized into three major groups: extradural cysts without spinal nerve roots (type I); extradural cysts with spinal nerve roots (type II); and intradural cysts (type III).

Extradural meningeal cysts without nerve roots (type I) are dural diverticula that are contiguous with the thecal sac by a narrow ostium.[28] The term encompasses those lesions previously preferred to as "extradural cysts, pouches, or diverticula" as well as "occult intrasacral meningoceles."[23, 29] Type I meningeal cysts in the thoracic spine are found commonly in adolescents where they arise from a dural pedicle near a dorsal nerve root[29, 30, 34] (Fig 10–3). Sacral type I cysts are found in adults and are connected to the tip of the caudal thecal sac by a pedicle[30] (Fig 10–4). Symptoms are related to location of a lesion with respect to cord and nerve roots and are usually shorter in duration for the thoracic lesions.

Meningeal cysts with nerve roots (type II) refers to those extradural lesions previously distinguished as (Tarlov) "perineurial cysts" and "nerve root diverticula."[30, 34, 35] While often seen as multiple incidental lesions in the lumbosacral spine of adults, they may occasionally be the cause of radiculopathy and/or incontinence (Fig 10–5). Despite the lack of a definable pedicle and ostium, both type I and type II cysts are suspected to produce pressure on adjacent structures and bone erosion via CSF pressure increases created by a valve-like mechanism.[33]

Type III meningeal cysts are intradural lesions most frequently found in the posterior subarachnoid space. Synonyms for these (primarily thoracic) lesions include "arachnoid diverticula" and "arachnoid cyst." They are

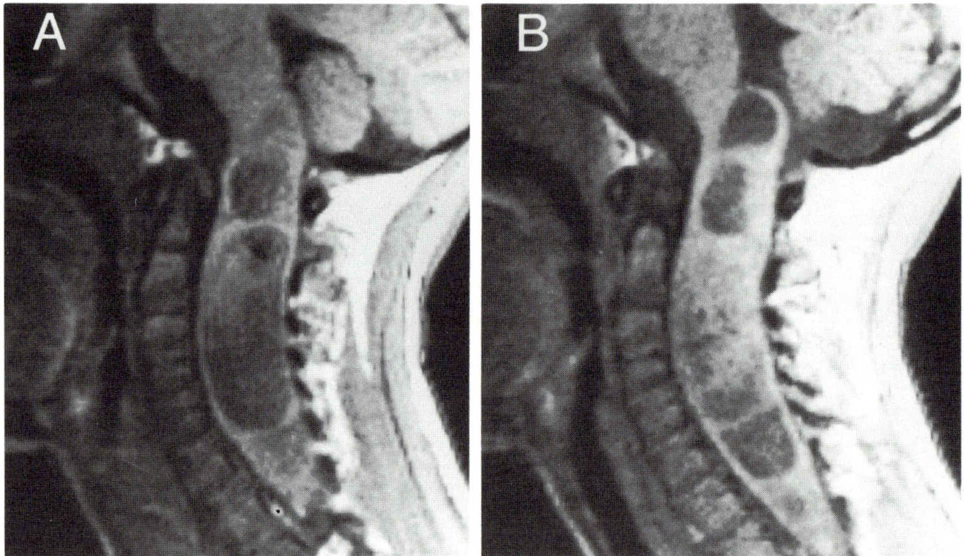

FIG 10–2.
500-msec TR/17-msec TE parasagittal (**A**) and sagittal (**B**) images of the cervical spine in a patient with a complicated syrinx cavity. Note the heterogeneity of the cyst contents, as well as the multiple septations throughout the cavity. The syrinx is poorly marginated and ill defined. Syrinxes such as these are difficult to distinguish from cavitary intramedullary neoplasms.

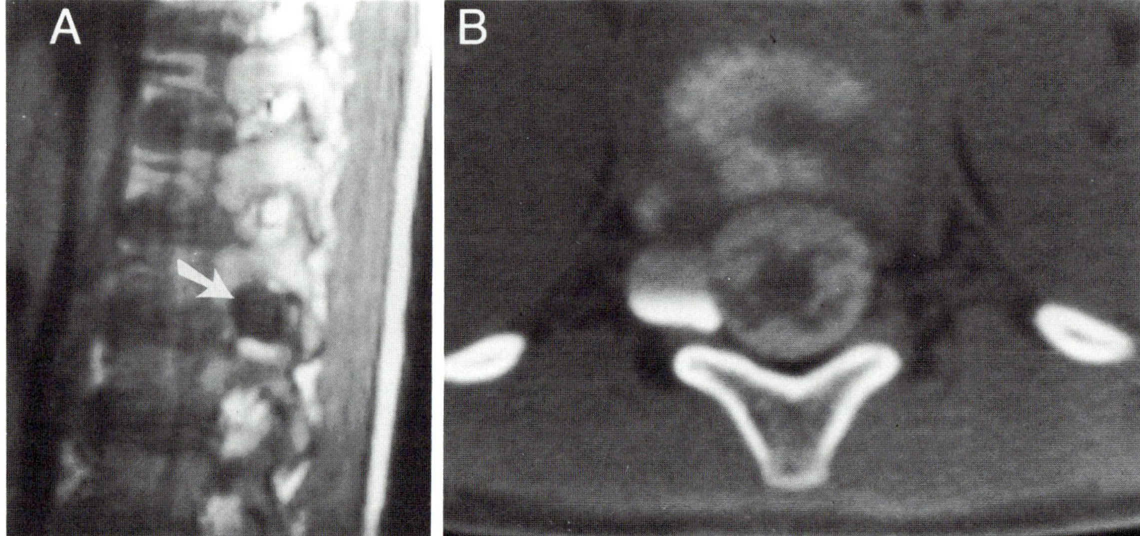

FIG 10–3.
A, 500-msec TR/17-msec TE parasagittal image through the lower thoracic spine in this adolescent demonstrates a focal area of low signal intensity within the neural foramen *(arrow).* Clinical suspicion was for a type I meningeal cyst. **B,** type I meningeal cyst was confirmed with a computed tomographic (CT) scan after water-soluble myelography.

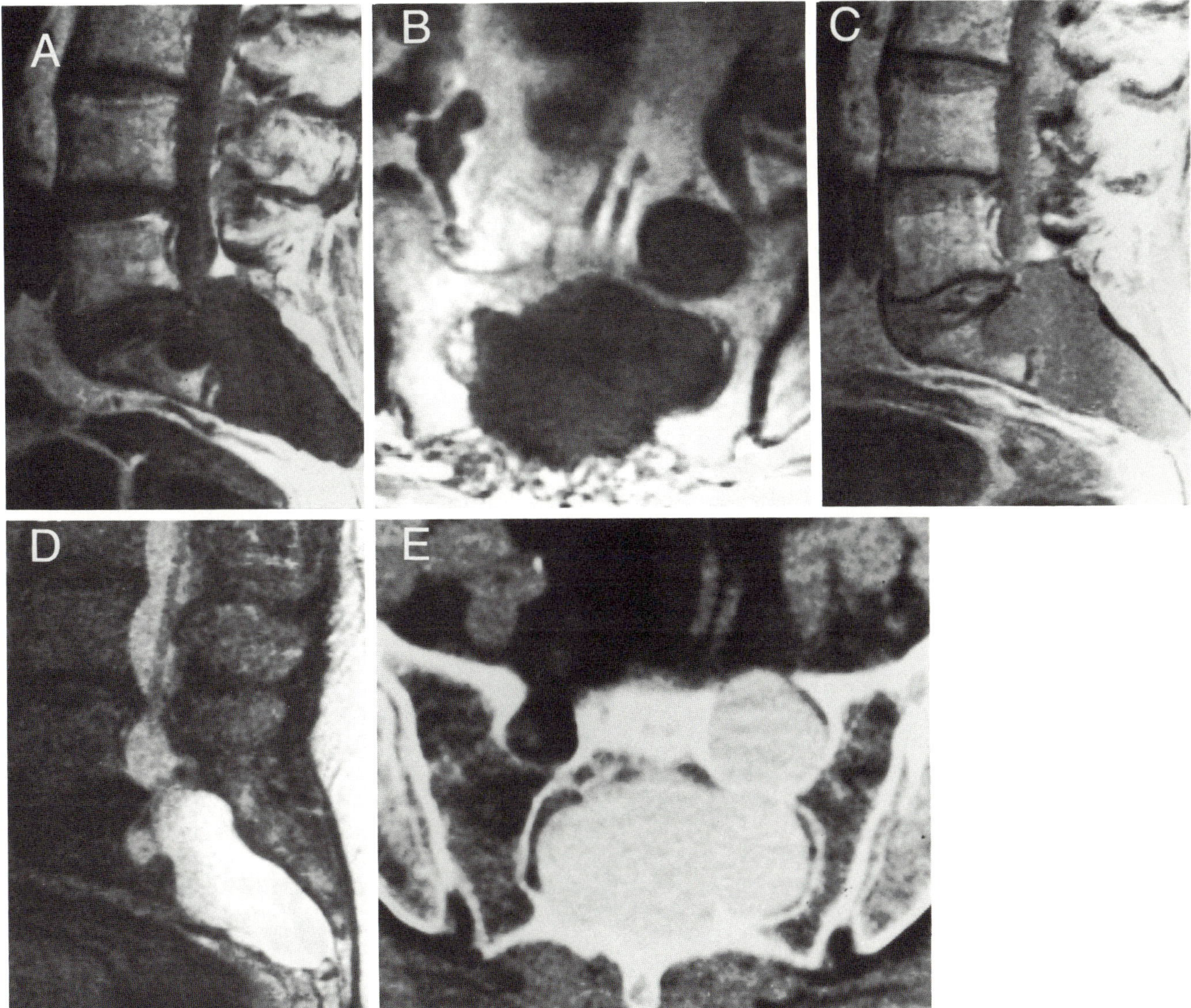

FIG 10–4.
500-msec TR/17-msec TE sagittal (**A**) and axial (**B**) images of a sacral type I cyst (previously referred to as occult intrasacral meningocele). Note the large, low signal, lytic process arising from the distal thecal sac and eroding the sacrum. **C,** 2,000-msec TR/30-msec TE sagittal image again demonstrates a large, cystic structure at the distal thecal sac eroding the sacrum. Notice that the signal intensity parallels that of CSF within the thecal sac on this long TR/short TE study. **D,** 2,000-msec TR/120-msec TE sagittal image of the lumbosacral spine again demonstrates a large cystic mass that parallels the signal intensity of CSF on this long TR/long TE study. **E,** delayed high-resolution CT scan through the sacrum following water-soluble myelography demonstrates the cystic mass within the sacrum that communicates with the thecal sac as evidence by the contrast material within it.

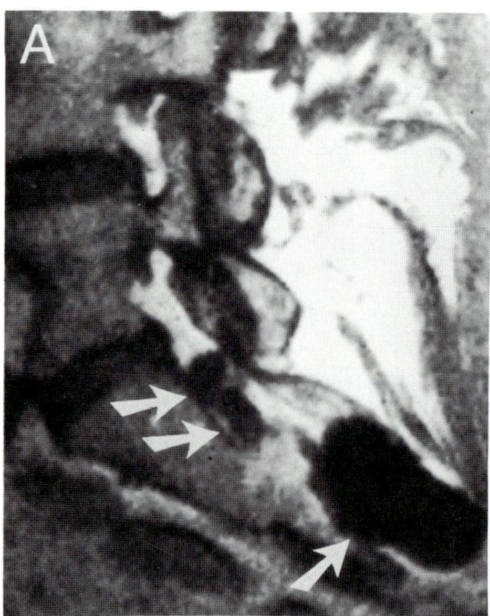

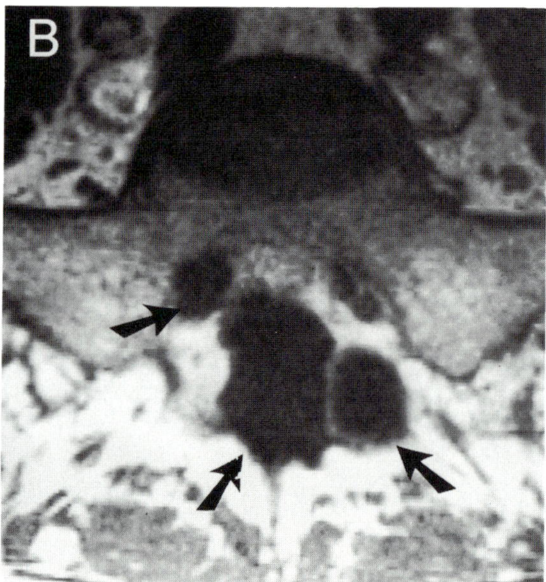

FIG 10–5.
500-msec TR/17-msec TE sagittal (**A**) and axial (**B**) images through the lumbosacral spine demonstrate multiple small, low signal intensity cystic areas *(arrows)* associated with various nerve root sleeves consistent with type II meningeal cysts (previously described as perineurial cyst or nerve root diverticula).

often multiple and clinically silent. When symptomatic, they typically present with signs suggesting posterior cord compression, although rare cases of anteriorly located cervical intradural cysts have been reported[37, 39, 40] (Fig 10–6).

Reports describing magnetic resonance findings in these lesions are few, but the imaging characteristics are by no means unexpected. Type I and type II lesions are typically anterior, posterior, or paraspinal lying within or outside of the vertebral canal and produce parallel CSF signal intensities on all spin-echo pulse sequences (see Fig 10–4). Depending on the force of CSF motion within the cyst, and on the use of gating, even echoes or refocussing gradients on the T_2-weighted study, signal intensity of the cyst may vary when compared to CSF signal within the canal. Bone erosion detectable as scalloping of the vertebral bodies or thinning of pedicles may be present. Type III cysts may be the most difficult to detect because they occur within the thecal sac and have very thin walls. They are often only recognizable by virtue of the mass effect and deformity that they produce on the spinal cord on T_1-weighted spin-echo images (see Fig 10–6).

VASCULAR MALFORMATIONS

In the past, vascular malformations of the spine and spinal cord have been categorized by investigators according to etiology and histologic configuration, angiographic pattern and relationship to the vascular supply of the spinal cord, and macroscopic appearance at the time of surgery.[41–43] Unfortunately, this diversity of classification criteria resulted in a wide variety of complex and confusing nomenclature for a group of relatively rare lesions. It is hoped that this section represents the distillation of the seminal features of each malformation that are important to its diagnosis and management.

Technically, vascular malformations of the spine and spinal cord are hemangiomas that can possess some neural tissue as an interstitial component, while vascular tumors (i.e., hemangioblastomas) do not.[41] In a manner analogous to similar malformations in the brain, such lesions may be further subdivided into (1) arteriovenous malformations (AVMs) (both dural and parenchymal), (2) cavernous angiomas (cavernous hemangiomas) and (3) capillary telangiectasias. One exception to this analogy are the venous angiomas, which represented a distinct entity in the brain. With respect to the spine, this term has been erroneously applied to the radiculomeningeal (dural) arteriovenous malformations; it is unclear as to whether venous angiomas exist as such in the spine and, if so, whether they are clinically significant.[44]

Arteriovenous Malformations

Arteriovenous malformations are comprised of fistulous communications between arteries and veins in the absence of an intervening capillary networks. Of

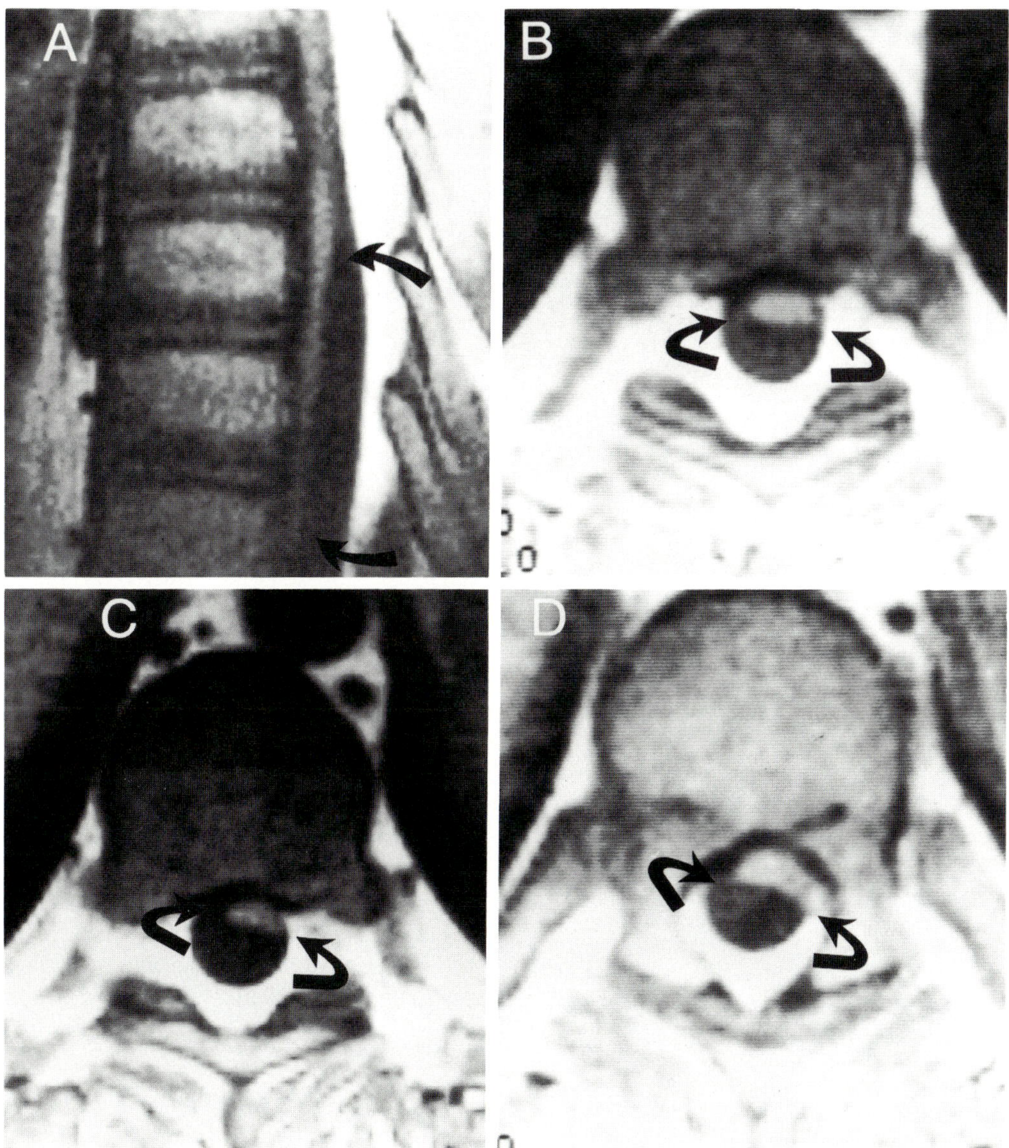

FIG 10–6.
A, midline 600-msec TR/17-msec TE sagittal image of the lower thoracic spine in this young female patient suggests a sudden, smooth tapering of the thoracic spinal cord *(arrows)* despite an apparent widening of the adjacent CSF space. **C–D,** serial 600-msec TR/17-msec TE, cranial-to-caudal axial images through the midthoracic and lower thoracic spine demonstrate severe effacement and flattening of the posterior surface of the spinal cord *(arrows)* despite an apparently "normal" appearance to the thecal sac. This case represents a surgically confirmed type III meningeal cyst ("arachnoid cyst").

paramount importance to the pathophysiology, presenting signs/symptoms, and diagnosis and treatment of these lesions is the location of the fistulous nidus with respect to the spinal cord and its vascular supply.[45] Consequently, these fistulas are designated as either intramedullary, extramedullary, or dural and are usually supplied by either anterior radiculomedullary, posterior radiculomedullary, or radiculomeningeal arteries, respectively. Of some clinical import is the presence of posterior or lateral cutaneous angiomas at the same segmental level as the AVM in 12% to 21% of such patients.[46–48] These are often referred to as metameric malformations indicating their common embryologic origin and can, by simple inspection, indicate the level of the intraspinal portion of the malformation.

Among patients with intramedullary and extramedullary malformations (i.e., those fed by radiculomedullary vessels), there is an approximately equal distribution among both sexes.[42, 49] Such lesions are more commonly cervical or cervicothoracic and possess a relatively large shunt volume fed by arteries that normally supply the cord.[42, 49, 50] Consequently, these lesions gen-

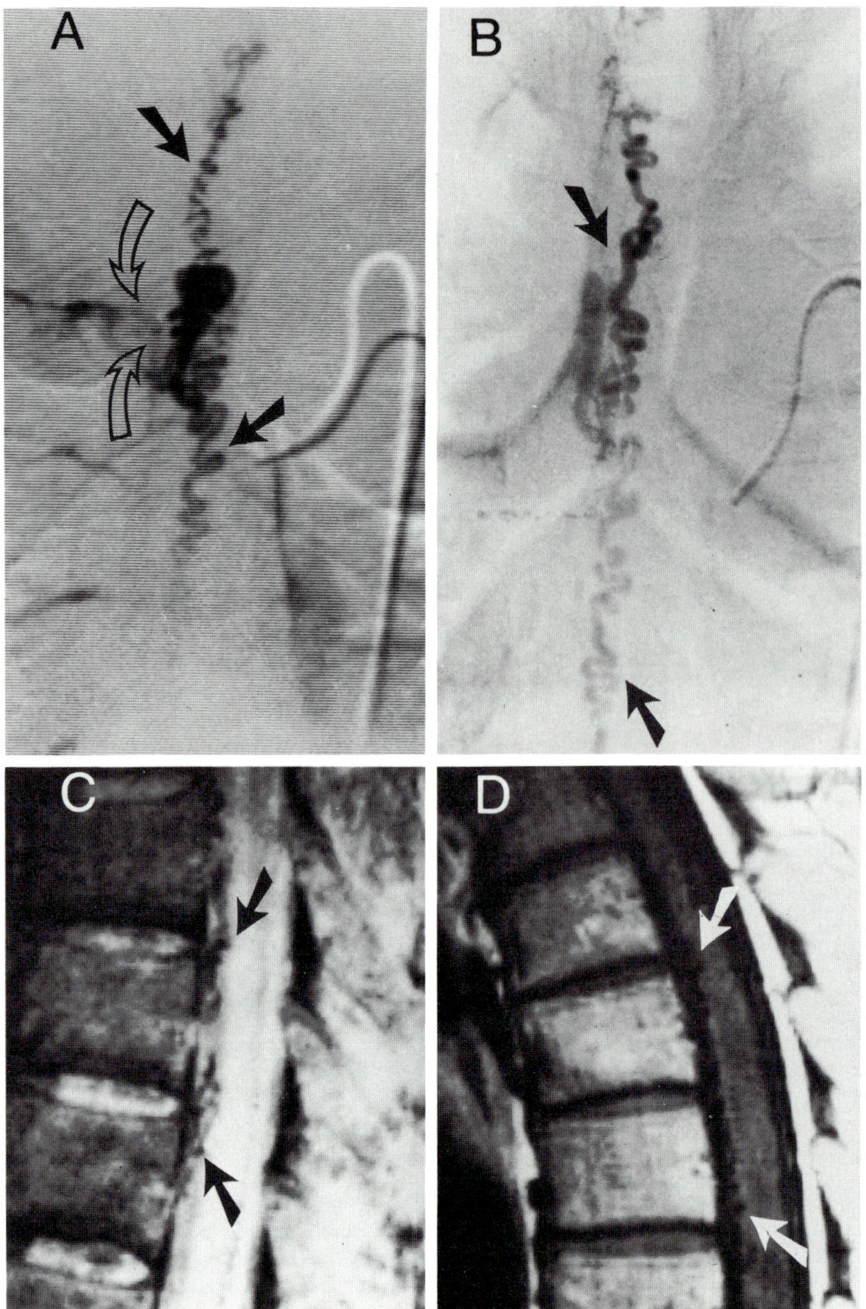

FIG 10–7.

A, early angiogram from selective injection of T5 intercostal artery on the right demonstrates washout of contrast material from the dural arteriovenous malformations (AVM) *(open arrows)* and the lateral nerve root sleeve and diffuse opacification of dilated coronal veins *(closed arrows).* **B,** later, venous film from the same T5 injection on the right demonstrates slow opacification *(arrows)* of additional coronal veins along the cord. **C,** midline 2,000-msec TR/90-msec TE sagittal examination of the midthoracic spine depicting serpentine areas of low signal intensity *(arrows)* outlined by high signal CSF thought to represent intradural, longitudinally oriented coronal veins. **D,** 500-msec TR/17-msec TE midline sagittal image at approximately the same level as **C** demonstrates small filling defects about the cord consistent with dilated coronal veins, but the defects are obviously not as conspicuous as those identified on the T_2-weighted image. *(Continued)*

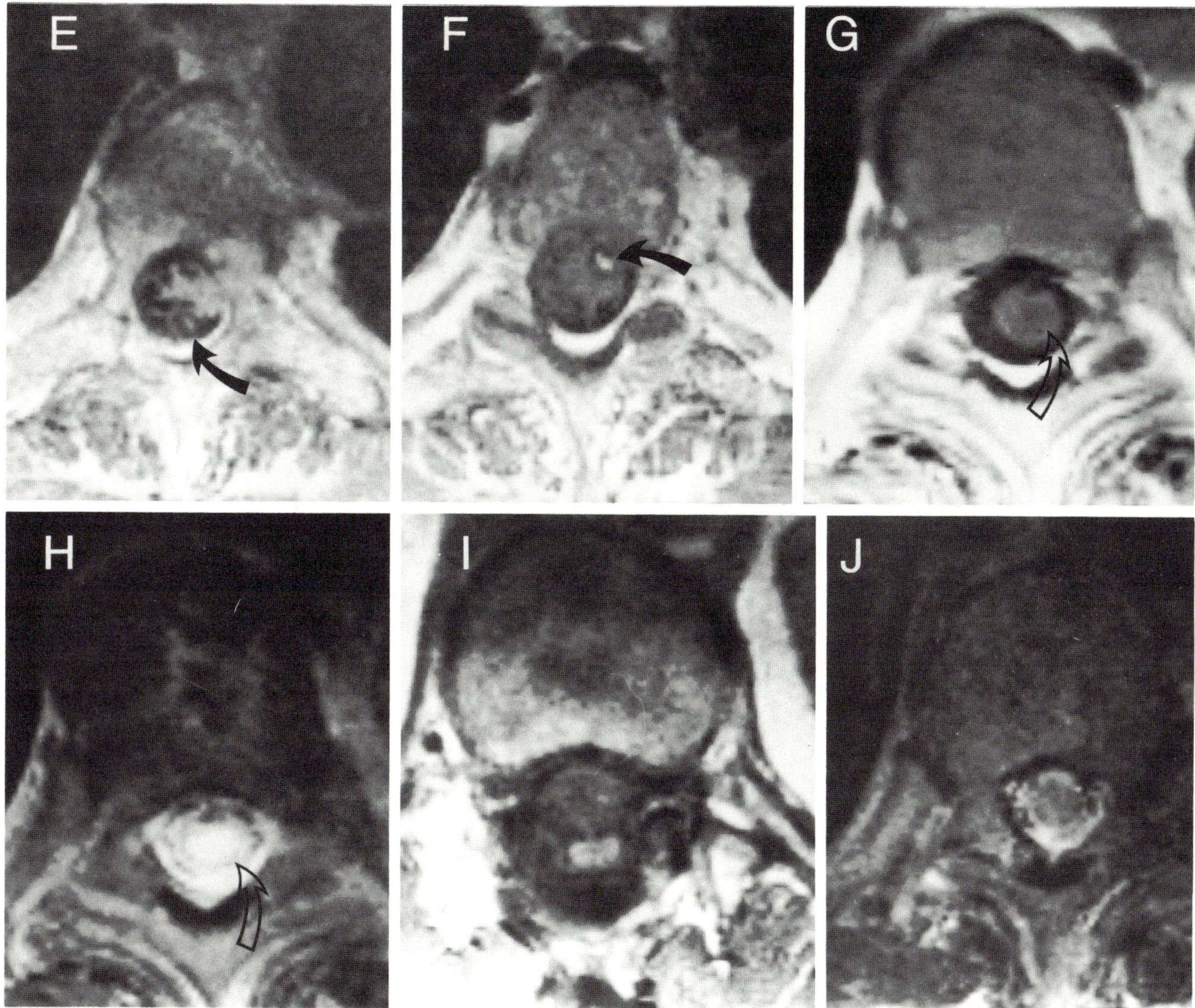

FIG 10–7 (cont.).
E and **F,** 600-msec TR/17-msec TE axial images through the upper thoracic spine demonstrate the circumferentially oriented coronal veins with several small areas of high signal intensity, possibly representing a thrombus *(arrows).* **G,** 600-msec TR/17-msec TE axial image through the lower thoracic spine suggests an ill-defined area of low signal intensity within the cord *(arrow).* **H,** 2,000-msec TR/90-msec TE axial image at approximately the same level as **G,** demonstrates high signal intensity within the cord at the same region where low signal intensity is identified on the T_1-weighted scan *(arrow).* These findings suggest intramedullary edema. **I** and **J,** T_1- and T_2-weighted axial scans, respectively, through the lower thoracic spine following surgery for this radiculomeningeal vascular malformation demonstrate partial resolution of the intramedullary signal-intensity changes noted on the preoperative scans.

erally present earlier (before 50 years of age) with symptoms of vascular steal (ischemia), subarachnoid hemorrhage, and/or hematomyelia.[42, 49–52] Possibly because of their high-flow state, such lesions may be accompanied by arterial aneurysms. While both lesions possess arterial supplies common to the spinal cord, intramedullary lesions are embedded deep within the anterior spinal cord and are considerably more difficult to treat. This is in contradistinction to the extramedullary lesions in which the nidus is located superficially on the dorsal aspect of the cord and thus remedial to surgical resection.[53] Experiences of Doppman et al.[53] and Di-Chiro et al.[54] indicate that MR may be useful in detecting such lesions by its ability to detect low signal feeding and draining vessels within the spinal cord on T_2-weighted images by virtue of the so-called flow-void phenomenon.[53, 54] Additionally, sagittal and/or coronal T_1-weighted images may further characterize the malformation by their ability to discern the low-signal nidus and enlarged anterior spinal artery in intramedullary lesions.[53,54] With this constellation of findings, MR is able to distinguish such lesions from spinal hemangioblastomas—a task that can be difficult with myelography, computed tomography, or even angiography.[54] It is also possible to document the response to therapy of such lesions with MR through its ability to detect thrombosis through the absence of flow void.[53]

Dural (radiculomeningeal) vascular malformations—long an enigmatic vascular spinal lesion—most frequently are recognized surgically and angiographically by the enlarged, arteriolized, slow-draining coronal veins of the spinal cord. Unlike their high-flow medullary counterparts, these lesions typically present in the thoracic and thoracolumbar spines of older patients (the large majority of which are male).[42,49] Also, the mode of presentation is quite different, commonly producing a slowly progressive myelopathy (rarely a sudden thrombophlebitis; the probable cause of the so-called Foix-Alajouanine syndrome).[55,56] Originally termed "extramedullary," the precise nature of these lesions came under serious scrutiny in 1974 when Aminoff et al.[57] argued that the myelopathic symptoms were the product of intramedullary edema and ischemia secondary to raised venous back pressure within the varicose coronal veins of the spinal cord. The dural site of arteriovenous shunting, however, remained to be discovered by Kendall and Logue[58] in 1977. Magnetic resonance is unlikely to replace myelography and angiography in the evaluation of such lesions; however, it is important to recognize the MR findings in patients being evaluated for myelopathy. Like the parenchymal arteriovenous malformations of the spinal cord, draining vessels of these dural lesions are identified as serpentine areas of low signal within the spinal canal on sagittal T_2-weighted images.[59] Axial T_1- and T_2-weighted images locate the low-signal, dilated coronal veins in their expected peripheral, circumferential location about the spinal cord.[59] Occasionally higher signal thrombi may be seen within these structures. Additionally, it is possible to appreciate the spinal cord edema first described by Aminoff in the lower spinal cord segments as areas of low signal on T_1-weighted images that progressively increase in signal with more T_2 weighting.[59] These intramedullary signal derangements may reverse following successful treatment (Fig 10–7).

Cavernous Hemangiomas

Cavernous hemangiomas are uncommon spinal vascular hemangiomas that consist of dilated endothelium-lined sinusoids separated by thin strands of fibrous tissue devoid of smooth muscle and elastic fibers.[44,60,61] These lesions are histologically distinguished from capillary telangiectasias by their abundance of hemosiderin and paucity of intervening normal neural tissue.[44,60,61] Histologic parallels and the reported presence of both lesions in the central nervous system of a single patient suggest that both are in fact representations of a spectrum of a single entity.[44,60–64]

The majority of spinal cavernous hemangiomas arise in the vertebral bodies with extension to the epidural space.[65] The MR appearance of these extradural lesions (high signal on T_1- and T_2-weighted images) is thought to be related to the presence of adipose and hematopoietic tissue (see Chapter 7).[66] Fontaine et al.[67] have recently described the MR appearance of intramedullary cavernous hemangiomas.[67] These lesions typically have a peripheral area of low signal intensity on T_1- and T_2-weighted spin-echo images thought to be secondary to the abundant hemosiderin contained within these lesions.[67] The central portion may have variable areas of increased and decreased signal secondary to the presence of calcifications and various forms of hemoglobin.[67] It should be remembered that the signal-intensity characteristics of hemoglobin and its breakdown products are variable depending on the concentration, magnetic field strength, and pulse sequence used (Fig. 10–8).[68,69] While the MR appearance of capillary telangiectasia of the spinal cord has yet to be reported, one might logically presume it to be similar to that of cavernous angiomas but without the peripheral ring of hemosiderin.

MULTIPLE SCLEROSIS/DEMYELINATING DISEASE

Multiple Sclerosis

Multiple sclerosis is a clinically variable disease characterized by multifocal destruction of myelin in the optic nerves, brain, and spinal cord. The disease usually begins in the second to fifth decades often manifesting with visual, sensory, and motor dysfunction.[70] Signs and symptoms characteristically wax and wane but often with less improvement and greater disability as time passes.[71] The prevalence of the disorder is higher in northern latitudes and among family members.[71,72] Emigrants from areas of high risk to areas of low risk have a lower incidence of the disease if they move before 15 years of age.[73,74] This familial and geographic tendency of multiple sclerosis suggests a possible environmental factor(s). Infectious agents, autoimmune disorders, or a combination of the two have been postulated as possible mechanisms. Pathologically, macroscopic lesions range in size from 1 mm to several centimeters and are scattered throughout the white matter; those involving the spinal cord tend to be more elongated.[75] Histologic

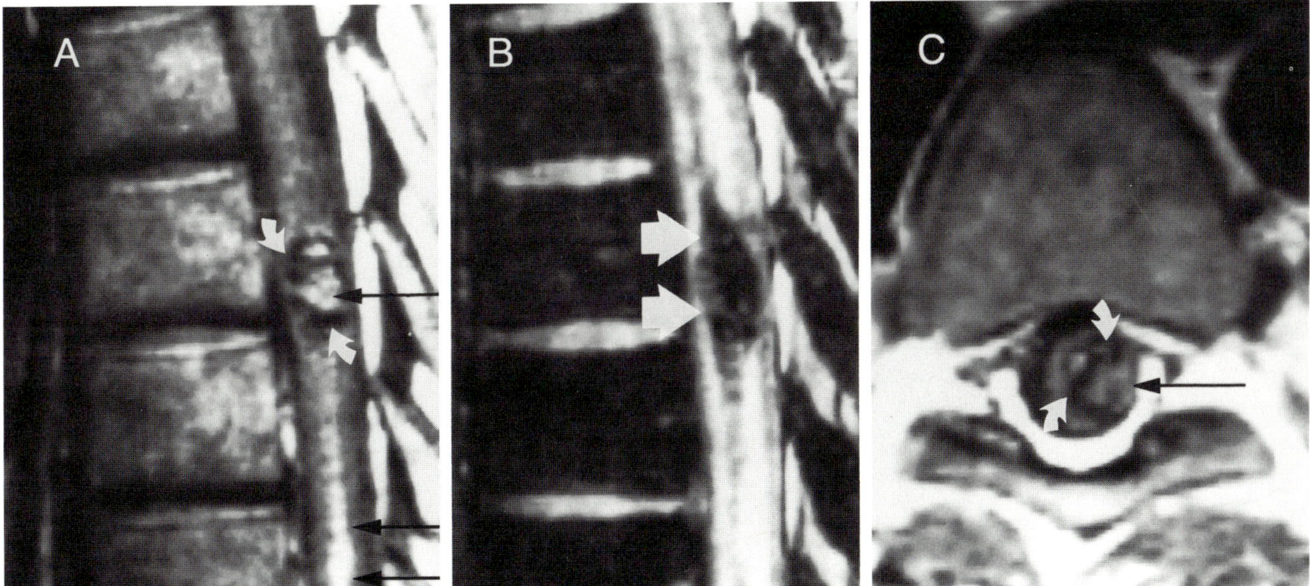

FIG 10–8.
A, 500 msec TR/17 msec TE sagittal spin-echo scan through the lower thoracic spine demonstrates a surgically proven cavernous hemangioma, represented by a low signal ring of hemosiderin *(curved white arrows)* surrounding a focal area of high signal intensity representing methemoglobin. Long linear area of high signal intensity beneath the lesion represents methemoglobin from recent hemorrhage *(long arrows).* **B,** midline sagittal FISP 10 degree image demonstrates the hemangioma as a large area of low signal *(white arrows)* because of the signal loss secondary to the magnetic susceptibility effect of the blood breakdown products. **C,** axial 500 msec TR/17 msec TE spin-echo scan through the cavernous hemangioma again demonstrates peripheral hemosiderin *(curved white arrows)* surrounding methemoglobin *(straight black arrow).*

sections demonstrate perivenous breakdown of the myelin sheath with sparing of adjacent axons.[76, 77] The plaques contain lymphocytes, plasma cells, and macrophages, which may contain myelin breakdown products.[76] Spinal cord involvement by multiple sclerosis often presents with weakness and/or paresthesias in one or more limbs, Lhermitte's sign, gait disturbance, and disorders of micturition. In association with optic nerve involvement, this syndrome has been referred to as "neuromyelitis optica" or Devic's disease.[71]

Primarily because of the variability in presentation, criteria for the diagnosis of multiple sclerosis have been developed on the basis of clinical and paraclinical (e.g., neuroimaging or laboratory) evidence of CNS lesions.[78] Magnetic resonance imaging has been found exquisitely sensitive to the presence of multiple sclerosis plaques involving the brain.[79, 80] The number and size of brain lesions detected by MR correlates well with the severity of disease.[81] These lesions are most frequently recognized as round or ovoid areas of low signal on T_1-weighted images that have increased signal on T_2-weighted scans, usually without mass effect. Whether these signal-intensity changes represent breakdown of blood-brain barrier, destruction of myelin, or both may be a reflection of the acuteness of the lesion.[82] It has been proposed that enhancement by paramagnetic contrast may reflect the level of clinical activity of a given lesion.[83] Reports of MR imaging of multiple sclerosis plaques in the spinal cord are few but generally depict similar signal-intensity changes on spin-echo images that are more linear or elongated[75, 80] (Fig 10–9 and 10–10). It must be noted that these reports have been limited to the cervical spinal cord in patients examined with a head coil; the use of surface coils, cardiac gating, and even echo rephasing or refocussing gradients has undoubtedly improved the recognition of lesions below the foramen magnum. It must also be kept in mind that the MR evaluation of patients with signs and symptoms of demyelinating disease is useful for not only what it shows, but what it does not.[71] Similar clinical presentations can be mimicked by brain stem glioma, epidermoid of the fourth ventricle, meningiomas and arachnoid cyst of the foramen magnum, brain stem and spinal cord vascular malformations, Chiari malformation, and cervical spondylosis.[71, 84–91] Consequently, even a negative MR examination of the spine and foramen magnum supplies useful clinical information.

Acute Disseminated Encephalomyelitis

Acute disseminated encephalomyelitis (ADEM) is pathologically indistinguishable from multiple sclerosis,

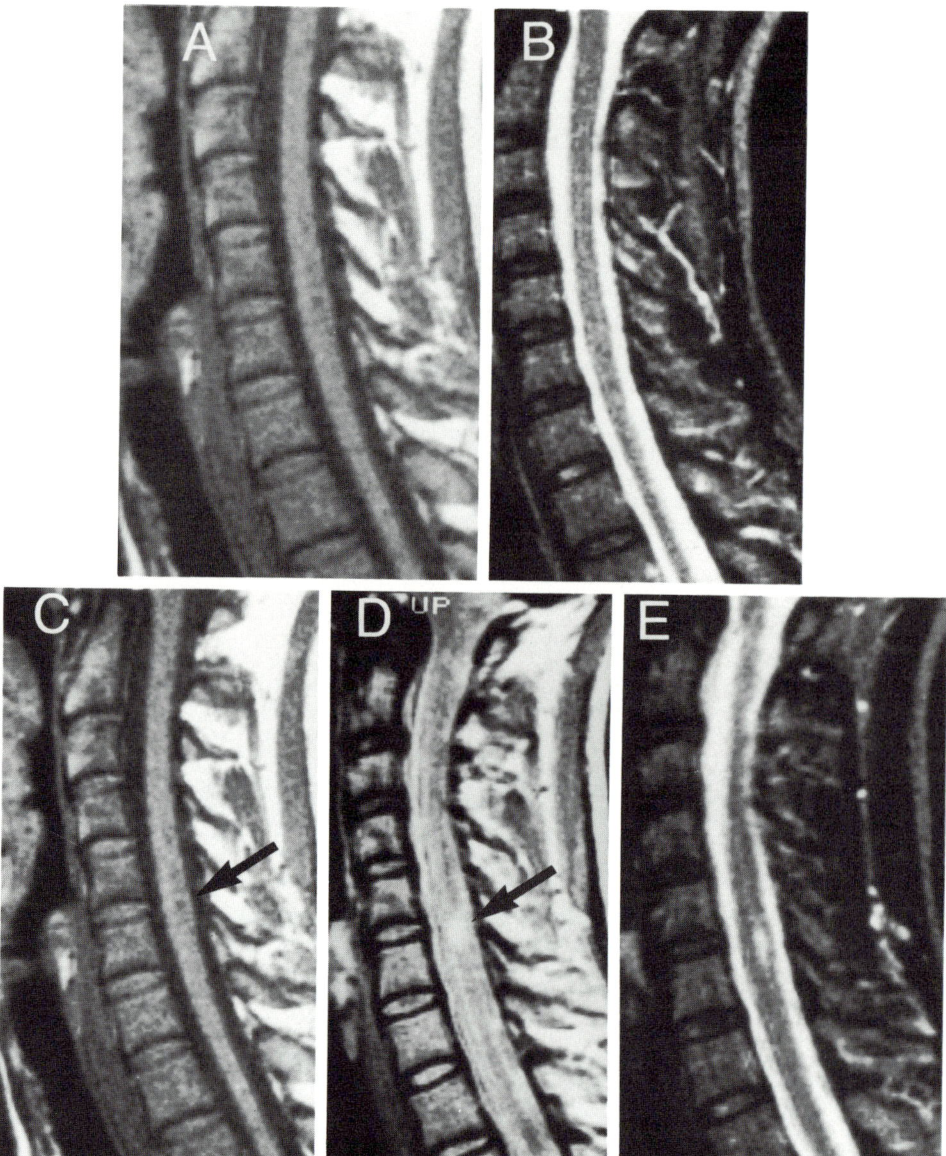

FIG 10–9.
A and **B,** 500-msec TR/17-msec TE and 2,000-msec TR/120-msec TE midline sagittal images of the cervical spine, respectively, in a patient suspected of having multiple sclerosis. These images are normal. **C–E,** 500-msec TR/17-msec TE, 2,000-msec TR/60–120-msec TE parasagittal images through the cervical spine on the same patient demonstrate a linear area of low signal intensity *(arrow)* on the T_1-weighted images that increases in signal with progressive T_2-weighting. The findings were consistent with a multiple sclerosis plaque capable of producing symptoms. This case serves to emphasize the spatial and contrast resolution requirements, particularly on T_2-weighted images, for the small lesions.

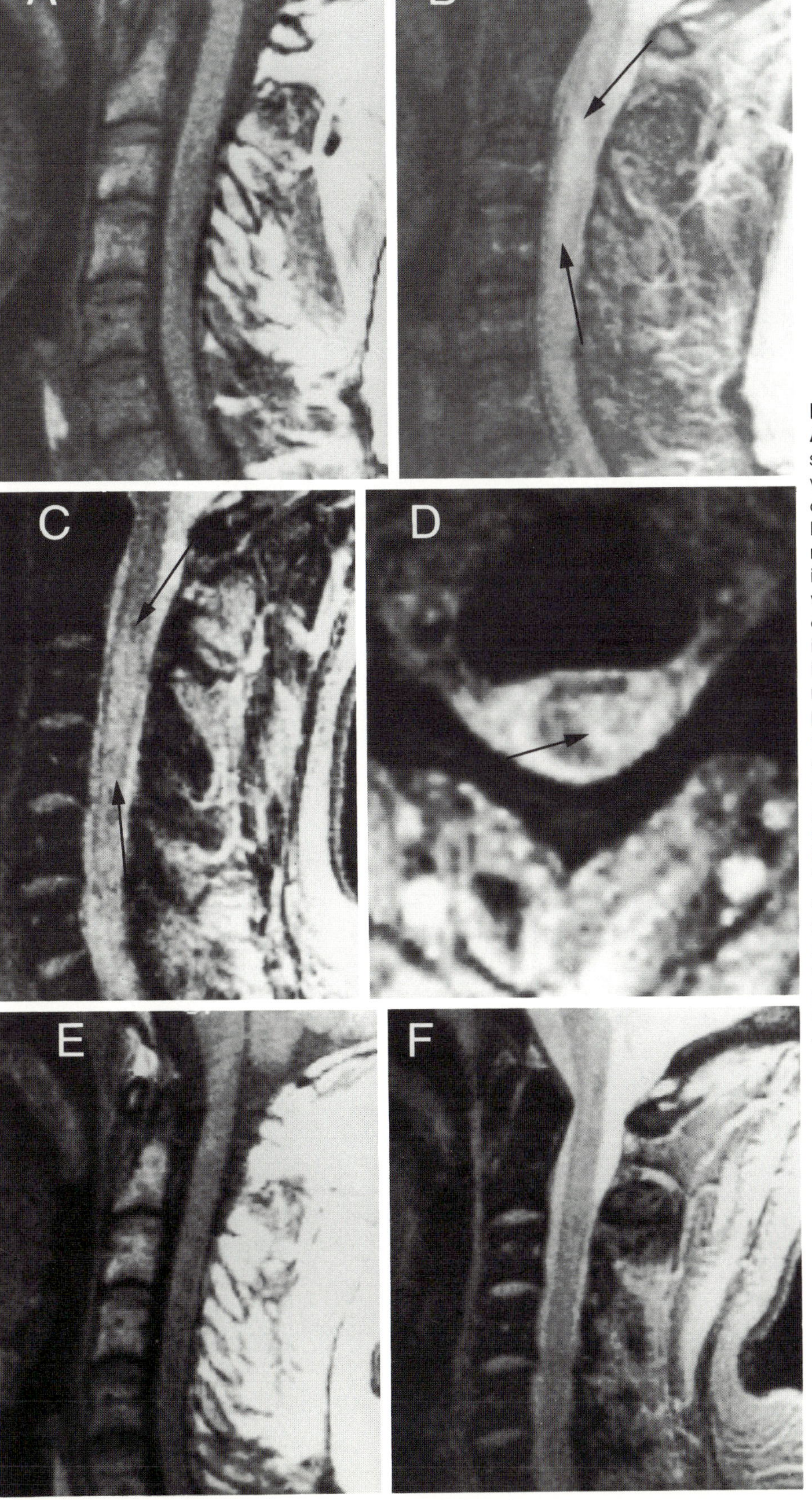

FIG 10–10.
A, 500-msec TR/17-msec TE midline sagittal image demonstrates mild widening of the cervical spinal cord at C2–3 with some ill-defined areas of low signal intensity within it. **B,** 2,000-msec TR/60-msec TE midline sagittal image again demonstrates cord widening as well as a large linear area *(arrows)* of increased signal intensity within it. Differential diagnosis includes primary intramedullary neoplasm vs. an acute demyelinating plaque. **C** and **D,** 200-msec TR/13-msec TE FISP 10-degree sagittal and axial images, respectively, confirm an abnormal area of high signal intensity *(arrows)* with cord widening at C2 and C3. **E,** following steroid treatment the patient was reimaged. 500-msec TR/17-msec TE midline sagittal images demonstrates that the overall size of the cord is returned to normal. **F,** repeat 200-msec TR/13-msec TE FISP 13-degree scan likewise shows a normal cord. Presumptive diagnosis was one of acute multiple sclerosis of the cervical spinal cord.

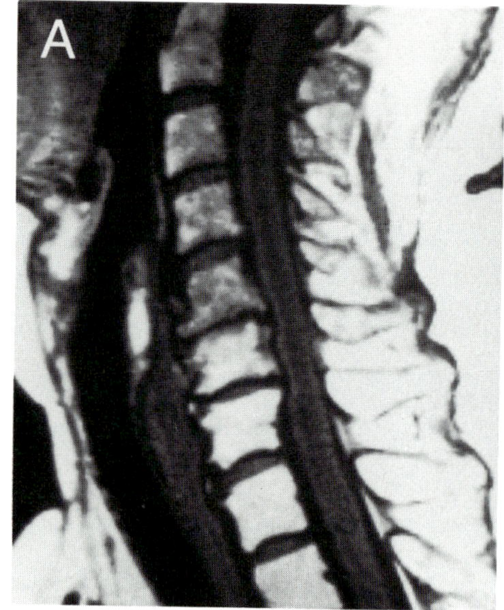

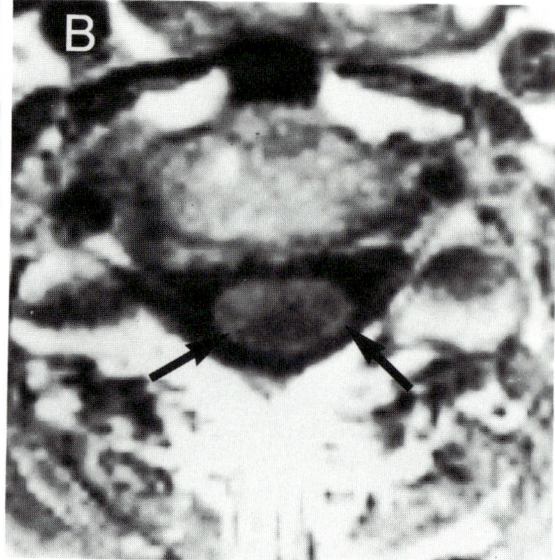

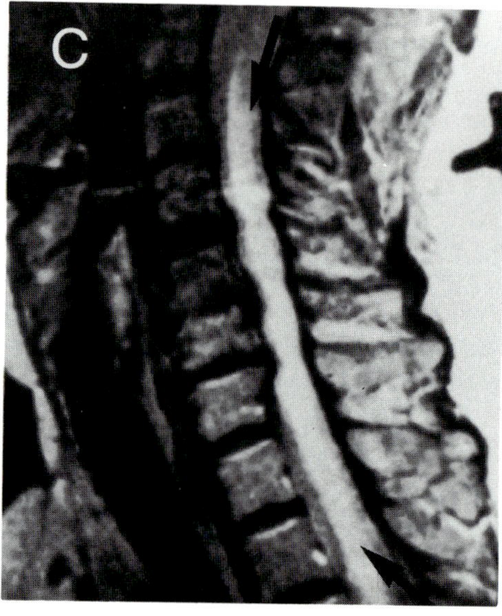

FIG 10–11.
A, 500-msec TR/17-msec TE midline sagittal image of the cervical spine on a patient previously irradiated for metastatic carcinoma of the breast to the cervical spine. Notice the high signal intensity of the lower cervical vertebral bodies and spinous processes consistent with the previous radiation therapy. Bony osteophytes are noted at the C5–6 and C6–7 levels. However, one can also appreciate an ill-defined decrease in the signal intensity of the central portion of the cervical spinal cord. **B,** 500-msec TR/17-msec TE axial image of the cervical spinal cord again confirms an abnormal area of low signal intensity within the cervical spinal cord, primarily noted posteriorly *(arrows)*. **C,** 2,000-msec TR/60-msec TE midline sagittal image of the cervical spine again demonstrates the bony osteophytes. However, notice the marked abnormal signal intensity througout the cervical spinal cord *(arrows)*, primarily within its central segment extending well above the level of radiation. Presumptive diagnosis was one of radiation myelitis.

i.e., perivenous demyelination.[92] However, clinically it occurs as a predominantly monophasic illness in children and is frequently preceded or accompanied by a viral infection or immunization. Neurologic signs point toward multiple focal lesions of the brain, spinal cord, and optic nerves. Permanent neurologic deficits are not infrequent (particularly with spinal cord involvement), and mortality is high.[93] Cases of relapsing ADEM are indistinguishable from multiple sclerosis.

Radiation Myelitis

Chronic progressive myelopathy following radiation therapy in the vicinity of the spinal cord is rare, estimated to be between 2% to 3% of cases.[94] Pallis et al.[95] recommends no more than 3,300 rads for treatment times of 42 days for greater than 10 cm of the spinal cord, and only 4,300 rads to fields less than 10 cm.[95] There is usually a latency period of at least 6 to 12 months followed by the slow onset of dysesthesia and paresthesia at and below the site of therapy. Subsequently, corticospinal and/or spinothalamic tracts become involved. Pathologically, there is coagulation necrosis involving the white matter to a greater extent than the gray matter, as well as hyaline thickening and thrombotic occlusion of arterioles.[96]

Magnetic resonance imaging will demonstrate abnormally high signal intensity of the vertebral bodies within the radiation port on T_1-weighted images secondary to replacement of normal hematopoietic elements by fat.[97] The spinal cord itself is also characterized by signal-intensity derangements with abnormally low signal on T_1-weighted images and high signal on T_2-weighted studies over the affected area (Fig 10–11).

REFERENCES

1. DeLaPaz RL, Brady TJ, Buananno FS, et al: Nuclear magnetic resonance (NMR) imaging of Arnold-Chiari type I malformation with hydromyelia. *J Comput Asst Tomogr* 1983; 7:126–129.
2. Han JS, Kaufman B, El Yousef SJ, et al: NMR imaging of the spine. *AJNR* 1983; 4:1151–1159.
3. Modic MT, Weinstein MA, Pavlicek W, et al: Nuclear magnetic resonance of the spine. *Radiology* 1983; 148:757–762.
4. Yeates A, Brant-Zawadzki M, Norman D, et al: Nuclear magnetic resonance imaging of syringomyelia. *AJNR* 1983; 4:234–237.
5. Modic MT, Weinstein MA, Pavlicek W, et al: Magnetic resonance imaging of the cervical spine. Techniques and clinical observations *AJR* 1983; 141:1129–1136.
6. Pojunas K, Williams AL, Daniels DL, et al: Syringomyelia and hydromyelia: Magnetic resonance evaluation. *Radiology* 1984; 153:679–683.
7. Kokmen E, Marsh WR, Baker HL: Magnetic resonance imaging in syringomyelia. *Neurosurgery* 1985; 17:267–270.
8. Quencer RM, Sheldon JJ, Post MJD: Magnetic resonance imaging of the chronically injured cervical spinal cord. *AJNR* 1986; 7:457–464.
9. Sherman JL, Barkovich AJ, Citrin CM: The MR appearance of syringomyelia: New observations. *AJR* 1987; 148:381–391.
10. Enzmann DR, O'Donohue J, Rubin JB, et al: CSF pulsations within nonneoplastic spinal cord cysts. *AJR* 1987; 149:149–157.
11. Castillo M, Quencer RM, Green B, et al: Syringomyelia as a consequence of compressive extramedullary lesions: Postoperative clinical and radiological manifestations. *AJR* 1988; 150:391–396.
12. Simon T: Uber syringomyelic und geschwulstbildung im Ruckenmark. *Arch Psychiatr Nervenkr* 1875; 5:120–163.
13. Gardner WJ: Hydrodynamic mechanism of syringomyelia—its relationship to myelocele. *J Neurol Neurosurg Psychiatry* 1965; 28:247–259.
14. Gardner LW, Angel J: The mechanism of syringomyelia and its surgical connection. *Clin Neurosurg* 1975; 6:131–140.
15. Ball MJ, Dayan AD: Pathogenesis of syringomyelia. *Lancet* 1972; 2:799–801.
16. Hughes JT, *Pathology of the Spinal Cord,* ed 2. Philadelphia, WB Saunders Co, 1978.
17. Feigin I, Ogata J, Buclzilovich G: Syringomyelia: The role of edema in its pathogenesis. *J Neuropathol Exp Neurol* 1971; 30:216.
18. Williams B: The distending force in the production of "communicating syringomyelia." *Lancet* 1969; 2:189–193.
19. Williams B: Current concepts in syringomyelia. *Br J Hosp Med* 1970; 4:331–342.
20. Williams B: On the pathogenesis of syringomyelia: A review. *J R Soc Med* 1980; 73:798–806.
21. Quencer RM, El Gammal T, Cohen G: Syringomyelia associated with intradural extramedullary masses of the spinal canal. *AJNR* 1986; 7:143–148.
22. Aboulker J: La syringomyelic et les liquides intra rachidiens. *Neurochirurgie* 1979; 25(suppl 1):9–144.
23. Aubin ML, Lignanel J, Jardin Bar D: Computed tomography in 75 clinical cases of syringomyelia. *AJNR* 1981; 2:199–204.
24. Bronskill MJ, McVeigh ER, Kucharczyk W, et al: Syrinx-like artifacts on MR images of the spinal cord. *Radiology* 1988; 166:485–488.
25. Levy LM, DiChiro G, Brooks RA, et al: Spinal cord artifacts from truncation errors during MR imaging. *Radiology* 1988; 166:479–483.
26. Rubin JM, Aisen AM, DiPietro MA: Ambiguities in MR imaging of tumoral cysts in the spinal cord. *J Comput Assist Tomogr* 1986; 10:395–398.
27. Williams AL, Haughton VM, Pojunas KW, et al: Differentiation of intramedullary neoplasms and cysts by MR. *AJR* 1987; 149:159–164.
28. Nabors MW, Pait TG, Byrd EB, et al: Updated assessment and current classification of spinal meningeal cysts. *J Neurosurg* 1988; 68:366–377.
29. Cloward RB: Congenital spinal extradural cysts: Case report with review of literature. *Ann Surg* 1968; 168:851–864.
30. Wilkins RH, Odom GL: Spinal extradural cysts, in Vinken PJ, Bruyn GW (eds): *Handbook of Clinical Neurology, Tumors of the Spine and Spinal Cord,* pt 2. vol 20, New York, Elsevier North-Holland, 1976, pp 137–175.
31. Fortuna A, LaTorre E, Ciapetta P: Arachnoid diverticula: A unitary approach to spinal cysts communicating with the subarachnoid space. *Acta Neurochir (Wien)* 1977; 39:259–268.
32. Lamas E, Lobato RD, Amor T: Occult intrasacral meningocele. *Surg Neurol* 1977; 8:181–184.
33. McCrum C, Williams B: Spinal extradural arachnoid pouches. Report of two cases. *J Neurosurg* 1982; 57:849–852.
34. Wilkins RH: Intraspinal cysts, in Wilkins RH, Rengacharry SS (eds): *Neurosurgery*. New York, McGraw-Hill Book Publishers, 1985, pp 2061–2070.
35. Tarlov IM: Spinal perineurial and messingeal cysts. *J Neurol Neurosurg Psychiatry* 1970; 33:833–843.
36. Cilluffo JM, Gomez MR, Reese DF, et al: Idiopathic ("congenital") spinal arachnoid diverticula. *Mayo Clin Proc* 1981; 56:93–101.
37. Kendall BE, Valentine AR, Keis B: Spinal arachnoid cysts: Clinical and radiological correlation with prognosis. *Neuroradiology* 1982; 22:225–234.
38. Swamy KS, Reddy AK, Srivastava VK, et al: Intraspinal arachnoid cysts. *Clin Neurol Neurosurg* 1984; 86:143–148.
39. Duncan A, Hoare RD: Spinal arachnoid cysts in children. *Radiology* 1978; 126:432–439.
40. Palmer JJ: Spinal arachnoid cysts. Report of six cases. *J Neurosurg* 1974; 41:728–735.

41. Aminoff MJ: Introduction: The nature of spinal angiomas, in Aminoff MJ (ed): *Spinal Angiomas*. Boston, Blackwell Scientific Publications, 1976, pp 1–4.
42. Doppman J, DiChiro G, Ommaya A: Arteriovenous malformations, in Doppman J, DiChiro G, Ommaya A (eds): *Selective Arteriography of the Spinal Cord*. St Louis, Warren H Green Inc, 1969, pp 59–124.
43. Teny P, Papatheodorou C: Myelographic appearance of vascular anomalies of the spinal cord. *Brit J Radiol* 1964; 37:358–366.
44. Rubinstein LJ: Tumors and malformation of blood vessels; Firminger HI (ed): *Tumors of the Central Nervous System*. Washington DC, Air Force Institute of Pathology, 1985, pp 235–256.
45. Doppman JL, DiChiro G, Oldfield EH: Origin of spinal arteriovenous malformation and normal cord vasculature from a common segmental artery: Angiographic and therapeutic considerations. *Radiology* 1985; 154:687–689.
46. Aminoff MJ: Associated lesions, in Aminoff MJ (ed): *Spinal Angiomas*. Boston, Blackwell Scientific Publications, 1976, pp 18–27.
47. Djindjian R: Neuroradiological examination of spinal cord angiomas, in Vinken PJ, Bruyn GW (eds): *Handbook of Clinical Neurology,* vol 12. New York, Elsevier North-Holland, 1972, pp 631–643.
48. Doppman JL, Wirth FP, DiChiro G, et al: Value of cutaneous angiomas in the arteriographic localization of spinal-cord arteriovenous malformations. *N Engl J Med* 1969; 281:1440–1444.
49. Aminoff MJ: Site, Sex, Age, in Aminoff MJ (ed): *Spinal Angiomas*. London, Blackwell Scientific Publications, 1976, pp 32–37.
50. Aminoff MJ: The volume of the shunt, in Aminoff MJ (ed): *Spinal Angiomas*. Boston, Blackwell Scientific Publications, 1976, pp 38–42.
51. Aminoff MJ: Spinal subarachnoid hemorrhage and hematomyelia, in Aminoff MJ (ed): *Spinal Angiomas*. Boston, Blackwell Scientific Publications, 1976, pp 43–53.
52. Riche MC, Modenesi-Freitas J, Djindjian M, et al: Arteriovenous malformations (AVM) of the spinal cord in children. *Neuroradiology (Berlin)* 1982; 22:171–180.
53. Doppman JL, DiChiro G, Dwyer AJ, et al: Magnetic resonance imaging of spinal arteriovenous malformations. *J Neurosurg* 1987; 66:830–834.
54. DiChiro G, Doppman JL, Dwyer AJ, et al: Tumors and arteriovenous malformations of the spinal cord: Assessment using MR. *Radiology* 1985; 156:689–697.
55. Aminoff MJ: Clinical features of spinal angiomas, in Aminoff MJ (ed): *Spinal Angiomas*. Boston, Blackwell Scientific Publications, 1976, pp 54–68.
56. Wirth FP, Post KD, DiChiro G, et al: Foix-Alajouanine disease. Spontaneous thrombosis of a spinal cord arteriovenous malformation: A case report. *Neurology* 1970; 20:1114–1118.
57. Aminoff MJ, Barnard RO, Logue V: The pathophysiology of spinal cord vascular malformations. *J Neurosci* 1974; 23:255–263.
58. Kendall BE, Logue V: Spinal epidural angiomatous malformations draining into intrathecal veins. *Neuroradiology* 1977; 13:181–189.
59. Masaryk TJ, Ross JS, Modic MT, et al: Radiculomeningeal vascular malformations of the spine: MR imaging. *Radiology* 1987; 164:845–849.
60. Jellinger K: Pathology of spinal vascular malformations and vascular tumors, in Pia HW, Djindjian R (eds): *Spinal Angiomas: Advances in Diagnosis and Therapy*. New York, Springer-Verlag 1978, pp 9–20.
61. McCormick WF: The pathology of vascular ("arteriovenous") malformations. *J Neurosurg* 1966; 24:807–816.
62. Bicknell JM, Carlow TJ, Kornfield M: Familial cavernous angiomas. *Arch Neurol* 1978; 35:746–749.
63. Heffner RR, Solitare GB: Hereditary hemorrhagic telangiectasia; neuropathological observations. *J Neurol Neurosurg Psychiatry* 1969; 32:604–608.
64. McCormick WF, Hardman JM, Boulter TR: Vascular malformations ("angiomas") of the brain with special reference to those occurring in the posterior fossa. *J Neurosurg* 1968; 28:241–251.
65. Guthkelch AN: Hemangiomas involving the spinal epidural space. *J Neurol Neurosurg Psychiatry* 1948; 11:199–210.
66. Ross JS, Masaryk TJ, Modic MT, et al: Vertebral hemangiomas: MR imaging. *Radiology* 1987; 165:165–169.
67. Fontaine S, Melanson D, Cosgrove R, et al: Cavernous hemangiomas of the spinal cord: MR imaging. *Radiology* 1988; 166:839–841.
68. Gomori JM, Grossman R, Zimmerman RA, et al: Intracranial hematoma imaging by high-field MR. *Radiology* 1985; 157:87–93.
69. Edelman RR, Johnson K, Buston R, et al: MR of hemorrhage: A new approach. *AJNR* 1986; 7:751–756.
70. McFarlin DE, McFarland HF: Multiple sclerosis. *N Engl J Med* 1982; 307:1183–1188.
71. McAlpine D, Lumsden CE, Acheson ED: Multiple sclerosis: A reappraisal. London, Churchill Livingstone Inc, 1972.
72. Kurtzke JF: Epidemiologic contributions to multiple sclerosis: An overview. *Neurology* 1980; 30:61–79.
73. Dean G, Kurtzke JF: On the risk of multiple sclerosis according to age at immigration to South Africa. *Br Med J* 1971; 3:725–729.
74. Alter M, Kahara E, Loewenson R: Migration and risk of multiple sclerosis. *Neurology* 1978; 28:1089–1093.
75. Maravilla KR, Weinreb JC, Suss R, et al: Magnetic resonance demonstration of multiple sclerosis plagues in the cervical cord. *AJNR* 1984; 5:685–689.
76. Prineas JW, Wright RG: Macrophages, lymphocytes and plasma cells in the perivascular compartment in chronic multiple sclerosis. *Lab Invest* 1978; 38:409–421.
77. Prineas J: Pathology of the early lesion in multiple sclerosis. *Hum Pathol* 1975; 6:531–554.
78. Poser CM, Paty DW, Scheinberg L, et al: New diagnostic criteria for multiple sclerosis: Guidelines for research protocols. *Ann Neurol* 1983; 13:227–231.
79. Bydder GM, Steiner RE, Young IR, et al: Clinical NMR imaging of the brain: 140 cases. *AJNR* 1982; 3:459–480; *AJR* 1982; 139:215–236.

80. Sheldon JJ, Siddharthan R, Tobias J, et al: MR imaging of multiple sclerosis comparison with clinical and CT examinations in 74 patients. *AJNR* 1985; 6:683–690.
81. Edwards MK, Farlow MR, Stevens JC: Multiple sclerosis: MRI and clinical correlation. *AJR* 1986; 147:571–574.
82. Poser CM, Kleefield J, O'Reilly GV, et al: Neuroimaging and the lesion of multiple sclerosis. *AJNR* 1987; 8:549–552.
83. Grossman RI, Gonzalez-Scarano F, Atlas SW, et al: Multiple sclerosis: Gadolinium enhancement in MR imaging. *Radiology* 1986; 161:721–725.
84. Sarkari NBS, Bickerstaff R: Relapses and remissions in brain stem tumors. *Br Med J* 1969; 2:21–23.
85. Cohen L, Macrae D: Tumors in the region of the foramen magnum. *J Neurosurg* 1962; 19:462–469.
86. Rosenbluth PR, Lichtenstein BW: Pearly tumor (epidermoid cholesteatoma) of the brain. Clinicopathological study of two cases. *J Neurosurg* 1960; 17:35–42.
87. Lehman RAW, Fieger HG: Arachnoid cyst producing recurrent neurological disturbances. *Surg Neurol* 1978; 10:134–136.
88. Howe JR, Taren JH: Foramen magnum tumors. Pitfalls in diagnosis. *JAMA* 1973; 225:1061–1066.
89. Stahl SM, Johnson KP, Malamud N: The clinical and pathological spectrum of brain-stem vascular malformations. Long-term course simulates multiple sclerosis. *Arch Neurol* 1980; 37:25–29.
90. Dhopesh VP, Weinstein JD: Spinal arteriovenous malformations simulating multiple sclerosis: Importance of early diagnosis. *Dis Nerv Sys* 1977; 38:848–851.
91. Banerji NK, Millar JHD: Chiari malformation presenting in adult life. *Brain* 1974; 97:157–168.
92. Lumsden CE: The neuropathology of multiple sclerosis, in Vinken PJ, Bruyn GW (eds): *Handbook of Clinical Neurology,* vol 9, New York, Elsevier North-Holland, 1978, p 305.
93. Miller HG, Shatnon JB, Gibbons JL: Acute disseminated encephalomyelitis and related syndromes. *Br Med J* 1957; 1:668–672.
94. Palmer JJ: Radiation myelopathy. *Brain* 1972; 95:109–122.
95. Pallis C, Louis C, Morgan RL: Radiation myelopathy. *Brain* 1961; 84:460–479.
96. Burns RJ, Jones AN, Robertson JS: Pathology of radiation myelopathy. *J Neurol Neurosurg Psychiatry* 1972; 35:888–898.
97. Ramsey RG, Zacharias CE: MR imaging of the spine after radiation therapy: Easily recognizable effects. *AJR* 1985; 144:1131–1135.

Index

D

E

F